Principles and Practice
of Intravenous Therapy

FOURTH EDITION

Principles and Practice of Intravenous Therapy

Revised by

Ada Lawrence Plumer, R.N.
Former Supervisor and Instructor, Intravenous Therapy Department
Massachusetts General Hospital, Boston

Cofounder of the National Intravenous Therapy Association, Inc.

Faye Cosentino, R.N., B.S., CRNI
Director, Intravenous Therapy Department
Lawrence Hospital, Bronxville, New York

LITTLE, BROWN AND COMPANY
Boston   Toronto

Library of Congress Cataloging-in-Publication Data

Plumer, Ada Lawrence.
　　Principles and practice of intravenous therapy.

　　Includes bibliographies and index.
　　1. Intravenous therapy.　I. Cosentino, Faye.
II. Title. [DNLM: 1. Infusions, Parenteral.
WB 354 P734p]
RM170.P57　1987　　　615'.63　　　86-15240
ISBN 0-316-71135-7

Copyright © 1987 by Ada Lawrence Plumer and Faye Cosentino

All rights reserved. No part of this book may be reproduced in any form or by any electronic or mechanical means including information storage and retrieval systems without permission in writing from the publisher, except by a reviewer who may quote brief passages in a review.

Library of Congress Catalog Card No. 86-15240

ISBN 0-673-39403-4

9　8　7　6　5

MV

Printed in the United States of America

Today quality intravenous therapy is being provided to countless patients because dedicated nurses have given their time and expertise to develop educational programs, standards of care, and criteria for certification. We respectfully dedicate this book to these professionals.

Preface

Principles and Practice of Intravenous Therapy, fourth edition, is intended to provide practical information to the nurses and other health care professionals who share the responsibility for providing quality care to the millions of patients receiving intravenous therapy each year.

Advances in medical science and modern technology have created tremendous changes and improvements in intravenous therapy in the five years since the publication of the third edition. Sophisticated devices and techniques that allow the patient to receive intravenous therapy in the home, unheard of until only a few short years ago, have opened a whole new area in home care. The development of totally implantable vascular access devices now allows drug therapy to be carried out in the home as well as in ambulatory centers, making the self-administration of intravenous medications the fastest growing area in intravenous therapy.

The fourth edition of this text has responded to these developments. In addition to updating throughout, a new chapter, Home Intravenous Therapy, discusses the selection, training, and monitoring of patients who use the new intravenous modalities. The chapter on intravenous equipment has been completely rewritten to include new devices made possible by modern-day technology. The selection and use of this new equipment are described in this updated and expanded chapter.

The fourth edition has also been reorganized, with chapters divided into six parts: Introduction to Intravenous Therapy; Fluids and Electrolytes; Equipment and Techniques; Blood and Intravenous Therapy; Hazards and Complications; and Specific Applications.

Part I, Introduction to Intravenous Therapy, includes a new chapter on risk management and quality assurance to help personnel better understand and meet the new JCAH (Joint Commission on Accreditation of Hospitals) requirements.

Specific Applications, Part VI, includes two new chapters about central venous catherization, now an everyday procedure. These chapters discuss areas such as catheter materials, designs, insertions, and complications in detail, and also includes step-by-step procedures for the use, maintenance, and care of all central venous catheter devices.

Many sections of the book have been completely rewritten or expanded. The National Guidelines established by the Center for Disease Control (CDC) and the Standards of Practice established by the National Intravenous Therapy Association (NITA) are referred to and adhered to throughout the book.

ACKNOWLEDGMENTS

We are deeply grateful to the following individuals for their cooperation, help, and interest in reading and critiquing specific chapters: *Lawrence B. Annes, M.D.*, Assistant Professor of Medicine, New York Medical College, Attending Cardiologist, Lawrence Hospital, Bronxville, New York (Intraarterial Therapy); *Charles Huggins, M.D.*, Director of Blood Transfusion Services, Massachusetts General Hospital, Associate Professor of Surgery, Harvard Medical School, Cambridge, Mass. (Transfusion Therapy; Therapeutic Phlebotomy); and *Margaret N. Kennedy, R.N.*, Special Assistant, Department of Nursing, Children's Medical Center of Dallas, Dallas, Texas (Unique Features of Pediatric Intravenous Therapy).

We are also thankful to the authors and publishers who have kindly allowed us the use of their copyrighted material and to the manufacturing companies of intravenous equipment for information and help.

Contributing Authors

We wish to express our deep appreciation to the following contributors for sharing their knowledge and expertise in particular highly specialized areas of intravenous therapy:

Rita Colley, R.N., B.A.
Senior Technical Development Manager, Travenol Laboratories, Deerfield, Illinois.

Vickie Phillips Duty, R.N., B.S.N.
Nurse Clinician, Hyperalimentation Unit, University of Cincinnati Medical Center, Cincinnati, Ohio

Suzanne Adelman Miller, R.N.
Oncology Nurse Consultant, Los Gatos, California

Betsy Cohen Teitell, R.N., M.S.
Southwest Clinical Manager, Healthdyne Company, Grand Prairie, Texas

Contents

PART I
Introduction to Intravenous Therapy 1

CHAPTER 1	**History of Intravenous Therapy**	3
	Ada Lawrence Plumer	
	Early History	3
	Twentieth-Century Advances	4
	Recent Milestones	6
CHAPTER 2	**Legal Implications of Intravenous Therapy**	8
	Ada Lawrence Plumer	
	Professional and Government Regulations	8
	Legal Guidelines	11
CHAPTER 3	**Organization of an Intravenous Department and Guide to Teaching**	15
	Ada Lawrence Plumer	
	The Value of Parenteral Teams	15
	Directorship of the Department	16
	Philosophy and Objectives	16
	Functions of an Intravenous Department	17
	Collection of Blood Samples	21
	Operational Activities of the Intravenous Department at the Massachusetts General Hospital	22
	Teaching Programs	24
CHAPTER 4	**Risk Management and Quality Assurance**	31
	Faye Cosentino	
	Risk Management	31
	Malpractice Claims	31
	Quality Assurance	32

Problem Identification 32
Problem Evaluation 33
Data Analysis and Interpretation 34
Implementation of Corrective Action 36
Problem Reevaluation (Follow-Up) 36
Problem Minimization or Solution 37
I.V. Therapy Quality Assurance 37
Quality Assurance Study #1 37
Quality Assurance Study #2 43
Quality Assurance Study #3 46

CHAPTER 5 The Staff Nurse's Responsibility in the Maintenance of Infusions 50
Ada Lawrence Plumer

Recommendations for Practice in the Use of I.V. Containers 50
Recommendations for Practice in the Use of Administration Sets 51
Recommended Practice (NITA) in Dressing Changes 51
Ambulating Patients with Infusions 52
Frequent Observation 52
Termination of Infusion 55

CHAPTER 6 Anatomy and Physiology Applied to Intravascular Therapy 57
Ada Lawrence Plumer

The Importance of Understanding Anatomy and Physiology 57
The Vascular System 58
The Skin 63
Superficial Fascia 64

PART II
Fluids and Electrolytes 67

CHAPTER 7 Fundamental Aspects of Fluid and Electrolyte Metabolism 69
Ada Lawrence Plumer

Introduction to Fluid and Electrolyte Balance 69
Fluid Content of the Body 70
Composition of Body Fluid 71
Body-Regulating Mechanisms 76
Electrolytes of Biological Fluids 77

CHAPTER 8 Rationale of Fluid and Electrolyte Therapy 83
Ada Lawrence Plumer

Objectives of Parenteral Therapy 83

	Maintenance Therapy	83
	Restoration of Previous Losses	85
	Replacement of Present Losses	85
	Electrolyte and Fluid Disturbances	88
	Parenteral Therapy for the Surgical Patient	88
	Parenteral Therapy for the Burned Patient	93
	Diabetic Acidosis	97

CHAPTER 9 Parenteral Fluids and Related Fluid and Electrolyte Abnormalities — 103

Ada Lawrence Plumer

Parenteral Fluids	103
Dextrose in Water Fluids	106
Isotonic Sodium Chloride Infusions	109
Isotonic Saline with Dextrose	111
Hypertonic Sodium Chloride Infusions	111
Hypotonic Sodium Chloride in Water	112
Hydrating Fluids	112
Hypotonic Multiple-Electrolyte Fluids	113
Isotonic Multiple-Electrolyte Fluids	114
Alkalizing Fluids	115
Acidifying Infusions	116
Evaluation of Water and Electrolyte Balance	117
Clinical Disturbances of Water and Electrolyte Metabolism	120

CHAPTER 10 Rate of Administration of Parenteral Infusions — 130

Ada Lawrence Plumer

Determining Factors for Infusion Rate	130
Computation of Flow Rate	132
Factors Affecting the Flow Rate	133

PART III

Equipment and Techniques 135

CHAPTER 11 Intravenous Equipment — 137

Ada Lawrence Plumer

Fluid Containers	137
Infusion Systems	138
Administration Sets	139
Pediatric Sets	141
Medication Sites	141
Check-Valve Sets	143
Controlled-Volume Sets	144

Y-Type Administration Sets	144
Positive-Pressure Sets	144
Blood Warmers	148
Y-Type Blood Component Sets	149
Filters	150
Final Filters	151
Infusion Pumps	155
Syringe Pumps	156
Controllers	164
Catheters	166

CHAPTER 12 Techniques of Intravenous Therapy — 172
Ada Lawrence Plumer

Approach to the Patient	172
Selecting the Vein	173
Selecting the Cannula	175
Securing Proper Lighting	177
Applying the Tourniquet	177
Preparation for Venipuncture	178
Techniques in Venipuncture	179
Basic Venipuncture	179
Anchoring the Steel Cannula and Securing the Armboard	181
The "Inside-the-Needle" Catheter and Associated Risks	183
The "Over-the-Needle" Catheter	184
The Cutdown Catheter	186

PART IV
Blood and Intravenous Therapy   189

CHAPTER 13 Transfusion Therapy — 191
Ada Lawrence Plumer

Basic Immunohematology	191
The Process of Immune Response	193
Blood Group Systems	193
Objectives of Transfusion Therapy	195
Whole Blood	195
Packed Red Cells	197
Frozen Blood	197
Plasma	198
Plasma Substitute: Dextran	203
$Rh_O(D)$ Immune Globulin	203
Blood Administration	204
Transfusion Reactions	207

CHAPTER 14	**Therapeutic Phlebotomy**	214
	Ada Lawrence Plumer	
	Blood for Transfusion Purposes	214
	Blood for Therapeutic Purposes	215
	Procedure for Bleeding	215
	Suggested Procedure for Therapeutic Phlebotomy	220
CHAPTER 15	**Laboratory Tests**	224
	Ada Lawrence Plumer	
	Collection of Venous Blood Samples	225
	Venipuncture for Withdrawing Blood	227
	The Vacuum System	228
	Drawing Blood via the Central Venous Catheter	229
	Withdrawing Blood and Initiating an Infusion	229
	Commonly Used Laboratory Tests	230
	Measurements of Electrolyte Concentration	231
	Venous Blood Measurement of Acid–Base Balance	233
	Enzymes	234
	Transaminase	235
	Liver Function Tests	236
	Kidney Function Tests	237
	Blood Sugar Tests	238
	Blood Typing	239

PART V
Hazards and Complications 267

CHAPTER 16	**Hazards and Complications of Intravenous Therapy**	269
	Ada Lawrence Plumer	
	Local Complications	269
	Thrombosis	269
	Thrombophlebitis	269
	Phlebothrombosis	270
	Infiltration	272
	Systemic Complications	273
CHAPTER 17	**Bacterial, Fungal, and Particulate Contamination**	280
	Ada Lawrence Plumer	
	Complications of Intravenous Therapy	280
	Sources of Bacteria	281
	Factors Influencing the Survival of Bacteria	283
	Factors Contributing to Contamination and Infection	284

Contents

Care of the Catheter	290
Intravenous-Associated Infections	290
Particulate Matter	291

PART VI
Specific Applications 299

CHAPTER 18 — Central Venous Catheterization — 301
Faye Cosentino

Vascular Anatomy	301
Central Venous Pressure	304
Central Venous Pressure Monitoring	307
Patient Preparation	310
Central Venous Cannulation	311
Insertion Sites	312
Central Insertion	312
Peripheral Insertion	313
Complications	314
Care and Maintenance of Central Venous Catheter Lines	317

CHAPTER 19 — Central Venous Catheters — 323
Faye Cosentino

Catheter Materials	323
Catheter Designs	324
Catheter Site Care	339
Catheter Maintenance and Operation	342
Totally Implanted Catheters	353
Implantable Pumps	364

CHAPTER 20 — Intravenous Administration of Drugs — 371
Ada Lawrence Plumer

Advantages	371
Hazards	372
Incompatibilities	372
Chemical Interactions	373
pH and Its Role in the Stability of Drugs	374
Vascular Irritation	375
Responsibility of the Hospital Committee	376
The Physician's Responsibility	377
The Intravenous Nurse's Responsibility	377
The Attending Nurse's Responsibility	378
Nurses' Intravenous Additive Station	378
Preparation of Intravenous Solutions and Additives	379
Intermittent Infusion	381

	The Heparin Lock	382
	The Intravenous Push	384
	Important Checkpoints in the Administration of I.V. Injections	385

CHAPTER 21   Total Parenteral Nutrition — Nursing Practice   389

Rita Colley   Vickie Phillips Duty

History	389
Indications	390
Solutions	390
Catheter Insertion	392
Air Embolism	396
Dressing Change Procedures	396
Intravenous Tubing and Filter Change	404
Infection Control	405
Metabolic Considerations	407
Urinary Glucose Measurement	408
Insulin Administration	408
Flow Rates	409
Accurate Charting	410
Hypoglycemia	410
Hyperglycemia and Hyperosmolarity	410
Intravenous Lipids	411
Home Hyperalimentation	413
General Considerations	424
Psychological Aspects	425
Future Trends	427
Hyperalimentation Nursing Standards of Practice	427

CHAPTER 22   Intravenous Cancer Chemotherapy Administration   439

Suzanne Adelman Miller

Nurse Preparation	439
Patient Education	442
Medication Preparation	444
Intravenous Technique	446
Venous Fragility	451
Localized Acute Allergic Reactions	451
Venous Spasm	453
Phlebitis	453
Generalized Anaphylactic Reaction	463
Extravasation	466

CHAPTER 23   Intraarterial Therapy   477

Faye Cosentino

Intraarterial Access	477
General Considerations	477

	One-Time Arterial Blood Gas Sampling	478
	Placement of an Indwelling Arterial Catheter	485
	Constant Arterial Pressure Monitoring	490
	Swan Ganz Catheters	494
	Arterial Blood Gas Parameters	495
	Four Primary Acid–Base Imbalances	500
	Mixed Acid–Base Imbalances	504
CHAPTER 24	**Unique Features of Pediatric Intravenous Therapy**	**506**
	Betsy Cohen Teitell	
	Preliminary Considerations in Pediatric I.V. Therapy	506
	I.V. Insertion	511
	Emotional Considerations	512
	Neonatal I.V. Therapy	513
	Total Parenteral Nutrition	517
CHAPTER 25	**Home Intravenous Therapy**	**527**
	Faye Cosentino	
	Home I.V. Therapy Procedures	528
	Patient Selection	528
	Patient Education	528
	Day of Discharge	533
	After Discharge	533
	Monthly Report to the Physician	533
	Follow-Up Care	533
	The Advantages of Home Treatment	534
	Answers to Review Questions	**539**
	Index	**553**

Principles and Practice
of Intravenous Therapy

NOTICE

The indications and dosages of all drugs in this book have been recommended in the medical literature and conform to the practices of the general medical community. The medications described do not necessarily have specific approval by the Food and Drug Administration for use in the diseases and dosages for which they are recommended. The package insert for each drug should be consulted for use and dosage as approved by the FDA. Because standards for usage change, it is advisable to keep abreast of revised recommendations, particularly those concerning new drugs.

PART I
Introduction to Intravenous Therapy

CHAPTER 1

History of Intravenous Therapy

Ada Lawrence Plumer

EARLY HISTORY

The idea of injecting various substances, including blood, into the circulatory system is not new; it has been in the human mind for centuries. In 1628 William Harvey's discovery of the circulation of the blood stimulated increased experimentation. In 1656 Sir Christopher Wren, with a quill and bladder, injected opium intravenously into dogs, and 6 years later, J. D. Major made the first successful injection in man [9].

In 1665 an animal near death from loss of blood was restored by infusion of blood from another animal. In 1667 a 15-year-old Parisian boy was the first human being to receive a transfusion successfully; lamb's blood was administered directly into the circulation by Jean Baptiste Denis, physician to Louis XIV [9]. The enthusiasm aroused by this success led to promiscuous transfusions of blood from animals to man with fatal results, and in 1687 by an edict of church and parliament animal-to-man transfusions were prohibited in Europe.

About 150 years passed before serious attempts were again made to inject blood into humans. James Blundell, an English obstetrician, revived the idea. In 1834, saving the lives of many women threatened by hemorrhage during childbirth, he proved that animal blood was unfit to inject into man and that only human blood was safe. Nevertheless, complications persisted; infections developed in donor and recipient. With the discovery of the principles of antisepsis by Pasteur and Lister, another obstacle was overcome, yet reactions and deaths continued.

The first attempt, recorded in 1821, to prevent coagulation during transfusion was by Jean Louis Prévost, a French physician, who, with Jean B. A. Dumas, used defibrinated blood in animal transfusions [9].

TWENTIETH-CENTURY ADVANCES

In 1900 Karl Landsteiner proved that not all human blood is alike; classifications were made [9]. In 1914 a chemical, sodium citrate, was found to prevent blood from clotting [9]. From then on rapid advance has taken place.

Hugh Leslie Marriot and Alan Kekwick, English physicians, introduced the continuous slow-drip method of blood transfusion; their findings were published in 1935 [9].

Administration of parenteral fluids by the intravenous route has become widely used only during the past 40 years. The difficulty in accepting this procedure was due to lack of safe solutions. The solutions used contained substances called pyrogens, proteins that are foreign to the body and not destroyed by sterilization. These caused chills and fever when injected into the circulation. About 1923, with the discovery and elimination of these pyrogens, the administration of parenteral fluids intravenously became safer and more frequent.

Until 1925 the most frequently used parenteral solution was normal saline solution. Water, because of its hypotonicity, could not be administered intravenously and had to be made isotonic; sodium chloride achieved this effect [5]. After 1925 dextrose was used extensively to make isotonic solutions and to provide a source of calories [5].

In the early 1930s administration of an intravenous injection was a major procedure reserved for the critically ill patient. The doctor performed the venipuncture assisted by a nurse. The success of intravenous therapy and the great increase in its use led to the establishment of a department of specially trained personnel for infusion therapy. In 1940 the Massachusetts General Hospital became one of the first hospitals to assign a nurse as Intravenous Therapist. The services of the intravenous nurse consisted in administering intravenous solutions and transfusions, cleaning infusion sets, and cleaning and sharpening needles. Emphasis was placed on the technical responsibility of maintaining the infusion and keeping the needle patent. The sole requisite of the intravenous nurse was the ability to perform a venipuncture skillfully.

As knowledge of electrolyte and fluid therapy grew, more solutions became available, and further knowledge was needed to monitor the fluid and electrolyte status of the patient. Normal saline was no longer the only electrolyte solution. Today over 200 commercially prepared intravenous fluids are available to meet every need of the patient.

A whole new approach to intravenous therapy and a respite to the starving patient evolved in 1965 when members of the Harrison Department of Surgical Research at the University of Pennsylvania showed that sufficient nutrients could be given to juvenile beagle dogs to support normal growth and development [4]. This led to what is known today as total parenteral nutrition.

In the middle 1940s disposable plastic sets became available and eventually replaced the reusable rubber tubings.

Glass containers were first used for intravenous solutions. Plastic bags were introduced in the 1970s; since air venting is not required, the risk of air embolism and airborne contamination was reduced. Today both plastic and glass containers are used for intravenous solutions.

Improvements and innovations in equipment have reduced hazards; sets and cannulas are now disposable, reducing risks of pyrogenic reactions and hepatitis. Prior to the Second World War, the metal needle was used extensively for infusing parenteral fluids. Frequent infiltrations as well as difficulties with the metal needle led to the development in 1945 of the flexible plastic tubing known as the intravenous catheter [3]. This tubing was introduced into the circulation by means of either a cutdown or a needle. These procedures were cumbersome and required the same aseptic techniques as a small surgical procedure. In 1952 Aubaniac [1] first described the percutaneous approach to the subclavian vein, a procedure vital for monitoring the central venous pressure. This procedure has been applied to administering total parenteral nutrition. In 1950 an innovation of the catheter, the Rochester needle, was introduced by Emil Gauthier, Head of Rochester Products Company, and David John Massa, Anesthesiologist at the Mayo Clinic [7, 10]. This device consisted of a resinous catheter on the outside of a steel needle; the catheter was slipped off the needle into the vein and the needle removed. In 1958 the Intracath,* a plastic catheter lying within the lumen of the needle, was introduced in individual sterile packaging [2]. This type of catheter has reduced the need for the surgical procedure, the cutdown.

The catheter is invaluable in lifesaving procedures; nevertheless serious complications have been documented in the use of both the percutaneous and the surgically placed catheter. Intravenous therapy was fast changing from a purely technical responsibility to one that required a broad range of knowledge. The first change in the steel needle appeared in 1957 when McGaw Laboratories introduced the first grips made out of rubber and looking like an inverted T on a small needle. Shortly after this, small vein sets appeared with foldable wings replacing the metal hub. The traditional steel needle gave way to the winged infusion needle since the latter provided more comfort and was less likely to infiltrate.

In spite of all the advances in scientific and medical technology, complications have increased to alarming proportions. Our expertise must now include the prevention of bacterial, fungal, and particulate contamination. Industry continues to provide equipment to increase the level of patient safety. Today filters are available that limit access of particulate matter, bacteria, fungus, endotoxins, and air to the bloodstream. Proper handling and use of this equipment are vital to the patient's safety.

In the past the subcutaneous and the intramuscular routes were preferred for the parenteral administration of drugs. Today medications are commonly given intravenously, with 60 to 80 percent of infusion fluids containing additives.

Transfusion therapy has moved ahead by leaps and bounds. Not until 1940 did Karl Landsteiner and Alexander Wiener discover the Rhesus system. By 1968 RhoGAM had been manufactured and made available to the physician. RhoGAM relegates Rh hemolytic disease to the past [8].

---

*Deseret Pharmaceutical Co., Inc., Sandy, Utah.

In the middle 1960s, Stanley Dudrick developed intravenous hyperalimentation, a method by which sufficient nutrients are administered into the vein to support life and maintain growth and development.

RECENT MILESTONES

The past 15 years have brought tremendous scientific, technological, and medical advances, and intravenous therapy has become recognized as a highly specialized field. Nurses are being called upon to perform many of the functions formerly reserved for the medical staff — intraarterial therapy, neonatal therapy, and chemotherapy. Professional organizations have been established to provide a forum for the interchange of ideas, information, experience, and knowledge, with the ultimate goal of raising standards and increasing the level of patient care.

The United States House of Representatives, on October 1, 1980, recognized and nationalized I.V. Nurse Day throughout the country. "Resolved, that I.V. Nurse Day be nationally celebrated in honor of the National Intravenous Therapy Association, Inc. on January 25 of each year," read a portion of the proclamation as presented by the Honorable Edward J. Mackey from the Fifth Congressional District of Massachusetts [6].

The National Intravenous Therapy Association (NITA) has established Nursing Standards of Practice that comprise the national guidelines used throughout the country. NITA's first national Certification Examination for Intravenous Nurses was offered at 17 sites across the United States on March 23, 1985.

Intravenous therapy has come a long way since the 1940s, when the sole requisite of the intravenous nurse was to be able to perform a venipuncture skillfully. Today, millions of patients are receiving highly specialized therapy.

Today widespread home I.V. therapy is being successfully accomplished in both private homes and nursing homes — I.V. therapy of all types, continuous, intermittent, involving central venous lines and peripheral lines.

Medical achievements will continue, industry will continue to keep pace by offering more complex equipment, and highly specialized nurses will be required to provide quality care.

REFERENCES

1. Aubaniac, L. L'injection intra veineuse sous-clariculaire: Advantages et technique. *Presse Medicale* 60:1456, 1952.
2. Burt, J. B. Personal communication, August 15, 1973.
3. Crossley, K., and Matsen, M. The scalp-vein needle. *J.A.M.A.* 220:985, 1972.
4. Dudrick, S. J. Rational intravenous therapy. *Am. J. Hosp. Pharm.* 28:83, 1971.
5. Elman, R. Fluid balance from the nurse's point of view. *Am. J. Nurs.* 49:222, 1949.
6. Gardner, C. United States House of Representatives honors the National Intravenous Therapy Association, Inc. *J. NITA* 14(1):5, 1985.
7. Massa, D. J., Lundy, J. S., Faulconer, A., Jr., and Ridley, R. W. A plastic needle. *Staff Meetings Mayo Clin.* July 5, 1950.

8. Queenam, J. T. Review of Rh Disease. In *RhoGAM One Year Later* (Proceeding of Symposium on RhoGAM Rho[D] Immune Globulin [Human], New York, April 17, 1969). Raritan, N.J.: Ortho Diagnostics, 1969.

9. Schmidt, J. E. *Medical Discoveries Who and When*. Springfield, Ill.: Thomas, 1959, pp. 59–62.

10. Smith, S. S., Jr. Personal communication, January 21, 1981.

CHAPTER 2

Legal Implications of Intravenous Therapy

Ada Lawrence Plumer

Because of the law and its interpretations, doubts and questions exist regarding the legal rights of nurses to administer intravenous therapy. The scope of intravenous therapy has become more complex and specialized. The nurse is now involved in administration procedures formerly performed solely by the physician and considered medical acts. Violation of the Medical Practice Act is considered a criminal offense.

PROFESSIONAL AND GOVERNMENT REGULATIONS

To alleviate the nurse's fears regarding possible liability for claimed violation of the Medical Practice Act, the medical profession has issued joint policy statements with nursing associations on a number of procedures, including intravenous therapy.

Joint statements are written when questions arise regarding the nurse's professional responsibility or obligation to perform specific therapeutic measures and these questions are not answered in existing statutes (i.e., nursing practice acts and medical practice acts). This is considered the most useful way to deal with procedures that are carried out by members of both professions.

Sponsors of joint statements are the state nurses' association, which is concerned with the area of nursing practice; the state medical society, which is concerned with therapeutic measures that were formerly considered solely the practice of medicine and which legally must be prescribed by the physician; and the state hospital association, which is concerned with the issue of institutional liability for therapeutic measures performed in member health care facilities.

Other ways of dealing with procedures are by rulings made by attorneys general, by state boards of nursing, and by the interpretation of the Nursing Practice Act. In some states the nurse practice acts relating to the definition of nursing are broad in wording and do not refer to specific procedures because it is believed that since practice changes rapidly it would be unfortunate if certain procedures had to be reviewed by state legislators before appropriate personnel could carry them out.

In 1985 a survey was made by the author to determine the status of intravenous therapy in the country as it pertained to nursing; the results were as follows:

1. Seventeen states have no policy or rulings.
2. Eight states have issued joint policy statements.
3. Eleven states have developed changes in the Nursing Practice Act to include statements on the practice of intravenous therapy.
4. Three states have opinions of the attorney general.
5. One state follows the Medical Practice Act.
6. Eighteen states have rulings applying to licensed practical nurses.
7. Two states have rulings applying to technicians.

Survey results show a growing trend to relax state statutes governing the administration of intravenous therapy by the registered nurse. In 1972, 34 states had issued joint policy statements compared to only 8 states in 1985. The reason given by some states is that they no longer feel that joint policy statements are necessary since intravenous therapy is considered usual nursing practice. Intravenous therapy is not, however, a part of the standard curriculum of most schools of nursing.

Increased use of intravenous therapy has resulted in its becoming commonplace but not without potential for serious hazards.

The 1985 survey showed that 18 states (up from 13 in 1981) have rulings allowing licensed practical nurses to administer intravenous therapy. Most states stipulate an adequate and appropriate educational preparation beyond the basic practice for as much as one year. The procedures that licensed practical nurses are allowed to perform are limited, and both the registered nurse who supervises the licensed practical nurse and the practical nurse herself are responsible for her actions. Other states surveyed believed that the broader scope of knowledge and understanding required for administering intravenous therapy cannot be built on basic practical nurse education nor can special preparedness training make it an appropriate function of a licensed practical nurse.

"The National Intravenous Therapy Association upholds the belief that only registered professional nurses who have met the requirements as described in the Registered Professional I.V. Nurses' Role Definition and who have completed the Educational Requirements adopted by this Association shall practice I.V. nursing."[3]

Professional nursing associations of intravenous nurses are taking an increasing role in decision making as it concerns the specialty. They established standards of education and practice which provide a criterion for judgment. These standards assure maximal safety for the patient and protect the physician, the nurse, and the health care facility.

In order to answer the question "Can I legally administer intravenous therapy?" each nurse must ask herself or himself:

1. Does the state law delegate this function to the nurse?
2. Does the particular institution's or agency's policy, with the approval of the medical staff, permit the nurse to perform this function?
3. Is the nurse limited in the types of fluids and medications he or she may administer by a list of fluids and drugs delineated by the hospital?
4. Is the order written by a licensed physician for a specific patient?
5. Is the nurse qualified by education and experience to administer intravenous therapy?

The nurse may properly refuse to perform intravenous therapy if in his or her professional judgment he or she is not qualified and competent. It has been established by law that in a question of negligence, individuals are not protected because they have "carried out the physician's orders." They are held liable in relation to their knowledge, skill, and judgment.

In hospitals and states in which no written opinion relevant to intravenous therapy exists, what is the registered nurse's responsibility when ordered by a licensed staff physician to administer intravenous therapy? "A nurse is legally required to carry out any nursing or medical procedure she is directed to carry out by a duly licensed physician unless she has reason to believe harm will result to the patient from doing so"[1]. In order to meet his or her legal responsibility to the patient, the nurse must be qualified by knowledge and experience to execute the medical procedure, otherwise that nurse may properly refuse to perform it. "Where there is no medical reason to question a physician's order, the nurse's failure to carry out such an order will subject her to liability for any consequent harm to the patient"[1].

States are recommending that schools of professional nursing include in their curriculum a course that will offer the student nurse clinical instruction and experience in intravenous therapy. The registered professional nurse would then be qualified to carry out the procedure when ordered by a licensed physician and determined as proper professional nursing practice of the employing health care facility.

Investigational Drugs

Today increasing numbers of investigational drugs are being administered intravenously. Investigational drugs are drugs that have not been approved for general use and have not been cleared for sale in interstate commerce by the Federal Food and Drug Administration. Hospitals have an obligation to their patients to see that specific guidelines, policies, and procedures for their use are established. A specific approved list should be available with basic information including dosage, strength available, actions and uses, side effects, and symptoms of toxicity. A patient consent is required.

Investigational drugs, if approved by the appropriate hospital policymaking committee for intravenous administration by the nurse, should be added to any approved list of medications provided by the committee.

The Private-Duty Nurse

A private-duty nurse, who works under the direction, supervision, and control of a hospital and private physician, is subject to the rules and regulations of the hospital concerning all matters relating to nursing care. If the hospital policy-making committee has rules regarding who may and may not give intravenous therapy, the private-duty nurse is subject to the same rules that apply to the staff nurse. To prevent any misunderstanding on the part of the private-duty nurse, a specific sentence may be added to the hospital's joint policy statement noting that the private-duty nurse who has complied with the criteria applicable to the administration of intravenous therapy may give an intravenous infusion.

The Agency Nurse

Agencies, whose purpose are to provide professional personnel for health care centers on a day-to-day basis, are increasing in number. They provide valuable help when a shortage of personnel occurs. However, health care centers must be aware of problems that exist: the agency nurse's unfamiliarity with the hospital, specific hospital policies, and possibly the functions performed by a specialized department. This is particularly true in the intravenous therapy department, where functions vary from hospital to hospital and have important legal consequence, functions with which the agency nurse may be unfamiliar. Hospitals and nursing departments have an obligation to recognize these problems and to take action to prevent potential risk to the patient as well as possible litigation.

LEGAL GUIDELINES

The fear of the intravenous nurse of involvement in malpractice suits is increasing with the increase in the complexity of therapy and in the numbers of intravenous specialists. Many of the functions performed by the nurse have important legal consequences. An understanding of the legal principles and guidelines involved is necessary if daily professional actions are not to result in unwanted malpractice suits. It will be easier to arrive at a clearer understanding of these guidelines if a few of the legal terms involved are first defined.

Definitions

Criminal law relates to an offense against the general public because of its harmful effect on the welfare of society as a whole. Criminal actions are prosecuted by a government authority, and punishment includes imprisonment or fine, or both. The administration of intravenous therapy, if performed in an unlawful manner, can involve the nurse in criminal conduct. Violation of the Nursing Practice Act or the Medical Practice Act by an unlicensed person is considered a criminal offense.

Civil law deals with conduct that affects the legal rights of the private person or corporation. When harm occurs the guilty party may be required to pay damages to the injured person.

A *tort* is a private wrong, by act or omission, which can result in a civil action by the harmed person. Common torts relevant to professional nursing practice include negligence, assault and battery, false imprisonment, slander and libel, and invasion of privacy. There are some defenses in civil actions, e.g., contributory negligence on the part of the plaintiff.

Coercion on a rational adult patient in order to insert a cannula constitutes assault and battery. If the patient refuses treatment, and explanation and encouragement fail, the physician should be notified.

Malpractice is the negligent conduct of professional persons. Negligent conduct is not acting in a reasonable and prudent manner, with resultant damage to a person or his or her property. It is not synonymous with carelessness, although a person who is careless is negligent.

If a nurse with no previous training administers an intravenous infusion, performs an arterial puncture, or adds medications to intravenous fluids, and does it as carefully as possible but harm results, a civil court may rule his or her conduct as negligent; that nurse should not have performed the act without previous training and experience. Such a negligent action is considered an act of malpractice because it involves a professional person. However, if the act of malpractice does not create harm, legal action cannot be initiated.

The rule of personal liability is "every person is liable for his own tortious conduct" [his own wrongdoing] [1]. No physician can protect the nurse from an act of negligence by bypassing this rule with verbal assurance. The nurse involved cannot avoid legal liability even though another person may be sued and held liable. The physician who orders an intracatheter cannot take responsibility for the nurse who is negligent in carrying out the procedure. If harm occurs, the nurse is liable for his or her own wrongdoing.

The rule of personal liability is relevant in medication errors. Medication errors are a common cause of malpractice claims against nurses [2]. Negligence results from the administration of a drug to the wrong patient, at the wrong time, in an incorrect dosage, or in an improperly prescribed manner. If the physician writes an incomplete or partially illegible order and the nurse fails to clarify it before administration and harm results, the nurse is liable for negligence. The same applies to the administration of intravenous fluids. Nurses have a legal and professional responsibility to know the purpose and effect of the intravenous fluids and medications which they administer. They must take care to ensure that patients receive the prescribed volume of fluid at the prescribed rate of flow. Fluid administered in an amount above or below that ordered constitutes an error that can result in fluid and electrolyte imbalances and lead to serious consequences for the patient and litigation for the nurse.

Approaches

The act of *observation* is the legal and professional responsibility of the nurse. Frequent observation is imperative for the early detection and prevention of complications. Complications that are not detected and are allowed to increase in severity because of failure to observe the patient constitute an act of negligence on the part of the nurse.

The rule of personal liability applies to supervisors and nurses under their supervision. Supervisors usually will not be held liable for the negligence of nurses under their supervision, since every person is liable for his or her own wrongdoing. However, a supervisor is expected to know if the nurse is competent to perform duties assigned without supervision. Supervisors who are negligent in the assignment of an inexperienced nurse or a nurse who requires supervision may be held liable for the acts of the nurse [1]. Nurses themselves are always held liable.

The nurse-patient relationship plays a significant role in influencing the patient in initiating legal liability against the nurse. The intravenous nurse must be particularly aware of and attentive to the emotional needs of the patient. Inserting cannulas can cause pain and apprehension in the patient. It is important for the specialist to develop an efficient interpersonal relationship. The nurse who is impersonal, aloof, and so busy with the technical process of starting an intravenous infusion that he or she has no time for establishing a kindly relationship with the patient is the suit-prone nurse whose personality may initiate resentment and later malpractice suits. The patient most likely to sue is the one who is resentful, frequently hostile, uncooperative, and dissatisfied with the nursing care. By demonstrating respect, care, and concern for the patient, as well as rendering skilled, efficient nursing care, the nurse may avoid malpractice claims.

Policies and procedures should be described in detail, and all intravenous nurses should be required to know and review them periodically. Policies and procedures should follow national guidelines established by the Center for Disease Control (CDC) and Nursing Standards of Practice established by the National Intravenous Therapy Association (NITA). These guidelines provide a model for intravenous nurses and optimal care and protection for the patient.

The impact of the National Intravenous Therapy Association is being seen as increased educational programs are being desired. Certification programs have been developed for specialty nursing practice. Certification is the process by which an association guarantees that a licensed individual has met specified standards and is found professionally and technically competent for specialty practice. Certification for the intravenous therapy nurse became available in the spring of 1985, when the first NITA professional credentialing examination took place. Recertification is required every three years by reexamination or by documented continuing education in intravenous nursing.

Evaluation of Adequate Performance

A standard must be carefully defined in order for the Health Care Institution or the nurse to evaluate adequate performance. Tools useful in this process include the following [2]:

1. Intravenous Nursing Standards of Practice (NITA)
2. State Agency Standards For Registered Nurses
3. Joint Commission on Accreditation of Hospitals' Standards For Registered Nurses
4. American Nurses' Association Standards of Nursing Practice
5. Policies and Procedures of the Employing Health Care Institution

REFERENCES

1. Bernzweig, E. P. *Nurses' Liability for Malpractice* (3rd ed.). New York: McGraw-Hill, 1981, pp. 68, 72, 114, 135.
2. Guarriello, D. L. Intravenous Therapy and the Law. NITA 6:278–281, 1983.
3. The National Intravenous Therapy Association, Inc., Philosophy:NITA 5:19, 1981.

CHAPTER 3

Organization of an Intravenous Department and Guide to Teaching

Ada Lawrence Plumer

THE VALUE OF PARENTERAL TEAMS

An intravenous department plays an important role in the services of a hospital. The quality of patient care is improved because specialized nurses, freed from other responsibilities, are able to focus attention on developing standards of performance; programs relevant to intravenous therapy are easier to maintain. These nurses, cognizant of potential dangers, are vigilant and meticulous in performing and maintaining intravenous therapy. Their continuous experience contributes to the performance of atraumatic venipunctures, conservation of veins, and reduction of complications. The knowledge, skill, and experience of these specialized nurses add to the safety of the blood bank program. The simultaneous administration of intravenous solutions and collection of blood samples does much to alleviate the anxiety of the patient and preserve the veins. The value of intravenous therapy teams has been well documented. In one hospital, despite the fact that the transfusion therapy service maintained 90 percent of the total number of catheters, it was responsible for only 11 percent of the transfusion-related infections [2]. This was attributed mainly to (1) the skill and experience of specially trained personnel in inserting catheters atraumatically and (2) the daily and twice-daily observation and care of catheter sites.

In a report of the National Coordinating Committee on Large Volume Parenterals, Baker [1] stated:

> With regard to nursing personnel, should functional specialization for IV administration be encouraged? An example of this would be the use of IV teams. Should their use be required? Certified? Should special or continuing education be required? There is a feeling that the answer is "yes" to all these questions. Any recommendations will probably stop short of making IV teams a requirement for the smaller hospital.

With the increasing complexity of intravenous therapy and the potential dangers associated with it, hospitals have come to recognize the value of intravenous therapy teams. Parenteral departments have been established in a great many hospitals. However since Diagnosis Related Groups (DRGs) have come into being, a number of hospitals have found it necessary to adopt a different approach to insure quality assurance in the provision of intravenous therapy. They have found it beneficial to employ one or more qualified, knowledgeable intravenous nurses to provide ongoing intravenous therapy education to the general nursing staff, to implement the quality control process, and to serve as resource for difficult intravenous procedures.

The National Intravenous Therapy Association (NITA) was established in 1973; in 1987 it has many chapters throughout the country. It has established nursing standards of practice to provide optimal care and protection for the patient. Certification is available to nurses working in the field of intravenous therapy. Hospitals should encourage their nurses to take every opportunity to further their education by participating in national organization and becoming Certified Registered Nurses in Intravenous Therapy (CRNI).

DIRECTORSHIP OF THE DEPARTMENT

Because the functions performed by the intravenous department are not generally classified as nursing procedures, the responsibility for this department is often allocated to the head of another department directly involved in the functions of intravenous therapy, such as the director of the blood bank, the pharmacy, or the anesthesia department. The intravenous department (1) fulfills an important function of the blood bank, administering bloods and blood components, (2) is in close alliance with the pharmacy, administering infusions of which 50 to 80 percent contain drugs, and (3) executes many of the functions performed by the anesthesiologist. Since some of these procedures may be considered medical functions it is advisable to have a physician share the responsibility or be available for counsel and advice.

PHILOSOPHY AND OBJECTIVES

In organizing a department the first consideration should be given to establishing a philosophy and the objectives necessary to support such a philosophy. An example follows:

Philosophy To administer safe and successful intravenous therapy in the best interests of the patient, the hospital, and the nursing profession.

Objectives The objectives of an intravenous department are as follows:

1. To develop skills and impart knowledge that will provide a high level of safety in the practice of intravenous therapy (embodies administration of solutions and drugs, administration of blood and blood components, placement of intravenous cannulas, and withdrawal of blood samples).
2. To encourage further education and knowledge in the field of intravenous therapy.

3. To assist in keeping the nursing staff educated in the maintenance of intravenous therapy and other nursing needs relevant to intravenous therapy.
4. To collaborate with orientation personnel in the development and implementation of continuing education in intravenous therapy.
5. To develop nursing judgment in intravenous therapy.
6. To keep abreast of the latest scientific and medical advances and their implications in the practice of intravenous therapy.

FUNCTIONS OF AN INTRAVENOUS DEPARTMENT

In organizing an intravenous department, one must first classify the functions to be performed. They may include the following:

1. Administration of parenteral fluids
2. Preparation and administration of drugs in solution
3. Administration of blood
4. Routine inspection and daily change of all infusion tubings and dressings
5. Bleeding of donors
6. Bleeding of patients under supervision of the physician
7. Collection of venous blood samples for all laboratories: chemistry, bacteriology, hematology, blood bank, and so on. This includes:
   a. Collection of blood samples routinely from all surgical admissions for typing and grouping in the blood bank
   b. Knowledge of the requirements of the various laboratory tests, including the proper collection and handling of blood samples

Subspecialty areas include:

1. Total parenteral nutrition
2. Intravenous cancer therapy
3. Intraarterial therapy
4. Pediatric intravenous therapy
5. Administration of intravenous push medications
6. Phlebotomies

Policies and Procedures

Policies and procedures play a basic and vital role in the functioning of a department, serving as a guide to its operations, providing the nurse with adequate instruction, and assuring the patient of a high level of nursing care. They may also provide legal protection in determining whether or not an individual involved in negligent conduct has had adequate instruction in performing the act.

Policies and procedures should comply with state and federal laws, and national guidelines should be followed. The Joint Commission on Accreditation of Hospitals (JCAH) provides a manual for hospital accreditation, the American Association of Blood Banks provides a technical manual with standards for care and administration of blood, the Center for Disease Control provides additional guidelines, and the National Intravenous Therapy Association provides Nursing Standards of Practice.

Policies describing the responsibilities of the intravenous nurse vary significantly among hospitals and should be outlined to prevent confusion or misunderstanding. Examples of a few such policies follow.

Administration of Parenteral Fluids

1. Intravenous nurses will, upon written order, initiate all infusions, with the exception of those not approved for administration by the nurse.
2. No more than two attempts at venipuncture will be allowed. If two attempts are unsuccessful, the supervisor must be notified.
3. Venipunctures should be avoided in the lower extremities except at a time when the patient's condition may necessitate this use, and this location has specifically been ordered by the physician.
4. All intravenous lines are to be changed every 24 to 48 hours depending upon hospital policy.
5. Solutions are to be labeled indicating the date and time the seal is broken. All intravenous solutions must be used or discarded within 24 hours of the time the container is opened.

Preparation and Administration of Intravenous Drugs

1. Nurses will, upon written order, prepare and administer only those solutions, medications, and combinations of drugs approved in writing by the pharmacy and the therapeutics committee.
2. Nurses must check the patient's chart and question the patient regarding sensitivity to drugs which may cause anaphylaxis. They must observe the patient following initial administration of such drugs. If a question of sensitivity exists, the drug should be administered by the physician.

Use of Force in Performing Venipuncture

No coercion will ever be used on a rational adult patient. If such a patient refuses an infusion or transfusion, the intravenous nurse will report the fact to the head nurse or physician.

Flushing and Irrigation of Intravenous Cannulas

1. Plugged cannulas are not to be irrigated or flushed. Positive pressure, either by the positive pressure chamber of the infusion set or by syringe, shall not be used to remove a stubborn clot.

2. Cannulas may be flushed or irrigated for the sole purpose of *maintaining* patency.

Procedures should provide in detail the step-by-step directions for performing each function.

Selection of Personnel

The intravenous nurse is usually a registered nurse who is specially hired and trained since intravenous therapy involves the administration of drugs, blood, and fluids requiring specialized judgment and skill. Because of the highly specialized therapy and the responsibility involved, the success of the department will depend upon the selection of its personnel. Not all nurses are successful as intravenous nurses.

The nurse, who will be drawing blood samples and giving transfusions where carelessness can mean a patient's life, must be conscientious. The importance of the job, the importance of being accurate, and the importance of careful patient identification must be realized by the nurse. Duties include mixing and administering drugs which, given intravenously, act rapidly. There is no margin for error.

Cooperation and teamwork are essential to the success of the department. No one individual's job is finished until the entire department has completed its work. If one nurse becomes involved in a time-consuming emergency, the others must show a readiness and willingness to help out and accomplish the remaining work.

Mental and emotional stability play an important part in the nurse's success as an intravenous therapist. Manual dexterity, necessary in administering an intravenous infusion, is greatly affected by the mental and emotional attitude of the nurse. The performance of few procedures is so easily affected by stress as is the execution of a difficult venipuncture.

An understanding and pleasant personality are other assets necessary to the success of the individual and the department. The nurse has unpleasant functions to perform. These unpleasant tasks are better tolerated by the patient if the nurse is understanding and congenial.

Tact is important. The nurse works in close conjunction with the hospital nursing staff, the blood bank, the various laboratories, and the patient. An inappropriate attitude and uncooperative personality can do much to impair the harmony of these departments.

The nurse in charge of the intravenous department, who must assume responsibility for the teaching, training, and successful functioning of this department, should have a voice in selecting its personnel.

Once the functions of this department are classified, the work load should start at a reasonable level. It may be desirable to start by performing only a few designated functions, such as the administration of blood and fluids. After this program has been successfully organized, other functions may be added. By so doing, the problems that may arise on initiating such a program may be met and remedied, and the success of the department may be guaranteed from the outset.

Before this department can go into operation, the hospital nursing staff must first be educated as to its functions.

Call System

A system for receiving calls must be organized, with special emphasis on emergency calls. Some systems work better than others under various conditions. The size of the hospital, number of patients, size and location of the department, and the functions to be performed must be taken into consideration in deciding which system would be most adaptable.

Requisitions
Requests for parenteral administrations and other functions may be filled out on requisitions and sent to the department. This system has the drawbacks of added paperwork, lost time involved, and the necessity of the intravenous therapist's having to return to the department to pick up the requisitions. It may prove successful in smaller hospitals, where calls are not as numerous as in a large hospital and where the nurses are stationed in the blood bank or laboratory.

Page System
The page operator lists the floor extensions as they are received. The intravenous nurse calls in every half hour to pick up calls. Any emergency call may be put through by means of voice page or by means of a radio pager.

Routine Rounds
Routine rounds may be made twice a day by the intravenous therapist. The requests for services are listed on a clipboard with the patient's name and room number. When orders have been filled they are checked off by the intravenous therapist. One nurse in each building is equipped with a radio pager. This is used only for emergency calls or requests that must be performed before the second round, or after rounds are completed.

This system involves less expenditure of time by the nursing staff. It eliminates the necessity for placing calls or sending out requisitions. The intravenous department is freed from unnecessary phone calls. The charge nurse, with a glance at the board, immediately knows what procedures have been performed.

Preparation of Equipment

Setting up the necessary equipment for procedures to be performed must be allotted to either the intravenous department or the nursing staff.

Preparation of Equipment by the Intravenous Department
When preparation of equipment becomes the responsibility of the intravenous department, an equipment cart must be provided on each floor. This cart carries all necessary equipment for parenteral administration as follows:

- Intravenous solutions
- Intravenous sets
- Armboards
- Poles

Tourniquet

Bandages

Adhesive tape

Alcohol

Syringes

Sterile sponges

Cannula assortment

Final filters

Antiseptic swabs and ointment

Broad spectrum antibiotic ointment

The nurse checks the orders directly from the doctor's order book and, by means of the equipment cart, sets up the procedures and initiates each order as he or she continues rounds.

Preparation of Equipment by Nursing Staff
The staff nurse distributes necessary equipment, solution, set, armboard, and pole for parenteral fluids. The intravenous nurse carries a prep tray. This system automatically places a double check on solutions and medications ordered and saves time. If each nurse is responsible for setting up the necessary equipment for the patient, little time is lost, whereas a great deal of time is utilized by the intravenous therapist in preparing all patients. This system eliminates the necessity for an equipment cart on each floor.

Cooperation of Interdepartmental Personnel

Before this department starts to function, a thorough explanation must be made to the staff of doctors, for only with cooperation in every department will success be guaranteed. The doctors should be requested to cooperate by writing intravenous orders early — before 9 A.M. when at all possible. This will assure that the physician's orders are initiated at a reasonable hour. This is particularly important when the intravenous department has inaugurated the system of making rounds.

COLLECTION OF BLOOD SAMPLES

Today, since intravenous therapy has become more specialized and time-consuming, the collection of blood samples is often allocated to the technician. In some health care facilities, collection of blood samples may be the function of the intravenous department, especially if the specimen is to be obtained from a specialized central venous catheter or from a totally implantable central venous system.

The program for collection of blood samples may be initiated and become an added function of the intravenous department only after:

1. The therapists have been adequately trained in the necessary laboratory procedures.

2. A system has been set up for receiving calls.
3. A method has been arranged for transportation of specimens to the laboratories.
4. The nursing staff and the departments have been made aware of their responsibilities.

Training of Therapists

Before this program is initiated, the intravenous therapist should visit the various laboratories. The nurse should be educated in the proper method of collecting, handling, and transporting blood specimens and must understand and be educated in the performance of the various laboratory tests.

Requisitions

A system for notifying the intravenous department of requests for blood samples must be arranged. Requisitions may (1) be sent directly to the intravenous department or (2) be left at a designated area on each floor to be picked up by the intravenous therapist on rounds. This system saves time and prevents the unnecessary handling and sorting of requisitions from all floors.

Transportation

A safe method of transporting the specimens to the various laboratories must be arranged. This duty may be allotted to: (1) ward helpers on each floor or (2) the intravenous nurse. This is impractical as many bloods must be delivered to laboratories within a limited time. The accuracy of some tests depends upon immediate analysis or proper refrigeration. Alternatively, specimens may be transported by a messenger service by routine pickup or by call system or by a direct specimen chute to the laboratories.

OPERATIONAL ACTIVITIES OF THE INTRAVENOUS DEPARTMENT AT THE MASSACHUSETTS GENERAL HOSPITAL

Call System

The intravenous department has inaugurated the system of routine rounds and makes use of the radio pager for urgent requests. The department services the wards by means of routine rounds twice a day plus early rounds for fasting blood samples only.

Requests for procedures to be performed are listed with the patient's name and room number on designated blackboards and clipboards. Orders executed are checked off by the therapist. Any orders written after first rounds are added to the board to be carried out on afternoon rounds.

One intravenous nurse in each building is equipped with a radio pager. This page system is used only when (1) emergency procedures are necessary, (2) urgent procedures are required that must be performed before second rounds, or (3) tests involving specific times must be made, e.g., blood samples to be drawn at a specific time after injection of dye. The page system is used full-time after last rounds are made.

A printed card reading INTRAVENOUS NURSE ON THE FLOOR is carried by each intravenous therapist. This card is left at the desk for the duration of time the nurse is on the ward.

Functions and Regulations

Administration of Parenteral Fluids
The intravenous nurse initiates all intravenous infusions, with the exception of those prepared by the doctor and containing drugs not on the authorized list. The intravenous nurse does not:

1. Administer intravenous infusions in the local extremities unless specifically ordered by the physician to do so, and the patient's condition warrants.
2. Apply positive pressure by pressure chamber in administering parenteral fluids.
3. Apply force in administering intravenous or other procedures on rational adult patients. Patients' refusal to comply with treatment is reported to the physician.

The intravenous nurse and the nursing service remove cannulas when infiltration occurs or infusion is terminated, on the order of the doctor.

Preparation and Administration of Drugs in Solution
The intravenous nurse prepares and administers all drugs on the authorized list only, affixing to the solution bottle a label containing the name of the patient, the name of the drug, dosage prepared, and the time and date. The intravenous nurse must realize that he or she is legally responsible for every medication he or she administers.

Administration of Transfusions
The intravenous department initiates transfusions. The following policies apply:

1. There must be an order by the physician on the date the transfusion is scheduled.
2. All transfusions require filters.
3. Bloods are not delivered to the wards until requested by the intravenous therapist.
4. Bloods are not to be placed in the ward refrigerator.
5. Bloods not used within a half hour are to be returned to the blood bank.
6. The intravenous therapist remains and observes the patient for the first 5 minutes after initiating the transfusion.
7. Transfusions are to be terminated at once if reactions occur. *Imperative:* Reaction slips are sent to the blood bank with a blood sample.
8. Positive pressure is never applied when administering blood except under the direct supervision of the physician.
9. Staff nurses are not allowed to attach blood to an intravenous infusion. This is the responsibility of the intravenous nurse.

Collection of Venous Blood Samples for All Hospital Laboratories
Collection of blood samples is now performed by technicians.

Program. Each ward has an allotted area designated for the use of the blood collection program. This area contains:

1. A large envelope in which blood requisitions are left for the intravenous nurse.
2. Blood collection equipment, including stock of various vacuum tubes and cannulas.
3. Containers (small wire baskets) to hold blood samples, labeled and painted different colors to designate the various laboratories.

Venous Blood Samples. All requisitions for venous blood are placed in the requisition envelope until 3 P.M. on weekdays and until noon on Saturdays. After 3 P.M. on weekdays only emergency requisitions and requisitions for the blood bank are honored. Each afternoon the technician draws blood samples on all surgical admissions, to be sent to the blood bank for typing.

TEACHING PROGRAMS

An adequate teaching program and criteria for the evaluation of the intravenous nurse must be established. The criteria will be dependent upon the role of the intravenous nurse as dictated by hospital policies. The competency of the nurse may be substantiated by answering questionnaires on intravenous therapy, transfusion therapy, and drug therapy and a demonstration of involved procedures, such as the administration of parenteral fluids using metal needles and plastic catheters, the administration of blood and its components, the preparation and administration of drug admixtures, and the collection of blood samples. The intravenous nurse receives on-the-job training. The length of time involved in teaching depends upon the individual and may range from 6 to 8 weeks. The following is a suggested outline for teaching intravenous, drug, and transfusion therapy.

Suggested Teaching Outline

I. Legal implications of intravenous therapy
   A. *State policy.* Review state rulings, joint policies related to intravenous therapy.
   B. *Hospital policy.* Review health institution's or agency's policy, which has been approved by the medical staff.
      1. Responsibilities of nurse in administering intravenous therapy
      2. List of fluids and drugs delineated by the hospital for administration by the nurse
   C. *National Standards.*
      1. CDC
      2. NITA
   D. Legal requirements
      1. Qualification by education and experience
      2. Adherence to hospital policy

3. Thorough knowledge of fluids and drugs: their effects, limitations, and dosages
            4. Order by licensed physician for specific patient
            5. Skilled judgment
        E. Review of policy and procedure books
            1. Policy statements do not provide immunity if the nurse is negligent.
            2. The nurse is legally responsible for his or her own acts.
II. Equipment
    A. Review all types of equipment, their characteristics and usage.
    B. Review procedures for the proper handling of equipment, changing of in-line administration sets, use of filters, etc.
    C. Adhere to established infection-control procedures and guidelines in the use of equipment.
        1. Aseptic technique in manipulation of equipment
        2. Inspection of parenteral fluids and containers
        3. Daily change of administration sets
III. Anatomy and physiology as applied to intravenous therapy
    A. Review names and locations of peripheral veins of the upper extremity.
    B. Differentiate between arteries and veins. Recognize an inadvertent arterial puncture.
    C. Recognize dangers associated with the use of veins of the lower extremities.
    D. Understand factors that influence the size and condition of the vein.
        1. Trauma
        2. Temperature
        3. Diagnosis of the patient
        4. Psychological outlook of the patient
    E. Choose veins suitable for venipuncture
        1. To infuse various fluids and medications, with preservation of veins in mind
        2. To draw blood samples
        3. To administer blood
IV. Intravenous Therapy
    A. Methods of infusion
        1. Constant
        2. Intermittent (by "piggyback" or heparin lock)
        3. Infusion by pump
    B. Manner and approach to the patient
        1. Explain the vasovagal reaction (an undesirable autonomic nervous system response).
        2. Alleviate fears.
            a. Make patient comfortable
            b. Explain procedure
            c. Reassure patient
            d. Appear confident

C. Methods of distending veins
   1. Apply a broad tourniquet above selected site
   2. Apply a blood pressure cuff inflated to 50 to 60 mm Hg or to just below diastolic pressure
   3. Have patient clench fist periodically.
   4. Allow arm to hang dependent over the side of the bed
   5. Tap lightly slightly distal to the proposed venipuncture site.
   6. Apply moist heat to entire extremity.
D. *Antiseptic and aseptic technique.* Skin flora have been implicated as an important source of organisms responsible for catheter-associated infection. Stress importance of handwashing. Adherence to aseptic and antiseptic technique is imperative, especially during preparation of the venipuncture site
E. Choice of cannula (straight metal needle, small-vein needle, catheter)
   1. Purpose of the infusion
   2. Condition and availability of the vein
   3. Gauge and length of cannula depend upon:
      a. Location of the vein
      b. Fluid employed
      c. Purpose of the infusion
F. Techniques of venipuncture
   1. Small-vein needle
   2. Syringe and needle
   3. Vacuum tube and needle holder (commercially supplied)
   4. Catheters (over-the-needle, through-the-needle). Complications associated with catheters included mechanical and chemical thrombophlebitis, infection, and catheter embolism.
G. Hazards and complications. Observing the patient, reporting reactions, and taking measures to prevent complications are the nurse's legal and professional responsibilities
   1. Systemic complications
      a. Infections (septicemia, fungemia)
         Preventive measures:
         (1) Use aseptic and antiseptic technique.
         (2) Inspect all fluids and containers before use.
         (3) Use fluids within 24 hours.
         (4) Change administration sets every 24–48 hours.
         (5) Do not irrigate plugged cannulas.
         (6) Remove nonfunctioning sets and needles.
      b. Pulmonary embolism (occurs when a substance, usually a clot, becomes free floating and is propelled by the venous circulation to the right side of the heart and on into the pulmonary artery)
         Preventive measures:
         (1) Use clot filters for infusing blood and blood components.
         (2) Use special blood filters of micropore size for infusing several units of stored bank blood.

(3) Avoid using veins of the lower extremities.
(4) Avoid irrigating plugged cannulas.
c. Air embolism (may be fatal when small bubbles accumulate dangerously and form tenacious bubbles that block the pulmonary capillaries)
Preventive measures:
(1) Vigilance in preventing fluid containers from emptying. Infusions through a central venous catheter carry greater risk of running dry as there is more likely to be a negative venous pressure.
(2) Vented Y-type infusions or piggyback infusions allowing solutions to run simultaneously may introduce air into line if container empties. Check valves, safety valves, and micropore filters (wet) reduce this risk.
d. Circulatory overload (a real hazard in patients with impaired renal and cardiac functions)
Preventive measures:
(1) Maintain infusion at prescribed flow rate. Do not play "catch-up" if infusion is behind schedule.
(2) Never apply positive pressure when infusing fluids and blood.
(3) Do not administer fluids in excess of quantity ordered to maintain a keep-open infusion.
(4) Be alert to signs of circulatory overload.
e. Speed shock (systemic reaction occurring when a substance foreign to the body is rapidly introduced into the circulation)
Preventive measures:
(1) Slow injection of drugs
(2) Use of controlled volume chambers
(3) Use of micropore drip sets
(4) Use of double clamps — an extra clamp ensures greater safety should the initial clamp let go.
(5) Ensure that intravenous fluid is flowing freely before regulating flow.
f. Fluid and medication error
Preventive measures:
(1) Be familiar with intravenous fluids.
(2) Know drug, dosage, and rate of administration.
(3) Clarify orders.
(4) Substantiate identity of the patient and the admixture.
2. Local complications
a. Phlebitis (mechanical, chemical, and septic)
Preventive measures:
(1) Do not use veins located over an area of joint flexion.
(2) Anchor cannulas well to prevent motion and reduce the risk of introducing microorganisms into puncture wound.
(3) Adequately dilute medications.
(4) Use a cannula relatively smaller than the vein.

(5) Use aseptic and antiseptic technique.
(6) Remove cannula within 72 hours.
(7) Remove cannula for:
  (a) Erythema
  (b) Induration
  (c) Tenderness by palpation of venous cord
  (d) Nonfunctioning needle
  b. Infiltration (recognize extravasation)
  (1) Check questionable extremity against normal extremity.
  (2) Apply a tourniquet tightly enough to restrict venous flow proximal to the injection site. If infusion continues regardless of this venous obstruction, extravasation is evident.
H. Intraarterial therapy
  1. Arterial puncture
    a. Syringe and needle
    b. Indwelling catheter
  2. Constant arterial pressure monitoring
    a. Set-up procedure
  3. Arterial blood gases (ABG)
    a. Collection
    b. Interpretation
  4. Swan Ganz catheter
    a. Basic knowledge
    b. Insertion
    c. Complications
V. Rationale of fluid and electrolyte therapy
  A. Fundamentals of fluid and electrolyte metabolism
    1. Body fluid compartments
    2. Electrolyte composition
    3. Acid-base balance
  B. Principles of fluid therapy
    1. Deficit
    2. Maintenance
    3. Replacement
  C. Intravenous fluids
    1. Classification and effect
      a. Isotonic
      b. Hypotonic
      c. Hypertonic
    2. Parenteral fluids
VI. Drug therapy
  A. Hazards
    1. Incompatibilities
      a. Therapeutic (undesirable reaction from overlapping effect of two drugs)

b. Physical (interaction which leads to a visible change such as color, precipitate, or gas bubbles)
c. Chemical (invisible interaction, with degradation of drug and loss of therapeutic activity)
2. Vascular trauma
3. Speed shock
4. Bacterial and fungal contamination
5. Particulate contamination
6. Medication errors

B. Knowledge of the drug
1. Dose and effect
2. Recommended rate of infusion
3. Reactions
4. Contraindications

C. Factors controlling stability and compatibility of admixtures
1. Pharmaceutical agents in drug formation (buffers, preservatives, and stabilizers)
2. Brand of drug (formulation varies)
3. pH of drug, pH of intravenous fluid
4. Concentration (degree of dilution)
5. Order of mixing
6. Diluent
7. Period of time solution stands
8. Light
9. Temperature

D. Preparation of admixture
1. Procedure for transcribing orders on medication label
2. Frequency with which medication order should be renewed
3. Reconstitution of drug using aseptic and antiseptic technique
   a. Correct diluent
   b. Correct volume
   c. Absence of particulate matter
4. Procedure for adding drug to fluid container
5. Stability of the admixture
6. Labeling

E. Administration of drugs
1. Substantiate identity of patient and admixture.
2. Check for sensitivities of patient to any drug that may cause anaphylaxis.
3. Observe patient for untoward reactions when administering an initial dose of an antibiotic.
4. Patients known to be sensitive to a drug require the presence of a physician.
5. Inspect admixture each time before administration.
6. Record drug, dosage, and amount of fluid on fluid intake chart and medication sheet.

VII. Transfusion therapy
    A. Fundamentals of immunohematology
        1. Factors governing red blood cell destruction
        2. ABO compatibility
        3. Rh compatibility
        4. Handling and storage of blood
    B. Blood and blood components
        1. Uses
        2. Methods of administration
        3. Reactions and protocol to follow
    C. Administration of blood and blood components
        1. Order for the transfusion must be written on the day the transfusion is scheduled.
        2. Substantiate identity of patient and blood.
        3. Inspect blood prior to administration.
        4. Follow proper technique in administration.
        5. Observe patient.
        6. Make documentation in patient's record.

REFERENCES

1. Baker, K. N. Interim report of National Coordinating Committee on Large Volume Parenterals. *Drug Intell. Clin. Pharm.* 7:477, 1973.
2. Bentley, D. W., and Lepper, M. H. Septicemia related to indwelling venous catheters. *J.A.M.A.* 206:1749, 1968.
3. Center for Disease Control. Guidelines for prevention of intravascular infection. *J. NITA* 5(1):39–50, 1982.
4. National Intravenous Therapy Association. (NITA). standards — I.V. therapy. *J. NITA* 5(1):24–29, 1982.

CHAPTER 4

Risk Management and Quality Assurance

Faye Cosentino

RISK MANAGEMENT

The general areas of potential risks for a hospital have been identified by malpractice claims. The hospital has the responsibility of creating and maintaining as safe an environment as possible for patients, visitors, and employees. The hospital is also responsible for the quality of care provided by the medical staff. It strives to protect the patient from injury as a result of negligence.

MALPRACTICE CLAIMS

The hospital and/or involved professional person may be charged with malpractice if an injury occurs AND (1) a standard of care or duty can be established, (2) the standard of care or duty was not met, (3) the patient was harmed or injured because the standard was not met, and (4) it is possible to foresee that injury or harm would result from not meeting the standards (depending on state law).

There are several systems used to identify, investigate, and control unfavorable situations, thus the term *risk management*.

Incident Reports An incident report is required for any accident or error resulting in actual or potential injury or harm. The report should contain only factual statements regarding the incident. Each report must be immediately followed up by a full investigation into all possible causes, and corrective action must be immediately taken to prevent its reoccurrence. Reporting all unexpected incidences, accidents, and errors can help identify pattern problems.

Safety Programs Establishment and monitoring of safety and security surveillance programs can be very effective in preventing unsafe or insecure environments which can result in injuries.

Patient-Family Resolution

Factors that contribute to patients filing malpractice claims include poor doctor–patient or nurse–patient relationships and inadequate communications in general. Potential claims can sometimes be avoided by sincere, honest discussions between the patient or family member and appropriate hospital personnel.

QUALITY ASSURANCE

The Joint Commission on Accreditation of Hospitals (JCAH) mandates an ongoing quality assurance program. The program must objectively and systematically monitor and evaluate the appropriateness and quality of patient care.

Opportunities to improve this care must be pursued. Any identified problems must be resolved. When problems or opportunities to improve care involve more than one department, necessary information must be communicated to all involved areas.

There must be follow-up of all identified problems to assure improvement or resolution.

At least annually, the quality assurance program must be evaluated, and revised if necessary, to assure that the objectives, scope, and organization result in an effective program.

The process of quality assurance focuses on (1) problem identification, (2) problem evaluation, (3) implementation of corrective action, (4) problem reevaluation (follow-up), and (5) problem minimization or solution.

PROBLEM IDENTIFICATION

Problems may be identified by many sources. These include incident reports, patient complaints, employee complaints, questionnaires, surveys, interviews, review of statistical data, and suggestions from patients, visitors, or other department members.

To determine if a problem warrants further investigation, the following questions need to be answered:

1. Is the problem related to quality of patient care?
2. Does the problem arise frequently enough to require correction?
3. Is there a possible solution to the problem?
4. Are the benefits to patient care from solving the problem worth the cost of investigation and solution?

Some problems are serious and require immediate solutions. Many will cross departmental lines and require cooperation from other department members. Priority-based decisions must be hospital-specific.

PROBLEM EVALUATION

Methods used for problem evaluation may include criterion-based studies, interviews with patients and/or staff members, surveys, and observations. Experimental designs can be an excellent method for problem evaluation. However, such designs can be complex and costly.

Criteria

Criteria act as a yardstick and refer to the standards on which the judgments will be based. They can be divided into three main categories: structure, process, and outcome. *Structure* refers to resources available, such as staffing capabilities, management, equipment, information systems, and facilities or building. *Process* refers to how the care should be delivered. Assumptions are made that some aspects of care should be provided in certain ways. *Outcome* is based on the principle that care is delivered in order to bring about certain results. For many studies structure, process, and outcome criteria may be combined.

Policy and procedure manuals are the hospital standards or criteria upon which procedure monitoring may be judged. Criteria may also be based on standards developed and tested by another hospital or listed in professional literature. To ensure an acceptable level of patient care, all manuals must be periodically revised and kept in accordance with national standards.

References for I.V. therapy national standards include: Center for Disease Control (CDC) *Guidelines for the Prevention and Control of Nosocomial Infections* [2], National Intravenous Therapy Association (NITA), *Intravenous Nursing Standards of Practice* [3], American Association of Blood Banks (AABB) *Safe Transfusion* [4], and Joint Commission on Accreditation of Hospitals (JCAH), *Accreditation Manual for Hospitals* [5].

When evaluating studies people tend to find what they are looking for. To minimize this effect of self-fulfilling prophecy, the criteria must be objective and measurable. To avoid subjectivity, care should be taken to use clear, concise terms that can be answered by yes or no, or by numbers. This objectivity must also be kept in mind when preparing a survey or an interview or performing an observation.

Regardless of what method of problem evaluation is used, to achieve meaningful results, standardization, reliability, and validity of the test are of utmost importance when selecting and designing any quality assurance study.

Standardization
Performing the study with standard directions under standard conditions to a sample group for whom the study is intended results in a standardized test. Using random sampling assures that every patient or event has an equal chance of being selected.

Random sampling may be achieved by selecting all patients whose hospital identification band ends in an odd number, or every other occurrence.

Reliability

The best method of estimating the reliability of a study is to perform that study with the same group on two different occasions. Correlating the results of the test–retest method takes into account different patient samples and errors caused by different conditions. If the study cannot be repeated without significant result variance, it cannot be considered reliable.

Validity

Validity of the study refers to whether or not it contains a fair sample of the multiple situations it is supposed to represent. For example, if the sample number is too small or if the proportion of critically ill patients varies, the test cannot be considered valid for a hospital-wide study.

DATA ANALYSIS AND INTERPRETATION

Once the study methodology and criteria have been established, data collection begins. Data are the results obtained from the study. Raw data are the individual results before these results have been compiled into a form that can be analyzed and interpreted.

Data are usually collected in a form that can be analyzed by statistics. This allows mathematical methods for analyzing, interpreting, and reporting these separate elements in summary form. The two main kinds of statistics are descriptive and inferential.

Compliance

Compliance refers to those situations in which the criteria are met. Noncompliance refers to the situations in which the criteria are not met. Both compliance and noncompliance are usually expressed in percentages. The expected compliance rate should be reasonable and achievable.

If the compliance rate appears high, one must carefully examine the conditions required for a standardized, reliable, and valid study of the identified problem. If all these conditions are being met, one must examine the criteria to assure that the identified problem is being addressed. Continuing with a study showing a high rate of compliance will not give the necessary information to solve an identified problem.

Descriptive Statistics

Descriptive statistics allow for meaningful reporting of findings in a small amount of space, even though a large amount of raw data may vary a great deal.

In summarizing study results, descriptive statistics are used to calculate: (1) the average result, (2) the difference between individual results and the average, and (3) the relationship between the average result on one part of the study and the average result on another part [6].

Comparing average results tells a good deal about the relationship between the two parts.

Chapter 4 | Risk Management and Quality Assurance

Arithmetic Mean
In statistical analysis the average result is called the mean. To find the mean, simply total all results and divide the answer by the total number in the study.

This is especially helpful when comparing performances of team members.

Median
Median is the result that falls exactly in the middle of all the score results. The same number of people scored above it as scored below it.

Mode
In any test or study situation, several people can achieve the same score or test result. The score or result that is seen most frequently is called the mode.

Standard Deviation
The difference between individual results and the mean indicates the extent to which figures in a given set vary from the mean. This tells how much variation is present between the group and the individual.

To calculate the standard deviation:

1. Calculate the mean for each score
2. Subtract the mean from each score and square the answer
3. Add all the squares together
4. Divide the sum by the total number of scores
5. Take the square root of that value

In most quality assurance studies it is not necessary to actually perform the mathematical calculations. It is sufficient to know that normally 68 percent of the scores will fall, plus or minus, within a given range from the mean. Calculating the difference between each score and the mean will identify those with abnormal deviations.

If the study design allows for measurement of two different factors, comparing data that pertain to each factor can provide additional information.

Inferential Statistics

Only from a well-designed experimental study can one expect to find that one thing causes another to occur. All other methods allow one to say only that there appears to be a correlation between two things.

Correlation
Correlation refers to an association between occurrences. A *high positive correlation* indicates that A has a high frequency of occurrence when it is associated with B. A *high negative correlation* indicates that A occurs rarely when it is associated with B.

Reporting the Study

Reporting studies to a central quality assurance committee enhances communications within the hospital. Such a committee encourages utilization of all information as efficiently as possible. It can also help a new participant by providing suggestions or assistance with all steps of a study.

Most quality assurance programs use standard hospital-wide forms for reporting the study. This form should be a very short summary of all the steps taken, study results, and what corrective action is planned. All raw data must be retained by the person performing the study.

Personal confidentiality of all participants in the study must be maintained. Copies of any study should be limited strictly to those demonstrating a need to know.

IMPLEMENTATION OF CORRECTIVE ACTION

Factors to consider when choosing a corrective action include identification of: (1) areas for change that the environment can best accommodate, (2) areas of potential barriers or constraints, (3) areas of potential support, and (4) the needed resources.

Each strategy must be analyzed for expected costs, advantages and disadvantages, anticipated benefits, and the feasibility of implementation.

Before developing the plan the following questions must be answered.

WHY is it being implemented?

WHAT must be done to operationalize the plan?

WHO will be involved with and responsible for accomplishing it?

WHERE will implementation take place?

WHEN will it be completed?

The best method of corrective action will depend upon each particular problem and individual situation.

Methods may include policy or procedure revision, equipment change, a new information system, continuous monitoring, or inservice education.

PROBLEM REEVALUATION (FOLLOW-UP)

After corrective action has been implemented, it is necessary to perform a reevaluation to determine if the applied corrective action results in minimization or solution of the problem. Without follow-up one cannot ensure the success of the entire evaluation process.

This evaluation should tell if the anticipated change did in fact occur. If so, is the change sufficient to solve the problem. One also needs to decide if any needs still remain and if so, how they will be met. If change did not occur, one must find the reasons and decide if a new strategy is required.

Frequently, reevaluation is performed by repeating the first evaluation and comparing preaction data with postaction data.

Any evaluation method may be used provided that it contains the necessary elements to obtain standardized, reliable, valid results.

PROBLEM MINIMIZATION OR SOLUTION

The final step is to develop a plan to assure the maintenance of the quality of care achieved with the corrective action. This may require periodic or continuous screening. Surveys, audits, questionnaires, or interviews may be used. Checklists incorporated into everyday care delivery procedures can provide an excellent source for quick identification of problems.

I.V. THERAPY QUALITY ASSURANCE

I.V. therapy quality assurance may be related to several different areas, including compliance with policy and procedure manuals, I.V. therapy-related complications, equipment evaluation, or documentation.

The quality assurance process may be performed by lengthy studies, short-term sampling, or simply solving a problem immediately with documentation and reporting of the quality process utilized.

The following three studies are examples of how the quality assurance process has been used to improve patient care.

QUALITY ASSURANCE STUDY #1

Problem Identification

I.V. therapists state that the number of restarts due to cannula clotting as a result of "run dry" containers is increasing. (Run dry occurs when the fluid container in use empties and air enters the tubing.)

Problem Evaluation

The problem requires a solution because the large number of restarts involved results in delays in medication administration as well as delays in performing other procedures.

Evaluation method: To document percentage of infusions requiring restarts due to run drys on each patient care unit.

Criteria for run dry restart: A completely full or totally empty I.V. container MUST be hanging on infusion. The tubing may be air blocked or the nurse may have withdrawn the air.

Presently available data: (1) Total number of infusions running, each day, on each nursing shift, for each patient care unit. (2) Total number infusions running in entire hospital each day, each unit.

Additional required data: Total number of restarts due to "run dry" containers, for each shift, on each patient care unit.

Time span of study: Must be long enough to allow for majority of nursing staff (who has responsibility of adding containers) to be included in study. Must be long enough to allow for all types of conditions and situations.

Instructions: To allow for standard conditions, nursing staff will not be informed of the study. The study will be performed by all I.V. therapists as they perform their daily procedures.

38 Part I | Introduction to Intravenous Therapy

Data Collection

1. A fill-in sheet was prepared to facilitate data collection (Exhibit 4.1).
2. All I.V. therapists will be involved in data collection.
3. The study will run for one work week (7 days) beginning on 3/10 at 24:00 and ending on 3/16 at 24:00.
4. Criterion for restart due to run dry is: Either a completely full or an entirely empty container MUST be present. The tubing may be air blocked or the nurse may have withdrawn the air.
5. Full instructions on completing the study fill-in sheet were given to each I.V. therapist. These instructions were also written on the sheet.

Data Analysis

The number of restarts, documented for the established criterion, was totaled for each shift of each patient care unit and placed on the study compilation sheet.

The total number of running infusions, for the same 7-day period, were obtained from existing data, totaled, and added to the compilation sheet.

The percentage of running infusions requiring restarts due to run drys was then computed for each shift on each unit.

The total number of possible occasions for run drys (the total of all infusions running on all shifts of all units) for the study period was 3,736. The number of required restarts was 392 (10%). This gives a daily mean of 56 restarts due to run dry infusions (Table 4.1).

Analysis of the compiled data shows that on the day shift, every unit is between 9% and 12%; 7 units have 11%, 6 units have 10%, 2 units have 9%, and 1 unit has 12%. The mean for the day shift is 10%.

On the evening shift, every unit is between 9% and 13%; 8 units have 11%, 6 units have 10%, 1 unit has 9%, and 1 unit has 13%. The mean for the evening shift is 11%.

On the night shift, every unit is between 10% and 12%; 12 units have 10%, 3 units have 11%, and 1 unit has 12%. The mean for the night shift is 10%.

Such slight variation from the total mean, for all shifts and all units, strongly suggests a hospital-wide problem.

Corrective Action

As the nursing staff were the responsible persons for replacing infusion containers, the first step in corrective action is to interview a sample of the nursing staff.

The first two nurses encountered on each shift of each unit were informed of the study and its results, and were asked the following questions:

1. Do you believe this was an accurate study?
2. Do you agree with the results?
3. How do you think run drys can be prevented?

Nursing Interview Results
Of the 96 nurses interviewed, 91 (95%) believed the study to be accurate. The same nurses also agreed with the results. The other 5 nurses believed the number of run drys requiring restarts should have been higher.

EXHIBIT 4.1
Data Collection Sheet for Documentation of Infusions Requiring Restarts Due to Run Drys

General Hospital I.V. Therapy Department Quality Assurance Study

Topic: I.V.s Requiring Restarts Due to Run Dry Containers

Unit	*Date:*			*Date:*			*Date:*		
	Day	Evening	Night	Day	Evening	Night	Day	Evening	Night
3 South									
3 North									
3 West									
3 East									
4 South									
4 North									
4 West									
4 East									
5 South									
5 North									
5 West									
5 East									
6 South									
6 North									
6 West									
6 East									

Instructions:

1. All I.V. therapists will perform study for a one week period, starting 24:00 on 3/10 until 24:00 on 3/16.
2. Criteria for run dry: Either a COMPLETELY FULL or TOTALLY EMPTY container MUST be present. Restart MUST be REQUIRED.
3. Obtain study sheet, use new sheet on fourth day.
4. Fill in date.
5. Opposite appropriate unit, fill in TOTAL NUMBER of I.V.s restarted DUE TO RUN DRYS, for EACH SHIFT.
6. Sign name to sheet. Leave completed sheets on office desk.
2. Add any additional comments below.

Comments:

Signature: _____

TABLE 4.1
Raw Data Compilation of Problem Evaluation Study

	Days			Evenings			Nights		
Unit	T	R	%	T	R	%	T	R	%
3 South	84	9	11	62	7	11	60	6	10
3 North	70	7	10	63	7	11	59	6	10
3 West	105	11	10	89	10	11	84	9	11
3 East	68	7	10	64	7	11	59	6	10
4 South	62	6	10	58	6	10	56	6	11
4 North	93	10	11	86	9	10	80	8	10
4 West	84	9	11	78	10	13	71	7	10
4 East	101	11	11	92	10	11	89	9	10
5 South	98	9	9	86	9	10	82	8	10
5 North	89	9	10	79	8	10	77	8	10
5 West	94	10	11	87	9	10	86	9	10
5 East	70	6	9	63	7	11	60	7	12
6 South	69	7	10	65	6	9	61	7	11
6 North	92	10	11	84	9	11	83	8	10
6 West	103	11	11	88	9	10	87	9	10
6 East	78	9	12	70	8	11	68	7	10
Total	1,360	141	Mean 10%	1,214	131	Mean 11%	1,162	120	Mean 10%

Code:
T = Total I.V.s in progress
R = Total restarts due to run drys
% = Percentage of I.V.s requiring restarts

Suggestions for prevention of restarts when the container ran dry were varied. Those most frequently mentioned were increasing nursing staff, using controllers on all infusions, shifting the responsibility of changing containers to the I.V. therapists, and providing some mechanism to prevent air blocking when the container empties.

All suggestions related to the fact that when a container completely empties, air occludes the tubing, preventing fluid from flowing when the next container is added. To reestablish flow rate, one must withdraw the air from the tubing *before* the cannula clots. On the average patient this must be done within 5 minutes. In the majority of run dry situations, the nurse knows that he or she does not have time to obtain the syringe and needle required to withdraw the air before the cannula clots.

Chapter 4 | Risk Management and Quality Assurance

Evaluations of Suggestions for Problem Solution
Due to budget restraints and availability of nurses, increasing the nursing staff is not appropriate. Purchasing controllers for all infusions is also not within the capital budget. Shifting the responsibility of adding containers to the I.V. therapists would require an increase in staffing for that department. This is not within the budget. The last suggestion of finding a method to prevent air blockage of the tubing appeared to be feasible and was investigated.

Implementation of Corrective Action
Hospital costs to restart infusions which ran dry were calculated. Study showed the daily mean is 56. Cost of supplies for each restart is $4.49. The daily hospital costs for restarts due to run drys is 56 × $4.49, or $251.44. In this situation, staff salaries are not included because staffing will not be decreased with the solution of this problem. Staff time will be used to perform other necessary procedures.

If the restart rate can be lowered to a reasonable 2%, monies saved can be transferred to another type of equipment (within the same budget) which would prevent air from entering the tubing when the container ran dry.

The study showed 3,736 possible occasions for run drys in a 7-day period, or a daily mean of 534. A 2% restart rate would result in 11 restarts daily. The reduction of 45 restarts would result in a daily cost savings of 45 × $4.49, or $202.05.

Existing data showed that with a 2% restart rate for run drys included, the daily mean for infusion starts and restarts would be 98. This results in the availability of $2.07 per start or restart, for equipment to prevent air from entering the tubing when the container empties.

Investigation of infusion equipment revealed an air-eliminating, particulate and bacterial retentive 0.2 micron filter. This filter would not only prevent air blocking but would also, as a result of particulate retention, decrease phlebitis and lower the number of restarts due to that complication. The filter is approved for 48-hour usage and would cost the hospital $1.25 each. As this is below the $2.07 allowance, this would also result in cost savings.

The filter manufacturer agreed to supply, free of charge, inservice education on the use of the filter and the required number of filters for a repeat of the original 7-day study.

The corrective action study was run from 24:00 on 4/1 to 24:00 on 4/7. All conditions, criteria, instructions, and data collection methods remained the same as for the original problem evaluation study.

Results of Corrective Action Study
Because we are dealing with very small numbers, the percentage rates are calculated to the tenth degree.

Data analysis was performed by the same methods used in the original study. The total number of possible occasions for run drys was 3,694. The

TABLE 4.2
Raw Data Compilation of Problem Reevaluation Study

Unit	Days			Evenings			Nights		
	T	R	%	T	R	%	T	R	%
3 South	82	2	2.4	60	1	1.7	58	1	1.7
3 North	71	1	1.4	65	1	1.5	55	1	1.8
3 West	108	2	1.9	90	2	2.2	86	2	2.5
3 East	65	1	1.5	61	1	1.6	58	1	1.7
4 South	60	1	1.7	52	1	1.9	50	1	2.0
4 North	95	2	2.1	85	2	2.4	78	2	2.6
4 West	86	1	1.2	80	2	2.5	72	2	2.8
4 East	98	2	2.0	91	2	2.2	86	2	2.4
5 South	103	2	1.9	89	2	2.2	80	2	2.5
5 North	90	2	2.2	80	1	1.3	76	2	2.6
5 West	96	2	2.0	84	2	2.4	84	2	2.4
5 East	68	1	1.5	60	1	1.7	58	1	1.7
6 South	70	1	1.4	63	1	1.6	60	1	1.7
6 North	93	2	2.2	82	2	2.4	80	2	2.5
6 West	98	2	2.0	85	2	2.4	82	2	2.4
6 East	82	2	2.4	74	1	1.4	65	1	1.5
Total	1,365	26	Mean 1.9%	1,201	24	Mean 2.0%	1,128	25	Mean 2.2%

Code:
T = Total I.V.s in progress
R = Total restarts due to run drys
% = Percentage of I.V.s requiring restarts

total number of required restarts was 75 (2.0%). This gives a daily mean of 10.7 restarts due to run dry infusions (Table 4.2).

Analysis of the compiled data shows that on the day shift, every unit is between 1.2% and 2.4%, with a mean of 1.9%. On the evening shift, every unit is between 1.3% and 2.5%, with a mean of 2.0%. On the night shift, every unit is between 1.5% and 2.8%, with a mean of 2.2%. Insignificant variations are shown.

The corrective action has achieved the desired 2% restart rate for clotted cannulae resulting from run dry containers. This has improved patient care and reduced hospital costs.

Problem Minimization or Solution

The solution of the problem will be assured by daily monitoring of all restarts due to run drys. A fill-in sheet is completed daily by each I.V. therapist. The sheet documents the total number of restarts required on each unit, each shift. The data is compiled on a monthly basis to identify any significant variations.

> **EXHIBIT 4.2**
> **Quality Assurance Activity Report of I.V. Restarts Due to Clotted Cannula Resulting from Run Drys**
>
> *General Hospital Quality Assurance Activity Report*
>
> Department/Service __I.V. Therapy__   Date __4/16/86__
>
> *Subject (identify specific problem or activity studied):* I.V. restarts due to clotted cannula resulting from run drys.
>
> *Problem Identified by:* I.V. Therapists
>
> *Data Sources:* I.V. containers and cannula patency
>
> *Study Results/Criteria:* completely full or entirely empty container with clotted cannula. Seven-day study. Total possible occasions = 3,736. Total run drys = 392 (10%). Day shift = 10%, evening shift = 11%, night shift = 10%.
>
> *Problem Resolution Proposed:* Air-eliminating filters added to I.V. system, to eliminate need to manually remove air from I.V. tubing when container runs dry.
>
> *Follow-Up of Problem Resolution:* With air-eliminating filters, the restart rate due to run drys was documented at 2.0%. Total possible occasions = 3,694. Total restarts = 75. Continuous monitoring will identify any future problems.
>
> Name: __Jane Smith, R.N.__
> Signature: *Jane Smith*
>
> Appropriate documentation and records must be retained by the department or service doing the study.

Reporting of Quality Assurance Study

The study is reported to the quality assurance committee, by completing a quality assurance activity report.

The report is a brief summary of the entire quality assurance process (Exhibit 4.2). All raw data (I.V. therapists' fill-in sheets, nursing interview results, and compilation sheets) from both studies are retained in the department, for future comparisons, discussions, or verifications.

QUALITY ASSURANCE STUDY #2

Problem Identification

Blood bank personnel state that I.V. therapists are not completing required documentation on transfusion forms when blood or blood components are administered.

Problem Evaluation

According to the American Association of Blood Banks (AABB), a complete record of each unit of blood or blood component must be retained within the blood bank. This is achieved by the use of a transfusion form, which is attached to each unit of cross-matched blood or blood component. This first copy of the form is kept with the patient's chart. The second copy is returned to the blood bank after the unit has been administered.

Evaluation Method: A check-off sheet was prepared for establishing how frequently incomplete documentation was occurring. The four areas requiring documentation are date, time, witness's signature, and transfusionist's signature.

The source for data collection was the copies of transfusion forms returned to the blood bank posttransfusion.

The study was performed by random sampling of all units administered in July. Every third unit on the blood sign-out sheet was selected.

Data Collection

The study sheet contains a column for blood donor numbers. Next to each number are 4 spaces, for date, time, transfusionist's signature, and witness's signature. If any of the four items was documented, an **X** was placed in the appropriate space (Exhibit 4.3).

Data Analysis

The number of units in the sample was 54. The number of DATE documented was 40 (74.1%). Number of TIME documented was 50 (92.6%). Number of TRAN (transfusionist's signature) was 48 (88.9%). Number of WITN (witness's signature) was 25 (46.3%).

These figures show that the hospital policy for documentation on transfusion forms, when blood or blood components are administered, is not being followed.

Corrective Action

Inservice education was given to all personnel administering blood or blood components. The requirements of the AABB were thoroughly discussed.

The benefits to patients by retaining complete documentation of all blood administered was emphasized.

The fact that there are four (4) areas which must be completed on each transfusion form was stressed.

Problem Reevaluation

To assure that inservice education had been appropriate corrective action to solve or minimize the problem, the first study was repeated on blood transfusions given in August. The data source sample selection and check-off sheet all remained the same.

Results of Corrective Study

Number of units in sample was 58. Number of DATE documented was 57 (98.3%). Number of TIME documented was 58 (100%). Number of TRAN documented was 58 (100%). Number of WITN documented was 56 (96.6%).

Inservice education had been appropriate corrective action to achieve a tolerable level of compliance.

Problem Minimization or Solution

To assure problem solution, a reminder note has been placed next to the blood sign-out sheet.

A small sample of blood transfusion forms will be checked quarterly, using the same criteria and study methods.

EXHIBIT 4.3
Check-Off Sheet for Documentation on Transfusion Form When Blood Is Administered

General Hospital I.V. Therapy Department Quality Assurance Study

Topic: Documentation on Transfusion Form When Blood Is Administered

Bld Unit	Date	Time	Tran	Witn	Bld Unit	Date	Time	Tran	Witn

Code:
Bld Unit = Blood unit number
Date = Date unit started
Time = Time unit started
Tran = Transfusionist signature
Witn = Witness signature

Instructions: If item documented on transfusion form, place X in appropriate box. If not documented on transfusion form, leave box blank.

EXHIBIT 4.4
Quality Assurance Activity Report of Incomplete Documentation of Transfusion Form

General Hospital Quality Assurance Activity Report

Department/Service __I.V. Therapy__   Date __9/20/86__

Subject (identify specific problem/activity studied): Incomplete documentation on transfusion form when blood started.

Problem Identified by: Blood bank personnel.

Data Sources: Laboratory copy of transfusion form.

Study Results: Study included every third unit on blood sign-out sheet, during July. Total = 54. Number "Date" documented = 40 (74.1%). Number "Time" documented = 50 (92.6%). Number "Witness Signature" = 25 (46.3%). Number "Transfusionist Signature" = 48 (88.9%).

Problem Resolution Proposed: Inservice education was given to all personnel who administer blood/blood components.

Follow-Up of Problem Resolution: Same study repeated on blood given in August. Total = 58. Number DATE = 57 (98.3%). Number TIME = 58 (100%). Number TRAN = 58 (100%). Number WITN = 56 (96.6%). Quarterly sampling will be done to assure problem solution.

Name: __Mary Black, R.N.__
Signature: __Mary Black__

Appropriate documentation and records must be retained by the department/service doing the study.

Reporting of Quality Assurance Study

The study is reported to the quality assurance committee, by completing a quality assurance activity report.

The report is a brief summary of the entire quality assurance process (Exhibit 4.4).

All raw data (check-off sheet and lab copy of transfusion form) must be retained by the appropriate departments, for any discussions, verifications, or future comparisons.

QUALITY ASSURANCE STUDY #3

Problem Identification

Intravenous therapists state that tubings are disconnecting from central line catheters.

Problem Evaluation

The problem requires an immediate investigation because a central catheter tubing disconnection can be life threatening. An air embolism or massive bleeding can occur.

Evaluation method: To document occurrences, each therapist was instructed to list all patients with central lines on the units he or she covers. Next to each patient's name and room number, the type of connection on the I.V.

system (Luer lock or non-Luer lock), and whether or not that patient's connection had ever separated.

All required data can be found on the patient's file cards. The therapist keeps a 3-by-5-inch file card on each patient receiving infusions. Card information includes whether the line is peripheral or central, type of connection on central lines, and any complications or unexpected occurrences. Cards are transferred to the I.V. therapist on the next shift.

Data Analysis

There were 24 patients with central lines; 6 disconnections had occurred. All 6 disconnections occurred when a non-Luer lock connection was present. There had never been a separation with a Luer lock connection.

There was a very high positive correlation between non-Luer lock connections and catheter tubing separations.

Corrective Action The Policy and Procedure Manual lacked a separate policy for central catheter tubing connections.

Because of the high positive correlation between separations and non-Luer lock connections, a policy was added to Luer lock all connections between the catheter and the filter on all central lines.

Because of the potential dangers of a disconnection, the policy was implemented immediately.

Problem Reevaluation No central catheter tubing separation has occurred since corrective action was taken.

Problem Solution Any separation of central catheter tubing connection is to be reported immediately.

Problem Reporting Whether or not this small, quickly solved problem requires a quality assurance activity report will be according to hospital policy.

It may require documentation only with an annual or biannual report, which is a summary of all quality assurance activity for that time period (Exhibit 4.5, p. 48).

EXHIBIT 4.5
Annual Review and Evaluation Report

General Hospital Review and Evaluation Report

Department or Service: __I.V. Therapy__

Date: __1/10/87__

Period Under Study: __January–December 1986__

Name: __Judy Smith, R.N.__

Signature: __Judy Smith__

Topic	Date Reviewed	Data Sources	Study Results	Corrective Action	Follow-Up
I.V. restarts due to clotted cannula resulting from Run Dry containers.	3/10/86 through 4/7/86	I.V. containers Cannula patency	7-day study Total = 3,736 Run Drys = 392 (10%)	Addition of air-eliminating filters	Repeat study Total = 3,694 Run Drys = 75 (2.0%)
Incomplete documentation on transfusion form when blood started.	7/1/86 through 8/31/86	Laboratory copies of transfusion forms	Total = 54 DATE = 40 (74.1%) TIME = 50 (92.6%) TRAN = 48 (88.9%) WITN = 25 (46.3%)	Inservice education	Repeat study Total = 58 DATE = 57 (98.3%) TIME = 58 (100%) TRAN = 58 (100%) WITN = 56 (96.6%)
Disconnection of tubing from central line catheters.	11/15/86	Patient file cards	Total study = 24 Total disconnections = 6 (25%). All 6 had non-Leur lock connections	Policy addition for Luer lock connections between filter and catheter	Any separation is to be immediately reported. None has occurred.

REFERENCES

1. Joint Commission on Accreditation of Hospitals. *Quality Review Bulletin: Special Edition.* Chicago, 1979.
2. Center for Disease Control. *Guidelines for the Prevention and Control of Nosocomial Infections.* Atlanta, 1983.
3. National Intravenous Therapy Association. Intravenous nursing standards of practice. *J. NITA* 5(1):19–34, 1982.
4. American Association of Blood Banks. *Safe Transfusion.* Washington, D.C., 1981.
5. Joint Commission on Accreditation of Hospitals. *Accreditation Manual for Hospitals.* Chicago, 1985. Pp. 149–152.
6. Colton, T. *Statistics in Medicine.* Boston: Little, Brown, 1974.

REVIEW QUESTIONS

1. The hospital strives to protect the patient from _____ as a result of _____.
2. An incident report should contain only _____ statements.

3. The two major factors which contribute to patients filing malpractice claims are _____ and _____ .
4. The process of quality assurance focuses on _____ , _____ , _____ , _____ and _____ .
5. Criteria are divided into three main categories. _____ , _____ , and _____ .
6. To minimize self-fulfilling prophecies, the criteria must be _____ and _____ .
7. To avoid subjectivity, criteria must be stated in terms which can be answered by _____ , _____ , or _____ .
8. Regardless of what method of problem evaluation is used, to achieve meaningful results, _____ , _____ , and _____ of the test are of utmost importance.
9. A _____ indicates that A occurs rarely when it is associated with B.
10. Without _____ one cannot ensure the success of the entire evaluation process.

CHAPTER 5

The Staff Nurse's Responsibility in the Maintenance of Infusions

Ada Lawrence Plumer

Safe, successful fluid therapy depends not only upon the knowledge and skill of the intravenous nurse, but also upon the role the staff nurse plays in maintaining the infusion. Policies describing the responsibilities of the staff nurse vary significantly among hospitals. It is important for the nurse to recognize this fact and be familiar with the hospital policies and procedures related to them.

National standards and guidelines have been established to protect the patient from potential hazards associated with intravenous therapy. The staff nurse, involved in the care of these patients, must be cognizant of the guidelines for quality control in the maintenance of intravenous therapy.

RECOMMENDATIONS FOR PRACTICE IN THE USE OF I.V. CONTAINERS [2]

There is great risk of infection if sterile technique is not observed.

1. Hands should be washed before parenteral fluids are opened and administered.
2. All fluid containers must be inspected prior to use for cracks, damaged caps, leaks, and expiration date. The solution must be inspected for discoloration, turbidity, and particulate matter. Questionable containers of parenteral fluids should never be used.
3. A label should be affixed to the container indicating the time and date the fluid container was opened.
4. Parenteral fluids should be discarded if not administered within 24 hours.
5. Lipid emulsions should be discarded if not administered within 12 hours.

RECOMMENDATIONS FOR PRACTICE IN THE USE OF ADMINISTRATION SETS [2]

1. Administration sets shall be changed every 24–48 hours and preferably at the time a new container of I.V. fluid is initiated.
2. Piggy-back administration sets shall be routinely changed every 24 hours; change should be made at the time a new container of I.V. fluid is being initiated.
3. Administration sets, including piggy-back sets, must be changed immediately after being used for infusions of blood, blood products, and lipid emulsions.
4. Administration sets used for total parenteral nutrition should be changed every 24 hours.
5. All additive devices, such as stopcocks and extension tubes, should be changed at the time the administration set is changed.
6. All tubing junctions should be securely attached in an appropriate manner, as with a Luer lock or clasping device.
7. The date the administration set is changed should be indicated on tape and affixed to the new set in a conspicuous place.
8. All I.V. systems should be maintained as closed systems whenever possible. Medications should be administered through injection ports after disinfecting them.
9. Blood specimens shall not be withdrawn through I.V. tubing.
10. I.V. systems shall not be flushed or irrigated to improve the flow.
11. The entire system, including the cannula, should be changed if purulent thrombophlebitis, cellulitis, or I.V.-related bacteremia are suspected (See Chapter 17).
12. The cannula and the administration set should be changed for phlebitis without concomitant signs of infection. The fluid should be cultured for a possible source of phlebitis.

RECOMMENDED PRACTICE (NITA) IN DRESSING CHANGES [2]

1. I.V. dressings should be changed every 24–48 hours and whenever the dressing becomes soiled, wet, or loose; at this time the site should be inspected for redness, swelling, and other signs of infection.
2. Aseptic technique must be used in changing dressings.
3. The injection site should be cleaned with 70% isopropyl alcohol or povidone-iodine solution and allowed to dry. This should be followed by the application of iodophor ointment, provided the patient is not allergic to iodine, and covered with a sterile dressing.

AMBULATING PATIENTS WITH INFUSIONS

Special precautions must be taken when ambulating patients with infusions. The fluid container must be kept sufficiently high at all times to maintain a constant flow. Any cessation in the rate must be detected immediately and remedied before a clot is allowed to plug the needle.

FREQUENT OBSERVATION

Fluid maintenance requires frequent observation of patients receiving infusions. The attending nurse should visit the patient frequently, checking the rate of flow, the amount of solution remaining, and the site of infusion, as described in the following sections.

Rate of Flow

Since the rate of flow, once established, is often difficult to maintain, the staff nurse should check and readjust the flow whenever necessary. Controllers assist the nurse in maintaining accurate flow rates. NITA advocates the use of controllers for the majority delivery of intravenous therapy; I.V. pumps, when a specified accuracy of administration is mandatory due to patient risk [2]. The registered professional nurse involved with these devices must be knowledgable in their use. Operating instructions should be affixed to each device; they should be carefully read and understood.

When Infusion Stops

When an infusion stops, the cause must be immediately investigated and remedied. The following procedure is to be used:

1. Check for infiltration.
2. Check the fluid level in the bottle.
3. Check for kinking of the tubing.
4. Open the clamp.
5. Check air vent. Has it been inserted if required and is it patent?
6. Check the cannula for patency by kinking the tubing a few inches from the cannula while pinching and releasing the tubing between the cannula and the kinked tubing. Resistance if encountered should be treated with caution as a clot may have plugged the cannula. If a patient complains of pain, a sclerosed vein may be the cause of the cessation of flow. In either case the cannula must be removed.
7. Is the cannula in line with the vein or up against the wall of the vein? A slight adjustment, by moving the cannula, may remedy the problem.
8. If the intravenous solution is cold, as in the case of blood, venous spasm may result. Heat placed directly on the vein will relieve the spasm and increase the flow of the infusion.
9. If the infusion is blood, check the filter; heavy sediment may be slowing the flow. Replace the filter if necessary.
10. Increase the height of the bottle to increase gravity.

11. If unable to restart the flow after these procedures have been followed, restart the infusion.

Amount of Solution in the Container

Air embolism and *blood embolism* are significant hazards of infusion therapy and may be associated with delay in changing solution bottles. A fresh bottle of solution should be added before the level of fluid falls in the drip chamber. Failure to do this results in the following problems:

Plugged Cannula
Intravenous solutions flow into the vein by means of gravity. Once the fluid level has dropped in the tubing to about the level of the patient's chest, the blood will be forced back into the cannula, occluding the lumen of the cannula. Occluded cannulas should be removed, not irrigated. Fibrinous material injected into the vein can propagate a thrombus, possibly resulting in an infarction. Irrigation may embolize small infected cannula thrombi, which could result in septicemia. Aspiration aimed at dislodging the fibrin may cause the vein to collapse around the cannula point traumatizing the vessel wall.

Trapped Air
If the bottle (in an air venting system) is changed after the level of fluid drops in the tubing and before the cannula plugs, the air is trapped in the tubing and forced into the patient by pressure of the fresh solution. Fatal air embolism can result. The use of plastic bags, containers which contain no air, and administration sets which have no junctions through which air can leak have reduced the risk of introducing air into the patient's veins. Air can be introduced at the beginning of an infusion by not completely clearing the set of air or when changing containers. Infusions through a central venous catheter carry an even greater risk of air embolism than do those through a peripheral vein. Air embolism can occur during tubing changes involving the central venous catheter (see air embolism, Chapter 16). It has been suggested, through animal experimentation, that a normal adult should tolerate air embolism of as much as 200 ml, but for persons in poor health smaller amounts may be fatal; less than 10 ml might be fatal in a gravely ill person [3].

Before the flow ceases and the bottle empties, replace the empty bottle with fresh solution using the following procedure:

1. Vent fresh bottle if vent is required.
2. Kink tubing to prevent air from being introduced into the flowing solution.
3. Change container. Hang solution bottle before unkinking tubing.
4. Readjust rate if necessary.

Nonfunctioning (leaking or plugged) sets should be removed.

The 0.22 Micron Air-Eliminating Filter

An 0.22 micron air-eliminating filter protects the patient from air embolism, bacteria, and particulate matter. NITA advocates the use of the 0.22 micron air-eliminating filters for routine administration of I.V. fluids [2].

Recommendations for the Use of 0.22 Micron Air-Eliminating Filters [2]

1. The filter should be placed at the terminal end of the administration set, that is, as close to the cannula as possible.
2. The filter should be changed every 24–48 hours.
3. Lipid emulsions, blood, and blood products should not be administered through the filter.
4. Consideration must be made to the administration of some drugs since their dosage may be affected by the filter; follow the manufacturer's recommendations.
5. The p.s.i. of the filter must be compatible with the electronic instrument used.

Infiltration or Inflammation at Injection Site

Failure to recognize an infiltration before the swelling has increased to a sizable degree may:

1. Cause damage to the tissues.
2. Prevent the patient from receiving necessary and urgent medication.
3. Limit veins available for future therapy.

If the question of infiltration exists, compare the questionable extremity with the normal extremity. An infusion has infiltrated if:

1. There is swelling about the site of the cannula.
2. A tourniquet applied above the cannula does not stop the flow of fluid.

Checking for an infiltration by a backflow of blood into the adapter is not a reliable method for the following reasons:

1. In small veins the cannula may approach the size of the vein, occluding the lumen and obstructing the flow of blood; the solution flows undiluted so that no backflow of blood is obtained.
2. The cannula may have punctured the vein, causing an infiltration, and at the same time be within the lumen of the vein, or the bevel may be only partially within the lumen of the vein, causing a swelling and still producing a backflow of blood on test.

Inspect the injection site for erythema, induration, or tenderness by palpation of the venous cord. If any of these signs occur, remove the cannula. When replacing it, sterile equipment should be used and the site changed, preferably to the opposite arm. Should infection be noted, the cannula and the infusion fluid should be cultured and lot numbers of sets and infusions recorded (see Chapter 9).

Outdated Sets and Cannulas

The Center for Disease Control (CDC) recommends changing intravenous tubing every 24–48 hours and needles and catheters every 48–72 hours, preferably every 48 hours (see Chapter 17).

For recommended procedures on intermittent infusions and heparin locks, see Chapter 20.

TERMINATION OF INFUSION

To terminate the infusion, use the following procedure:

1. Stop flow by clamping off tubing.
2. Remove all tape from cannula. Do not use scissors.
3. With a dry sterile sponge held over the injection site, remove cannula. The cannula must be removed nearly flush with the skin. This prevents the point from damaging the posterior wall of the vein, thus encouraging the process of thrombosis. Visually ascertain that the length of the cannula removed corresponds with length inserted. Information should be noted on the dressing.
4. Apply pressure instantly and firmly. Do not rub. Hematomas occur from cannulas carelessly removed and render veins useless for future use.

Small adhesive bandages, such as Band-Aids, should not be used unless specifically ordered. It must be emphasized that such a bandage is not used to stop bleeding and does not take the place of pressure. If ordered, it should be applied only after pressure has been applied and the bleeding stopped.

REFERENCES

1. Center for Disease Control. Guidelines for prevention of intravascular infection. *J. NITA* 5(1):39–50, 1982.
2. National Intravenous Therapy Association. NITA standards — I.V. therapy. *J. NITA* 5(1): 24–29, 1982.
3. Fireitag, J., and Miller, L. (eds.). *Manual of Medical Therapeutics* (23rd ed.). Boston: Little, Brown and Company, 1980, p. 293.

REVIEW QUESTIONS

1. To minimize the risk of phlebitis, the intravenous tubing should be changed every _____ hours.
2. How is the needle checked for patency should the infusion stop?
3. What procedure is used to increase the rate of flow when venospasm, due to a change in temperature, stops the infusion?
4. For what two reasons is it important to remove an occluded cannula rather than attempt to irrigate it?
5. Why do infusions via the central venous catheter carry a greater risk of embolism than those through a peripheral line?

6. A reliable method of confirming an infiltration is to note the absence of blood in the adapter when back pressure is exerted. True or false?
7. Observing a backflow of blood in the adapter is a true indication that infiltration has not occurred. True or false?
8. Name three signs of phlebitis, any one of which should be cause for removal of the cannula.

CHAPTER 6

Anatomy and Physiology Applied to Intravascular Therapy

Ada Lawrence Plumer

THE IMPORTANCE OF UNDERSTANDING ANATOMY AND PHYSIOLOGY

Intravascular therapy consists of the introduction of fluids, blood, and drugs directly into the vascular system; that is, into arteries, into bone marrow, and into veins. The *arteries* are used as a route to introduce radiopaque material for diagnostic purposes, such as arteriograms for cerebral disorders, as well as for monitoring blood pressure, drawing arterial blood gases, and administering cancer chemotherapy. The dangers of arterial spasm and subsequent gangrene present problems that make this type of therapy hazardous for therapeutic use. The *bone marrow,* because of its venous plexus, can be utilized for intravascular therapy. However, because infusions into the bone marrow can be dangerous, this route should be used only if other channels are unavailable. Repeated intramarrow injections could result in osteomyelitis. The *veins,* because of their abundance and location, present the most readily accessible route.

Applied to intravascular therapy, knowledge of the anatomy and physiology of veins and arteries is essential to the proficiency of the therapist and the welfare of the patient. Through a study of the superficial veins, the therapist acquires a sense of discrimination in the choice of veins for intravenous use. Many factors must be considered in selecting a vein; the anatomical characteristics offer a basis for good judgment. The size, location, and resilience of the vein affect its desirability for infusion purposes.

Familiarity with the principles underlying venous physiology is also of prime value to the therapist. An understanding of the reaction of veins to the nervous stimulation of the vasoconstrictors and vasodilators enables the therapist to (1) increase the size and visibility of a vein before attempting venipuncture and (2) relieve venous spasm and thus assist in infusion maintenance.

With proficiency of the therapist, the primary goal of intravenous therapy is achieved: the welfare of the patient. Painless and effective therapy is desirable, promoting the patient's comfort and well-being, and often his complete recovery from disease or trauma as well. An integral part of this goal is the recognition and prevention of complications. Therapists, through their knowledge of anatomy and physiology, can reduce these risks.

Phlebitis and *thrombosis* are by far the commonest complications resulting from parenteral therapy. Although seemingly mild, they do present serious consequences: (1) they cause moderate to severe discomfort, often taking many days or weeks to subside, and (2) they limit the veins available for further therapy. Injury to the endothelial lining of the vein contributes to these local complications. A thorough understanding of the peripheral veins alerts the therapist to observe precautions in technique in performing venipunctures. Proper technique in venipuncture minimizes the trauma to the vessel wall and provides an entry as painless and safe as possible. Examination of the superficial veins of the lower extremities alerts the therapist to the dangers resulting from their use. By avoiding venipunctures in veins susceptible to varicosities and sluggish circulation, the likelihood of phlebitis and thrombosis is decreased and the secondary risk of *pulmonary embolism* is reduced.

Awareness of the characteristics that differentiate veins from arteries assists the therapist in reducing the risk of *necrosis* and *gangrene*; these serious complications occur when a medication is inadvertently injected into an artery.

An understanding of the anatomy and physiology of the veins and arteries enables the therapist to recognize the existence of an *arteriovenous anastomosis*; failure to recognize this condition results in repeated and unsuccessful venipunctures performed in an attempt to initiate the infusion. These repeated punctures compound the trauma to the inner lining of the vein and increase the risk of the local complications already described, any of which limits the number of available veins, interrupts the course of therapy, and causes unnecessary pain and even dire consequences for the patient.

THE VASCULAR SYSTEM

The circulatory system is divided into two main systems, the pulmonary and the systemic, each with its own set of vessels. The *pulmonary system* consists of the blood flow from the right ventricle of the heart to the lungs, where it is oxygenated and returned to the left atrium. The *systemic system*, the larger of the two, is the one which concerns the intravenous therapist. It consists of the aorta, arteries, arterioles, capillaries, venules, and veins through which the blood must flow. The blood leaves the left ventricle, flows to all parts of the body, and returns to the right atrium of the heart via the vena cava. The *systemic veins* are divided into three classes: (1) superficial, (2) deep, and (3) venous sinuses [1].

Superficial Veins The superficial or cutaneous veins are those used in venipuncture. They are located just beneath the skin in the superficial fascia. These veins and the deep veins sometimes unite; in the lower extremities they unite freely [2]. For example, the small saphenous vein, a superficial vein, drains the dorsum of the foot and the posterior section of the leg; it ascends the back of the leg and empties directly into the deep popliteal vein. Before the small saphenous vein terminates in the deep popliteal, it sends out a branch which, after joining the great saphenous vein, also terminates in a deep vein, the femoral vein. Because of these deep connections, great concern arises when it becomes necessary to use the veins in the lower extremities. Thrombosis may occur which could easily extend to the deep veins and cause pulmonary embolism. Understanding this, the nurse should refrain from the use of these veins.

Varicosities occurring in the lower extremities, although readily available to venipuncture, are not a satisfactory route for parenteral administration. The relatively stagnant blood in such veins is likely to clot, resulting in a superficial phlebitis. Medication injected below a varicosity may result in another potential danger, a collection of the infused drug in the varicosity. This is caused by the stagnant blood flow. This "pocket" of infused medication may delay the effect of the drug when immediate action is desired; another concern is the danger of untoward reactions to the drug which may occur when this accumulation reaches the general circulation.

Arteriovenous Anastomosis

Deep veins are usually enclosed in the same sheath with the arteries. Occasionally an arteriovenous anastomosis may occur on a congenital basis or as the result of past penetrating injury of the vein and adjacent artery. When such trauma occurs, the blood flows directly from the artery into the vein; as a result, the veins draining an arteriovenous fistula are overburdened with high-pressure arterial blood. These veins appear large and tortuous. In these unusual circumstances the therapist's quick recognition of an arteriovenous fistula may prevent pain, complications, and loss of time due to repeated unsuccessful attempts to start the infusion.

Arteries and Veins

Knowledge of the characteristics differentiating veins from arteries and the position of each is important to the therapist so that he or she may avoid the complications of an inadvertent arterial puncture. Arteries and veins are similar in structure; both are composed of three layers of tissue. A close examination of these layers reveals their differing characteristics.

Tunica Intima, or the Inner Layer
The first layer consists of an inner elastic endothelial lining which also forms the valves in veins. These valves are absent in arteries. The endothelial lining is identical in the arteries and the veins, consisting of a smooth layer of flat cells. This smooth surface allows the cells and platelets to flow through the blood vessels without interruption under normal conditions. Care must be taken to avoid roughening this surface when performing a venipuncture or removing a needle from a vein. Any trauma that roughens the endothelial lining encourages the process of thrombosis whereby cells and platelets adhere to the vessel wall.

Many veins contain valves which are semilunar folds of the endothelium. These valves are found in the larger veins of the extremities; their function is to keep the blood flowing toward the heart. Where muscular pressure would cause a backing up of the blood supply, these valves play an important role. They occur at points of branching and often cause a noticeable bulge in the veins. Applying a tourniquet to the extremity impedes the venous flow. When suction is applied, as occurs in the process of drawing blood, the valves compress and close the lumen of the vein, preventing the backward flow of the blood. These valves thus interfere with the process of withdrawing blood. Recognizing the presence of a valve, the nurse may resolve the difficulty by slightly readjusting the needle.

These valves are absent in many of the small veins, which can therefore be utilized when, owing to obstruction from a thrombus in the ascending vein, they would otherwise prove useless. The cannula may be inserted below the thrombosis, with its direction toward the distal end of the extremity; this results in a rerouting of the fluid and avoidance of the thrombosed portion.

Tunica Media, or the Middle Layer

The second layer consists of muscular and elastic tissue. The nerve fibers, both vasoconstrictors and vasodilators, are located in this middle layer. These fibers, constantly receiving impulses from the vasoconstrictor center in the medulla, keep the vessels in a state of tonus. They also stimulate both arteries and veins to contract or relax. The middle layer is not as strong and stiff in the veins as in the arteries, and therefore the veins tend to collapse or distend as the pressure within falls or rises. Arteries do not collapse.

Stimulation by a change in temperature or by mechanical or chemical irritation may produce spasms in the vein or artery. For instance, interrupting a continuous infusion to administer a pint of cold blood may produce vasoconstriction; this results in spasm, impedes the flow of blood, and causes pain. Application of heat to the vein promotes vasodilation, which will relieve the spasm, improve the flow of blood, and relieve the pain. The same results are obtained by heat when an irritating drug has caused vasoconstriction. In this situation, heat serves a twofold purpose: it (1) relieves the spasm and increases the blood flow and (2) protects the vessel wall from inflammation caused by the medication — with heat dilating the vein and increasing the flow of blood, the drug becomes more diluted and less irritating. The use of heat to achieve vasodilation is also an aid when it becomes necessary to use veins that are small and poorly filled.

Spasms produced by a chemical irritation in an artery may result in dire consequences. A single artery supplies circulation to a particular area. If this artery is damaged, the related area will suffer from impaired circulation and possibly from necrosis and gangrene. If a chemical agent is introduced into the artery, a spasm may result — a contraction that could shut off the blood supply completely. This problem is not as serious when veins are used, since many veins supply a particular area; if one is injured, others will maintain the circulation.

Tunica Adventitia, or the Outer Layer

The third layer consists of areolar connective tissue; it surrounds and supports the vessel. In arteries this layer is thicker than in veins because it is subjected to greater pressure from the force of blood within.

Arteries need more protection than veins and are so placed that injury is less likely to occur. Whereas veins are superficially located, most arteries lie deep in the tissues and are protected by muscle. Occasionally an artery is located superficially in an unusual place; this artery is then called an *aberrant artery*. An aberrant artery must not be mistaken for a vein. If a chemical which

Chapter 6 | Anatomy and Physiology Applied to Intravascular Therapy

causes spasm is introduced into an aberrant artery, permanent damage may result.

Arteries pulsate and veins do not, a helpful differentiating characteristic.

Superficial Veins of the Upper Extremities

The superficial veins of the upper extremities are shown in Figures 6.1 and 6.2. They consist of the following: digital, metacarpal, cephalic, basilic, and median veins.

The Digital Veins

The dorsal digital veins flow along the lateral portions of the fingers and are joined to each other by communicating branches [1]. At times these veins are available as a last resort for fluid administration. In some patients they are prominent enough to accommodate a 21-gauge small vein needle. With adequate taping the fingers can be completely immobilized, thereby preventing the needle from puncturing the posterior wall of the vein and causing extravasation of fluid.

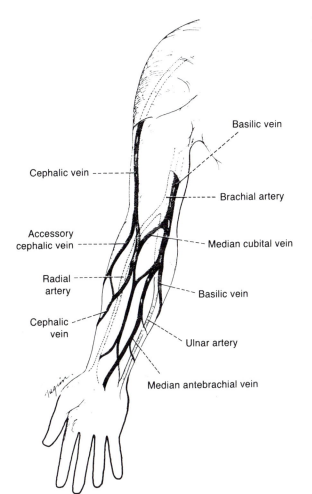

FIGURE 6.1
The superficial veins of the forearm.

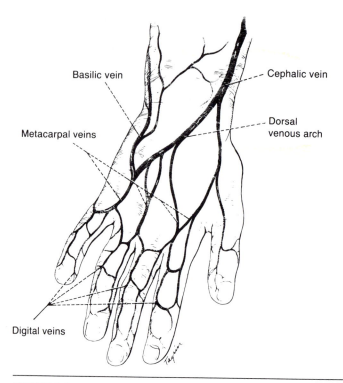

FIGURE 6.2
The superficial veins of the dorsal aspect of the hand.

The Metacarpal Veins

The three metacarpal veins are formed by the union of the digital veins [1]. The position of these veins makes them well adapted for intravenous use; the needle and adapter, in most cases, lie flat between the joints and the metacarpal bones of the hand, the bones themselves providing a natural splint. The early use of the metacarpal veins is important in a course of parenteral therapy. Irritating fluid passing through a vein traumatized by previous puncture causes inflammation and pain. Therefore performing venipunctures for fluid administration at the distal end of the extremity, early in the course of therapy, is beneficial; it enables the nurse to initiate each successive venipuncture above the previous puncture site. Unnecessary inflammation and pain are avoided and opportunity for multiple venipunctures is provided.

Occasionally the use of the metacarpal veins in the elderly is contraindicated. Owing to inadequate tissue and thin skin in this area, extravasation of blood on venipuncture may readily occur.

The Cephalic Vein

The cephalic vein has its source in the radial part of the dorsal venous network formed by the metacarpal veins. Receiving tributaries from both surfaces of the forearm, it flows upward along the radial border of the forearm [1]. Because of its size and position, this vein provides an excellent route for transfusion administration. It readily accommodates a large cannula and, by virtue of its position in the forearm, a natural splint is provided for the cannula and adapter.

The *accessory cephalic vein* originates from either one of two sources; a plexus on the back of the forearm or the dorsal venous network. Ascending the arm, it joins the cephalic vein below the elbow. Occasionally it arises from that portion of the cephalic vein just above the wrist and flows back into the main cephalic vein at some higher point [1]. The accessory cephalic vein readily receives a large cannula and is a very good choice for use in blood administration.

The Basilic Vein

The basilic vein has its origin in the ulnar part of the dorsal venous network and ascends along the ulnar portion of the forearm. It diverges toward the anterior surface of the arm just below the elbow, where it meets the median cubital vein. During a course of intravenous therapy this large vein is often overlooked because of its inconspicuous position on the ulnar border of the hand and forearm; when other veins have been exhausted, this vein may still be available. By flexing the elbow and bending the arm up, the basilic vein is brought into view.

The Median Veins

The *median antebrachial vein* arises from the venous plexus on the palm of the hand and extends upward along the ulnar side of the front of the forearm; it empties into the basilic vein or the median cubital vein. This vein, when prominent, affords a route for parenteral fluid administration. However, there are frequent variations of the superficial veins of the forearm, and this vein is not always present as a well-defined vessel.

The *median cephalic* and *median basilic veins* in the antecubital fossa are the veins most generally used for withdrawal of blood. Because of their size and superficial location, they are readily accessible for venipuncture. They receive a large-sized cannula and, owing to the muscular and connective tissue supporting them, have little tendency to roll.

Since the median cephalic vein crosses in front of the brachial artery, care must be taken during venipuncture to avoid puncturing the artery. Accidental intraarterial injection of a drug could result in permanent damage.

The basilic vein, outside the antecubital fossa on the ulnar curve of the arm, is the least desirable for venipuncture. On removal of the cannula a hematoma may readily occur if the patient flexes his or her elbow to stop the bleeding rather than elevating the arm in the preferred manner.

THE SKIN

The skin is made up of two layers, the epidermis and the dermis. The *epidermis* is the uppermost layer which forms a protective covering for the dermis. Its degree of thickness varies in different parts of the body. It is thickest on the palms of the hands and the soles of the feet and thinnest on the inner surface of the limbs. Its degree of thickness also varies with age. In an elderly patient the skin on the dorsum of the hand may be so thin that it does not adequately support the vein for venipuncture when parenteral infusions are required.

The *dermis*, or underlayer, is highly sensitive and vascular. It contains many capillaries and thousands of nerve fibers. These nerve fibers are of different types and include those which react to temperature, touch, pressure, and pain. The number of nerve fibers varies in different areas of the body. Some areas of the body skin are highly sensitive; other areas are only mildly sensitive. The insertion of a needle in one area may cause a great deal of pain, while another area may be virtually painless. In my experience the inner aspect of the wrist is a highly sensitive area. Venipunctures are performed here only when other veins have been exhausted.

SUPERFICIAL FASCIA

The superficial fascia, or subcutaneous areolar connective tissue, lies below the two layers of skin and is, in itself, another covering. It is in this fascia that the superficial veins are located. It varies in thickness. When a cannula is inserted into this fascia, there is free movement of the skin above. Great care in aseptic technique must be observed, as an infection in this loose tissue spreads easily. Such an infection is called *cellulitis* [2].

REFERENCES

1. Warwick, R., and Williams, P. L. (eds.). *Gray's Anatomy of the Human Body* (28th ed.). Philadelphia: Lea & Febiger, 1973. Pp. 700–703.

2. Kimber, D. C., Gray, C. E., and Stackpoles, C. E. *Textbook of Anatomy and Physiology* (15th ed.). New York: Macmillan, 1966. Pp. 69, 398, 423–431.

REVIEW QUESTIONS

1. What is the reason for concern when the veins of the lower extremities are used for parenteral administration?
2. What potential dangers may occur when varicosities are used as a route for fluid and drug administration?
3. What is an arteriovenous fistula?
4. What characteristic of the arteriovenous fistula makes it impracticable for fluid administration?
5. What is an aberrant artery?
6. What potential harm may result from an inadvertent arterial injection of a drug?
7. Name the layer of tissue in which the vasodilator and vasoconstrictor nerve fibers are located.
8. What factors stimulate the vasoconstrictor nerve fibers to produce spasm, impeding the flow of fluids and causing pain?
9. _____ applied to the vein promotes vasodilation to aid in relieving spasms, improving blood flow, and relieving pain.
10. Name the superficial veins of the upper extremity.

Chapter 6 | Anatomy and Physiology Applied to Intravascular Therapy

11. The _median cephalic_ and the _median basilic_ veins in the antecubital fossa are the veins most generally used for withdrawal of blood.
12. Why is the basilic vein the least desirable of the median veins for venipuncture? _hematoma may develop on removal of cannula_
13. The skin is made up of two layers, called the _dermis_ and the _epidermis_.
14. Name the subcutaneous connective tissue which lies between the two layers of skin and contains the veins. _Superficial fascia_
15. An infection involving the connective tissue is called _cellulitis_

PART II
Fluids and Electrolytes

CHAPTER 7

Fundamental Aspects of Fluid and Electrolyte Metabolism

Ada Lawrence Plumer

INTRODUCTION TO FLUID AND ELECTROLYTE BALANCE

Over the past 25 years our knowledge of fluid and electrolyte balance has increased to the extent that we now recognize an imbalance as a threat to life. With this increased knowledge has come an increase in the nurse's responsibility in parenteral therapy. Not only is accurate recording of the patient's intake and output important, but so too is the ability to recognize symptoms of imbalance; prompt recognition of an imbalance may indicate adjustment in therapy which may be crucial to the safety of the patient.

Today electrolyte therapy is used extensively. At least 70 percent of all fluids administered contain some electrolytes. Electrolyte therapy is often a lifesaving procedure; its safe and successful administration is essential. Knowledge of the fundamentals of fluid and electrolyte metabolism contributes to safe electrolyte therapy. This knowledge alerts the nurse to (1) the necessity for accurate fluid and electrolyte administration, (2) the potential dangers of electrolyte therapy, and (3) a change in the patient's condition which could alter the therapy prescribed.

Abnormalities of body fluid and electrolyte metabolism present certain therapeutic problems. When the mechanisms normally regulating fluid volume, electrolyte composition, and osmolality are impaired, therapy becomes complicated. An understanding of these metabolic abnormalities enables the nurse to understand the problems involved. Such problems exist in patients with renal insufficiency, adrenal insufficiency, adrenal hyperactivity, and other kinds of impaired organ function. For example, correction of a severe potassium deficit resulting from vomiting and diarrhea presents a problem in the dehydrated patient. Potassium replacement is imperative. However, potassium administered to patients with renal insufficiency results in potassium toxicity; the kidneys are unable to excrete electrolytes. The adverse effects of excess potassium on the heart muscle are arrhythmia and heart block. The nurse must recognize the importance of (1) hydrating the patient before potassium can be administered safely and (2) watching for diminished diuresis which could necessitate a change in therapy. Once antidiuresis occurs, the potassium infusion must be interrupted and the physician notified.

Therapeutic problems also exist in patients with impaired liver function. Gastric replacement is necessary when there has been an excessive loss of gastric fluid. Most deficits caused by gastric suction, unless severe, are treated with 0.9% sodium chloride in 5% dextrose in water. However, severe loss may call for gastric replacement solutions containing ammonium chloride, which can be potentially dangerous when administered to patients with impaired liver function. Ammonium chloride administered to a patient with severe liver damage may result in ammonia intoxication because of the liver's inability to convert ammonia to hydrogen ion and urea.

These examples illustrate how knowledge of fluid and electrolyte metabolism contributes to safe, successful therapy in the critically ill patient.

FLUID CONTENT OF THE BODY

The total body water content of an individual varies with age, weight, and sex. The amount of water is dependent upon the amount of body fat. Body fat is essentially water-free; the greater the fat content, the less is the water content. In a normal male with an average amount of fat, the water weight is about 60 percent of the body weight. In a female, because of the normally larger degree of body fat, the proportion of water weight to body weight is less, about 54 percent of body weight.

Compartments

The total body fluid is functionally divided into two main compartments: the intracellular and the extracellular compartments. The intracellular compartment consists of the fluid inside the cells and comprises about two-thirds of the body fluid, or 40 percent of the body weight. The extracellular compartment consists of the fluid outside the body cells — the plasma representing 5 percent of the body weight and the interstitial fluid (fluid in tissues) representing 15 percent of the body weight. See Figure 7.1 for a schematic representation of compartments.

In newborn infants the proportion is approximately three-fifths intracellular and two-fifths extracellular. This ratio changes and reaches the adult level by the time the infant is about 30 months old.

There is one additional compartment, the transcellular compartment. The transcellular fluid is the product of cellular metabolism and consists of secretions such as gastrointestinal secretions and urine. Analysis of the secretions may assist the physician in tracing lost electrolytes and prescribing proper fluid and electrolyte replacement. Excessive fluid and electrolyte loss must be replaced to maintain fluid and electrolyte balance in the two main compartments. The amount of body water loss is easily computed by weighing the patient and noting loss of weight: 1 liter of body water is equivalent to 1 kg, or 2.2 pounds, of body weight. Up to 5 percent weight loss in a child or adult may signify moderate fluid volume deficit — over 5 percent may indicate severe fluid volume deficit [4]. Weight changes are also valuable as indicators of body water gains — acute weight gain may indicate water excess.

COMPOSITION OF BODY FLUID

The body fluid contains two types of solutes (dissolved substances): the electrolytes and the nonelectrolytes (see Figure 7.1). The *nonelectrolytes* are molecules which do not break into particles in solution but remain intact. They consist of (1) dextrose, (2) urea, and (3) creatinine.

Electrolytes are molecules which break into electrically charged particles called ions. The ion carrying a positive charge is called a cation, the ion with a negative charge, an anion. Potassium chloride is an electrolyte which, dissolved in water, yields potassium cations and chloride anions. Chemical balance is always maintained; the total number of positive charges equals the total number of negative charges. The quantity of charges and their concentration is expressed as milliequivalents (mEq) per liter of fluid. As the number of negative charges must equal the number of positive charges for chemical balance, the milliequivalents of cations must equal the milliequivalents of anions [1] (see Table 7.1).

Electrolyte Composition

Each fluid compartment has its own electrolyte composition (see Figure 7.1). The extracellular compartment (plasma and interstitial fluid) contains a high concentration of sodium, chloride, and bicarbonate and a low concentration of potassium. The composition of the intracellular fluid is quite different; the concentrations of potassium, magnesium, and phosphate are high, whereas the sodium and chloride concentrations are relatively low.

Electrolyte composition of the intracellular fluid is in part related to electrolyte composition of the plasma and interstitial fluids. Disturbances in the extracellular fluid are reflected in the patient's symptoms. These facts, combined with the accessibility of plasma, make the analysis of plasma a valuable guide to therapy. Occasionally, however, the electrolyte determination of plasma may be misleading. For example, concentration of potassium in plasma may be high while there is a body deficit. This surplus is due to the shift of potassium from intracellular to extracellular fluid in the process of large potassium losses through the kidneys. Determination of plasma sodium may also present a false picture. In the case of an edematous cardiac patient, the plasma

TABLE 7.1
Plasma Electrolytes Illustrating Total mEq of Cations Equaling Total mEq of Anions

Cations	mEq/L	Anions	mEq/L
Na^+	142	HCO_3^-	24
K^+	5	Cl^-	105
Ca^{2+}	5	HPO_4^{2-}	2
Mg^{2+}	2	SO_4^{2-}	1
		Organic acid$^-$	6
		Proteinate$^-$	16
Total	154		154

Source: Baxter Laboratories. *Fundamentals of Body Water and Electrolytes.* Morton Grove, Ill., 1977, pp. 5, 21. Reprinted with the permission of Travenol Laboratories, Inc., Parenteral Products Division, Deerfield, Ill.

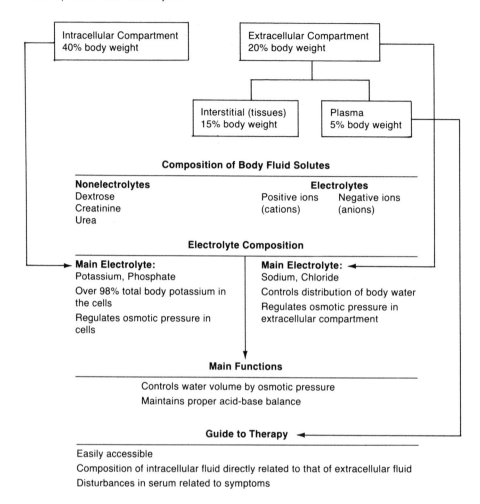

FIGURE 7.1
Total body water composition.

concentration may be low in spite of excess body sodium. This is due to the fact that total body sodium is equal to the sum of the products of volume times concentration in the various compartments.

Electrolytes serve two main purposes: (1) to act in controlling body water volume by osmotic pressure and (2) to maintain the proper acid–alkaline balance of the body.

Osmolality

Osmolality is the total solute concentration and reflects the relative water and total solute concentration since it is expressed per liter of serum. The osmotic pressure is determined by the number of solutes in solution. If the extracellular fluid contains a relatively large number of dissolved particles and the intracellular fluid contains a small amount of dissolved particles, the osmotic pressure would cause water to pass from the less concentrated fluid to the more concentrated. Therefore fluid from the intracellular compartment would pass into the extracellular compartment until the concentration became equal.

The unit of osmotic pressure is the osmole and the values are expressed in milliosmoles (mOsm). Normal blood plasma has an osmolality of about 290 mOsm/kg water. The determination of serum osmolality is sometimes used to detect dehydration or overhydration. Because sodium chloride is the principal solute in the extracellular fluid, the osmolality reading usually parallels the sodium reading or is very close to two times the serum sodium plus 10. Therefore measurement of sodium concentration also indicates the water needs of the body. At times the osmolality reading may falsely indicate dehydration. Because the osmolality is the total solute concentration, nonelectrolytes are included in the reading. An elevated level of blood urea can therefore increase the osmolality without exerting osmotic pressure. A determination of blood urea nitrogen may supply a correction to the osmolality reading in cases of increased serum urea.

Acid–Alkaline (Base) Balance

The alkalinity or acidity of a solution depends upon the degree of hydrogen ion concentration. An increase in the hydrogen ions results in a more acid solution; a decrease, in a more alkaline solution. Acidity is expressed by the symbol pH, which refers to the amount of hydrogen ion concentration. A solution having a pH of 7 is regarded as neutral.

The extracellular fluid has a pH ranging from 7.35 to 7.45 and is thus slightly alkaline. When the pH of the blood is higher than 7.45, an alkaline condition exists; when lower than 7.35, an acid condition exists.

The biological fluids, both extracellular and intracellular, contain a buffer system which maintains the proper acid–alkaline balance. This buffer system consists of fluid with salts of a weak acid or weak base. A base or hydroxide neutralizes the effect of an acid. These weak acids and bases maintain pH values by soaking up surplus ions or releasing them; acids yield hydrogen ions, bases accept hydrogen ions.

The carbonic acid–sodium bicarbonate system is the most important buffer system in the extracellular compartment. The normal ratio is 1 part of carbonic acid to 20 parts of base bicarbonate, which represents 1.2 mEq carbonic acid to 24 mEq base bicarbonate [4].

Acid–Base Imbalance

Acid–base imbalances are normally the result of an excess or a deficit in either base bicarbonate or carbonic acid. Deviations of pH from 7.35 to 7.45 are combated by the buffer system and by the respiratory and renal regulatory mechanisms. There are two types of disturbance that can affect the acid–base balance: respiratory and metabolic. Refer to Figure 7.2 for a diagrammatic presentation of the material that follows.

Respiratory Disturbances

Respiratory disturbances affect the carbonic side of the balance by increasing or decreasing carbonic acid; when carbon dioxide unites with extracellular fluid, carbonic acid is produced.

Respiratory alkalosis is caused when excess carbon dioxide is exhaled

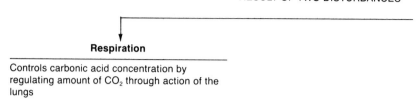

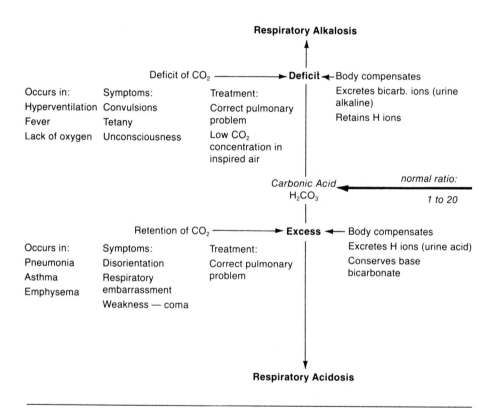

FIGURE 7.2
Acid-base imbalances as a result of respiratory or metabolic disturbances.

during rapid or deep breathing. Carbonic acid is depleted, owing to the carbon dioxide loss. Respiratory alkalosis may occur as the result of emotional disturbances, such as anxiety and hysteria, and also from lack of oxygen or from fever [4].

Symptoms are convulsions, tetany, and unconsciousness. Laboratory determination is a urinary pH above 7 and a plasma bicarbonate below 24 mEq per liter [4]. The body attempts to restore the ratio to normal by depressing the bicarbonate so as to compensate for the deficit in the carbonic acid.

Respiratory acidosis occurs when exhalation of carbon dioxide is depressed; the excess retention of carbon dioxide increases the carbonic acid. It

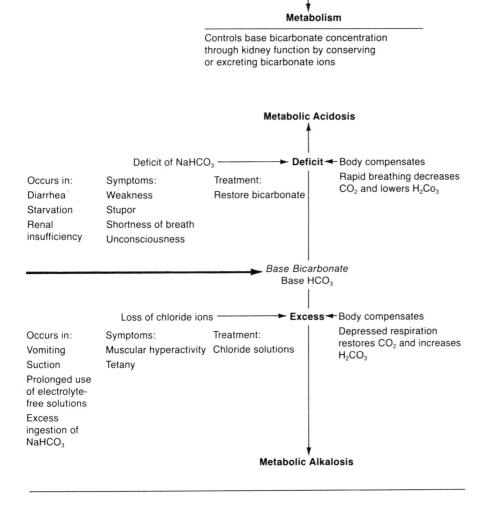

may occur in conditions that interfere with normal breathing: emphysema, asthma, and pneumonia [4].

Symptoms are weakness, disorientation, depressed breathing, and coma. Urinary pH is below 6, and plasma bicarbonate is above 24 mEq per liter. The increase of the bicarbonate is due to the body's attempt to restore the carbonic acid–bicarbonate ratio [4].

Metabolic Disturbances
Metabolic disturbances affect the bicarbonate side of the balance. Kidney function controls the bicarbonate concentration by regulating the amount of

cations (hydrogen, ammonium, and potassium) in exchange for sodium ions to combine with the reabsorbed bicarbonate in the distal tubular lumen. As hydrogen ions are excreted, bicarbonate is generated, maintaining the proper acid–base balance of the blood. Ammonia excretion is increased in response to a high acidity; bicarbonate replaces the ammonia.

Metabolic alkalosis is a condition associated with excess bicarbonate. This condition occurs when there is loss of chloride. Chloride and bicarbonate are both anions, which must equal the total number of cations. When the chloride anions are lost, the deficit must be made up by an equal number of anions to maintain electrolyte equilibrium; bicarbonate increases in compensation and alkalosis occurs.

Metabolic alkalosis is also associated with decreased levels of intracellular potassium. Potassium escapes from the cell into the extracellular fluid and is lost through the transcellular fluid. When body potassium is lost, the shift of the sodium and hydrogen ions from the extracellular fluid causes alkalosis, while the increase of hydrogen ions in the intracellular fluid causes acidosis of the cells.

Muscular hyperactivity, tetany, and depressed respiration are symptoms of metabolic alkalosis. The muscular hyperactivity and the tetany are symptoms of the deficit in ionized calcium which exists in alkalosis. Laboratory determinations are urinary pH above 7, plasma pH above 7.45, and bicarbonate above 24 mEq per liter [4].

Treatment consists of the administration of solutions containing chloride to replace bicarbonate ions. Excess of bicarbonate ions is accompanied by potassium deficiency, so potassium must also be replaced.

Metabolic acidosis is a condition associated with a deficit in the bicarbonate concentration. This occurs when (1) excessive amounts of ketone acids accumulate, as in uncontrolled diabetes or starvation, (2) inorganic acids like phosphate and sulphate accumulate, as in renal disease, and (3) excessive losses of bicarbonate occur from gastrointestinal drainage or diarrhea. Acidosis may occur also from intravenous administration of excessive amounts of sodium chloride or ammonium chloride, causing chloride ions to flood the extracellular fluid.

Stupor, shortness of breath, weakness, and unconsciousness are the symptoms of metabolic acidosis. Laboratory determination of urinary pH is below 6, plasma pH below 7.35, and plasma bicarbonate below 24 mEq per liter [4].

Therapy consists of increasing the bicarbonate level. Solutions of sodium lactate are often employed, but since lactate ion must be oxidized to carbon dioxide before it can affect the acid–base balance, it is advisable to use sodium bicarbonate solutions which are effective even when the patient is suffering from oxygen lack.

BODY-REGULATING MECHANISMS

The body contains regulating mechanisms which maintain the constancy of body fluid volume, electrolyte composition, and osmolality. These mechanisms consist of the renocardiovascular, endocrine (adrenal, pituitary, and parathyroid), and respiratory systems. The kidneys, skin, and lungs are the main regulating agents [4].

The *kidney* plays a major role in fluid and electrolyte balance. To function adequately, the kidney depends upon its own soundness as well as on the coordination of all the regulating organs. The distal renal tubules in the kidney are important in regulating the body fluid. They selectively retain or reject electrolytes and other substances to maintain normal osmolality and blood volume; sodium is retained and potassium is excreted [1].

The kidneys also play an important part in acid–base regulation. The distal tubule has the ability to form ammonia and exchange hydrogen ion (in form of ammonia) for bicarbonate to maintain the carbonic acid–bicarbonate ratio.

The *lungs* and the *skin* play an important role in fluid balance — the skin in loss of fluid through insensible perspiration and the lungs in loss of fluid by expiration. It has been noted [2] that normal intake of 2,500 ml from all sources will deliver a loss of about 1,000 ml in breath and perspiration, 1,400 ml in urine, and 100 ml in feces.

The *renocardiovascular system* maintains fluid balance by regulating the amount and composition of urine. Renal disease, cardiac failure, shock, postoperative stress, and alarm impair this regulating mechanism.

The *adrenal glands* influence the retention or excretion of sodium, potassium, and water. These glands secrete aldosterone, a hormone that increases the reabsorption of sodium from the renal tubules in exchange for potassium, thus maintaining normal sodium concentration [4]. Any stress, such as surgery, increases the secretion of aldosterone, thus increasing the reabsorption of sodium bicarbonate. Adrenal hyperactivity also increases the secretions of the hormone and causes excess sodium retention. Excess loss of sodium occurs with adrenal insufficiency.

The *pituitary gland* is another important organ in the control of fluid and electrolyte balance. The posterior lobe of the pituitary releases antidiuretic hormone (ADH). This hormone inhibits diuresis by increasing water reabsorption in the distal tubule. Increased concentration of sodium in the extracellular fluid stimulates the pituitary to release ADH. This hormone increases the reabsorption of water to dilute the sodium to the normal level of concentration. Increased body fluid osmolality, decreased body fluid volume, stress, and shock are conditions which increase ADH secretions. Increased body fluid volume, decreased osmolality, and alcohol inhibit ADH secretions.

The *pulmonary system* regulates acid–base balance by controlling the concentration of carbonic acid through exhalation or retention of carbon dioxide.

ELECTROLYTES OF BIOLOGICAL FLUIDS

Potassium

Potassium is one of the most important electrolytes in the body. An excess or deficiency of potassium can cause serious impairment of body function and even result in death.

Potassium is the main electrolyte in the intracellular compartment, which houses over 98 percent of the body's total potassium. The healthy cell requires a high potassium concentration for cellular activity. When the cell dies, there is an exchange of potassium into the extracellular fluid with a transfer of sodium into the cell. This process also occurs to some degree when cellular metabolism is impaired, as in catabolism (breaking down) of cells from a crushing injury.

Plasma concentration of potassium is 4.0–5.5 mEq per liter. In the cell, the normal concentration is 115–150 mEq per liter of fluid. Variations from either of these levels can produce critical effects. When a repeated potassium level is above 5.6 mEq per liter, a potassium excess is indicated; renal impairment will usually be shown by renal function studies. High serum concentrations have an adverse effect on the heart muscle and may cause cardiac arrhythmias; elevation to two to three times the normal level may result in cardiac arrest. The electrocardiogram may detect signs of potassium excess with peaked and elevated T waves; P waves later disappear, and finally, "biphasic deflections [result] from fusion of the QRS complex, RST segment, and the T waves" [4]. *Hypokalemia* is the term that expresses serum potassium concentration below normal; *hyperkalemia* denotes serum potassium above normal.

Hypokalemia

Hypokalemia (serum potassium level below 4 mEq per liter) may result when any one of the following conditions occurs: (1) total body potassium is below normal, (2) concentration of potassium in cells is below normal, or (3) concentration of potassium in serum is below normal [3].

These conditions are often caused by variations in the intake or output of potassium. A decreased intake of potassium from prolonged fluid therapy (lacking potassium replacement) may result in hypokalemia. It may also occur during a "starvation diet," as the kidneys do not normally conserve potassium. An increased loss of potassium usually results from polyuria, vomiting, gastric suction (prolonged), diarrhea, and steroid therapy [3].

On the other hand, these conditions of potassium deficiency may be unrelated to intake and output. They can be caused by a sudden shift of potassium from extracellular fluid to intracellular fluid, such as that occurring from (1) anabolism (building up of cells), (2) healing processes, or (3) the use of insulin and glucose in the treatment of diabetic acidosis [3]. The shifts resulting from anabolism and healing processes are not usually of severe consequence unless accompanied by intervening factors. In the treatment of diabetic acidosis, the potassium shift may occur suddenly with grave consequences. When cells are anabolized, potassium shifts into the cells. During the use of glucose in the treatment of diabetic acidosis, the glucose in the cells is quickly metabolized into glycogen for storage, causing a sudden shift of potassium from the extracellular fluid to the intracellular fluid [3]. This process results in hypokalemia.

The signs and symptoms of hypokalemia are malaise, skeletal and smooth muscle atony, apathy, muscular cramps, and postural hypotension. Treatment consists of administration of potassium orally or parenterally.

Chapter 7 | Fundamental Aspects of Fluid and Electrolyte Metabolism

Hyperkalemia

Hyperkalemia may result from renal failure with potassium retention or from excessive or rapid administration of potassium in fluid therapy. It may also occur in conditions unrelated to retention or excessive intake. A sudden shift of potassium from intracellular to extracellular fluid results when catabolism of cells takes place, as in a crushing injury; potassium shifts from cells to plasma.

The signs and symptoms of hyperkalemia are similar to those of hypokalemia. In addition to those signs already listed, the patient may experience tingling or numbness in the extremities, and the heart rate may be slow. A serum potassium level above 5.5 mEq per liter confirms the diagnosis.

Treatment consists of stopping the potassium intake. Dialysis may be necessary for a long-term renal problem. If the cause is a shift of potassium from cells to plasma, glucose and insulin therapy may be used.

Sodium

Sodium is the main electrolyte in the extracellular fluid; its normal concentration is 135–145 mEq per liter of plasma. The main role of sodium is to control the distribution of water throughout the body and to maintain a normal fluid balance. Alterations in sodium concentration markedly influence the fluid volume: the loss of sodium is accompanied by loss of water and dehydration; the gain of sodium, by retention of fluid.

The body, by regulating the urinary output, normally maintains a constant fluid volume and isotonicity of the plasma. The urinary output is controlled by ADH, secreted by the pituitary gland. If a hypotonic concentration results from a low sodium concentration, the fluid is drawn from the plasma into the cells. The body attempts to correct this process; the pituitary inhibits ADH and diuresis results, with a loss of extracellular fluid. This loss of fluid increases sodium concentration to a normal level.

If a hypertonic concentration results from increased concentration of extracellular sodium, fluid is drawn from the cells. Again the body reacts, and the pituitary is stimulated to secrete ADH. This causes a retention of fluid that dilutes sodium to normal concentrations.

Therefore increased sodium concentration stimulates the production of ADH, with retention of water thus diluting sodium to the normal level; a decrease in sodium concentration inhibits the production of ADH, resulting in a loss of water which raises the concentration of sodium to the normal level.

In the kidneys sodium is reabsorbed in exchange for potassium. Therefore with an increase in sodium there is loss of potassium; with a loss of sodium there is an increase in potassium.

A *sodium deficit* may be present when plasma sodium falls below 135 mEq per liter. It is caused by (1) excessive sweating with large intake of water by mouth (salt is lost and fluid increased, thus reducing sodium concentration), (2) excessive infusion of nonelectrolyte fluids, (3) gastrointestinal suction plus water by mouth, and (4) adrenal insufficiency, which causes large loss of electrolytes.

The symptoms of a sodium deficit are apprehension, abdominal cramps, diarrhea, and convulsions.

Dehydration results from loss of sodium and leads to peripheral circulatory failure. When sodium and water are lost from the plasma, the body attempts to replace them by a transfer of sodium and water from the interstitial fluid. Eventually the water will be drawn from the cells and circulation will fail; plasma volume will not be sustained.

Sodium excess may be present when the plasma sodium rises above 147 mEq per liter. Its causes are (1) excessive infusions of saline, (2) diarrhea, (3) insufficient water intake, (4) diabetes mellitus, and (5) tracheobronchitis (excess loss of water from lungs because of rapid breathing).

The symptoms of sodium excess are dry sticky mucous membranes, oliguria, excitement, and convulsions.

Calcium

Calcium is an electrolyte constituent of the plasma which is present in a concentration of about 5 mEq per liter. Calcium serves several purposes. It plays an important role in formation and function of bones and teeth. As ionized calcium, it is involved in (1) normal clotting of the blood and (2) regulation of neuromuscular irritability.

The parathyroid glands, located within the thyroid gland, control calcium metabolism. The parathyroid hormone, acting on the kidneys and bones, regulates the concentration of ionized calcium in the extracellular fluid. Impairment of this regulatory mechanism alters the calcium concentration. Hyperparathyroidism causes an elevation in the serum calcium level and a decrease in the serum phosphate level.

Calcium deficit may occur in patients with diarrhea or with problems in gastrointestinal absorption, in extensive infections of the subcutaneous tissue, and in burns [4]. This deficiency can result in muscle tremors and cramps, in excessive irritability, and even in convulsions.

Calcium ionization is influenced by pH; it is decreased in alkalosis and increased in acidosis. With no loss of calcium a patient in alkalosis may develop symptoms of calcium deficit: muscle cramps, tetany, and convulsions. This is due to the decreased ionization of calcium caused by the elevated pH.

A patient in acidosis may have a calcium deficit with no symptoms because the acid pH has caused an increased ionization of available calcium. Symptoms of calcium deficit may appear if acidosis is converted to alkalosis.

Other Electrolytes

Magnesium's primary role is in enzyme activity, contributing to the metabolism of both carbohydrates and proteins. Its serum concentration is 1.7–2.3 mEq per liter. A deficit in magnesium is not common but may occur from impaired gastrointestinal absorption.

Chloride, the chief anion of the extracellular fluid, has a plasma concentration of 100–106 mEq per liter. A deficiency of chloride leads to a deficiency of potassium, and vice versa. There is also a loss of chloride with a loss of sodium, but because this loss can be compensated for by an increase in bicarbonate, the proportion will differ [1].

Phosphate is the chief anion of the intracellular fluid; its normal level in plasma is 1.7–2.3 mEq per liter.

Chapter 7 | Fundamental Aspects of Fluid and Electrolyte Metabolism

REFERENCES

1. Baxter Laboratories. *Fundamentals of Body Water and Electrolytes*. Morton Grove, Ill., 1977, Pp. 5, 21.
2. Burgess, R. E. Fluids and electrolytes. *Am. J. Nurs.* 65:90–95, 1965.
3. Crowell, C. E., and Staff of Educational Design, Inc., N.Y. Potassium imbalance. *Am. J. Nurs.* 67:343, 1967.
4. Metheny, N. M., and Snively, W. D., Jr. *Nurses' Handbook of Fluid Balance* (4th ed.) Philadelphia: Lippincott, 1983. Pp. 8, 9, 17, 51, 54, 68–81, 282.

REVIEW QUESTIONS

1. Total body fluid is functionally divided into two main compartments: the _intracellular_ and the _extracellular_ compartments.
2. The plasma represents 5 percent of the body weight and is present in the _extracellular_ compartment.
3. The body contains two types of solutes: the _electrolytes_ and the _nonelectrolytes_.
4. Name the nonelectrolytes found in body fluid. _dextrose, urea, creatinine_
5. Define the term *electrolytes*. _molecules which break into electrically-charged ions_
6. What is the osmolality of normal blood plasma? _290 +0-50_
7. What electrolyte controls the distribution of body water and regulates osmotic pressure in the extracellular compartment? _Na Cl ?_
8. What electrolyte regulates osmotic pressure in cells? _K_
9. What are the two main functions of electrolytes? _(1) act in control body water volume by osmotic pressure (2) maintain acid-alkaline balance_
10. What is the symbol expressing acidity? _pH_
11. What is the normal pH of the blood? _7.35 7.45_
12. What is the most important buffer system of the extracellular compartment? _Carbonic acid - sodium bicarbonate_
13. Which side of the acid–alkaline balance is affected by respiratory alkalosis? _pH ↑_
14. What would the following signs and symptoms suggest: weakness, disorientation, depressed breathing, and coma, urinary pH below 6, plasma bicarbonate above 24 mEq per liter? _resp-acidosis_
15. Why is the plasma bicarbonate above 24 mEq per liter in respiratory acidosis? _body trying to restore carbonic-acid base ratio_
16. Why may a patient in alkalosis develop symptoms of calcium deficit?
17. What side of the acid–alkaline balance do metabolic disturbances affect?
18. How does kidney function control the bicarbonate concentration?
19. Why does metabolic alkalosis occur when there is loss of chloride?
20. Metabolic acidosis is a condition associated with a deficit in the _____ concentration.
21. What conditions or types of therapy cause metabolic acidosis?
22. Name the homeostatic mechanisms that maintain the constancy of body fluid volume, electrolyte composition, and osmolality.

23. What organ secretes aldosterone?
24. What is the function of aldosterone?
25. What hormone released by the pituitary gland controls the urinary output?
26. What three conditions can cause hyperkalemia?
27. What is the main role of sodium?
28. What is the normal plasma concentration of sodium?
29. What hormone is stimulated by increased sodium plasma concentration?
30. How does ADH correct the sodium concentration?
31. What is the normal calcium plasma concentration?
32. What functions are ionized calcium involved in?
33. What homeostatic mechanism controls calcium metabolism?
34. What causes a calcium deficit?
35. Why may a patient in acidosis have a calcium deficit yet show no symptoms of the calcium deficit?
36. What is the primary role of magnesium?
37. What is the normal concentration of chloride in the plasma?
38. A deficiency of chloride leads to a deficiency of potassium, and vice versa. True or false?

CHAPTER 8

Rationale of Fluid and Electrolyte Therapy

Ada Lawrence Plumer

OBJECTIVES OF PARENTERAL THERAPY

Parenteral therapy has three main objectives: (1) to maintain daily body fluid requirements, (2) to restore previous body fluid losses, and (3) to replace present body fluid losses.

MAINTENANCE THERAPY

Maintenance therapy consists of provision of all the nutrient needs of the patient: water, electrolytes, dextrose, vitamins, and protein. Of these needs, water has the priority. The body may survive for a prolonged period without vitamins, dextrose, and protein, but without water, dehydration and death occur.

Water

Water is needed by the body to replace the insensible loss which occurs with evaporation from the skin and evaporated moisture from the expired air. An average adult loses from 500 to 1,000 ml of water per 24 hours through insensible loss [5]. The skin loss varies with the temperature and humidity.

Water must also be provided for kidney function; the amount needed depends upon the amount of waste products to be excreted as well as the concentrating ability of the kidneys [5]. Protein and salt increase the need for water.

Until 1925 parenteral fluids consisted solely of isotonic saline solutions [5]. Because water is hypotonic and cannot be given intravenously, salt was added to attain isotonicity. If given intravenously, distilled water causes hemolysis; the distilled water is drawn into the blood cells owing to the greater solute concentration, causing them to swell and burst. After 1925 glucose began to be used extensively to make water isotonic and to provide calories [5].

An individual's fluid requirements are based on age, height, weight, and amount of body fat. Because fat is water-free, a large amount of body fat contains a relatively low amount of water; as body fat increases, water decreases in inverse proportion to body weight [7]. The normal fluid and electrolyte requirements based on body surface area have been found to be more constant than when expressed in terms of body weight. Many of the essential physiological processes such as heat loss, blood volume, organ size, and respiration have a direct relationship to the body surface area [7]. The fluid and electrolyte requirements are also proportionate to surface area, regardless of the age of the patient [7]. These requirements are based on square meter of body surface area and calculated for a 24-hour period. Nomograms are available for determining surface area (see Figure 8.1). Pocket nomograms* for I.V. fluid therapy determine surface area by weight alone with adjustments for obese or thin individuals. Calculations by weight alone give only an approximate surface area and are not accurate when used for individuals of other than average build.

Balanced solutions are available for maintenance. An estimate is made of the average requirements of fluid and electrolytes in a healthy person and applied to the patient. The balanced solutions contain electrolytes in proportion to the daily needs of the patient, but not in excess of the body's tolerance, as long as adequate kidney function exists. When a patient's water needs are provided by these maintenance solutions, the daily needs of sodium and potassium are also met. For maintenance, 1,500 ml per square meter of body surface is administered over a 24-hour period [7].

Glucose

Glucose, a necessary nutrient in maintenance therapy, has important functions. As it is converted into glycogen by the liver, it improves hepatic function. By supplying necessary calories for energy, it spares body protein and minimizes the development of ketosis occasioned by the oxidation of fat stores for essential energy in the absence of added glucose.

The basic daily caloric requirement of a 70-kg adult at rest is about 1,600 calories. However, the administration of 100 gm glucose a day is helpful in minimizing the ketosis of starvation [7]; 100 gm is contained in 2 liters 5% dextrose in water or 1 liter 10% dextrose in water.

Protein

Protein is another nutrient important to maintenance therapy. Though a patient may be adequately maintained on glucose, water, vitamins, and electrolytes over a limited time, protein may be required to replace normal protein losses over an extended period of time. It is necessary for cellular repair, healing of wounds, and synthesis of vitamins and some enzymes. The usual daily requirement for a healthy adult is 1 gm protein per kilogram of body weight [7]. Protein is available as amino acids; taken orally, it is broken down into amino acids before being absorbed into the blood.

Vitamins

Vitamins, though not nutrients in the true sense of the word, are necessary for the utilization of other nutrients. Vitamin C and the various B complex vitamins are the most frequently used in parenteral therapy. As these vitamins are water soluble, they are not retained by the body but lost through urinary ex-

---

*Cohn Fluid Calculator (for I.V. Fluid Therapy): Travenol Laboratories, Inc., Deerfield, Ill. Designed by Bertram D. Cohn, M.D., F.A.A.P., F.A.C.S.

cretion. Because of this loss, larger amounts are required parenterally to ensure adequate maintenance than may be required when administered orally. Vitamin B complex vitamins play an important role in the metabolism of carbohydrates and in maintaining gastrointestinal function. As vitamin C promotes wound healing, it is frequently used for the surgical patient.

Vitamins A and D are fat-soluble vitamins, better retained by the body and not generally required by the patient on maintenance therapy.

RESTORATION OF PREVIOUS LOSSES

Restoration of previous losses is essential when past maintenance has not been met — when the output has exceeded the intake. Severe dehydration may occur from failure to replace these losses. Therapy consists of replacing losses from previous deficits in addition to providing fluid and electrolytes for daily maintenance. The status of the kidneys must be considered before electrolyte replacement and maintenance can be initiated; urinary suppression may result from decreased fluid volume or renal impairment. A hydrating solution such as 5% dextrose in 0.2% (34.2 mEq) sodium chloride is administered. Urinary flow will be restored if the retention is functional. The patient must be rehydrated rapidly to establish an adequate urinary output. Only after kidney function is proved adequate can large electrolyte losses be replaced. Potassium chloride must be used with considerable caution and is considered potentially dangerous if administered when renal function is impaired. A buildup of potassium, owing to the kidney's inability to excrete salts, can prove hazardous; arrhythmia and heart block can result from the effect of excess potassium on the heart muscle.

REPLACEMENT OF PRESENT LOSSES

Replacement of present losses of fluid and electrolytes is as necessary as daily maintenance and replacement of previous losses. The importance of accurate measurement of all intake and output cannot be underestimated as a means of calculating fluid loss. Fluid loss may also be estimated by determining loss of body weight; 1 liter body water equals 1 kg, or 2.2 pounds, body weight. An osmolality determination may indicate the water needs of the body. If necessary a corrective blood urea nitrogen determination may be done in conjunction with the osmolality.

The type of replacement is dependent upon the type of fluid being lost. A choice of appropriate replacement solutions is available. Excessive loss of gastric fluid must be replaced by solutions resembling the fluid lost, such as gastric replacement solutions. Excessive loss of intestinal fluid must be replaced by an intestinal replacement fluid. Examples of conditions that may result from current losses are alkalosis and acidosis (see Figure 7.2, pp. 74–75).

Alkalosis

Alkalosis may occur from an excessive loss of gastric fluid, either by vomiting or suction. Gastric juices, with a pH of 1 to 3, are the most acid of the body secretions [7]. Excess loss of chloride causes an increase in the bicarbonate

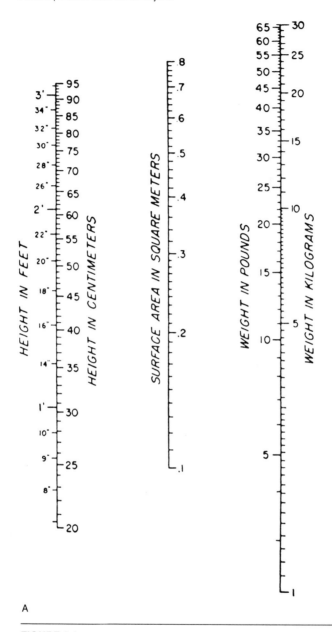

FIGURE 8.1
Body surface area nomograms for (A) infants and young children, and (B) older children and adults. To determine the surface area of the patient, draw a straight line between the point representing height on the left vertical scale to the point representing weight on the right vertical scale. The point at which the line intersects the middle vertical scale

Chapter 8 | Rationale of Fluid and Electrolyte Therapy

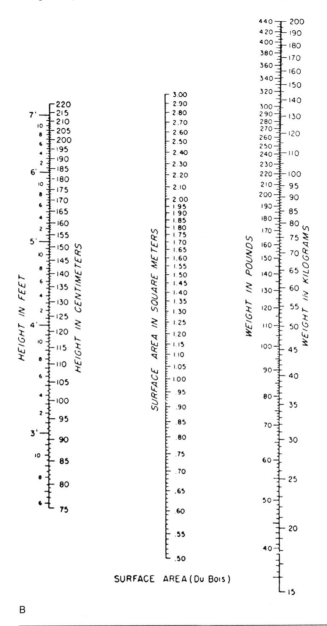

B

represents the patient's body surface area in square meters. Reprinted by permission of the publishers from *Functional Endocrinology from Birth Through Adolescence* by N. B. Talbot, E. H. Sobel, J. W. McArthur, and J. D. Crawford, Cambridge, Mass.: Harvard University Press, © 1952, 1980 by the President and Fellows of Harvard College.

ions; total anions must always equal total cations. The patient's respiration becomes slow and shallow; the body attempts to correct alkalosis by retaining carbon dioxide. Because of the body's inability to ionize calcium in the presence of a high pH, muscular hyperactivity and tetany occur. The patient may become irritable, uncooperative, and disoriented.

Prompt recognition of symptoms is important for early treatment or for altering current treatment. Most alkalotic states secondary to gastric suction are corrected by sodium chloride and potassium chloride solutions. Special gastric replacement solutions are available. They contain ammonium chloride, which replaces the chloride without increasing the sodium. The hydrogen ions, liberated by urea in the conversion of ammonium chloride, correct alkalosis. These solutions, invaluable in certain conditions, can be potentially dangerous if given to patients with impaired liver or kidney function. Ammonia, metabolized by the liver, is converted into urea and hydrogen ion. If the liver fails to convert the ammonia to urea, ammonia retention and toxicity will result. Symptoms of ammonia toxicity include pallor, sweating, tetany, and coma, and death may ensue.

Acidosis

Acidosis may occur when the excessive fluid loss is alkaline, as are intestinal secretions, bile, and pancreatic juices. Intestinal secretions contain large amounts of bicarbonate ions; with the loss of these ions, there is an increase in the chloride ions — and acidosis occurs. Symptoms include shortness of breath with rapid breathing (respiratory compensation to reduce carbon dioxide and correct acidosis). Weakness and coma occur. In order to replace lost alkaline secretions and correct acidosis, specific parenteral solutions containing base salts, such as sodium lactate or sodium bicarbonate, are employed.

ELECTROLYTE AND FLUID DISTURBANCES

Fluid and electrolyte imbalances occurring in the ill patient are serious complications which can threaten life. The correction of these imbalances is of vital concern to the welfare of the patient. A discussion follows of a few of the most common clinical cases in which fluid disturbances contribute to serious complications, with emphasis on the physiological changes accompanying these imbalances and the parenteral therapy necessary to correct them.

PARENTERAL THERAPY FOR THE SURGICAL PATIENT

A knowledge of the endocrine response to stress assists the nurse in a better understanding of imbalances and problems associated with them. It also contributes to safe and successful parenteral therapy: the nurse knows what to expect, is alert to the possible dangers of imbalances, and recognizes early symptoms.

Endocrine Response to Stress

The endocrine homeostatic controls are affected by stress. At times stress from preoperative apprehension triggers an undesirable endocrine response, making it necessary to postpone an operation. Apprehension, pain, and duration and severity of trauma give rise to surgical stress and cause an increased endocrine

Chapter 8 | Rationale of Fluid and Electrolyte Therapy

response during the first 2–5 days following surgery. On the whole the stress reaction is normal and is nature's way of protecting the body from hypotension resulting from trauma and shock. Correction is often unnecessary and may, in fact, be harmful.

The two major endocrine homeostatic controls affected by stress are the pituitary gland and the adrenal gland (see Figure 8.2). The posterior pituitary controls quantitative secretions of ADH (antidiuretic hormone); the anterior pituitary controls secretions of ACTH (adrenocorticotropic hormone). ACTH stimulates the adrenal gland to increase (1) mineralocorticoid secretions (aldosterone) and (2) glucocorticoid secretions (hydrocortisone) [7]. The adrenal

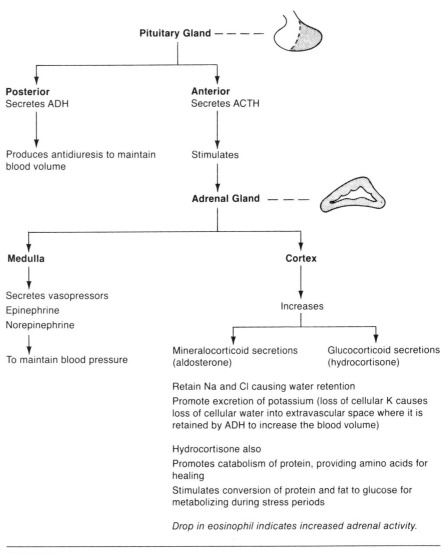

FIGURE 8.2
Endocrine response to stress.

medulla secretes vasopressors (epinephrine and norepinephrine) to help maintain the blood pressure.

A direct physiological effect is produced when stress increases the secretions of these various hormones. When the posterior pituitary increases ADH secretions, antidiuresis is effected, thus helping maintain blood volume. When the anterior pituitary increases ACTH secretions, the adrenal gland is stimulated to increase the secretions of aldosterone and hydrocortisone. These two adrenal hormones help maintain blood volume by (1) causing the retention of sodium ions and chloride anions, thereby causing water retention, and (2) promoting the excretion of potassium (loss of cellular potassium ions causes loss of cellular water into extracellular space, where it is retained by ADH to maintain blood volume) [7].

Hydrocortisone also promotes the catabolism of protein to provide necessary amino acids for healing and stimulates the conversion of protein and fat to glucose for metabolism during the stress period. This metabolic activity may elevate the blood sugar level, a finding which may mistakenly suggest diabetes mellitus. A drop in the eosinophil count and an elevated level of serum 17-hydroxycorticosteroid hormones indicate increased adrenal activity [7].

Fluid Therapy

Accurate records of intake and output measurements are important for assessing the proper fluid requirements and preventing serious fluid imbalances during the early postoperative period. The daily requirement of 1,500 to 2,000 ml varies with the patient's needs. Caution must be taken not to overhydrate the patient — the intake should be adequate but should not exceed the fluid losses.

We have seen how the adrenocortical secretions, increased by trauma and stress of surgery, cause some water and sodium retention. This retention may be severe enough to give a false picture of oliguria. Excessive quantities of nonelectrolyte solutions, such as 5% dextrose in water, administered at a time when antidiuresis is occurring may cause a serious fluid imbalance, hyponatremia.

Hyponatremia

Hyponatremia is a condition in which the serum sodium concentration is less than normal. Water-yielding solutions, infused in excess of the body's tolerance, expand the extracellular compartment, lowering the electrolyte concentration. By the process of osmosis water invades the cells, with a resulting excess accumulation of intracellular fluid. Usually there is no edema, as edema is the result of an excess accumulation of fluid in the extracellular compartment [2].

Symptoms of water excess include confusion, hallucinations, delirium, weight gain, hyperventilation, muscular weakness, twitching, and convulsions. If these occur during the early postoperative stages, the nurse should suspect water excess. This is of particular concern in the young and the aged. Serious consequences, even death, can result.

Restricting the fluid intake may correct mild water excess, but for the more severe cases the administration of high concentrations of sodium chloride may be indicated. The electrolyte concentration of the plasma, increased by the concentrated saline, causes an increase in the osmotic pressure, drawing fluid from the cells for excretion by the kidneys.

Often parenteral therapy during the stress period consists of administering conservative amounts of 5% dextrose in water. As some sodium retention results from the endocrine response to stress, caution is taken to avoid administration of excessive quantities of saline at a time when there is an interference in the elimination of salt. During this early period, the physician frequently gives 5% dextrose in quarter- or half-strength saline to avoid sodium excess.

Hypernatremia

Hypernatremia is a condition in which the serum sodium concentration is higher than normal. This excess can cause (1) expanded extracellular fluid volume or edema and (2) possible disruption of cellular function (in potassium-depleted patients the sodium may replace the intracellular potassium).

Symptoms of sodium excess include flushed skin, elevation in temperature, dry sticky mucous membranes, thirst, and a decrease or absence of urinary output. Treatment consists of reducing the intake of salt and water and promoting diuresis to eliminate the excess of salt and water from the plasma.

Nutrients

Carbohydrates

Carbohydrates provide an indispensable source of calories for the postoperative patient unable to receive oral sustenance. When carbohydrates are inadequate, the body will utilize its own fat to supply calories; the by-products are ketone bodies. These acid bodies neutralize bicarbonate and produce metabolic acidosis. The only by-products excreted in the utilization of carbohydrates are water and carbon dioxide.

Carbohydrates, by providing calories for essential energy, also reduce catabolism of protein. During the stress response the renal excretion of nitrogen (from the catabolism of protein) exceeds the intake. By reducing the protein breakdown, glucose helps prevent a negative nitrogen balance.

Carbohydrates do not provide adequate calories for the patient receiving prolonged therapy. One liter of 5% dextrose in water provides 170 calories. Many liters, a volume too great for most patients to tolerate, would be required to provide a patient with 1,600 calories. Greater concentrations of glucose, 20% and 50%, may be administered to provide calories for patients unable to tolerate large volumes of fluid (e.g., patients with renal insufficiency). The concentrated solutions must be administered slowly for utilization of the glucose to take place. Rapid administration results in diuresis; the concentrated glucose acts as a diuretic, drawing interstitial fluid into the plasma for excretion by the kidneys.

Alcohol

Alcohol solutions may be administered to the postoperative patient for nutritional and physiological benefits. Nutritionally the alcohol supplements calories provided by the glucose, 1 gm ethyl alcohol yielding 6 to 8 calories [7]. Because alcohol is quickly and completely metabolized, it provides calories for essential energy, sparing fat and protein. Metabolized in preference to glucose, alcohol allows the infused glucose to be stored as glycogen.

Physiologically, alcohol produces a sedative effect, reducing pain; 200–300 ml of a 5% solution per hour produces sedation without intoxication in the average adult [7]. Alcohol also inhibits the secretion of ADH, promoting water excretion.

It is well to bear in mind that the solutions containing alcohol, particularly hypertonic solutions, can cause phlebitis. These solutions, if allowed to infiltrate, may cause tissue necrosis. The needle should be carefully inserted within the vein and inspected frequently to detect any infiltration.

Protein

Patients who receive parenteral fluid therapy for a prolonged period of time require protein for cellular repair, wound healing, and growth. Stress states accompanying surgical procedures and trauma frequently result in protein deficiency.

During the stress period, increased secretions of glucocorticoids from the adrenal cortex cause protein breakdown and the conversion of protein and fat to glucose for energy. More urinary nitrogen is lost than normal. When nitrogen loss exceeds intake, the patient is said to be in a *negative balance*. This response to stress is normal. However, protein losses must be counteracted; preservation of body cell mass is essential. A depleted body cell mass can be restored only by hyperalimentation.

Protein preparations, commercially available as crystalline amino acids* and protein hydrolysates,† are administered by peripheral infusion. Providing sufficient calories is essential to prevent breakdown of protein for energy. Approximately 1 gram of protein per kilogram of body weight is required by a healthy adult to replace normal protein loss [7].

Infusion of protein hydrolysates should be started slowly and cautiously (2 ml per minute or less). Adverse reactions — nausea, vomiting, fever, chills — require termination of the infusion. The rate should not exceed 4 ml per kilogram of body weight per hour [7].

Because of the high NH_4 level, extreme caution is required if administered to patients with hepatic insufficiency or emaciation. Patients with metabolic disorders that impair nitrogen metabolism, such as hepatic coma or severe renal failure, should not receive amino acids.

Supplemental medications added to the solution may result in incompatibilities. Always check with the pharmacist before adding any medication to solutions.

Solutions, once opened, must be used immediately. Storing a partially used container of solution in the refrigerator for future use provides a culture medium for the growth of bacteria.

No solutions that are cloudy or that contain precipitate should be used.

---

*Novamine (KabiVitrum, Inc.); Alemeda, Calif.

†Aminosyn (Abbott Laboratories); North Chicago, Ill.

Fat Emulsions

Fat emulsions provide a source of calories and essential fatty acids for metabolic processes. They provide a high caloric yield, 9 Kcal per gram as compared with 4 Kcal per gram from carbohydrates. See Chapter 21 for more complete information.

Potassium

Once the stress period is past, adrenal activity decreases and diuresis begins. At this time, usually after the second to the fifth postoperative day, potassium is given daily to prevent a deficit; potassium is not conserved by the body but is lost in the urine. Electrolyte maintenance fluids may be used or potassium may be added to parenteral solutions. When potassium is added to parenteral fluids, the container, bag, or bottle should be thoroughly shaken to mix and dilute the potassium. Potassium should *never* be added to a hanging container while the infusion is running; such action could result in a bolus injection of the drug. Rapid injection, which increases the drug concentration in the plasma, can result in trauma to the vessel wall and even in cardiac arrest. Potassium should never be given by I.V. push or bolus administration.

The status of the kidneys must be considered. If kidney function is inadequate, the patient must be rehydrated. During this infusion, the nurse must watch for diminished diuresis and notify the physician if antidiuresis occurs.

Potassium 40 mEq per liter is usually sufficient to replace normal loss. It is usually infused over an 8-hour period.

In extreme cases of hypokalemia, when the plasma potassium is less than 2.5 mEq per liter, it may be necessary to infuse potassium at a much faster rate, not faster than 40 mEq per hour [7]. Continuous monitoring by electrocardiogram is required when high doses of potassium are infused. The solution containing potassium should be conspicuously labeled and must never be used when positive pressure is indicated — rapid infusion may result in cardiac arrest.

Potassium is irritating to the vein and may cause a great deal of pain, especially if infused into a vein where a previous venipuncture has been performed. Slowing the rate may decrease the pain.

Vitamins

Vitamins B complex and C are usually added to parenteral solutions if, after 2 or 3 days, the patient is unable to take fluids orally. Vitamin C is important in promoting healing in the surgical patient, and vitamin B complex aids carbohydrate metabolism.

PARENTERAL THERAPY FOR THE BURNED PATIENT

The body mechanisms that regulate fluid and electrolyte balance are altered when severe burns occur. The changes that take place during the first 48 hours must be recognized and dealt with. Fluid and electrolyte therapy sufficient to replace losses and maintain a status quo increase the patient's chances of

Fluid and Electrolyte Changes

survival. Awareness of these physiological changes contributes to intelligent therapy and aids in the patient's recovery.

Intravascular to Interstitial Fluid Shift
The shift from intravascular to interstitial fluid, followed by shock, begins immediately following the burn. This fluid shift represents the water, electrolyte, and protein that are lost through the damaged capillaries, resulting in edema and a marked reduction in plasma volume. The severity of the shift depends upon the degree and extent of the burn. In an adult with a 50 percent burn, the edema may exceed the total plasma volume of the patient. Parenteral fluids must be given immediately to replace the fluid loss and combat shock.

Dehydration
In the early phases of fluid shift from plasma to tissues, water and electrolytes are lost in larger quantities than is the protein (protein, because of its larger molecular size, does not readily pass through the capillary walls). The osmotic pressure, increased by the higher protein concentration of the plasma, draws fluid from the undamaged tissues and generalized tissue dehydration occurs.

A much more significant fluid loss occurs as (1) exudate from the burned area, (2) water in the form of vapor at the burned area, and (3) blood lost through the damaged capillaries. These losses further contribute to dehydration and hypovolemia.

Decreased Urinary Output
Decreased urinary output occurs when the lowered blood volume causes a diminished renal blood flow. Increased endocrine secretions further contribute to the decrease in urinary output; adrenal cortical secretions cause sodium and water absorption; ADH causes increased water reabsorption by the kidneys.

In deep burns free hemoglobin, released by destruction of red cells, may produce renal damage.

Potassium Excess
When excessive amounts of potassium build up in the extracellular fluid, potassium excess occurs; cell destruction releases potassium and decreased renal flow obstructs normal excretion of potassium. Plasma potassium concentrations may rise to a dangerously high level. Because of the tendency to plasma potassium excess and the uncertainty of the extent of renal impairment in the burned patient, administration of potassium is contraindicated.

Sodium Deficit
When plasma is lost in edema and exudate, sodium, the chief electrolyte of the extracellular fluid, is lost with the plasma, and sodium deficit occurs. Further loss may occur as sodium moves into the cells to replace lost potassium.

Metabolic Acidosis
Acidosis results from a loss of bicarbonate ions accompanying the loss of sodium ions as well as from altered aerobic metabolized tissue destruction.

Fluid Therapy

When moderate or severe burns occur, immediate fluid therapy is necessary to combat hypovolemic shock and prevent renal depression. A large-gauge indwelling venous catheter is inserted to ensure parenteral therapy during this critical period. As the measurement of venous pressure is an important guide against overinfusion, a second catheter may be inserted for venous pressure determination.

In small burns that require parenteral therapy, solutions such as isotonic saline, Ringer's solution, or 5% dextrose in water or saline may be sufficient, but in severe burns a colloid is usually employed. Colloids, because of their tendency to hold fluids in the vascular compartment, are used to maintain blood volume and combat shock. Plasma, albumin, and dextran are the most common of the colloidal solutions used. Whole blood is added when indicated.

Fluid therapy consists in supplying (1) the normal daily fluid requirements and (2) additional amounts of fluid for replacement of burn losses. The amount of fluid necessary to replace burn losses is calculated in relation to the extent and severity of the burn. The "rule of nines" has been commonly used to estimate the burned area. The surface area of the body is divided into areas of 9 percent or its multiples (see Table 8.1). This method must be used cautiously or dangerously high estimates may occur. Charts that give a more detailed breakdown of surface area provide greater accuracy and are more beneficial.

During the first 24 hours, caution must be taken to avoid overzealous fluid therapy. Later, when fluid shifts back into the plasma, excess parenteral fluid can cause overburdened circulation and pulmonary edema. If smoke and heat damage have impaired lung capacity to function, the threat of pulmonary edema is further increased. Only enough fluid to maintain blood volume and urinary output is administered.

The shift from interstitial fluid to plasma begins on the second to third day after the burn and accounts for the large reduction in parenteral fluids. An increase in the urinary output should alert the nurse to the edema mobilization taking place and the need to decrease fluid therapy.

Massachusetts General Hospital's Principles of Fluid Replacement

Various formulas based on fluid needs for the first 24 hours have been developed to serve as a guide to fluid therapy. Such estimates are helpful in reducing the danger of overhydration or underhydration that exists during the critical period.

TABLE 8.1
"Rule of Nines" for Estimating Burned Body Area in Adults

Part of Body	Percentage of Body
Head and neck	9
Anterior trunk	18
Each arm	9
Posterior trunk	18
Genitalia	1
Each leg	18

In the years following the fire in 1942 at the Coconut Grove (a Boston nightclub), the Massachusetts General Hospital made great strides in introducing theory and principles beneficial to burn therapy. Immediately after a burn, edema begins to develop in the involved area. The description of the nature of this fluid and protein loss into the interstitial compartment was accomplished to a great extent by Oliver Cope.

The Massachusetts General Hospital and the Shriners Institute, in general, follow the revised Parkland formula as a method for first estimation for fluid resuscitation of burn-injured patients. This formula generally is adequate for small-to-moderate injury in good-risk patients [3].

Revised Parkland formula [3] is as follows:

First 24 hours

Adults

2 ml/kg/% BSA deep partial/full-thickness burn

Children

3 ml/kg/% BSA deep partial/full-thickness burn

One-half of the first 24-hour total amount is infused in the first 8 hours. The fluid used is lactated Ringer's. It is not usually required in burns smaller than 15 percent in adults and 10 percent in children. Calculations of the percentage of total body surface burn are made by using the Lund-Browder estimation of BSA percent burned [6] for children and adults. Changes in the above estimation may be necessary depending upon the patient's clinical status (urinary output or hemodynamic parameters). If the patient's circulatory response to resuscitation is inadequate, colloid is frequently added in the first 24 hours. Extensive injury and significant injury in the young or elderly require colloid support with fresh frozen plasma in the first 24 hours; an attempt is made to keep the plasma albumin above 3 gm per 100 ml plasma [3].

After the first 24 hours colloid support depends upon the clinical indications, and fluid requirements are usually confined to normal maintenance fluids depending on plasma electrolytes, osmolality, and urine production.

Whole blood transfusions, if required, are usually administered after the fluid resuscitation and remobilization phase. A decreased red blood cell volume usually is not apparent until 48 hours after the burn, when the red cells damaged by the heat become increasingly more fragile and hemolyze. Slow administration of blood during the critical period may delay the urgent need for the more vitally needed fluid.

Many formulas are available for calculating the estimated fluid requirement during the first 24 hours postburn. Because it is believed that each patient should be treated on an individual basis, formulas give only a rough approximation of the amount of fluid that should be infused and are used only while the critical period exists. The Brooke formula is used frequently with lactated Ringer's injection replacing the nonelectrolyte fluid.

The Brooke Army Hospital formula [4] that follows is one of the most widely used.

First 24 hours

Normal fluid requirements

2,000 ml of nonelectrolyte solution (5% dextrose in water)

Replacement of burn loss

Colloid and electrolyte solution in ratio of 1 to 3 with amount of replacement fluid equaling 2 ml × kg body weight × percentage of body area burned

One-half of this total amount infused in first 8 hours and the rest in 16 remaining hours

Second 24 hours

Normal fluid requirements

2,000 ml of 5% dextrose in water

Replacement of burn loss

One-half the amount of colloid and electrolyte solution of the first 24 hours

The Evans formula is probably one of the best known. It is much the same as the Brooke formula with the exception that equal proportions of colloid and electrolyte solutions are used. This ratio was originally based on the belief that the fluid lost in edema contained 50 percent plasma.

DIABETIC ACIDOSIS

Diabetic acidosis is an endocrine disorder causing complex fluid and electrolyte disturbances. It occurs when a lack of insulin prevents the metabolism of glucose, and essential calories are provided instead by the catabolism of fat and protein. Acidosis results from the accumulation of acid by-products. Knowledge of the physiological changes in diabetic acidosis aids the nurse in early detection of imbalances and in an understanding of the treatment involved.

Physiological Changes

Lack of insulin prevents cellular metabolism of glucose and its conversion into glycogen. Glucose accumulates in the bloodstream *(hyperglycemia)*. When the blood sugar rises above 180 mg per 100 ml, glucose spills over into the urine *(glycosuria)*. The kidneys require 10 to 20 ml water to excrete 1 gm glucose; water excretion increases *(polyuria)*.

The body's fat and protein are utilized to provide necessary calories for energy. Ketone bodies, metabolic by-products, reduce plasma bicarbonate, and acidosis occurs.

Fluid and Electrolyte Disturbances

Dehydration

Dehydration results from excessive fluid and electrolyte losses. Cellular fluid deficit occurs when water is drawn from the cells by the hyperosmolality of the blood. Extracellular deficit occurs when (1) glycosuria increases the urinary output, (2) ketone bodies increase the load on the kidneys and the water to excrete them, (3) vomiting causes loss of fluid and electrolytes, (4) oral intake is reduced because of the patient's condition, and (5) hyperventilation is induced by the acidotic state.

Decreased Kidney Function

Dehydration lowers the blood volume, decreasing renal blood flow, and the kidneys produce less of the ammonia needed to maintain acid–base balance. Severe dehydration may lower the blood volume enough to cause circulatory shock and oliguria.

Ketosis

Ketosis is the excessive production of ketone bodies in the bloodstream. Ketone bodies are the end products of oxidation of fatty acids. Ketosis occurs when a lack of insulin results in (1) excessive fatty acids being converted by the liver to ketones, and (2) the decreased utilization of ketones by the peripheral tissues. Electrolytes and ketone bodies, retained in high serum concentration, increase the acidosis; the increase in the number of hydrogen ions, from the retention of ketone bodies, may drop the blood pH to 7.25 and lower. The bicarbonate anions decrease to compensate for the increase in ketone anions and may drop the bicarbonate level to 12 mEq per liter or less [7].

Electrolyte Changes

Cellular potassium deficit occurs when cells, unable to metabolize glucose, break down and release potassium into the serum. Normal or high serum potassium concentration may exist in spite of a body deficit (98 percent of the body's potassium is contained in the cells). Increase in the concentration of serum potassium is the result of the large amounts of potassium released from the cells plus the increased retention of potassium due to impaired kidney function. In severe diabetic acidosis, serious sodium and chloride deficits may occur when these electrolytes are lost through diuresis, vomiting, and gastric dilatation.

Signs and Symptoms of Diabetic Acidosis

The nurse should be familiar with the signs and symptoms that characterize diabetic acidosis. By recognizing impending diabetic acidosis, early treatment may be initiated and complications prevented.

1. *Hyperglycemia* occurs when a lack of insulin prevents glucose metabolism; glucose accumulates in the bloodstream.
2. *Glycosuria* occurs when the accumulation of glucose exceeds the renal tolerance and spills over into the urine.
3. *Polyuria.* Osmotic diuresis occurs when the heavy load of nonmetabolized glucose and the metabolic end products increase the osmolality of the blood, and the increased renal solute load requires more fluid for excretion.
4. *Thirst* is prompted by cellular dehydration due to the osmotic effect produced by hyperglycemia.

5. *Weakness* and *tiredness* come from the inability of the body to utilize glucose and from a potassium deficit.
6. *Flushed face* results from the acid condition.
7. *Rapid deep breathing* is the body's defense against acidosis; expiration of large amounts of carbon dioxide reduces carbonic acid and increases the pH of the blood.
8. *Acetone breath* results from an increased accumulation of acetone bodies.
9. *Nausea* and *vomiting* are caused by distention due to atony of gastric muscles.
10. *Weight loss* accompanies an excess loss of fluid (1 liter of body water equals 2.2 pounds, or 1 kg, body weight) and a lack of glucose metabolism.
11. *Low blood pressure* results from a severe fluid deficit.
12. *Oliguria* follows the decreased renal blood flow that results from a severe deficit in fluid volume.

Parenteral Therapy

Insulin is given to metabolize the excess glucose and combat diabetic acidosis. Since absorption is quickest by the bloodstream, insulin is administered intravenously. When given subcutaneously or intramuscularly, the slower rate of absorption of insulin may be further decreased by peripheral vascular collapse in the presence of shock. The dose of insulin, when administered by continuous infusion, is usually 4–8 units per hour [7]. There are many types of infusion pumps available to assure accurate and continuous administration of medications.

Parenteral fluids are administered to increase the blood volume and restore kidney function. Early treatment of the hypotonic patient usually consists of the administration of sodium chloride (0.9% NaCl) to replace sodium and chloride losses and to expand the blood volume. Later hypotonic fluids with sodium chloride may be employed. Bicarbonate replacement may be necessary when severe acidosis is present.

Potassium administration is contraindicated in the early treatment of diabetic acidosis. During the later stages (10–24 hours after treatment) the plasma potassium level falls; improved renal function increases potassium excretion and, in anabolic states, as the glucose is converted into glycogen, a sudden shift of potassium from extracellular fluid to intracellular fluid further lowers the plasma potassium level. If the patient is hydrated, potassium should be administered when the plasma potassium concentration falls.

A severe potassium deficit may occur if symptoms are not recognized and early treatment begun. Symptoms include weak grip, irregular pulse, weak picking at the bedclothes, shallow respiration, and abdominal distention.

REFERENCES

1. Adriani, J. Venipuncture. *Am. J. Nurs.*, 62:66, 1962.
2. Burgess, R. E. Fluid and electrolytes. *Am. J. Nurs.* 65:90, 1965.

3. Burke, J. F. Assessment and Initial Care of Burn Patients. Paper read at the American College of Surgeons, Committee on Trauma, Chicago, 1979.
4. Collentine, G. E., Jr. How to calculate fluids for burned patients. *Am. J. Nurs.* 62:77, 1962.
5. Elman, R. Fluid balance from the nurse's point of view. *Am. J. Nurs.*, 49:222, 1949.
6. Lund, C. C., and Browder, N. C. The estimation of areas of burns. *Surg. Gynecol. Obstet.* 79:352, 1944.
7. Metheny, N. M., and Snively, W. D., Jr. *Nurses' Handbook of Fluid Balance* Philadelphia: Lippincott, 4th ed. 1985, pp. 18, 19, 91, 147–154, 161, 185–192, 293–297.
8. Talbot, N. B., Sobel, E. H., McArthur, J. W., and Crawford, J. D. *Functional Endocrinology from Birth Through Adolescence.* Cambridge, Mass.: Harvard University Press, 1952.

BIBLIOGRAPHY

DelVecchio, A. Intravenous therapy considerations in the burn patient. *J. NITA* 2(4):117, 1979.

Goldfarb, W., Gaisford, J. C., and Slater, H. Concepts in catheter placement and nutritional support in burn victims. *J. NITA* 3(6):208, 1980.

REVIEW QUESTIONS

Parenteral Therapy

1. The three objectives of parenteral therapy are _____ , _____ , and _____ .
2. What does the amount of water needed for kidney function depend upon?
3. The normal fluid and electrolyte requirements based on _____ have been found to be more constant than when expressed in terms of body weight.
4. Balanced solutions are used for _____ .
5. How many milliliters of balanced solutions per square meter of body surface must be administered over a 24-hour period to provide the patient's water, sodium, and potassium requirements?
6. What are the three important functions of glucose?
7. What are the three important functions of protein?
8. Name the water-soluble vitamins not retained by the body.
9. What role does vitamin B complex play?
10. Why is vitamin C frequently given to the surgical patient?
11. Which electrolyte is considered potentially dangerous if administered when renal function is impaired?
12. Fluid loss may be estimated by determining loss of body weight. One liter of body water equals _____ of body weight.

Stress Related to Surgery

13. The adrenal medulla secretes the vasopressors _____ and _____ to help maintain the blood pressure.

Chapter 8 | Rationale of Fluid and Electrolyte Therapy

14. Two adrenal hormones, _____ and _____ , help maintain blood volume.
15. What type of fluids, if administered in excessive amounts at a time when antidiuresis is occurring, may cause hyponatremia, a serious fluid imbalance?
16. What do the following symptoms occurring during the early postoperative period suggest: confusion, delirium, hallucinations, weight gain, hyperventilation, muscular weakness, twitching, and convulsions?
17. The treatment to correct mild water excess consists of _____ .
18. What parenteral fluids, administered in the first few postoperative days, predispose the patient to hyponatremia?
19. What is the direct effect of a rapid administration of concentrated glucose, such as 20% and 50%?
20. What benefits to the postoperative patient may be derived from the administration of an alcohol solution?
21. When alcohol is infused with carbohydrates, the alcohol is metabolized in preference to glucose. What occurs with the infused glucose?
22. What role do B complex and C vitamins play in treating the surgical patient?

Burns

23. What fluid shift begins immediately following severe burns?
24. What causes the fluid losses that contribute to dehydration and hypovolemia?
25. What factors contribute to a decreased urinary output?
26. Why is a sodium deficit likely?
27. What causes metabolic acidosis in the severely burned patient?
28. Why is immediate fluid therapy essential when moderate or severe burns occur?
29. Why is it of utmost importance to avoid overzealous fluid therapy during the first 24 hours following the burn?
30. What fluid shift begins on the second to third day after the burn?
31. What should an increase in the urinary output occurring on the second or third day after the burn alert the nurse to?
32. Why is it important to use whole blood cautiously during the first 48 hours after the burn?

Diabetic Acidosis

33. What are the physiological changes that occur from a lack of insulin?
34. What causes deficits in the cellular fluid and extracellular fluid?
35. What is the reason for decreased kidney function?
36. Define the term *ketosis*.
37. What are the signs and symptoms of diabetic acidosis?

38. What solutions may be administered during the first 4–6 hours to restore kidney function and increase the blood volume?
39. Why is potassium contraindicated in the early treatment of diabetic acidosis?

CHAPTER 9

Parenteral Fluids and Related Fluid and Electrolyte Abnormalities

Ada Lawrence Plumer

PARENTERAL FLUIDS

A knowledge of parenteral fluids is essential if the patient is to be protected from the rapid and critical changes in fluid and electrolyte balance caused by infusions.

Until the 1930s, intravenous fluids consisted of dextrose and saline; little was known about electrolyte therapy. Today, with over 200 types of commercially prepared fluids available and with the great increase in their use, fluid and electrolyte disturbances are more common. Intravenous fluids are being taken for granted. It is assumed that the nurse who works daily with infusions is familiar with them; yet bottles of fluid are being hung daily by nurses who know little of the chemical composition and the physical effects of the infusions they administer. With the increase in fluids and in the knowledge concerning them, more rational intravenous therapy must be practiced.

Nurses have a legal and professional responsibility to know the normal amount and the desired and untoward effects of any intravenous infusion they administer. The type of fluid, the amount, and the rate of flow are arrived at only after the physician has carefully assessed the patient's clinical condition. Mudge [10] stated, "The physician must examine the details of management as carefully as in any other therapeutic regimen in clinical medicine." Nurses must follow the orders as carefully as they would in administering a medication, thereby ensuring that the patient receives only the quantity of fluid ordered at the rate of flow prescribed.

Definition of Intravenous Infusion

An infusion is usually regarded as an amount of fluid in excess of 100 ml designated for parenteral infusion, since the volume must be administered over a long period of time. However, when medications are administered by "piggyback" minibags (50–100 ml), a shorter period of time (usually 30 min–1 hour) may be required, whereas 150–200 ml volumes may require over an hour.

Intravenous fluids are mistakenly referred to as *intravenous solutions*. The term *solution* is defined in the U.S.P. (United States Pharmacopeia) [12] as "liquid preparations that contain one or more soluble chemical substances usually dissolved in water. They are distinguished from injection, for example, because they are not intended for administration by infusion or injection." They may vary widely in methods of preparation. The U.S.P. refers to parenteral fluids as injections, and methods of preparation must follow standards for injection.

Official Requirements of Intravenous Fluids

Intravenous injections must meet the tests, standards, and all specifications of the U.S.P. applicable to injections. This includes quantitative and qualitative assays of infusions, including tests for pyrogens and sterility.

Particulate Matter

Each container must be carefully examined to detect cracks and the fluid examined for cloudiness or presence of particles. The final responsibility falls on the pharmacist and the nurse who administers the fluid. Tests to detect the presence of particulate matter and standards for an acceptable limit of particles have been established by the U.S.P. "The large-volume injection for single-dose infusion meets the requirements of the test if it contains not more than 50 particles per ml that are equal to or larger than 10.0 µm and not more than 5 particles per ml that are equal to or larger than 25.0 µm in effective linear dimension" [11].

pH

The pH indicates hydrogen ion concentration or free acid activity in solution [8]. All intravenous fluids must meet the pH requirements set forth by the U.S.P. Most of these requirements call for a solution that is slightly acid, usually ranging in pH from 3.5 to 6.2.

Dextrose requires a slightly acid pH to yield a stable solution. Heat sterilization, used for all commercial solutions, contributes to the acidity. The pH is often adjusted by the manufacturer to even lower levels during processing to yield a more stable solution. A few intravenous fluids have a more physiological pH.

It is important to know the pH of the commonly used intravenous fluids since it may affect the stability of an added drug and cause the drug to deteriorate. The acidity of dextrose solutions has been criticized for its corrosive effect on veins (see Chapter 16).

Tonicity

Parenteral fluids are classified according to the tonicity of the fluid in relation to the normal blood plasma. The osmolality of blood plasma is 290 mOsm per liter. Fluid that approximates 290 mOsm per liter is considered isotonic. Intravenous fluids with an osmolality significantly higher than 290 mOsm (+50 mOsm) are considered hypertonic, while those with an osmolality significantly lower than 290 mOsm (−50 mOsm) are hypotonic [2]. Parenteral fluids range largely from approximately one-half isotonic (0.45% sodium chloride) to five to ten times isotonic (25–50% dextrose).

The tonicity of the fluid when infused into the circulation has a direct physical effect on the patient. It affects fluid and electrolyte metabolism and may result in disastrous clinical disturbances. Hypertonic fluids increase the osmotic pressure of the blood plasma, drawing fluid from the cells; excessive infusions of such fluid can cause cellular dehydration. Hypotonic fluids lower the osmotic pressure, causing fluid to invade the cells; when such fluid is infused beyond the patient's tolerance for water, water intoxication results. Isotonic fluids cause increased extracellular fluid volume, which can result in circulatory overload. By knowing the osmolality of the infusion and the physical effect it produces, the nurse is alerted to the potential fluid and electrolyte imbalances.

The choice of veins used for an infusion is affected by the tonicity of the fluid; hyperosmolar fluids must be infused through veins with a large blood volume in order to dilute the fluid and prevent trauma to the vessel.

The tonicity of the fluid affects the rate at which it can be infused; hypertonic dextrose infused rapidly may result in diuresis and dehydration.

Because of the direct and effective role osmolality plays in intravenous therapy, it is helpful for the nurse involved in the administration of intravenous fluids to be able to determine their osmolality. The osmotic pressure is proportional to the total number of particles in the fluid. The milliosmole is the unit that measures the particles or the osmotic pressure. By converting milliequivalents to milliosmoles, an approximate osmolality may be determined. A quick method for approximating the tonicity of intravenous injections follows [13].

Fluids Containing Univalent Electrolytes
Each milliequivalent is approximately equal to a milliosmole since univalent electrolytes, when ionized, carry one charge per particle. Normal saline injection (0.9% sodium chloride) contains 154 mEq of sodium and 154 mEq of chloride per liter, making a total of 308 mEq per liter, or approximately 308 mOsm per liter.

Fluids Containing Divalent Electrolytes
Since each particle carries two charges when ionized, the milliequivalents per liter or the number of electrical charges per liter when divided by the charge per ion (2) will give the approximate number of particles or milliosmoles per liter. As an example, when 20 mEq of magnesium sulfate is introduced into a liter of fluid, each particle ionized will carry 2 charges. By dividing 20 mEq or 20 charges by 2, an approximate 10 particles or 10 mOsm per liter is reached for each component, or 20 mOsm per liter total.

The osmolality of electrolytes in solution may be accurately computed, but involves the use of the atomic weight and the concentration of the given electrolytes in milligrams per liter. The methods for accurately computing the osmolality of an electrolyte in solution and a whole electrolyte in solution follow [11].

Osmolality of a Given Electrolyte in Solution

Formula: $\dfrac{\text{milligrams of electrolyte/liter}}{(\text{atomic weight})(\text{valence})} = $ milliosmoles/liter

Example: 39 mg K/liter

$$\dfrac{39}{39 \times 1} = 1 \text{ mOsm/liter}$$

Example: 40 mg Ca/liter

$$\dfrac{40}{40 \times 2} = \tfrac{1}{2}\text{mOsm/liter}$$

Osmolality of a Whole Electrolyte in Solution

The milliosmolar value of the whole electrolyte in solution is equal to the sum of the milliosmolar values of the separate ions. For example, determine the number of milliosmoles in 1 liter of a 0.9% sodium chloride (NaCl) solution.

Formula (atomic) weight of NaCl = 58.5 gm (58,500 mg)

1 millimole NaCl $\frac{1}{1,000}$ formula weight = 58.5 mg

Assuming complete dissociation,

1 millimole NaCl

= 2 mOsm of total particles *or*

each 58.5 mg of the whole electrolyte (NaCl)

= 2 mOsm of total particles.

To calculate the osmotic activity (expressed as milliosmoles) for 9,000 mg (0.9% NaCl), use the following proportion:

$$\dfrac{58.5 \text{ mg (weight of 1 mOsm of whole electrolytes)}}{9,000 \text{ mg (weight of whole electrolyte/liter)}}$$

$$= \dfrac{2 \text{ mOsm (number of particles from whole electrolyte)}}{X \text{ (mOsm)}}$$

X = 307.7 mOsm

DEXTROSE IN WATER FLUIDS

When glucose occurs as a part of parenteral injections it is usually referred to as *dextrose*, a designation by U.S.P. for glucose of requisite purity. Dextrose is available in concentrations of 2.5, 5, 10, 20, and 50% in water. In order to determine the osmolality or the caloric value of a dextrose solution, it is necessary to know the total number of grams or milligrams per liter. Because 1 ml water weighs 1 gm, and 1 ml is 1 percent of 100 ml, milliliters, grams, and percentages can be used interchangeably when calculating solution strength. Thus, 5% dextrose in water = 5 gm dextrose in 100 ml = 50 gm dextrose in 1 liter.

Calories	"It should be noted that hexoses (glucose or dextrose and fructose) do not yield 4 calories per gram as do dietary carbohydrates (e.g., starches) but only 3.75 calories per gram. Thus one liter of a 10% solution yields 375 calories. In addition, U.S.P. standards require the use of monohydrated glucose in glucose solutions, per se, so that only 91 percent is actually glucose, i.e., one liter of 10% glucose solution will yield $0.91 \times 375 = 340$ calories" [14].
Tonicity of 5% Dextrose in Water	Dextrose 5% in water is considered an isotonic solution because its tonicity approximates that of normal blood plasma, 290 mOsm per liter. Since dextrose is a nonelectrolyte and the total number of particles in solution does not depend upon ionization, the osmolality of dextrose solutions is determined differently from that of electrolyte solutions. One millimole (one formula weight in milligrams) of dextrose represents 1 mOsm (unit of osmotic pressure). One millimole of monohydrated glucose is 198 mg, and 1 liter of 5% dextrose in water contains 50,000 mg. Thus, $$\frac{50{,}000 \text{ mg}}{198 \text{ mg}} = 252 \text{ mOsm/liter.}$$
pH	The U.S.P. requirement for pH of dextrose solutions is 3.5–6.5. This broad pH range may at times contribute to an incompatibility in one bottle of dextrose and not in another when an additive is involved (see Chapter 20).
Metabolic Effect of Dextrose [7]	1. Provides calories for essential energy. 2. Since glucose is converted into glycogen by synthesis in the liver, it improves hepatic function. 3. Spares body protein (prevents unnecessary breakdown of protein tissue). 4. Prevents ketosis or excretion of organic acid which frequently occurs when fat is burned by the body without an adequate supply of glucose. 5. When deposited intracellularly in the liver as glycogen, dextrose causes a shift of potassium from the extracellular to the intracellular fluid compartment. This effect is used in the treatment of hyperkalemia by infusing dextrose and insulin.
Indications for Use	*Dehydration* Dextrose 2.5% in water and dextrose 5% in water provide immediate hydration to the dehydrated patient and are often used for hydrating the medical and surgical patient. Dextrose 5% in water is considered isotonic only in the bottle; once infused into the vascular system, the dextrose is rapidly metabolized, leaving the water. The water decreases the osmotic pressure of the blood plasma and invades the cells, providing immediately available water to dehydrated tissues.

Hypernatremia
If the patient is not in circulatory difficulty with extracellular expansion, 5% dextrose may be administered to decrease the concentration of sodium.

Vehicle for Administration of Drugs
Many of the drugs for intravenous use are added to infusions of 5% dextrose in water.

Nutrition
Concentrations of 20% and 50% dextrose in conjunction with electrolytes provide long-term nutrition. Insulin is frequently added to prevent overtaxing of the islet tissue of the pancreas.

Hyperkalemia
Infusions of dextrose in high concentration with insulin cause anabolism (buildup of body cells), which results in a shift of potassium from the extracellular to the intracellular compartment, thereby lowering the serum potassium concentration.

Undesirable Effects

Hypokalemia
Since the kidneys do not store potassium, prolonged fluid therapy with electrolyte-free fluids may result in hypokalemia. When cells are anabolized by the metabolism of glucose, a shift of potassium from extracellular to intracellular fluid may occur, resulting in hypokalemia.

Dehydration
Osmotic diuresis occurs when dextrose is infused at a rate faster than the patient's ability to metabolize it. A heavy load of nonmetabolized glucose increases the osmolality of the blood and acts as a diuretic; the increased solute load requires more fluid for excretion. A normal, healthy individual with a urinary specific gravity of 1.029 to 1.032 requires 15 ml water to excrete 1 gm solute, whereas individuals with poor kidney function or low concentrating ability of the kidneys require much more water to excrete the same amount of solute [9].

Hyperinsulinism
This condition may occur from a rapid infusion of hypertonic carbohydrate solutes. In response to a rise in blood sugar, extra insulin pours from the beta islet cells of the pancreas in its attempt to metabolize the infused carbohydrate. Termination of the infusion may leave excess insulin in the body, causing such symptoms as nervousness, sweating, and weakness due to the severe hypoglycemia that may be induced. Frequently, after infusion of hypertonic dextrose, a small amount of isotonic dextrose is administered to cover the excess insulin [9].

Water Intoxication
This imbalance results from an increase in the volume of the extracellular fluid from water alone. Prolonged infusions of isotonic or hypotonic dextrose in

water may cause water intoxication. This condition is compounded by stress, which leads to inappropriate release of antidiuretic hormone and fluid retention. The average adult can metabolize water at a rate of about 35–40 ml per kilogram per day, and the kidney can safely metabolize only about 2,500 to 3,000 ml per day in an average patient receiving intravenous therapy [6]. Under stress, the patient's ability to metabolize water is decreased.

Administration Isotonic dextrose may be administered through a peripheral vein. Hyperosmolar fluids such as 50% dextrose in water should be infused into the superior vena cava through a central venous catheter or a subclavian line. Hypertonic dextrose administered through a peripheral vein with small blood volume may traumatize the vein and cause thrombophlebitis; infiltration can result in necrosis of the tissues.

Sodium-free dextrose injections should not be administered by hyperdermoclysis. Dextrose solutions, by attracting body electrolytes in the pooled area of infusions, may cause peripheral circulatory collapse and anuria in sodium-depleted patients.

Electrolyte-free dextrose injections should not be used in conjunction with blood infusions. Dextrose mixed with blood causes hemolysis of the red cells.

The amount of water required for hydration depends upon the condition and the needs of the patient. The average adult patient requires 1,500–2,500 ml water per day. In patients with prolonged fever, the water requirement depends upon the degree of temperature elevation. The 24-hour fluid requirement for a temperature between 101 and 103°F increases by at least 500 ml while a prolonged temperature above 103°F increases by at least 1,000 ml [4].

The rate of administration depends upon the condition of the patient and the purpose of therapy. When the infusion is used to supply calories, the rate must be slow enough to allow complete metabolism of the glucose (0.5 gm per kilogram per hour in normal adults). When the infusion is used to produce diuresis, the rate must be fast enough to prevent complete metabolism of the dextrose, thereby increasing the osmolality of the extracellular fluid.

ISOTONIC SODIUM CHLORIDE INFUSIONS

Sodium Chloride Injection (0.9%), U.S.P. (normal saline), contains 308 mOsm per liter (Na, 154 mEq per liter; Cl, 154 mEq per liter), has a pH between 4.5 and 7.0, and is usually supplied in volumes of 1,000, 500, 250, and 100 ml. The term *normal* or *physiological* is misleading since the chloride in normal saline is 154 mEq per liter, compared to the normal plasma chloride value of 103 mEq per liter, while the sodium is 154 mEq per liter, or about 9 percent higher than the normal plasma value of 140 mEq per liter. Since the other electrolytes present in plasma are lacking in normal saline, the isotonicity of the solution depends upon the sodium and chloride ions, resulting in a higher concentration of these ions.

Indications for Use
1. Extracellular fluid replacement when chloride loss has been relatively greater than or equal to sodium loss.

2. Treatment of metabolic alkalosis in the presence of fluid loss; the increase in chloride ions provided by the infusion causes a compensatory decrease in the number of bicarbonate ions.
3. Sodium depletion. When there is an extracellular fluid volume deficit accompanying the sodium deficit, normal saline or an isotonic solution of sodium chloride is used to correct the deficit [9].
4. Initiation and termination of blood transfusions. When isotonic saline is used to precede a blood transfusion, the hemolysis of red cells, which occurs with dextrose in water, is avoided.

Dangers

Normal sodium chloride provides more sodium and chloride than the patient needs. Marked electrolyte imbalances have resulted from the almost exclusive use of normal saline. Untoward effects include the following.

Hypernatremia
An adult's dietary requirement for sodium is about 90–250 mEq per day, with a minimum requirement of 15 mEq and a maximum tolerance of 400 mEq [3]. When 3 liters of normal saline or 5% dextrose in normal saline is administered, the patient receives 462 mEq of sodium (154 mEq per liter $\times$ 3), a level that exceeds normal tolerance. Such an infusion at a time when sodium retention is occurring, as during stress, can result in hypernatremia.

There is an increased danger in the elderly, in patients with severe dehydration, and in patients with chronic glomerulonephritis; these patients require more water to excrete the salt than do patients with normal renal function. Isotonic saline does not provide water but requires most of its volume for the excretion of salt.

Acidosis
One liter of normal saline contains one-third more chloride than is present in the extracellular fluid; when infused in large quantities, the excess chloride ions cause a loss of bicarbonate ions and result in an acidifying effect.

Hypokalemia
Infusion of saline increases potassium excretion and at the same time expands the volume of extracellular fluid, further decreasing the concentration of the extracellular potassium ion.

Circulatory Overload
Continuous infusions of isotonic fluids expand the extracellular compartment and lead to circulatory overload.

Requirements

In an average adult, the daily requirements of sodium chloride are met by infusing a liter of 0.9% sodium chloride, but the dosage is dependent upon the patient's size, needs, and clinical condition.

ISOTONIC SALINE WITH DEXTROSE

Dextrose 5% in Normal Saline

Dextrose 5% in normal saline contains 252 mOsm of dextrose (Cl, 154 mEq per liter; Na, 154 mEq per liter), has a pH of 3.5–6.0, and is available in volumes of 1,000, 500, 250, and 150 ml.

When normal saline is infused, the addition of 100 gm dextrose prevents formation of ketone bodies and the increased demand for water the ketone bodies impose for renal excretion. The dextrose prevents catabolism and, consequently, loss of potassium and intracellular water.

Indications for Use

1. Temporary treatment of circulatory insufficiency and shock due to hypovolemia in the immediate absence of a plasma expander.
2. Early treatment along with plasma or albumin for replacement of loss due to burn.
3. Early treatment of acute adrenocortical insufficiency.

Dangers
The hazards are the same as those for normal saline (see preceding section).

Dextrose 10% in Normal Saline

Dextrose 10% in normal isotonic saline contains 504 mOsm per liter of dextrose (Na, 154 mEq per liter; Cl, 154 mEq per liter), has a pH of 3.5–6.0 and is usually supplied in volumes of 1,000 and 500 ml.

Indications for Use
This fluid is used as a nutrient and an electrolyte (Na and Cl) replenisher.

Dangers
Hypernatremia, acidosis, and circulatory overload may result when normal saline is administered in excess of the patient's tolerance.

Administration
Dextrose 10% in normal saline, because of its hypertonicity, must be administered intravenously, preferably through a vein of large diameter to dilute the fluid and reduce the risk of trauma to the vessel. Close observation and precautions are necessary to prevent infiltration and damage to the tissues.

HYPERTONIC SODIUM CHLORIDE INFUSIONS

These infusions include 3% sodium chloride (Na, 513 mEq per liter; Cl, 513 mEq per liter) and 5% sodium chloride (Na, 850 mEq per liter; Cl, 850 mEq per liter).

Indications for Use

Severe Dilutional Hyponatremia (Water Intoxication)
Hypertonic sodium chloride, upon infusion, increases the osmotic pressure of

the extracellular fluid, drawing water from the cells for excretion by the kidneys.

Severe Sodium Depletion
Infusions of hypertonic saline replenish sodium stores. An estimate of the sodium deficit can be made by taking the difference between the normal sodium concentration and the patient's current sodium concentration and multiplying it by 60 percent of the body weight in kilograms; sodium depletion is based on total body water and not on extracellular fluid [10].

Administration

Hypertonic saline infusions must be administered carefully and slowly to prevent pulmonary edema. Frequent reevaluation of the clinical and electrolyte picture during administration is advised. A 3% or 5% solution of sodium chloride is used to correct the deficit if the fluid volume is normal or excessive; the amount of sodium administered is dependent upon the sodium deficit in the plasma [9].

Hypertonic saline solutions should be infused slowly (such as 200 ml over a minimum of 4 hours) [9], and the patient should be observed constantly. The fluid must be infused by vein, with great care to prevent infiltration and trauma to the tissues.

HYPOTONIC SODIUM CHLORIDE IN WATER

One-half hypotonic saline (0.45% saline containing 77 mEq Na per liter and 77 mEq Cl per liter) is used as an electrolyte replenisher. When there is a question regarding the amount of saline required, hypotonic saline is preferred over isotonic saline. In general, 0.45% sodium chloride is preferable to normal saline.

HYDRATING FLUIDS

Since solutions consisting of dextrose with hypotonic saline provide more water than is required for excretion of salt, they are useful as hydrating fluids. These solutions include 2.5% dextrose in 0.45% saline (126 mOsm dextrose per liter, with 77 mEq Na per liter and 77 mEq Cl per liter), 5% dextrose in 0.45% saline (252 mOsm dextrose per liter, with 77 mEq Na per liter and 77 mEq Cl per liter), and 5% dextrose in 0.2% saline (252 mOsm dextrose per liter, with 34.2 mEq Na per liter and 34.2 mEq Cl per liter).

Indications for Use

1. Commonly called *initial hydrating solutions,* hypotonic saline dextrose infusions are used to assess the status of the kidneys before electrolyte replacement and maintenance are initiated.
2. Hydration of medical and surgical patients.
3. Promotion of diuresis in dehydrated patients.

Administration

To assess the status of the kidneys, the fluid is administered at the rate of 8 ml per square meter of body surface per minute (see the nomograms in Figure 8.1,

Chapter 9 | Parenteral Fluids and Related Abnormalities

pp. 86–87) for 45 minutes. The restoration of urinary flow shows that the kidneys have begun to function; the hydrating fluid may be replaced by more specifically needed electrolytes. If after 45 minutes the urinary flow is not restored, the rate of infusion is reduced to 2 ml per square meter of body surface per minute for another hour. If this does not produce diuresis, renal impairment is assumed [9].

Initial hydrating fluids must be used cautiously in edematous patients with cardiac, renal, or hepatic disease. Once good renal function is obtained, appropriate electrolytes should be administered to prevent hypokalemia.

HYPOTONIC MULTIPLE-ELECTROLYTE FLUIDS

Hypotonic multiple-electrolyte fluids (Table 9.1) are patterned after the type devised by Butler. Butler, with his co-workers at the Massachusetts General Hospital, was the first to emphasize the fact that basic water and electrolyte requirements are proportionate to the body surface area. Butler-type fluids are one-third to one-half as concentrated as plasma. They provide fluid to meet the patient's fluid volume requirement and in so doing provide cellular and extracellular electrolytes in quantities balanced between the minimal needs and the maximal tolerance of the patient. These fluids, because of their hypotonicity, provide water for urinary and metabolic needs and take advantage of the body's hemeostatic mechanisms to retain the electrolytes and reject those not needed, thus maintaining water and electrolyte balance [9].

Hypotonic fluids should contain 5% dextrose for its protein-sparing and antiketogenic effect [5]. The dextrose will increase the tonicity of the fluid "in the bottle," but once infused the dextrose will be metabolized, leaving the water and salt. Whether the patient has received too much or too little water depends upon the tonicity of the electrolyte and not the osmotic effect of dextrose.

A balanced solution of hypotonic electrolytes is ideal for routine maintenance. There are several modifications of the Butler-type fluids. Those containing 75 mEq of total cation per liter are used for older infants, children, and adults.

Administration

A useful formula for maintenance water requirements, based on studies by Crawford, Butler, and Talbot, is

Maintenance water = 1,600 ml./square meter of body surface area/day [5].

TABLE 9.1
Individual Electrolyte Composition of Hypotonic Multiple-Electrolyte Fluids (mEq/L)

Fluid	Manufacturer	Na	K	Ca	Mg^{2+}	Cl	Lactate	Acetate
Isolyte R	McGaw	40	16	5	3	40	12	12
Normosol-M	Abbott	40	13	0	3	40	0	16
Plasma-Lyte M	Travenol	40	16	5	3	40	12	12

In the case of obese or edematous patients this should be calculated on ideal weight rather than actual weight. The water requirement must be patterned after the condition of the patient. When infection, trauma involving the brain, or stress lead to inappropriate release of antidiuretic hormone, maintenance requirements are less. Excessive fluid losses through urine, stool, expired air, and so forth require increased water. The rate of infusion is usually 3 ml per square meter of body surface per minute.

Dangers

Hyperkalemia
When renal function is impaired, intravenous potassium should be used cautiously. The nurse should be alert to signs of hyperkalemia. If such signs develop, the physician should be notified and the fluid replaced by more appropriate electrolytes.

Water Intoxication
The patient's tolerance limits for water can be exceeded. Care should be exercised in maintaining the prescribed flow rate and in ensuring that the patient receives the prescribed volume of fluid. Water intoxication is more likely to occur when inappropriate release of antidiuretic hormone, in response to stress, causes water retention. These patients should be carefully watched to detect any early signs of an imbalance, so that a change in therapy can be initiated before the condition becomes precarious. Weighing the patient is the best way to monitor the status of water balance. Daily weights are extremely important in following the state of hydration in very ill patients.

ISOTONIC MULTIPLE-ELECTROLYTE FLUIDS

Many types of commercial replacement fluids are available; three such fluids are listed in Table 9.2. When severe vomiting, diarrhea, or diuresis result in a heavy loss of water and electrolytes, replacement therapy is necessary. Balanced fluids of isotonic electrolytes (Plasma-Lyte* and Isolyte E†) having an ionic composition similar to plasma are used.

Administration

Rapid initial replacement is seldom necessary. However, if impaired circulation and renal function of a severely dehydrated patient become evident and it is necessary to restore the patient's blood pressure quickly, 30 ml per kilogram of an isotonic fluid may be provided in the first hour or two [5]. Fluid overload must be prevented. Central venous pressure monitoring is especially helpful in the elderly patient and in patients with renal or cardiovascular disorders.

Extracellular replacement can generally be assumed to be complete after 48 hours of replacement therapy unless proved otherwise by clinical or laboratory evidence. To continue replacement fluids after deficits have been corrected may result in sodium excess leading to pulmonary edema or heart failure

---

*Travenol Laboratories, Deerfield, Ill.
†McGaw Laboratories, Irvine, Calif.

Chapter 9 | Parenteral Fluids and Related Abnormalities

TABLE 9.2
Individual Electrolyte Composition of Isotonic Multiple Electrolyte Fluids (mEq/L)

Fluid	Manufacturer	Na	K	Cl	HCO₃	Ca	Mg	NH₄	pH
Plasma-Lyte	Travenol	140	10	103	55	5	3	0	0
Isolyte E Electrolyte No. 3	McGaw Travenol	63	17	150	0	0	0	70	3.3–3.7
Lactated Ringer's injection (Hartmann's)		130	4	109	28	3	0	0	6.75

[5]. Patients receiving replacement therapy should be observed closely to detect any signs of circulatory overload.

Gastric replacement fluids, such as Electrolyte No. 3 by Travenol, provide the usual electrolytes lost by vomiting or gastric suction. They contain ammonium ions which are metabolized in the liver to hydrogen ions and urea, replacing the hydrogen ion lost in gastric juices. They are useful in metabolic alkalosis due to excessive ingestion of sodium bicarbonate. The usual adult dose is 500–2,000 ml and the infusion should not be faster than 500 ml per hour (check with physician).

Gastric replacement fluids are contraindicated in the presence of hepatic insufficiency or renal failure. They require the same precautions as any fluid containing potassium, and should be avoided in patients with renal damage or Addison's disease. Also, the low pH causes incompatibilities with many additives.

Lactated Ringer's injection is a popular fluid and is considered safe in certain conditions. Since the electrolyte concentration very closely resembles that of the extracellular fluid, it may be used to replace fluid loss from burns and fluid lost as bile and diarrhea. Lactated Ringer's injection has been useful in mild acidosis, the lactate ion being metabolized in the liver to bicarbonate.

Dangers Three liters contains about 390 mEq of sodium, which can quickly elevate the sodium level in a patient who is not deficient [3]. Lactated Ringer's injection is contraindicated in severe metabolic acidosis or alkalosis and in liver disease or anoxic states which influence lactate metabolism.

ALKALIZING FLUIDS

When anesthesia or disorders such as dehydration, shock, liver disease, starvation, and diabetes cause retention of chlorides, ketone bodies, or organic salts, or when excessive bicarbonate is lost, metabolic acidosis occurs. Treatment consists of infusion with an appropriate alkalizing fluid. These fluids include one-sixth molar isotonic sodium lactate (1.9%, with 167 mEq Na per liter, 167 mEq lactate ions per liter, and a pH of 6.0 to 7.3), one-sixth molar Sodium Bicarbonate Injection, U.S.P. (1.5%, with 178 mEq Na per liter, 178 mEq bicarbonate per liter, and a pH of 7.0–8.0), and hypertonic sodium bicarbonate injection (7.5% or 5%).

One-Sixth Molar Sodium Lactate

The lactate ion must be oxidized in the body to carbon dioxide before it can effect acid–base balance; the complete conversion of sodium lactate to bicarbonate requires about 1–2 hours [1]. Since oxidation is necessary to increase the bicarbonate concentration, sodium lactate is not used for patients suffering from oxygen lack, as in shock or congenital heart disease with persistent cyanosis. It is also contraindicated in liver disease as the lactate ions are improperly metabolized.

One-sixth molar sodium lactate is used when acidosis results from a sodium deficiency in such disorders as vomiting, starvation, uncontrolled diabetes mellitus, acute infections, and renal failure [1].

The usual dose is 1 liter of a one-sixth molar solution, but the dosage depends upon the patient's condition and the serum sodium level. One-sixth molar infusion may be administered by venoclysis or hyperdermoclysis and usually at a rate not greater than 300 ml per hour [1]. The patient should be observed closely for any evidence of alkalosis.

Sodium Bicarbonate

Sodium Bicarbonate Injection, U.S.P. (1.5%, with 178 mEq per liter Na, 178 mEq per liter bicarbonate), is an isotonic solution that provides bicarbonate ions in conditions in which excess depletion has occurred. It is used for severe hyperpnea early in the treatment of severe acidosis until the signs of dyspnea and hyperpnea are relieved. The bicarbonate ion is released in the form of carbon dioxide through the lungs, leaving an excess of sodium cation behind to exert its electrolyte effect [1].

The usual dose is 500 ml in a 1.5% solution. The dosage is dependent upon the patient's weight, condition, and carbon dioxide content. If the isotonic infusion is not available it may be made by adding two 50-ml ampules containing 3.75 gm each of sodium bicarbonate to 400 ml hypotonic saline. The fluid should be infused slowly intravenously. Rapid injection may induce cellular acidity and death. The patient should be watched for signs of hypocalcemic tetany, and calcium supplement should be administered if required; calcium does not ionize well in an alkaline medium.

ACIDIFYING INFUSIONS

Normal saline (0.9% sodium chloride injection, U.S.P.) is not usually listed among the acidifying infusions. However, since metabolic alkalosis is a condition associated with excess bicarbonate and loss of chloride, isotonic saline provides conservative treatment. When the chloride ions are infused, the bicarbonate decreases in compensation and the alkalosis is relieved.

Ammonium chloride, the usual acidifying agent, is available as isotonic 0.9% ammonium chloride injection (167 mEq NH_4 per liter and 167 mEq Cl per liter) and hypertonic 2.14% ammonium chloride injection (400 mEq NH_4 per liter and 400 mEq Cl per liter). The pH range is 4.0–6.0. Both concentrations are supplied in 1-liter bottles.

Chapter 9 | Parenteral Fluids and Related Abnormalities

Indications for Use Ammonium chloride is used as an acidifying infusion in severe metabolic alkalosis due to loss of gastric secretions, pyloric stenosis, or other causes. The ammonium ion is converted by the liver to hydrogen ion and to ammonia, which is excreted as urea.

Administration The 2.14% ammonium chloride is usually used in the treatment of the adult patient; 0.9% ammonium chloride is used for children [9].

The dosage depends upon the condition of the patient and upon an accurate chemical picture, including plasma carbon dioxide-combining power. Ammonium chloride must be infused at a very slow rate to enable the liver to metabolize the ammonium ion. Rapid injection can result in toxic effects causing irregular breathing, bradycardia, and twitching [1].

Precautions Since its acidifying effect depends upon the liver for conversion, ammonium chloride must not be administered to patients with severe hepatic disease or renal failure. It is contraindicated in any condition with a high ammonium level.

EVALUATION OF WATER AND ELECTROLYTE BALANCE

A rational approach is necessary if the patient is to receive safe and successful intravenous therapy. In the past, emphasis was placed on the technical responsibility of the nurse in maintaining the infusion and in keeping the needle patent. With the increase in the use of intravenous therapy, clinical disturbances in fluid and electrolyte metabolism are more common. Changes can occur quickly and in the absence of the physician. Today the nurse's responsibility consists of monitoring the fluid and electrolyte status of the patient as well as the progress of the infusion. Greater emphasis must be placed on the causes and effects of fluid and electrolyte abnormalities so that these imbalances may be anticipated and recognized before they become disastrous. The nurse should be familiar with the parameters used in evaluating fluid and electrolyte imbalances and in supplying fluid and electrolyte requirements.

Central Venous Pressure Monitoring of the central venous pressure provides a simple, accurate, and valuable guide in detecting changes in blood volume and in assessing fluid requirements. It is particularly valuable in assessing the ability of the heart to tolerate the infusion. The importance of a properly functioning central venous pressure line must be stressed; many erroneous conclusions are drawn from false values recorded when the line is not properly responsive to right atrial pressures.

A normal venous pressure indicates an adequate circulatory blood volume.

An elevated venous pressure may mean an increase in circulatory volume and right heart pressure, with the possibility of circulatory overload. It may also indicate other problems such as a pulmonary embolus, myocardial infarction, or lack of digitalis. Determination of the hematocrit value will supplement clinical information [6].

A low venous pressure, too low to measure, indicates that the patient has probably lost fluid or blood. One must not overlook the fact that fluid loss can result from the improper administration of intravenous fluids. If rapid infusion of dextrose exceeds the patient's tolerance, massive diuresis with dehydration and diminished circulatory volume may occur. The decreased venous blood return into the right atrium is reflected by a decrease in the central venous pressure.

Pulse

The quality and the rate of the pulse provide clinical information valuable in assessing fluid and electrolyte changes in the patient. A high pulse pressure, bounding and not easily obliterated by pressure, indicates a high cardiac output caused by circulatory overload. A regular pulse, easily obliterated by pressure, indicates low cardiac output resulting from a lowered blood volume. A bounding, easily obliterated pressure signifies a drop in blood pressure with a wide pulse pressure, indicative of impending circulatory collapse. As the patient's condition deteriorates the pulse will become rapid, weak, thready, and easily obliterated, signifying circulatory collapse.

Peripheral Veins

Examination of the peripheral veins provides a means of evaluating the plasma volume. The peripheral veins will usually empty in 3–5 seconds when the hand is elevated and will fill in the same length of time when the hand is lowered to a dependent position. Peripheral vein filling takes longer than 3–5 seconds in patients with sodium depletion and extracellular dehydration [9]. Slow emptying of the peripheral veins indicates overhydration and an excessive blood volume, while slow filling indicates a low blood volume and often precedes hypotension. Peripheral veins which become engorged and clearly visible indicate an increase in the plasma volume secondary to an interstitial-to-vascular fluid shift or an increase in extracellular fluid volume [9].

Weight

A sudden gain or loss in weight is a significant sign of a change in the fluid volume. A change in the volume of body fluid can be computed by weighing the patient daily at the same time of day, on the same scales, with the same amount of clothing. A loss or gain of 1 kilogram body weight reflects a loss or gain of 1 liter body fluid. A weight loss of up to 5 percent in a child or an adult indicates a moderate fluid volume deficit, and a weight loss of over 5 percent indicates a serious fluid volume deficit [9].

Weisburg [15] stated:

> The weight in pounds can be converted to kilograms by a simple mental calculation. Divide pounds by 2; 10 percent of this quotient is subtracted from the quotient to obtain the weight in kilograms. For example, a 180 pound patient weighs 81 kg; 180 divided by 2 equals 90, and 10 percent of 90 is 9, which is subtracted from the 90 to give 81 kg.

Thirst

Thirst is an important and valuable symptom denoting a deficit in body fluid or, more specifically, cellular dehydration. This type of dehydration occurs when the extracellular fluid becomes hypertonic, either as a result of water deprivation or the infusion of hypertonic saline. The increase in osmotic pres-

Chapter 9 | Parenteral Fluids and Related Abnormalities

sure causes fluid to be drawn from the cells, resulting in cellular dehydration, the stimulus to thirst.

Normally thirst governs the need for water, but in certain conditions the lack of thirst may accompany dehydration. This is especially true in the aged, in whom thirst is not urgent. These patients may lose their thirst and as a result become severely dehydrated before the condition is recognized.

In the severely burned patient, the great thirst experienced may lead to ingestion of excess water and to a serious sodium deficit.

Intake and Output   Water intake and output should be carefully measured and recorded. Hourly urine output measurements may be particularly important. A urine output of 200 ml per hour indicates that too much water is being infused too rapidly. Dudrick [6] stated, "By regulating the urine output between 30 and 50 ml./hr. the patient receives at least enough fluid for his kidneys to work efficiently."

A decreased urinary output accompanies a decreased blood volume; changes in the arterial pressure and pressure in the glomeruli result in the oliguria or anuria of profound shock. The increase in urinary output accompanying an increase in blood volume is primarily due to changes in arterial pressure and pressure in the glomeruli [9].

Skin   Observing changes in skin turgor (elasticity) and texture is helpful in assessing the state of water balance. To test skin turgor, pinch the skin over the sternum or forehead in the adult and/or the medial aspects of the thigh in the child, and then release it; in the normal individual, the pinched skin will return to its original position. Skin that remains in a raised position for several seconds indicates a deficit in fluid volume.

A dry, leathery tongue may indicate a fluid volume deficit or mouth breathing. To differentiate between the two, the mucous membrane may be checked for moisture by running the finger between the gums and the cheek; dryness indicates a fluid volume deficit.

Edema   Edema reflects an increase in the extracellular fluid volume outside the circulating intravascular compartment. It depends upon an imbalance or a disturbance in (1) the exchange of water and electrolytes between the patient and the environment or (2) the exchange of water and electrolytes between the compartments of the body. The fluid and electrolyte exchange between the body compartments may be affected by an alteration in (1) the circulatory system, (2) the lymphatic system, or (3) the concentration of albumin in the serum; water and electrolytes escape from the circulation faster than they enter, and edema ensues. Edema may be (1) generalized, as in congestive failure, (2) localized, as with ascites, or (3) peripheral.

By detecting edema early, a clinical imbalance may be corrected before the patient's condition deteriorates. Early peripheral edema may be detected by finger printing, a procedure in which the finger is rolled over the bony prominence of the sternum or tibia. As edema increases, pitting edema will occur and may be detected by pressure of the fingers on the subcutaneous tissue.

In generalized edema, such as that seen in cardiac failure, there is an increase in total extracellular water volume as well as interstitial edema. Symptoms such as venous engorgement, restlessness, dyspnea, cyanosis, and pulmonary rales indicate generalized edema.

Laboratory Values

Laboratory values, when used to supplement clinical observations, aid in forming diagnostic and therapeutic guidelines.

Electrolyte studies (serum sodium, potassium, chloride, bicarbonate, and pH) performed daily are important in assessing the fluid and electrolyte status of the patient receiving intravenous fluids. In patients with massive electrolyte losses such studies may be required two or three times a day.

Blood cell count and hematocrit determinations are helpful in detecting hemoconcentration or hemodilution; hemoconcentration reflects a diminished plasma volume due to dehydration, and hemodilution, an increased volume from overtreatment with water.

Measurement of *serum protein with the albumin–globulin ratio* helps in detecting a change in fluid volume; large quantities of parenteral fluid rapidly administered dilute and decrease the serum protein concentration. This determination is helpful when used to supplement clinical observation — otherwise it may be misleading and interpreted as showing actual depletion. A decrease in serum protein reduces the osmotic pressure of the extracellular compartment, causing some edema and loss of plasma volume.

Blood urea nitrogen should be measured frequently to evaluate kidney function, an important parameter in treating fluid and electrolyte imbalances.

CLINICAL DISTURBANCES OF WATER AND ELECTROLYTE METABOLISM

Most of the common clinical disturbances in water and electrolyte balance result from changes in the volume of total body water or in one or more of the fluid compartments of the body. Clinical disturbances in water and electrolyte metabolism have been classified into six types: isotonic, hypertonic, and hypotonic expansion and isotonic, hypertonic, and hypotonic contraction. These are discussed in the following pages and are summarized in Tables 9.3 and 9.4.

Isotonic Expansion

Isotonic expansion (circulatory overload) occurs when fluids of the same tonicity as plasma are infused into the vascular circulation. Because solutions isotonic to plasma do not affect the osmolality, there is no flow of water from the extracellular compartment to the intracellular compartment. The extracellular compartment expands in proportion to the fluid infused and is the only compartment affected. The increase in the volume of fluid dilutes the concentration of hemoglobin and lowers the hematocrit and total protein levels, but the serum sodium level remains the same.

Isotonic expansion is a critical complication of intravenous therapy. Patients who receive isotonic fluids around the clock are prime targets and should be observed closely for early signs of circulatory overload. Normal saline or solutions containing balanced isotonic multiple electrolytes are used for preexisting or continuing fluid and electrolyte losses and are not the ideal fluids for maintenance therapy. The electrolyte isotonicity of these solutions causes expansion of the extracellular compartment and does not provide the extra water

TABLE 9.3
Comparison of Three Types of Dehydration

	Isotonic	Hypertonic	Hypotonic
Cause	Loss of blood or isotonic fluid	Excess loss of water or insufficient intake	Loss of salt
Effect on fluid compartments	ECF volume ↓	ICF and ECF volume ↓	ICF volume ↑ ECF volume ↓
Clinical signs			
Weight	↓	↓	↓
Rate of H_2O excretion	↓	↓	↑
Rate of Na excretion	↓	↓	↓
Thirst	—	Early sign, due to cellular dehydration	—
Pulse rate	Regular, easily obliterated by pressure	Regular and normal in early stages	Increased, weak and thready, easily obliterated by pressure
Hand vein filling time (normal = 3–5 sec)	May ↑	May be normal	Normal to ↑
Behavior	—	Irritability, restlessness, possibly confusion	Possibly vomiting and cramps
Signs in late stages	Developing shock with pulse weak and thready	Skin turgor diminished; dry, furrowed tongue; death, possibly due to rise of osmotic pressure	Skin turgor may be diminished; thready pulse; possibly confusion and apathy; death from peripheral circulatory failure
Laboratory values			
Hematocrit	↑	↑	↑
Hemoglobin	↑	↑	↑
Total protein and albumin-globulin ratio	↑	↑	↑
Sodium concentration	—	↑	↓

that balanced hypotonic solutions provide for the kidney to retain or secrete as needed [3].

The early postoperative or posttrauma patient is susceptible to this critical complication. The increased endocrine response to stress during the first 2–5 days following surgery results in retention of sodium chloride and water

TABLE 9.4
Comparison of Three Types of Fluid Expansion

	Isotonic	Hypertonic	Hypotonic
Cause	Infusion of excess quantities of isotonic fluids	Infusion of excess quantities of hypertonic saline	Increased intake or infusion of water in excess of patient's tolerance
Effects on fluid compartments	ECF volume ↑	ECF volume ↑ ICF volume ↓	ECF and ICF volume ↑
Clinical signs			
Weight	↑	↑ depending on amount infused	↑
Rate of H_2O excretion	↑	↓	↑
Rate of Na excretion	↑	↑	↑
Thirst	—	Present	—
Pulse rate	Bounding, not easily obliterated by pressure	Full, bounding (significant)	May be regular and not easily obliterated by pressure
Hand vein emptying time (normal = 3–5 sec)	↑	↑	↑
Edema	May be present	Early, tibial edema; later, pitting edema; diminished skin turgor	Tibial edema with finger printing
Signs of intracranial pressure	—	—	Irritability, headache, confusion
Signs in late stages	Hoarseness, pulmonary edema, cyanosis, coughing, dyspnea	Water rales, pulmonary edema	Pulmonary edema
Other signs	—	Hoarseness (a frequent early sign)	Cramping of exercised muscles
Laboratory values			
Hematocrit	↓	↓	↓
Hemoglobin	↓	↓	↓
Total protein and albumin-globulin ratio	↓	↓	↓
Sodium concentration	—	↑	↓

[9]. When a patient under stress is receiving isotonic infusions, the nurse must anticipate and watch for signs of circulatory overload.

Elderly patients receiving isotonic fluids must be carefully monitored as they have a lower tolerance to fluids and electrolytes. Because they are also likely to have some degree of cardiac and renal impairment, the ability of the kidneys to eliminate fluid is likely to be diminished. The status of these patients can change quickly.

In the patient who has had a craniotomy, large-volume isotonic infusions can increase the intracranial pressure and prove detrimental.

Patients who are potential candidates for isotonic expansion must be watched carefully and turned frequently to prevent fluid from settling in the lungs. Pulmonary edema can result from the cardiac and pulmonary side-effects of intravenous therapy. Dudrick [6] stated, "The apices of the lungs which are high will tend to be fairly dry, but the bases of their lungs, posteriorly and inferiorly, can be fairly wet." As a result, hypostatic pneumonia secondary to gravity may develop.

Manifestations

The nurse who monitors intravenous infusions must be familiar with the early clinical manifestations that accompany isotonic expansion in order to recognize and prevent its development; mild pulmonary edema progressing to severe pulmonary edema is a late stage that must be prevented. Early clinical manifestations consist of: (1) weight gain; (2) increase in fluid intake over output; (3) a high pulse pressure, bounding and not easily obliterated, showing signs of high cardiac output; (4) increase in central venous pressure; (5) peripheral hand vein emptying time longer than normal 3–5 seconds when the hand is elevated from a dependent position; (6) peripheral edema, depending on the extent of fluid expansion; and (7) hoarseness. If intravenous therapy is allowed to continue, isotonic expansion becomes more apparent and dangerous, with easily recognized signs: cyanosis, dyspnea, coughing, and neck vein engorgement.

Laboratory characteristics include a drop in the hematocrit value and reduced concentrations of hemoglobin and of total protein.

Treatment

Treatment for circulatory overload when detected early is relatively simple and consists of withholding all fluids until excess water and electrolytes have been eliminated by the body. After the condition is rectified, hypotonic maintenance fluids will provide the patient with fluid and a minimum daily requirement of electrolytes. The hypotonicity of the fluid allows the kidneys to maintain the needed amount and selectively retain or excrete the excess.

Isotonic Contraction

Isotonic contraction occurs when there is loss of fluid and electrolytes isotonic to the extracellular fluid, such as whole blood or large volumes of fluid from diarrhea or vomiting. The extracellular compartment contracts. Since the fluid lost is isotonic, the osmolality of the extracellular compartment remains unchanged and there is no movement of water between the compartments; only the extracellular volume is affected.

Manifestations

Because of the loss of fluid, the hematocrit level and the concentration of hemoglobin and total protein are increased. There is no change in the serum sodium concentration.

Clinical manifestations are: (1) weight loss; (2) negative fluid balance (a decrease in urinary output but a greater output than total fluid intake); (3) pulse that is regular in rate, easily obliterated by pressure, and as the patient's condition deteriorates the pulse becomes weak and thready; and (4) possible increase in peripheral hand filling time above the normal 3–5 seconds when the hand is moved from an elevated to a dependent position.

Treatment

Treatment consists of replacing the fluid loss with isotonic solutions containing balanced electrolytes (see Table 9.2).

Hypertonic Expansion

Hypertonic expansion occurs when the volume of body water is increased by the intravenous infusion of hypertonic saline. Sodium chloride 3% or 5% is used to replace a massive sodium loss or to remove excess accumulation of body fluids, but if it is rapidly infused hypertonic expansion can result. The saline increases the osmotic pressure of the extracellular compartment, causing water to be drawn from the intracellular compartment until both compartments are isosmotic. There is an increase in the volume of the extracellular compartment and a decrease in the volume of the cellular compartment. The osmolality of the extracellular fluid is higher than before the infusion but lower than the high level after the infusion because of the increased extracellular fluid volume [10].

Caution must be used in the intravenous administration of hypertonic saline. Circulatory overload with hypernatremia can occur. The nurse must understand the reason for the infusion, the condition of the patient, the proper rate of administration, and the signs and symptoms of hypertonic expansion.

Manifestations

Clinical manifestations include a gain in body weight dependent upon the volume infused. A small volume (500 ml) will not contribute to a significant weight gain [13]. An increased sodium load results in a decreased rate of water excretion; however, the abrupt increase in plasma volume may cause an increase in the rate of water excretion as the body attempts to excrete the excess salt and water. The degree of thirst will be dependent upon the hypertonicity of the plasma and consequently the amount of cellular dehydration. Peripheral hand vein emptying time may be increased beyond the normal 5 seconds when the hand is elevated, but is dependent upon the degree of expansion of the extracellular compartment. A bounding pulse is significant in detecting hypertonic expansion. The serum sodium concentration is increased. The hematocrit level and the concentration of hemoglobin and total serum protein are decreased as a result of the expanded fluid volume in the extracellular compartment.

Treatment
Treatment consists of stopping the infusion to allow the kidneys to eliminate the overload of salt and water. If there are no cardiovascular side-effects, 5% dextrose in water may be infused slowly to reduce the tonicity of the extracellular fluid and replace body water.

Hypertonic Contraction

Hypertonic contraction (hypertonic or cellular dehydration) occurs when there is a loss of water without a corresponding loss of salt. This condition occurs in patients who are unable to take sufficient fluid for a prolonged period of time or in patients with excess insensible water loss through the lungs and skin.

In the elderly, hypertonic dehydration is a common clinical disturbance; there is frequently a decrease in the thirst stimuli in response to hypertonicity of body fluids, and adequate intake of fluid is not met. In the unconscious or incontinent, frequency and excess urination may go undetected or may be recognized as a sign of good renal function. A loss of tubular ability to concentrate urine in the aged will result in a large urinary volume when an increased solute load is presented to the patient [9]. Elderly patients also have a diminished response to ADH. Large amounts of dilute urine may be lost, resulting in hypertonic dehydration.

To prevent fluid imbalance, the nurse must recognize that individuals differ widely in the water they require; patients whose kidneys do not concentrate well require more water than those whose kidneys concentrate well. The daily fluid requirement must be met.

In hypertonic contraction, the loss of water from the extracellular compartment results in an increase in the osmolality, causing water to flow from the cells to the extracellular compartment. Cellular dehydration occurs as water leaves the cellular compartment to replace the plasma volume. Both compartments, the intracellular and the extracellular, are affected by the water loss; there is a decrease in volume and an increase in osmolality in both compartments. In contrast, in isotonic contraction only the extracellular compartment is affected and the contraction is more serious.

Because signs of hypertonic contraction are not obvious in the early stages, the nurse must anticipate such an imbalance and be alert to any changes.

Manifestations
Clinically, thirst is an early and reliable sign of hypertonic contraction but may be absent in the elderly, complicating early recognition of this imbalance. Weight loss occurs. Negative fluid balance (output greater than intake) is present. Hourly output measurements show a decrease in the rate of excretion of water. The pulse has a normal quality and is regular in the early stages of hypertonic contraction. The hand vein filling time may be within the normal limits; cellular fluid has partly replenished the plasma. Irritability, restlessness, and possibly confusion may be present. Skin turgor diminishes and is a sign of dehydration in the later stages. A dry mouth with a furrowed tongue indicates dehydration.

Laboratory studies show an increase in serum sodium concentration, hematocrit level, hemoglobin concentration, and total serum protein concentration.

Treatment
Treatment consists of hydrating the patient by administering a balanced hypotonic solution such as the Butler-type solutions; 2,400 ml per square meter of body surface per day for moderate preexisting deficit and 3,000 ml per square meter of body surface per day for severe preexisting deficit [9]. The usual rate for intravenous administration is 3 ml per square meter of body surface area. A therapeutic test for functional renal depression may be necessary before infusing water and electrolytes for maintenance.

Hypotonic Expansion

Hypotonic expansion (water intoxication, dilutional hyponatremia) occurs when the increase in the volume of body fluids is due to water alone. Water expands the extracellular compartment, causing a decrease in the concentration. Water then diffuses into the cells until both compartments are isosmotic. Both the extracellular and the intracellular compartments are affected; the volume is increased and the concentration is decreased. The serum sodium concentration and the hematocrit, hemoglobin, and total serum protein levels are reduced.

Hypotonic expansion occurs in patients who are receiving large quantities of electrolyte-free water to replace excessive fluid and electrolytes lost from gastric suction, vomiting, diarrhea, or diuresis, or insensibly through the skin.

Patients receiving continuous infusion of 5% dextrose in water are particularly susceptible to water intoxication. This solution contains 252 mOsm dextrose per liter, making it an isotonic solution in the bottle. Once introduced into the circulation, the dextrose is quickly metabolized, leaving the water free to dilute and expand the extracellular compartment. With the decreased osmolality of the extracellular fluid, water diffuses into the cells and hypotonic expansion occurs.

The patient's tolerance to water can be exceeded by infusion of excess amounts of hypotonic fluids. The kidneys of the normal adult can metabolize water in amounts of 35–45 ml per kilogram per day, but the kidneys of the average patient can metabolize only 2,500–3,000 ml per day; above these volumes abnormal accumulation of water occurs [6].

Hypotonic expansion is more likely to occur during the early postoperative period, when retention of water is being affected by the response to stress. It is particularly likely in the elderly patient, in whom the response to stress is compounded by impairment in renal function. Small amounts of adjusted hypotonic saline (sodium 90 mEq, chloride 60 mEq, and lactate 30 mEq per liter) have a real place in the early postoperative management of the aged.

Manifestations
When acute onset of behavioral changes, such as confusion, apathy, and disorientation, occurs in the elderly patient postoperatively, overhydration should be suspected. Central nervous system disturbances such as weakness, muscle twitching, and convulsions are seen, as are headaches, nausea, and vomiting.

There is an increase in fluid intake over fluid output. Weight gain is always present. Blood pressure usually is normal but may be elevated. Peripheral hand veins are usually full, and hand emptying time is increased beyond the normal 5 seconds when the hand is elevated from a dependent position. The pulse may be regular and not easily obliterated when pressure is applied.

Treatment

Treatment consists of withholding all fluids until the excess water is excreted. In severe hyponatremia it may be necessary to administer small quantities of hypertonic saline to increase the osmotic pressure and the flow of water from the cells to the extracellular compartment for excretion by the kidneys. Hypertonic saline must be used cautiously and must not be administered to patients with congestive heart failure.

Hypotonic Contraction

Hypotonic contraction (hypotonic dehydration) occurs when fluids containing relatively more salt than water are lost from the body. This loss results in a decrease in the effective osmolality of the extracellular compartment. Water is drawn into the cells until osmotic equilibrium is established. Owing to the invasion of water the intracellular compartment is expanded and the extracellular compartment is contracted.

This imbalance may result from the loss of salt from any one of several sources: urine of patients receiving diuretics, fistula drainage, severe burns, vomitus, and sweat. The elderly are affected by the loss of small quantities of sodium.

Manifestations

Clinical manifestations include (1) weight loss; (2) negative fluid balance; (3) pulse rate increased, weak or thready, and easily obliterated; (4) increased hand filling time; and (5) decreased skin turgor.

Laboratory studies show a decrease in serum sodium concentration and an increase in hematocrit, hemoglobin, and total serum protein levels.

Treatment

Treatment of hypotonic contraction consists of replacing the fluids and electrolytes that have been lost. Because other electrolytes are usually lost along with the sodium loss, a balanced electrolyte solution may be administered.

REFERENCES

1. American Society of Hospital Pharmacists. *Am. Hosp. Form. Serv.* Washington, D.C., 1980, pp. 40:04, 40:08.
2. Burgess, R. E. Fluid and electrolytes. *Am. J. Nurs.* 65:90, 1965.
3. Burns, W. Indications for I.V. therapy (Proceedings of Clinical Seminar, San Francisco, 1968). In *Health Care World Wide*. North Chicago, Ill.:Abbott Laboratories, 1972, pp. 7, 8, 12.
4. Condon, R., and Nyhus, L. (Eds.). *Manual of Surgical Therapeutics* (3rd ed.) Boston: Little, Brown, 1975, p. 203.
5. Drug and Therapeutic Information, Inc. Parenteral water and electrolyte solutions. *Med. Lett.* 12(19):77, 1970.
6. Dudrick, S. J. Rational I.V. therapy. *Am. J. Hosp. Pharm.* 28:83–85, 1971.

7. Elman, R. Fluid balance from the nurse's point of view. *Am. Nurs.* 49:223, 1949.
8. Lebowitz, M. H., MaSuda, J. V., and Beckerman, J. H. The pH and acidity of intravenous infusion solutions. *J.A.M.A.* 215:1937, 1971.
9. Metheny, N. M., and Snively, W. D., Jr. *Nurses' Handbook of Fluid Balance* (4th ed.). Philadelphia: Lippincott, 1983, pp. 16, 17, 41, 95, 96, 105, 110, 147, 157, 159, 192.
10. Mudge, G. H. Agent Affecting Volume and Composition of Body Fluids. In L. Goodman and A. Gilman (Eds.), *The Pharmacological Basis of Therapeutics* (6th ed.). New York: Macmillan, 1980, pp. 762, 763, 848, 851, 859.
11. Stoklosa, M. J. *Pharmaceutical Calculations* (6th ed.). Philadelphia: Lea & Febiger, 1974, pp. 236, 237.
12. *United States Pharmacopeia* (20th ed.). Easton, Pa.: Mack Publishing, 1980, pp. 803, 1027.
13. Voda, A. M. Body water dynamics. *Am. J. Nurs.* 70:2597, 2598, 2600, 2601.
14. Weisberg, H. F. Pitfalls in fluid and electrolyte therapy. *J. St. Barnabas Med. Center* 2:106, 1964.
15. Weisberg, H. F. Parenteral Fluid Therapy in Adults. In H. F. Conn (Ed.), *Current Therapy*. Philadelphia: Saunders, 1969, p. 414.

REVIEW QUESTIONS

1. Define the term *osmotic pressure*.
2. Isotonic fluids are fluids that have the same tonicity as the plasma. True or false?
3. In milliosmols, what is the approximate osmolality of (a) hypotonic fluids and (b) hypertonic fluids?
4. _____ fluids increase the osmotic pressure, drawing fluid from the cells; _____ fluids lower the osmotic pressure, causing fluids to invade the cells; _____ fluids cause increased extracellular fluid volume, which can result in circulatory overload.
5. The tonicity of fluid does not affect the choice of veins for infusion purposes. True or false?
6. Normal saline is a hypertonic fluid. True or false?
7. How many grams of dextrose are in 250 ml 20% dextrose in water?
8. Give the metabolic effects of dextrose.
9. What undesirable effects can result from prolonged or rapid infusion of dextrose in water?
10. How much water can the kidney safely metabolize in the average patient receiving intravenous therapy?
11. What untoward effects may arise from the use of normal isotonic sodium chloride solution?
12. What are the indications for use of hypertonic sodium chloride solutions?
13. Give three reasons for the use of hydrating fluids.
14. Why are solutions of dextrose and hypotonic saline considered hydrating fluids?
15. Why are balanced solutions of hypotonic electrolytes, such as Butler-type fluids, considered ideal for maintenance?
16. What potential dangers may occur when balanced hypotonic electrolyte fluids are administered to (a) a patient with impaired renal function or (b) a patient whose tolerance for water has been exceeded?

Chapter 9 | Parenteral Fluids and Related Abnormalities

17. When are isotonic multiple electrolyte fluids indicated?
18. Gastric replacement fluids replace the hydrogen ion lost in gastric juices because they contain _____ which are metabolized in the liver to _____ and _____ .
19. What type of fluids are indicated when a retention of chlorides, ketone bodies, or organic salts occurs as in shock, liver disease, and starvation?
20. Why is sodium lactate contraindicated for acidosis in patients suffering from oxygen lack, such as in congenital heart disease with persistent cyanosis?
21. Normal isotonic saline provides conservative treatment for metabolic alkalosis. True or false?
22. Improper administration of intravenous fluids may result in fluid loss. True or false?
23. List the clinical parameters that provide valuable information in assessing fluid and electrolyte changes.
24. What simple mental calculation can be used to convert pounds to kilograms?
25. Describe the test for skin turgor.
26. How is early peripheral edema detected?
27. What condition does hemoconcentration suggest?
28. Which patients are potential candidates for isotonic expansion (circulatory overload)?
29. What causes isotonic contraction?
30. What causes hypertonic expansion?
31. Why is hypertonic contraction (cellular dehydration) a common clinical disturbance in the elderly?
32. What fluid imbalance may result from the continuous infusion of 5% dextrose in water?

CHAPTER 10

Rate of Administration of Parenteral Infusions

Ada Lawrence Plumer

One of the prime considerations in the administration of parenteral solutions is the rate of flow. Ideally the physician orders the rate of flow since in determining the rate he or she must consider the solution, the patient's condition, and the desired effect. The nurse who initiates the infusion or who cares for its maintenance is responsible for regulating and maintaining the proper rate of administration.

DETERMINING FACTORS FOR INFUSION RATE

To determine the flow rate intelligently, the nurse must have a knowledge of parenteral solutions, their effect, and rate of administration. The nurse must also understand other factors that influence the speed of the infusion. These factors include (1) surface area of the body, (2) condition of the patient, (3) age of the patient, (4) composition of the fluid, and (5) the patient's tolerance to the infusion.

Surface Area of the Body

The body surface area is proportionate to many essential physiological processes (organ size, blood volume, respiration, and heat loss) and therefore to the total metabolic activity. It provides a helpful guide for determining the amount of fluids and electrolytes and for computing the rate of infusions. The larger an individual, the more fluid and nutrients are required and the faster they can be utilized. The usual infusion rate is 3 ml per square meter of body surface per minute (see nomograms for determining surface area, Figure 8.1, pp. 86–87). This rate applies to maintenance and replacement fluids. However, the speed must be carefully adjusted to each individual.

Condition of Patient

Since the heart and the kidneys play a vital role in the utilization of infused solutions, the cardiac and renal status of the patient affects the desired rate of administration. An expanded blood volume may occur when fluids, rapidly infused, overtax an impaired heart and renal damage causes retention of fluid.

Patients suffering from hypovolemia must receive plasma and blood rapidly, but the desired speed of the infusion may be affected by impairment of the homeostatic controls. Therefore the rate should be specified by the physician. Vital signs must be carefully observed and the speed of the infusion decreased as the blood pressure rises.

Age of Patient

Because there is usually some degree of cardiac and renal damage in the elderly, fluids are administered slowly to prevent an increase in venous pressure which could result in pulmonary edema and cardiovascular disturbances [1]. Infants and small children are particularly susceptible to pulmonary edema when excessive quantities of fluid or rapidly infused fluids expand the vascular system. The rate of administration must be determined by the physician and all precautions observed to ensure steady maintenance at the required rate of flow. If difficulty is encountered in controlling a constant rate, it should be reported and corrected at once.

The special pediatric infusion sets which deliver a smaller size drop (50–60 drops per milliliter) provide precision control of the rate of flow. There are a variety of mechanical controlling devices available to assist the nurse in maintaining a constant accurate flow rate (see Chapter 11). NITA Nursing Standards advocate I.V. controllers for use with the majority of infusions.

Composition of Fluid

The composition of the fluid affects the rate of flow. When the solution is used as a vehicle for administering drugs, the speed of the infusion depends upon the drug and the effect the physician wishes to produce. Potassium, because of its deleterious effect on the heart when infused at a rapid rate, should be administered with caution. About 20–40 mEq potassium in a liter of solution infused over an eight-hour period is an average rate for administering potassium parenterally [1].

Concentration of solutions must be considered since the flow rate may alter the desired effect. When dextrose is administered for caloric benefits it is infused at a rate that will ensure complete utilization. Dextrose has been administered at a maximum speed of 0.5 gm per kilogram of body weight per hour without producing glycosuria in a normal individual. At this rate it would take approximately 1½ hours to administer a liter of 5% dextrose to an individual weighing 70 kg or twice as long for a liter of 10% dextrose. This maximum rate is faster than usual and is not customarily used except in an emergency.

When a diuretic effect is desired a more rapid infusion is necessary. If the solution is too rapidly infused for complete metabolism, the glucose accumulates in the bloodstream, increases the osmolality, and acts as a diuretic.

When oliguria or anuria occurs, the status of the kidneys must be determined before solutions containing potassium can be administered. Urinary suppression may be due to a blood volume deficit or to kidney damage. An initial hydrating solution, to test kidney function, is usually administered at a rate of 8 ml per square meter of body surface per minute for 45 minutes [1]. If urinary flow is not accomplished the rate is slowed to about 2 ml per square meter of body surface per minute for another hour. If urinary output has not occurred after this period, it is presumed that kidney damage is present [1].

Tolerance

Tolerance to solutions varies with individuals and influences the rate of infusion. A 5% solution of alcohol has been administered at the rate of 200–300 ml per hour to sedate without intoxication in an average adult. However, when such a solution is to be administered, the rate must be titrated to the individual and prescribed by the physician.

When protein hydrolysates are infused, a slower rate of administration, 2 ml per minute, is necessary to test the patient's sensitivity to the protein [1]. Nausea and a feeling of warmth may occur from excessively rapid administration; if these symptoms do not subside when the rate of administration is decreased, the infusion should be stopped [1].

COMPUTATION OF FLOW RATE

Frequently the physician orders a total volume of fluid to be infused over a 24-hour period. If the nurse knows the volume and the flow rate of the administration set in use, he or she can easily compute the required rate of flow. A quick, easy formula for computing flow rate in drops (gtt) per minute is:

$$\frac{\text{gtt/ml of given set}}{60 \text{ (min in hour)}} \times \text{total hourly volume} = \text{gtt/min}$$

If a set delivers 15 drops per milliliter and 240 milliliters are to be infused in 1 hour.

$$\frac{15}{60} \times 240 = \frac{1}{4} \times 240 = 60 \text{ gtt/min}$$

Whenever a set is used that delivers 15 drops per milliliter, merely divide the hourly volume to be infused by 4 and the number of drops per minute will be obtained.

If the set delivers 10 drops per milliliter, divide the number of milliliters to be infused by 6 for drops per minute:

$$\frac{10}{60} \times \text{hourly volume} = \frac{1}{6} \times \text{hourly volume} = \text{gtt/min}$$

Manufacturers of parenteral solutions have devised convenient calculators to assist the nurse in accurate rate determinations.

The Travenol Minislide* provides the nurse with a handy, quick device for computing fluid rates. It consists of a slide rule containing four scales:

Top, scale A: total milliliters to be infused
Bottom, scale D: flow rate in drops per minute

The insert slides between scales A and D and contains:

Scale B: number of drops per milliliter (10–60) a given set delivers
Scale C: time in hours for infusion

---

*Copyright 1978, American Slide-Chart Corp., Wheaton, Ill. Designed by Harry F. Weisberg, M.D.

Chapter 10 | Rate of Administration of Parenteral Infusions

The flow rate or the infusion time at the prescribed rate may be determined by sliding the insert until the number of drops that the set delivers is aligned with total milliliters to be infused. Opposite the time (hours) for infusion, see drops required per minute; opposite the prescribed flow rate, see the infusion time (hours).

The opposite side of the Minislide contains the Cohn Fluid Calculator.* Since the body surface area is an important criterion for determining the rate of infusion, this calculator is a helpful aid in determining the surface area and the total amount of fluid required. Total milliliters to be infused in 24 hours is determined by sliding the insert until the weight of the patient in kilograms is reached; consideration is given to the body size of the patient — thin, average, or obese. Once the weight in kilograms is set, the surface area in square meters and the total amount of fluid to be infused in 24 hours is indicated.

No guide to safe flow rates is as important as is the patient's reaction to the infusion, which should, therefore, be checked frequently.

FACTORS AFFECTING THE FLOW RATE

The infusion should be checked frequently to maintain the required rate of flow. Because of certain factors, the rate is subject to change.

Height of the Solution Bottle

Intravenous fluids run by gravity. Any change in gravity by raising or lowering the infusion bottle will change the rate of flow. When patients receiving infusions are ambulated or transported to X ray, the solution bottle should be retained at the same height, or the speed of the infusion readjusted to maintain the prescribed rate of flow.

Clot in the Cannula

Any temporary stoppage of the infusion, such as a delay in changing infusion bottles, may cause a clot to form in the lumen of the cannula, partially or completely obstructing it. Clot formation may also occur when an increase in venous pressure in the infusion arm forces blood back into the cannula. This results from restriction of the venous circulation and is most commonly caused by (1) the blood pressure cuff on the infusion arm, (2) restraints placed on or above the infusion cannula, and (3) the patient's lying on the arm receiving the infusion.

Change in Position of the Cannula

A change in the cannula's position may push the bevel of the cannula against or away from the wall of the vein. Special precautions should be taken to prevent speed shock or overloading of the vascular system by making sure that the solution is flowing freely before adjusting the rate.

Other Changes

Stimulation of the vasoconstrictors from any infusion of cold blood or irritating solution may cause venous spasm, impeding the rate of flow. A warm pack placed on the vein proximal to the infusion cannula will offset this reaction.

---

*Travenol Laboratories, Inc., Deerfield, Ill. Designed by Bertram D. Cohn, M.D., F.A.A.P., F.A.C.S.

Part II | Fluids and Electrolytes

Trauma to the Vein Any injury such as phlebitis or thrombosis which reduces the lumen of the vein will decrease the flow of the solution.

Clogged Vent A clogged air vent in the administration set used with air-dependent containers will cause the infusion to stop. Check the vent needle for patency.

If there is any question as to the rate of administration, the therapist should check with the physician. This applies to intravenous administration of drugs in solution. The rates should also be established on patients receiving two or more infusions simultaneously. Any change in the rate from that normally used should be ordered by the attending physician.

The nurse should never exert positive pressure (manual pressure) to infuse solutions or blood. This should be the responsibility of the physician.

REFERENCE

1. Metheny, N. M., and Snively, W. D., Jr. *Nurses' Handbook of Fluid Balance* (4th ed.). Philadelphia: Lippincott, 1983. pp. 16, 144–149, 161.

REVIEW QUESTIONS

1. What factors determine the rate of infusion? *age, wt, medical condition of the, tolerance composition of the*
2. The usual infusion rate for maintenance and replacement fluids is *3 ml* ml per square meter of body surface per minute.
3. The larger an individual is, the more fluid and nutrients are required and the faster they can be utilized. (True) or false?
4. What is the most commonly occurring danger from fluid too rapidly infused? *pulmonary edema*
5. Name two devices that can be used to provide precision control of the rate of flow. *volume control (pediatric infusion) or pump*
6. What is the average length of time taken to infuse one liter of solution containing 40 mEq potassium? *8 hrs*
7. The concentration of the solution is an important factor to be considered in regulating the rate of infusion. (True) or false?
8. Glucose has a *diuretic* effect when infused too rapidly.
9. What is the usual rate of administration of hydrating fluid when initially used to determine if urinary suppression is due to blood volume deficit or kidney disease? *8 ml*
10. a. What is the rate of administration for protein hydrolysates, when it is initially infused? *2 ml*
    b. Why? *to test sensitivity to protein*
11. What is the quick, easy formula for computing flow rate in drops (gtt) per minute? $\frac{gtt \text{ of ml set}}{60 (\text{min}/\text{hr})} \times \text{vol. for 1 hr} = gtt/\text{min}$
12. What is the rate of administration for 240 ml fluid to be infused in 1 hour if the set delivers 15 drops per minute? *60 gtts/min*
13. What factors affect the flow rate? *ht. of bottle, position of cannula, clot, trauma, clogged vent, trauma to vein*

PART III
Equipment and Techniques

CHAPTER 11

Intravenous Equipment

Ada Lawrence Plumer

Rapidly changing technology has kept pace with the advances in medical science and has provided many improved, sophisticated devices for the administration of intravenous therapy. Specialized equipment is available to meet the patient's every need: positive-pressure pumps for intravenous and intraarterial therapy; controllers and monitors for regulating and monitoring the rate of infusion; air-venting microbe-retentive filters, catheters, and administration sets. Nurses' knowledge in the selection and use of these devices is vital to the comfort and safety of the patient.

FLUID CONTAINERS

Sterile evacuated glass containers with premixed fluids first became available in 1929. Later, plastic containers became available for the storage and delivery of blood products. Travenol was the first to develop the plastic bag for parenteral fluids. Today all manufacturers provide plastic containers as well as glass containers. The plastic container, the popular container for parenteral fluids, is easily transported with minimal risk of damage and is easily disposed of. Because it contains no rubber bushings, coring is eliminated and particulate matter reduced. Air venting is not required, thus the risk of air embolism and airborne contamination is reduced.

Plastic bags are susceptible to accidental puncture, which creates a port of entry for microorganisms. Because punctures may not be evident, the container should be squeezed prior to use and visually checked for leakage.

The *Viaflex* Plastic Container* series offer hospitals a complete line of parenteral fluids of various volumes, whereas the Viaflex Plus Plastic Containers offer a complete line of the most commonly used I.V. medications, premixed in unit-dose in both large volume and mini-bag plastic containers.

---

*Travenol Laboratories, Inc., Parenteral Products Division, Deerfield, Ill.

The *Accumed I.V. Delivery System** consists of the semirigid plastic bottle, which stands upright and rigid. It is a closed system that collapses in a symmetrical manner, making calculations easily readable. Made of polyolefin, it contains no plasticizers and is as inert as glass. Its two rigid ports, one for admixtures and the other for administration sets, are protected by a quick and easy snap cap, which also carries a solution description for on-side storage of the container. I.V. medications, premixed in solutions, are available.

The *Life Care Plastic Container*† is a plastic bag that features easy-to-use ports. The large target area for adding medications is readily accessible on the side of the container. This series of containers is available in large volume containers, piggyback partial-fills, empties, and premixed I.V. solutions.

INFUSION SYSTEMS

There are basically three types of infusion systems currently available in the United States: (1) the plastic bag and plastic bottle, (2) the closed system, and (3) the open system. The plastic bag and plastic bottle contain no vacuum, and, since the containers are flexible and collapsible, they need no air to replace fluid flowing from the containers. All other systems employ glass bottles with a partial vacuum requiring air vents. The Abbott‡ system is a closed system since only filtered air is admitted to the container; the air vent, containing the filter, is an integral part of the administration set. The open system is used by Travenol§ and McGaw**; air enters through a plastic tube in the container and collects in the air space in the bottle.

Methods for adding medications to the fluid containers vary with each system. The plastic bag contains a resealable latex medication port through which the medication is injected. Since the plastic bag lacks a vacuum, medications must be added with a syringe and needle. A unit for creating a vacuum in the container is available to the pharmacist and provides speed and ease to the admixture program. When medications are added to the plastic containers during the infusion, special precautions must be taken to make certain that the clamp on the administration set is completely closed and the flow interrupted before the medication is added. This prevents an undiluted, toxic dose of medication from entering the administration set and being infused. Medications and solutions should always be mixed thoroughly before administration, regardless of the system used.

In the closed system, medication may be added to the solution bottle during the infusion by using the air vent located in the administration set as a

---

*American McGaw Laboratories, Inc., Irvine, Calif.; Division of American Hospital Supply Corporation.

†Abbott Laboratories, Hospital Products Division, North Chicago, Ill.

‡Abbott Laboratories, Hospital Products Division, North Chicago, Ill.

§Travenol Laboratories, Inc., Deerfield, Ill.

**American McGaw Laboratories, Inc., Irvine, Calif.; Division of American Hospital Supply Corporation.

medication port. The filter is removed and the syringe is attached. Meticulous care must be observed to maintain sterility of the filter when removing the filter, adding the medication, and replacing the filter. The fluid bottle contains a solid rubber stopper through which medications may be added prior to infusion.

In the open system, bottles have a removable metal disk under which a sterile latex disk provides a closed method for aseptically adding a medication and for a visible check for vacuum. The vacuum is noted by the depression in the seal and must be present to ensure sterility. Before the latex disk is removed, the medication is added through the outlet port with a syringe and needle; the vacuum draws the medication into the bottle. During infusion, the medication may be added through the designated area on the rubber bushing after the clamp on the administration set has been closed. The medication and solution must be mixed thoroughly by agitating the fluid before administration.

ADMINISTRATION SETS

An important factor in the administration set is the rate of flow which the given set is gauged to produce. Commercial sets vary — they may deliver from 10 to 20 drops per milliliter, depending upon the nature of the fluid. Increased viscosity causes the size of the drop to increase, so that a set that delivers 15 drops per milliliter will deliver 10 drops per milliliter when blood is administered. This information is of vital concern to the accurate control of the rate of infusion.

Most conventional sets use the roller clamp or slide clamp for controlling the flow rate. Changes in the drop rate invariably occur after the rate is regulated and require time-consuming readjustments of the clamp to establish and maintain flow rates. Now there are alternatives to the roller clamp that save nursing time and that are valuable in maintaining the rate of parenteral solutions.

The *CorrectFLO** bridges the gap between roller clamps and electronic flow devices (Figure 11.1). It is equipped with an adjustable valve which regulates and maintains a constant flow rate. As easy to use as a roller clamp, it provides greater safety in the routine administration of intravenous solutions as well as critical applications where pumps are not used. It is available on administration sets, extension sets, and custom configurations.

The *Accudot Administration Set*† uses a flow-metering system which eliminates drifting flow rates (Figure 11.2). The metering device consists of "an adjustable dam" controlled by a knob. Because it is connected on the entry and exit ports, the intravenous tubing is isolated from the metering device and does not affect changes in the flow rate. The rate can be set and it will stay until the infusion is complete, eliminating "free flow" runaway I.V.s and helping prevent I.V. flow-rate variations.

---

*Biomedical Dynamics Corporation, Minneapolis, Minn.
†IMED Corporation, San Diego, Calif.

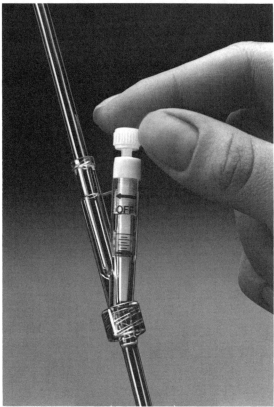

FIGURE 11.1
CorrectFLO™, an alternative to the roller clamp. It provides consistant and reliable fluid administration without the need for constant adjustment. Courtesy of Biomedical Dynamics Corp., Minneapolis, Minn.

Nonpolyvinylchloride Intravenous Administration Sets

Nonpolyvinylchloride intravenous administration sets are available for gravity infusion and for volumetric pumps. Now nitroglycerine, fat emulsions, and other drugs can be administered without lowering the dosage of the drug through absorption into the walls of the PVC tubing.

Non-PVC Accuset* Administration Sets consist of tubing containing polyethelene on the inside and ethylene vinyl acetate on the outside. They provide a PVC-free path for infusion of nitroglycerin, fat emulsions, and other drugs. This set can be used with the IMED Volumetric Infusion Pump.

The *I.V. 7A01 Nitroglycerine Delivery Set*† contains especially formulated tubing that minimizes the absorption of nitroglycerine into the tubing. It contains a universal spike for use with all parenteral fluid containers and a patented blue ball in the drip chamber which seats itself once the container empties, preventing air from entering the system and the need to reprime the set if the infusion is to continue.

---

*IMED Corporation, San Diego, Calif.
†Valleylab Inc. Boulder, Co.

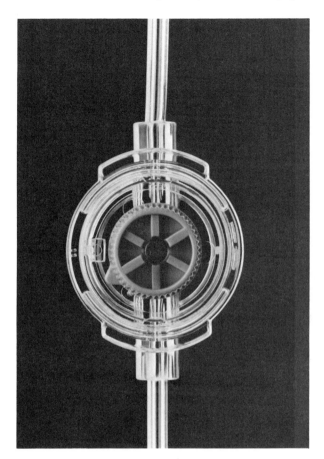

FIGURE 11.2
Accudot® Administration Sets use a precision valve to control flow, assuring precise I.V. flow control until infusion is complete. Courtesy of IMED Corporation, San Diego, Calif.

PEDIATRIC SETS

It is frequently necessary to maintain the flow at a minimal rate. One method is to reduce the size of the drop by the use of special sets, originally designed for pediatric infusions. These sets are valuable for use in parenteral therapy for the adult patient as well, since by reducing the size of the drop it is possible to maintain a constant intravenous flow with a minimal amount of fluid. These sets deliver 50–60 drops per milliliter, depending upon the viscosity of the solution; at the rate of 60 drops per minute it would take 1 hour to infuse 60 ml.

MEDICATION SITES

Various devices are available for adding medications through the infusion needle or for setting up a secondary infusion. Some sets contain Y-type injection sites which facilitate this procedure. Twin-site supplementary sets are available (Figure 11.3) for attaching to regular sets lacking these injection sites. Three-way stopcocks provide another method of introducing drugs through

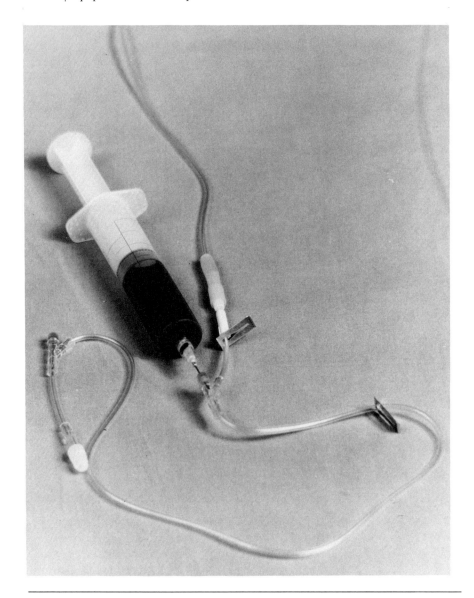

FIGURE 11.3
Venotube Twin-Site Extension Set. Supplementary set containing Y-type injection sites. The needle is inserted directly through the medication site. (Dye added to facilitate photography.) Courtesy of Abbott Laboratories, North Chicago, Ill.

the infusion cannula. These are especially valuable for anesthesia and for the operating room when supplementary medications are required, and when transfusions and secondary infusions are necessary.

Any opening into the tubing may permit air to be sucked into the infusion, with the danger of resultant air embolism. If three-way stopcocks are used, caution must be exercised to see that the inlet which is not in use is completely shut off. The nurse should ever be on the alert for any faulty opening that allows air bubbles to escape into the flowing solution.

Injection ports are provided by various extension sets and injection caps.

The *Jelco* Intermittent Injection Cap* makes a secure Luer lock attachment to I.V. catheters and provides a resealable injection site with a hold-up volume capacity of only 0.14 cc. The cap is removable, allowing attachment of an administration set.

The T-Port Extension Set,† with a Luer lock collar and a slide clamp, contains an injection port immediately adjacent to the catheter connection site. This is a short extension set.

The *Micro-Volume Doubleline Extension Set‡* eliminates the problem that arises when two fluids or medications are infused in one line. It consists of a 36-inch length of separable PVC tubing. Two lines — one a drug-delivery line containing a 0.22 micron air-eliminating, bacteria-retentive filter with a maximum pressure of 40 psi; the other a primary line suitable for blood — connect to a male Luer lock connector chamber in which the two fluids meet. The male Luer lock connector chamber holds less than 0.06 ml fluid, minimizing drug interaction. There are female Luer lock connectors on both lines. The priming volume is only 0.63 ml.

The Miniloop Connector§ is a valuable accessory to the intravenous administration set. A rigid loop, which connects the catheter to the administration set, eliminates kinking at the catheter connection and provides a method for securely taping the connection to the patient's body. The low-volume, pressure-monitoring tubing makes this connector applicable for pressure-monitoring devices.

CHECK-VALVE SETS

Sets are available with an in-line check valve, which provides a more convenient and safer method for administering medications and fluids. A secondary infusion or a single dose of medication can be administered "piggyback" into the injection site located below the check valve. The valve automatically shuts off the main-line infusion while the admixture is running and automatically allows the main infusion to start when the medication has run in. This valve prevents mixing of the two fluids, eliminates the risk of air entering the line when the secondary bottle empties, and prevents the cannula from becoming occluded by an interruption in the infusion. Since the rate of flow must be regulated by one clamp, the rate of administration remains the same for both fluids.

---

*Critikon, Inc., a Johnson and Johnson Company, Tampa, Fl.

†Burron Medical Inc., Bethlehem, Pa.

‡Auto Syringe Division, Travenol Laboratories, Inc., Hooksett, N.H.

§Medex Inc., Hillard, Oh.

CONTROLLED-VOLUME SETS

With the increasing use and number of solutions containing drugs and electrolytes, greater accuracy in controlling the volume of intravenous fluids is necessary. There are several devices that permit accurate administration of measured volumes of fluids.

Sets contain vented, calibrated buret chambers that control the volume from 100 to 150 cc (Figure 11.4). The buret chamber of some sets contains a rubber float which prevents air from entering the tubing once the infusion is completed.

Some calibrated buret chambers contain a microporous filter to block the passage of air when the chamber empties. Refilling these chambers requires a specific procedure. The word OSCAR will help recall the procedure: O — Open clamp; S — Squeeze drip chamber and hold; C — Close clamp close to drip chamber; A — And; R — Release drip chamber.

Most chambers contain an injection port which allows medications to be added. The NCCLVP (National Coordinating Committee for Large Volume Parenterals) does not recommend the chamber for intermittent administration of antibiotics because of the high risk of contamination. If this chamber is used, fluid should be placed in the chamber first to prevent the antibiotic from being absorbed in the float membrane.

Y-TYPE ADMINISTRATION SETS

A variety of commercial sets are available for alternate or simultaneous infusion of two solutions. Some sets contain a filter and a pressure unit for blood infusions.

There may be a significant hazard of air embolism when the Y-type administration set is used ignorantly or carelessly with vented containers. Constant vigilance is necessary if both solutions are administered simultaneously. If one container is allowed to empty, large quantities of air can be sucked into the tubing; the empty bottle becomes the vent owing to the greater atmospheric pressure in the empty bottle and tube over the pressure below the partially constricted clamp in the tubing of the flowing solution [7].

POSITIVE-PRESSURE SETS

Positive-pressure sets (Figure 11.5) are designed to increase the rapidity of infusions and are an asset when rapid replacement of fluid becomes necessary. They permit fluid to be administered by gravity, with a built-in pressure chamber available for rapid administration of blood should emergency arise. When used with the collapsible plastic blood unit, this system avoids the danger of air embolism; because the bag collapses, the need for air is eliminated. In contrast to the collapsible bag, the glass container must be vented to allow the fluid to flow; air pressure must be used when blood or fluid is forced into the bloodstream. As the last portion of blood from the container is forced into the bloodstream, the air under pressure may rapidly enter the vein before the clamp can be applied, resulting in a fatal embolus. According to Adriani [1],

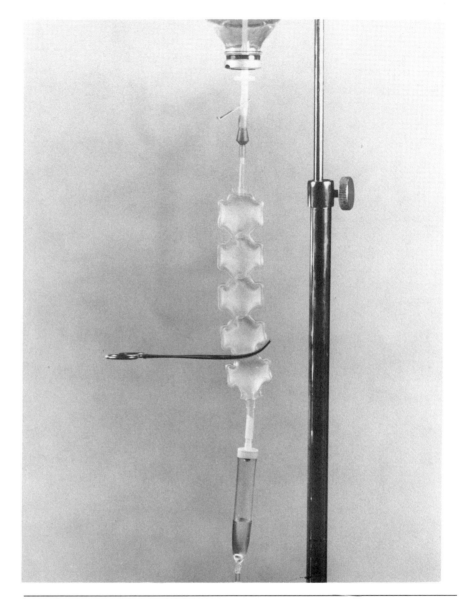

FIGURE 11.4
Metriset. Calibrated chamber controls volume to 100 ml. Medications are added directly into the chamber through the medication plug. Courtesy of American McGaw, Division of American Hospital Supply Corporation, Irvine, Calif.

"Air pressure should not be used to force blood and other fluids into the blood stream."

The pump chamber must be filled at all times. The nurse should never apply positive pressure to infuse fluids; this is the responsibility of the physician.

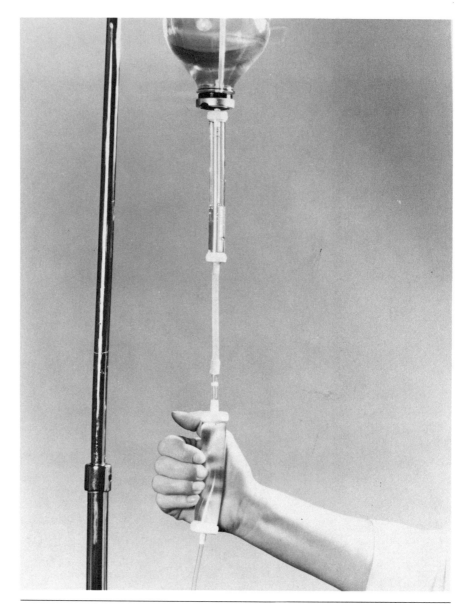

FIGURE 11.5
Positive pressure set permits fluids to run by gravity, with pressure unit available for rapid infusion should emergency arise. Courtesy of American McGaw, Division of American Hospital Supply Corporation, Irvine, Calif.

The pressure cuff (Figure 11.6) is another device that provides rapid infusion of blood. This cuff, with a pressure gauge calibrated in millimeters of mercury, fits over the plastic blood unit. Application of external pressure to the blood container permits rapid infusion of blood. This closed system avoids the inherent danger of air embolism.

Large-bore tubing sets are now available for trauma care. They provide

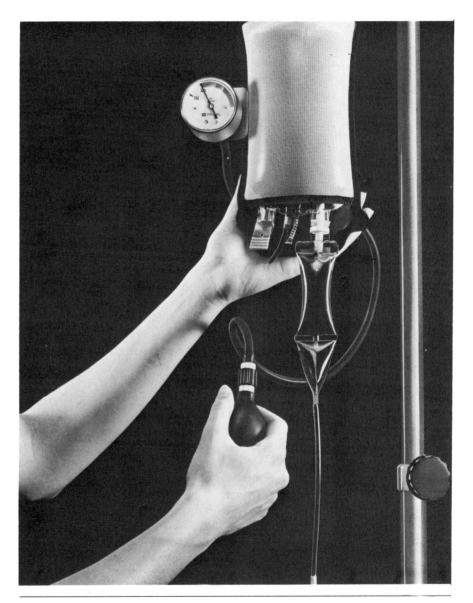

FIGURE 11.6
Blood cuff, by means of external pressure, provides rapid infusion of blood. In-line filter is used. Courtesy of Fenwal Laboratories, Division of Travenol, Inc., Deerfield, Ill.

rapid flow rates when seconds count, up to 514 ml per minute and with a 55% faster packed-cell flow rate than standard blood administration sets. The straight set and the Y-type set are both available with either the standard blood filter or with a 20 Micron High Capacity Transfusion Filter (ENTERPRISE H.C.).*

---

*Fenwal Laboratories, Division of Travenol Laboratories, Inc., Deerfield, Ill.

BLOOD WARMERS

Prewarmed blood may be indicated when conditions (such as massive hemorrhage) exist that warrant large and rapid transfusions; cold blood administered under such conditions may produce effects of cardiac and general hypothermia. Boyan [3] cited results of observations carried out in the operating rooms of Memorial (Sloan-Kettering Cancer Center) Hospital, New York, which showed that the incidence of cardiac arrest during massive blood replacement (3,000 ml or more per hour) dropped from 58.3 percent to 6.8 percent when cold bank blood was warmed to body temperature during infusion. He stated: "To avoid the effects of cardiac and general hypothermia during massive hemorrhage, cold bank blood should be warmed to body temperature when administered rapidly and in large amounts." Warm blood is usually required in exchange transfusions of newborns and in transfusions of patients with potent cold agglutinins.

Several manufacturing companies* have devised units consisting of blood-warming coils that are placed in warm-water baths. In one unit the blood is warmed at an approximate rate of 150 ml per minute in the adult coil and at approximately 50 ml per minute in the pediatric coil. Some units contain a water bath automatically controlled to maintain a desired temperature of between 39° and 40°C, warming the blood to about 35°C.

An alternative to the water bath is the *Fenwal Dry Heat Blood Warmer* (Figure 11.7).† This device contains two warming plates, which hold and warm the disposable plastic warming bag containing integral tubing and a connector on the inlet side for connection to a recipient set. The blood is warmed as it flows from the transfusion administration set through the tubing in the warming bag and through integral tubing to the recipient. It contains a digital temperature display and an audible temperature alarm and shut-off.

Another blood fluid warmer, the *FloTem*,‡ is a portable solid-state unit weighing 2 pounds. It is particularly useful in emergency rooms, operating rooms, and ambulances because it can be attached to a standard I.V. pole and does not interfere with nursing care. The warmer uses standard blood tubing and, because there are no connectors and sterilization is not required, potential contamination of the blood is eliminated. The safety features include an independent audio-alarm, an automatic power cut-off to the heater, and monitoring lights.

Warming devices must undergo careful and continuing quality-control procedures. In many hospitals, this is carried out by the medical engineering department. Extra caution in use of the warm water method may be observed by placing a thermometer in the water before administering the blood.

---

*Dupaco Inc., San Marcos, Calif., among them.
†Fenwal Laboratories, Division of Travenol Laboratories, Inc., Deerfield, Ill.
‡DataChem Inc., Indianapolis, Ind.

Chapter 11 | Intravenous Equipment

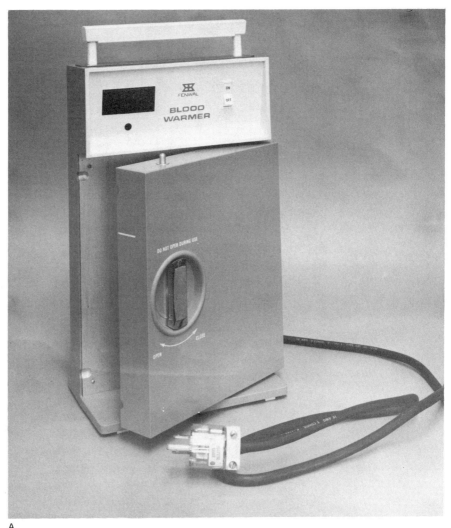

A

FIGURE 11.7
(A) Dry Heat Blood Warmer. (B) Disposable plastic warming bag which is positioned between two warming plates within the Dry Heat Blood Warmer (p. 150). Courtesy of Fenwal Laboratories, Division of Travenol, Inc., Deerfield, Ill.

Y-TYPE BLOOD COMPONENT SETS

Y-type blood component sets are available for the direct administration of platelets or cryoprecipitate (Figure 11.8). One arm of the Y contains a spike for introducing into the component bag; the other arm, an adapter for attaching a 50-cc syringe. The blood component is aspirated into the syringe; the main clamp is then opened, the air expelled, and the main line filled. A small mesh filter is enclosed within the adapter. The venipuncture is made and the

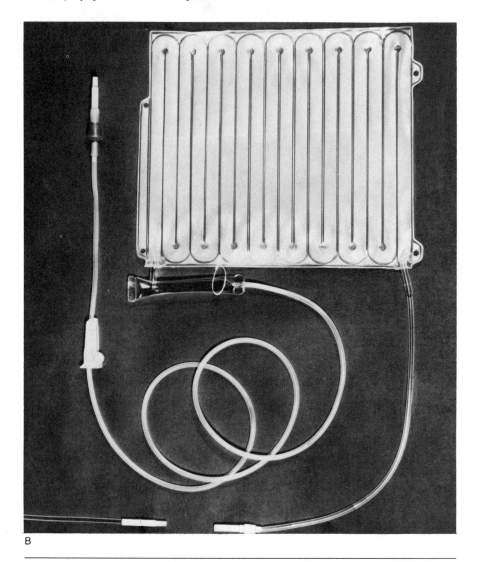

B

FIGURE 11.7 (*continued*)

component administered by syringe. The necessity for starting an initial infusion is eliminated, and loss of components in the tubing is avoided.

FILTERS

Administration sets with the standard clot filter of 170 microns are available for infusion of blood and blood components. The supplementary filter can be added to an in-use administration set, permitting infusion of blood; easy replacement of the filter, should clogging occur, allows multiple infusions of blood. Several manufacturers design blood filters with a pore size of 40 microns or less to trap microaggregates and protect the lung from this particulate matter. Evidence has demonstrated that cellular degradation develops with

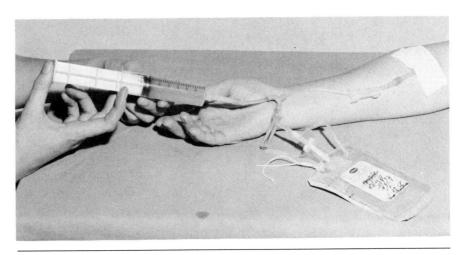

FIGURE 11.8
Platelet recipient set. Platelets being infused through Y-type blood component set. Courtesy of Fenwal Laboratories, Division of Travenol, Inc., Deerfield, Ill.

storage of banked blood. This debris has been implicated as a cause of respiratory insufficiency when large quantities of stored bank blood are infused (see Chapter 17). The small-pored filter is recommended for use when several units of stored bank blood are to be infused.

One such filter (Figure 11.9) is a 40 micron screen, low-priming volume filter. It has a large 161 cm² filter surface area that provides a high-unit filtering capacity of 10 units of CPD whole blood (see Chapter 13).

FINAL FILTERS

Final filters are available in a variety of forms, sizes, and materials. Two commonly used in-line filters are the depth filter and the membrane filter. The depth filter consists of fibers or fragmented material that have been pressed or bonded to form a tortuous maze. Fluid flows through a random path which absorbs and traps the particles. Because the pore size is not uniform, "depth filters cannot properly be given an absolute rating. Instead, they are assigned a nominal rating which, by definition, is the particle size above which 98 percent of the contaminants will be retained; for instance, a depth filter rated at 5 microns will retain 98 percent of all particles larger than 5 microns, though 2 percent will pass through" [2]. Depth filters are efficient in removing particles; they do not block the passage of air.

Membrane filters are screen-type filters with uniformly sized pores which provide an absolute rating. A 5 micron screen-type filter will retain on the flat membrane all particles greater than 5 microns.

The U.S.P. has established an acceptable limit of particles for single-dose infusion as not more than 50 particles per milliliter that are equal to or larger than 10.0 μm and not more than 5 particles per milliliter that are equal to or larger than 25.0 μm in effective linear dimension [6].

Porosity filters of 0.22 micron are bacteria-, fungus-, and air-retention

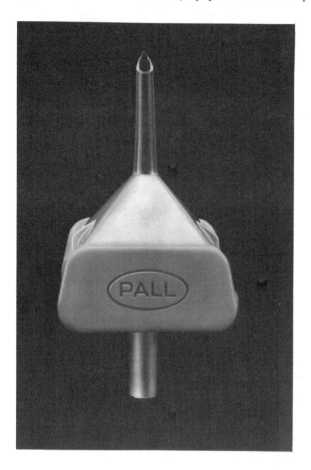

FIGURE 11.9
Pall SQ-405. Microaggregate Blood Transfusion Filter, a 40 micron screen filter with the large 161 cm^2 surface area to provide high unit filtering capacity of 10 units of CPD whole blood. Courtesy of Pall Biomedical Products Corp., Glen Cove, N.Y.

filters. The 0.22 micron air-venting filters automatically vent air through a nonwettable (hydrophobic) membrane and permit uniform high-gravity flow rates via large wettable (hydrophilic) membranes. They prevent an air block, which could ultimately result in a plugged cannula.

Filters are also rated according to the psi (pounds per square inch) of pressure they will withstand, an important consideration in selecting the proper filter. The filter should withstand the psi exerted by the infusion pump or rupture may occur. If the psi rating of the housing is less than that of the membrane, excess force will break the housing, leaving the filter intact.

There are two schools of thought relevant to the use of 0.22 micron filters. National Intravenous Therapy Association (NITA) standards recommend the routine use of 0.22 micron air-eliminating filters for delivering routine I.V. therapy to protect the patient from particulates, air embolism, and microorganisms, and to minimize the risk of I.V.-related complications and sepsis [5].

The Center for Disease Control (CDC) does not recommend in-line filters as a routine infection control [4]. In-line filters provide infection control and protect the patient groups who are at a greater risk of infection, those patients who are immunocompromised.

Optimal filters should (1) automatically vent air; (2) retain bacteria, fun-

Chapter 11 | Intravenous Equipment

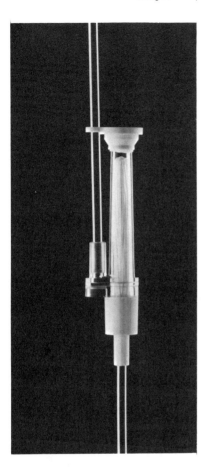

FIGURE 11.10
Travenol® Hollow Fiber Filter. An in-line 0.22 micron porosity filter with many advantages; fast and easy to prime with a filter life of 48 hours. Also available as an add on unit. Courtesy of Travenol Laboratories, Inc., Deerfield, Ill.

gi, and endotoxins; (3) be nonbinding of drugs; (4) allow high gravity flow rates; and (5) have a pressure tolerance to withstand the psi of the infusion pump. Pressure rating of the housing, when less than that of the filter membrane, may provide added protection.

A large number of various types of filters are available; they may vary in shape, in media composition, in pore size, in pressure, and in length of filter life. The shape may affect the rate of flow; the media composition, the retention of endotoxins; the pore size, the retention of bacteria and particulates; the pressure, the ability of the filter to withstand pressure exerted by infusion pumps; in addition, the filter life may vary in length.

The *Travenol Hollow Fiber Filter** is a 0.22 micron sterilizing filter that offers definite advantages over flat membrane filters (Figure 11.10). Its innovative design provides a larger filter area, which makes it fast and easy to prime and which helps to prevent clogging and drug binding for an extended 48-hour filter-set life. It may be used with a wide range of drugs and TPN solutions, and its nonclogging filter provides uninterrupted flow rates in routine

---

*Travenol Laboratories, Inc., Parenteral Products Div., Deerfield, Ill.

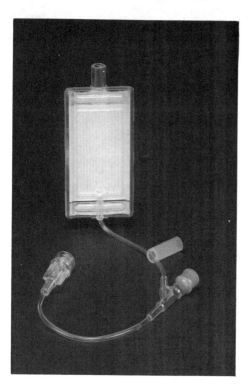

FIGURE 11.11
Pall ELD-96 (Extended Life Disposable) Final Filter can remove endotoxins as well as microbial contaminants, particulate matter, and air. It can be used safely for periods up to 96 hours allowing I.V. tubing also to be used for extended periods of time. Courtesy of Pall Biomedical Products Corp., Glen Cove, N.Y.

antibiotic therapy. Its high pressure allows its use under conditions where the pressure generated is not greater than 45 psi.

The *ELD-96 (Extended Life Disposable Filter).** features a unique membrane able to remove endotoxins as well as microbial contaminants, particulate matter, and air (Figure 11.11). Bacteria retained on the filter may break down after 24 hours and release bacterial toxin confined within the body of a bacterium. This new filter, a technological advance, provides protection for the patient and a longer filter life of 96 hours. The I.V. tubing is also allowed to be used for the extended period of time. These filters maintain a high level of quality assurance exceeding that of conventional infection control procedures by protecting both the administration system and the patient from contamination due to in-use manipulation. The ELD-96 connects directly to the catheter, acting as a protective extension set. It reduces the risk associated with frequent catheter manipulation, and extends the safe useful life of the administration set. The filter, 0.2 micron, has a psi of 30.

The *SCF-96 (Solution Container Filter)** is designed for routine use, such as intermittent piggyback and heparin-lock therapies (Figure 11.12). It also provides automatic venting of solution containers and prevention of run-drys. This 0.2 micron filter provides the same protection as the ELD-96, removing endotoxins as well as microbial contaminants and particulate matter, and having an extended life of 96 hours.

---

*ELD-96 and SCF-96 filters, both Pall Biomedical Products Corporation, Glen Cove, N.Y.

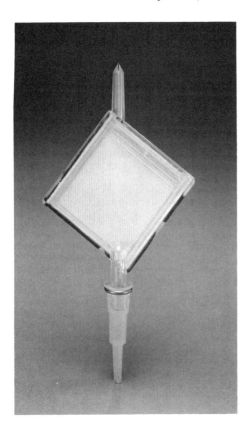

FIGURE 11.12
Pall SCF-96 (Solution Container Filter) is designed for routine use such as piggyback and heparin-lock therapies. It removes endotoxins as well as other contaminants and has a filter life of 96 hours. Courtesy of Pall Biomedical Products Corp., Glen Cove, N.Y.

IMED Filtersets* are available both as a 5 micron porosity filter and as a 0.22 micron filter. They contain a hydrophobic membrane for eliminating air from the line. They use quick-priming, kink-resistant micropore tubing and can resist back pressures because of a strong nylon-supported filter medium.

INFUSION PUMPS

Infusion pumps have proved invaluable in neonatal, pediatric, and adult intensive care units, where critical infusions of small volumes of fluid or doses of high-potency drugs are indicated.

These pumps have increased the level of safety in parenteral therapy. In some models, the risk of air embolism is reduced by alarm systems and by the automatic interruption of the infusion when the container empties. A controlled rate of flow reduces the risk of circulatory overload.

Infusion pumps have saved valuable nursing time; the uniform control of fluid eliminates the need to count drops and adjust flow rates. Plugging of the cannula which occurs when blood backs into the cannula owing to an increase in venous pressure due to coughing, crying, or strain, is eliminated; the pressure generated by the pump exceeds the maximum venous pressure.

---

*IMED Corporation, San Diego, Calif.

Pumps are finding increasing uses in keep-open arterial lines and infusions of drugs, bloods, and viscous fluids such as hyperalimentation solutions.

Advances in technology have provided the medical field with more sophisticated positive-pressure devices. Many kinds and models of pumps have become available. They can be divided into three classes; (1) the syringe pump, (2) the nonvolumetric pump, and (3) the volumetric pump [5]. The nonvolumetric pump measures drop rate and the volumetric pump, as the name implies, measures volume.

Pressure exerted by the pump is expressed in psi (pounds per square inch) of mmHg (millimeters of mercury); one psi and 51.7 mmHg exert the same amount of pressure [9]. The psi of a pump is important in that it may affect the type of filter being used or the ability of the pump to infuse fluids through arterial lines. The psi must not exceed the pressure the filter can withstand or a rupture may occur; when the pump is used for arterial infusion, the psi must be high enough to overcome arterial pressure.

A wide assortment of features, varying with the brand or model of pump, are available, including a tamper-proof design (which eliminates the possibility of a change in the flow rate by someone inadvertently pushing the control knobs); a KVO (keep vein open), which automatically changes to a slower rate when a low volume is reached; standard intravenous tubing with allowance for removal to gravity flow; and batteries, which allow ambulation of the patient. All pumps feature alarms and lights which alert the user to possible problems such as air in line, occlusion, infusion complete, low battery, and so forth.

Reading the literature, familiarizing oneself with the pump, and observing all precautions are imperative measures to ensure safe, efficient operation. Serious problems may occur if the staff is not adequately informed of the distinctive functional characteristics of the selected pump.

SYRINGE PUMPS

Syringe pumps provide precise infusion by controlling the rate by drive speed and syringe size, thus eliminating the variables of the drop rate. Syringe pumps are valuable for critical infusions of small doses of high-potency drugs; they may provide constant or intermittent flow.

The *Harvard Mini-Infuser** syringe pump, weighing less than 2 pounds and battery operated, provides unrestricted mobility for the patient. It is the ideal pump for controlled intermittent delivery of medications, including most antibiotics, for the patient in either the hospital or the home setting. It is simple to use; with the snap of the syringe on the pump and the touch of the "on" switch, the medication is delivered at a precisely controlled predetermined rate. The syringe plunger is delivered by a lever, electronically controlled, to maintain a constant flow rate. The infusion time is determined by the amount of fluid and the size of the syringe. When an infusion ends or an occlusion occurs, the pump automatically shuts off. With syringe pump accuracy, a selected concentrated dilution of the drug is accurately delivered over a desired time period

---

*Bard MedSystems Division, C. R. Bard Inc., North Reading, Mass.

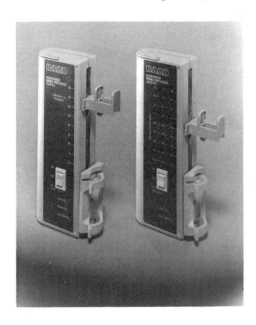

FIGURE 11.13
Harvard Mini-Infuser™ is designed for the controlled intermittent I.V. administration of medications, including most antibiotics. Small, with a battery life of up to 6 months, it is ideal for ambulatory patients. Courtesy of Bard MedSystems Div., C. R. Bard, Inc., North Reading, Mass.

directly into a heparin lock or a calibrated volume-control chamber or as a piggyback in combination with a primary line.

The Harvard Mini-Infuser provides the pharmacy with ultimate control over both drug dosage and rate of administration. Standard disposable syringes and microbore extension sets are used. The extension set is available with a 0.2 micron acrylic membrane filter. The Mini-Infuser system consists of 3 single-speed models which deliver medications in 35 minutes or less, and a 3-speed model that infuses in up to 70 minutes. Two new models, 150XL and 300XL (Figure 11.13) are being introduced with a 5–60cc syringe capacity. One model will accept any of 5 different syringes and provides a choice of delivery times.

The *Auto-Syringe** represents a unique line of portable and semiportable infusion pumps that can be used for subcutaneous, intravenous, intraarterial, or epidural infusions. Fluids can be delivered continuously or intermittently. These pumps may be used in neonatology and pediatrics for the administration of blood, fat, emulsions, and antibiotics, and with keep-open lines; as well as in chemotherapy, anesthesia, analgesia, and labor and delivery, and other areas of the hospital. The Auto-Syringe is made more versatile with the use of Auto Syringe's Micro-Volume Doubleline Extension Set. It contains Luer lock connectors and a 0.22 micron air-eliminating, bacterial-retentive filter with a maximum intermittent pressure of 40 psi. Drug interaction is minimized by the small volume (0.06 ml) contained in the male Luer lock where the two fluids meet. The primary line is suitable for whole blood. The Auto-Syringe AS8MP, newest of the pumps, is small enough to fit in a shirt pocket, and, from a 1–3 ml reservoir, delivers U40 or U100 insulin. It is programmable and offers the ability to preprogram bolus delivery.

---

*Auto Syringe Division, Travenol Laboratories, Inc., Hooksett, N.H.

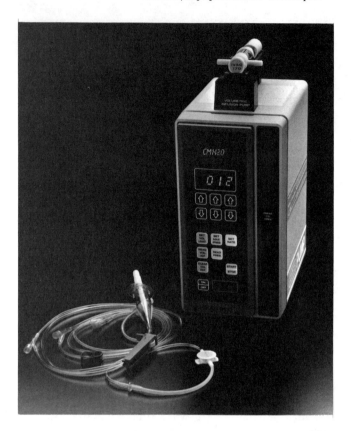

FIGURE 11.14
IVAC Variable Pressure Volumetric Pump-Model 560. Recommended for volume-critical applications requiring adjustable occlusion limits and low output pressure. Courtesy of IVAC Corp., San Diego, Calif.

Volumetric Pumps

Most pumps are volumetric; they measure the volume being delivered in milliliters rather than in drops. Volumetric pumps utilize either the peristaltic (roller) device or the piston cylinder unit (also called syringe cassette).

The *IVAC Variable Pressure Volumetric Pump Model 560** is a peristaltic pump, a unique pump in that it displays peripheral and central venous pressures in mmHg or cmH$_2$O as well as provides volume accuracy of flow from 1 to 499 ml per hour (Figure 11.14). An adjustable I.V. stand allows easy zero-point leveling to the patient's right atrium, and a built-in pressure transducer allows peripheral and central venous pressure readings for vascular assessment. The operator, with a flick of the switch, can identify the infusion site pressure or view the total volume infused. This pump is recommended for volume-critical infusions that require adjustable occlusion limits and low output pressure; an output pressure of 0–499 mmHg or 0–699 cmH$_2$O can be selected. The volume limit range is 1–9,999 ml. A "Keep Open" rate of 5 ml per hour will automatically be maintained after the selected volume has been infused. An alarm will alert air in line when the air-in-line detector is used.

An information display assists in the starting procedure. Its numeric display shows selected infusion rate, pressure readout, volume limit setting, maximum pressure limit, and volume infused. The maximum occlusion pressure

---

*IVAC Corporation, San Diego, Calif.

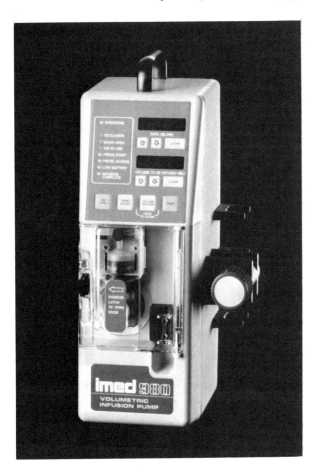

FIGURE 11.15
IMED® 980 Volumetric Pump has the unique ability for high-rate capacity of up to 2000 ml per hour and yet will deliver a flow rate as low as 1 ml per hour. Courtesy of IMED Corp., San Diego, Calif.

can be set for quick detection of fluid restriction. The flow sensor detects fluid in the drip chamber. This display provides valuable information and assistance in the fluid administration of cardiovascular drugs, antibiotics, anticoagulants, chemotherapeutic agents, and infusions requiring various output pressures such as arterial infusions, total parenteral nutrition (TPN), blood, and filtered lines.

The *IMED 980 Volumetric Pump** utilizes the piston cylinder unit (Figure 11.15). It is unique in that it has a high-rate capability, up to 2,000 ml per hour, and yet will deliver a flow rate as low as 1 ml per hour. Using the *IMED Accuset Cassette* (Figure 11.16), the delivery of fluid is constant and accurate because each stroke is divided into several hundred pulses. By not allowing an open uncontrolled line between the fluid container and the patient, the possibility of free flow is virtually eliminated. This pump will easily adapt to syringes as flow containers, making it adaptable for a variety of applications, including I.V. pushes, blood, fat emulsions, or TPN delivery. It has a nonoptional air-in-line detector capable of detecting 0.05 cc or more air in all fluids including blood and blood products, opaque solutions, and three-in-one TPN

*IMED Corporation, San Diego, Calif.

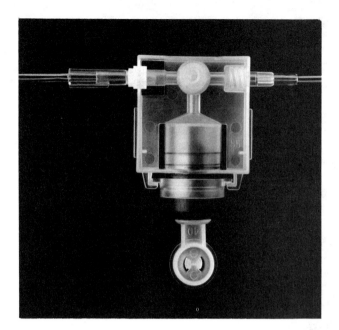

FIGURE 11.16
IMED® Accuset® cassette used with IMED Volumetric Infusion pumps divides each stroke into several hundred pulses for constant and accurate delivery at set infusion rate. Courtesy of IMED Corp., San Diego, Calif.

mixtures. It will alarm "Infusion Complete" when it senses an empty container and provide 1 ml per hour KVO rate. It has a broad occlusion pressure rate. Its automatic priming, touch-sensitive selector button, facilitating set-up, and easy-to-read rate and volume displays make this pump easy to use.

The Valleylab Infutrol 7000* is a new pump specifically designed for use in intensive care and other specialty areas (Figure 11.17). It is ideal for infusing minute amounts of critical drugs, the wide infusion dose range being 0.1–699.9 ml per hour in 0.1 ml increments. It has an automatic KVO of less than 1 ml per hour. This is a microprocessor-controlled, adjustable, positive-pressure device which, through its exclusive Patient Occlusion Monitor, has the unique ability to detect early warning of occluded or disconnected lines, thereby reducing complications. It provides positive pressure but at the same time can sense and automatically deliver at the minimum operating pressure.

Right on the front panel is the Patient Occlusion Monitor. The left side of the monitor contains a green light bar on a 1–10 scale which indicates, at a glance, the relative operating pressure of that specific patient. The other side contains a yellow limit light, also on a 1–10 scale. The pressure limits are adjustable from 2 to 10 psi above the required operating pressure of the patient. The unit automatically senses when the operating pressure reaches the adjustable limit set and immediately alarms. The pump adapts readily for ambulatory use with its battery life of 8 hours. It is an easy-to-use infusion pump with many safety features and clear signals and readouts.

Another unique pump is the *AccuPro Volumetric Infusion Pump*,† which

---

*Valleylab, Inc., Boulder, Co.

†American McGaw Laboratories, Inc., Irvine, Calif.; Division of American Hospital Supply Corporation.

Chapter 11 | Intravenous Equipment

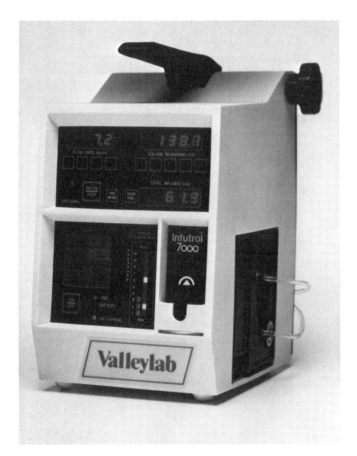

FIGURE 11.17
Valleylab Infutrol™ 7000 is a pump that automatically senses when the operating pressure reaches your adjustable pressure limit and immediately alarms. Courtesy of Valleylab, Inc., Boulder, Colo.

has unique piggyback capabilities that not only allow delivery of primary and piggyback infusions but can also deliver these infusions at different rates. The pump will recall primary infusion when in the piggyback mode.

*The Omni-Flow 4000,** a single pump, provides a completely programmable, multiple infusion system for delivery of up to 4 solutions in the exact dosages, sequence, and times. There is an automatic flush following delivery of a solution when required. Syringes or multiple-dose containers can replace piggyback containers.

The *Travenol Infusor*† is a totally new concept in infusion devices (Figure 11.18). It is completely self-powered; when a drug solution is injected into the infusor, the elastomeric balloon reservoir creates constant internal pressure. As the reservoir deflates, the medication is delivered through a filter and a controlled-size orifice, providing a continuous constant rate. Rates of drug administration are achieved by varying the concentration of the solution. The

---

*Omni-Flow, Woburn, Mass.

†Travenol Laboratories, Inc., Parenteral Products, Morton Grove, Ill.

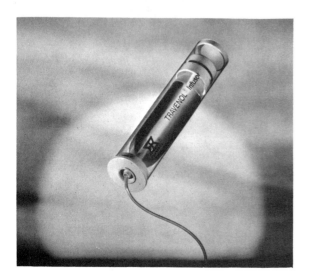

FIGURE 11.18
Travenol® Infusor. This total infusion system is completely self-powered for patients requiring slow, continuous intravenous administration of drug solutions. Contents are delivered through a filter and a controlled size orifaie. Courtesy of Travenol Laboratories, Inc., Deerfield, Ill.

infusion times (1–24 hours per Infusor) are achieved by adjusting the total volume. The Infusor operates, when filled, with a sustained internal pressure of approximately 490 mmHg. The flow may be stopped by securing a Luer Cap into the Luer locking adaptor. This small (just 6.5 inches long), lightweight (less than 3 oz filled), portable, and totally disposable device can deliver a continuous flow of 48 ml medication over approximately 24 hours. It is engineered to accommodate a wide range of drugs, dosage rates, and infusing times, providing slow continuous administration of drug solution, especially convenient for ambulatory patients.

The *IVAC Neo-Mate Variable Pressure Microinfusion Pump Model 565** is a microinfusion pump which uses a microbore burette volume administration set (Figure 11.19). It provides delivery rates of from 0.1 ml to 99.9 ml per hour at 0.1 ml increments. The output pressure can be adjusted from 0 to 499 mmHg or 0 to 699 cmH$_2$O to provide appropriate pressure for various applications; lower settings help detect flow restriction whereas higher settings may be required for arterial infusions. The volume limit range is 0.1–999.9 ml in 0.1 ml increments. An important feature is the automatic "Keep Open" rate; after a selected volume is infused an automatic "keep open" rate (1.0 ml per hour or selected rate, whichever is less) continues the infusion. Battery life is approximately 8 hours when fully charged (at 25 ml per hour). An alarm indicates a low battery. Among features designed for patient protection are a 2-piece Luer lock which secures the I.V. site connection and an air detector.

The *IMED 965 Micro-Volumetric Infusion Pump*† delivers fluid precisely at up to 99.9 ml per hour in 0.1 ml increments. It is flexible in that it has a unique capability for syringe application. The pump administers opaque fluids as well as clear fluids, including fat emulsions, blood, and blood components,

---

*IVAC Corporation, San Diego, Calif.
†IMED Corporation, San Diego, Calif.

Chapter 11 | Intravenous Equipment 163

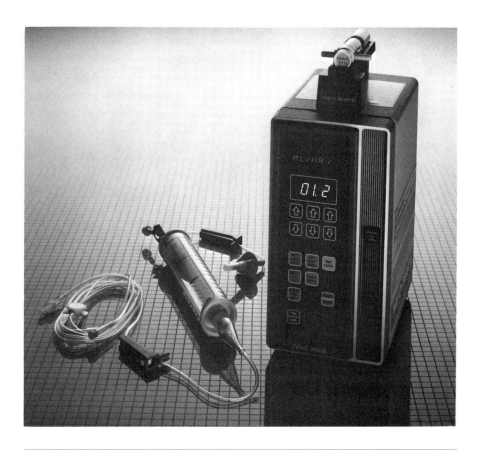

FIGURE 11.19
IVAC Neo-Mate Variable Pressure Microinfusion Pump-Model 565 provides both convenient medication administration and accurate volume control. Courtesy of IVAC Corp., San Diego, Calif.

as well as critical drugs. A nonoptional air detector system detects air of 0.05 ml or larger in all fluids. The IMED 965 uses Microset Administration Sets with a patented cassette, eliminating free flow. The set offers Luer lock fittings and microbore tubing. Non-PVC Microsets allow infusion of nitroglycerin, fat emulsions, and other drugs without the loss of drug absorption which has been documented to occur in PVC tubing. This pump is ideal for emergency use because it is portable and has a battery life of 22 hours at 50 ml per hour.

The Abbott/Parker Life Care 1500* is an ambulatory microinfuser. Smaller than a business card and weighing less than 2.5 oz, this tiny pocket-sized pump is useful in patient-controlled analgesia, antibiotic, chemotherapy, and other therapies.

---

*Parker Hannifin Corporation, Irvine, Calif., marketed by Abbott Laboratories, Inc.

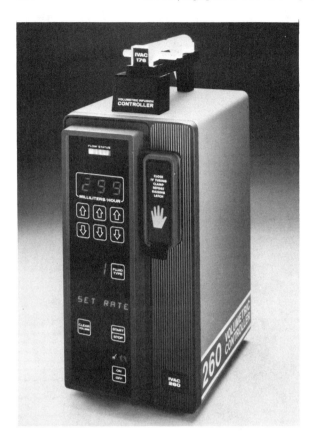

FIGURE 11.20
IVAC Volumetric Controller Model 260, with its new advanced microprocessor, provides set-up and alarm messages and displays early warnings of restrictions within the I.V. line and I.V. site. Courtesy of IVAC Corp., San Diego, Calif.

CONTROLLERS

Controllers operate strictly on gravity flow, unlike pumps. Gravity flow of fluid is regulated by a drop sensor and electric feedback mechanism. The alarm is activated when established flow rates are violated. Controllers reduce the potential for runaways and empty bottles, and they prevent unnecessary venipunctures. Infiltrations may be detected; back pressure from the infiltrating fluid is indicated by a reduced flow rate, which activates an alarm. Controllers assist the nurse in maintaining a constant, accurate flow rate, valuable when accuracy of fluid administration is required. Turco [8] indicates that the choice of device for 80 percent of intravenous fluid and drug administrations that require closely regulated flow may be the controller.

IVAC originated the controller concept in 1972 and is still a leader in this field. The *IVAC Volumetric Controller Model 260** is valuable for infusions that require site-monitoring capability in general care areas as well as

---

*IVAC Corporation, San Diego, Calif.

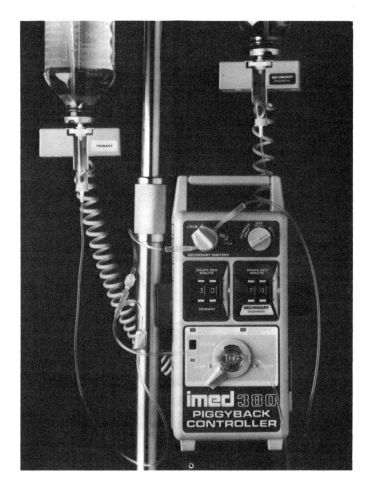

FIGURE 11.21
The IMED® 380 Piggyback Controller is a unique controller that delivers a second fluid at an independent rate automatically. Courtesy of IMED Corp., San Diego, Calif.

specialty care areas such as pediatrics, oncology, and neurology (Figure 11.20). This controller provides volumetric accuracy, delivering from 1 to 299 ml per hour. Simple to use, it detects most infiltrations and positionals as well as occlusions. It requires IVAC 60 drops per milliliter Blue Spike primary and secondary Solution Administration Sets. The alarm is activated by empty container, occlusion, most positionals and infiltrations, unobtainable rate, and low battery. It has the ability to prevent air from entering the infusion. The I.V. rate and the amount infused are displayed.

The *IMED 380 Piggyback Controller*† was the first piggyback controller to deliver a second fluid at an independent rate automatically (Figure 11.21). It runs the secondary fluid at one rate; when the container empties it automatically switches to an independent rate for the primary fluid. The flow-rate change is 1–99 drops per minute with independent selection of primary and secondary rates. It electronically monitors the I.V. site and the flow rates.

---

†IMED Corporation, San Diego, Calif.

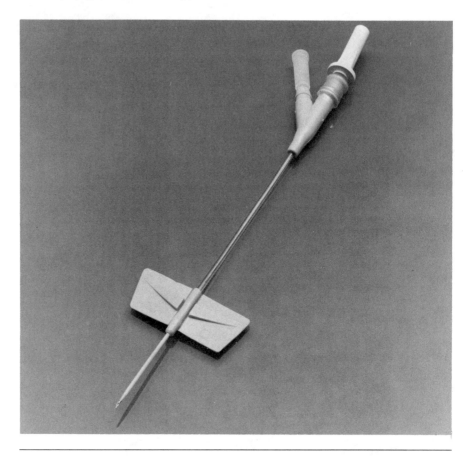

FIGURE 11.22
Angio-Set with "Y" adapter. Courtesy of the Deseret Company, Sandy, Utah.

CATHETERS

Innovations in catheter technology have produced catheters to meet the patient's every need, from peripheral infusion to the most sophisticated therapy; see also Chapters 18 and 19.

Catheters vary in gauge, length, composition, and design. The composition may be polyvinylchloride, polyurethane, or silicone. Thin-wall designed catheters provide increased flow rates which allow smaller sized catheters to be used. Most catheters are radiopaque or contain a stripe of radiopaque material for x-ray visualization.

Catheters may be over-the-needle (OTN), where the catheter, mounted on the needle, is slipped off the needle into the vein and the needle is removed; or inside-the-needle (INC), where the catheter is pushed through the needle until the desired length is in the vein, and the cutting edge is protected by a shield.

Some catheters are provided with wings and all the advantages of a small-vein needle on insertion and on taping (Figure 11.22). The adapter of the I.V. set connection is located a few inches from the catheter and provides ease and

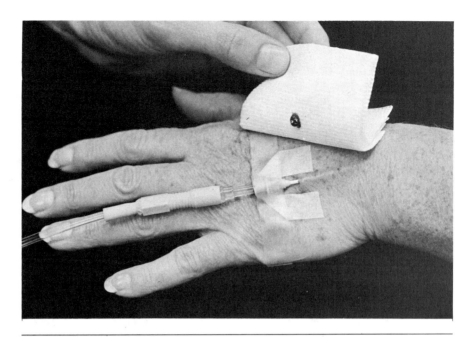

FIGURE 11.23
Quik-Cath® Radiopaque Intravascular over-the-needle Teflon catheter with a tapered, flat-bottomed hub and security extensions, interlocking notch and pin with preoriented bevel position indicator, and flashback chamber. Courtesy of Travenol Laboratories, Inc., Deerfield, Ill.

better technique when changing sets, reducing the potential for mechanical phlebitis and contamination. Such catheters are available with injection sites as an integral part of the catheter; the mixing of drugs or blood components with primary parenteral fluid is reduced to a minimum (0.4 ml), minimizing the potential of incompatibilities.

The *Jelco I.V. Catheter** is a thin-wall virgin Teflon† catheter. It is available as a radiopaque cannula or as a Transparent Virgin Teflon cannula with encapsulated stripes. The latter provides a visible flashback of blood when the cannula is introduced into the vein, and the stripes allow x-ray detection. The color-coded hub indicates the catheter gauge.

The *Accucath Intravenous Catheter*‡ is an over-the-needle catheter which features a bonded silicone lubricant for smooth entry, an antikink sleeve, a bevel-indicator lock, and optional stabilizing wings.

The *Quick-Cath*§, a radiopaque thin-wall over-the-needle Teflon catheter with a double-tapered tip and a siliconized short-bevel needle provides a smooth vessel entry (Figure 11.23). The hub, tapered and flat-bottomed with

---

*Critikon, a Johnson and Johnson Company, Tampa, Fla.

†Trademark DuPont Company.

‡Burron Medical Inc. Bethlehem, Pa.

§Parenteral Products Division, Travenol Laboratories, Deerfield, Ill.

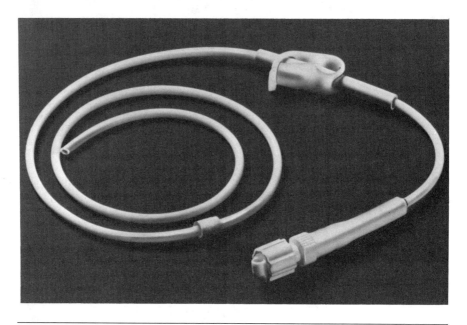

FIGURE 11.24
Corcath™ Vascular Catheter, silicone elastomer, designed for chemotherapy, hyperalimentation, or other long-term therapy. Courtesy of CORMED,™ Inc., Medina, N.Y.

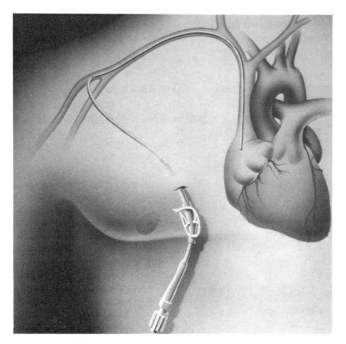

FIGURE 11.25
Corcath™ Vascular Catheter in place. Note the tunneling of the catheter before it enters the vasculature. Courtesy of CORMED,™ Inc., Medina, N.Y.

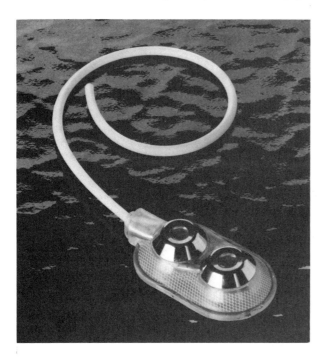

FIGURE 11.26
MediPort®-DL. The first double lumen implantable vascular access port with a separate septum/reservoir bodies allowing infusion of incompatible drugs, blood sampling, and continuous infusion plus many other possibilities. Courtesy of CORMED,™ Inc., Medina, N.Y.

winglike extensions, provides taping support; an interlocking notch and pin with preoriented bevel position indicator indicates the needle bevel position; and the clear flashback chamber permits detection of blood flashback on entry of the catheter into the vein. The wings allow periodic inspection of the puncture site since the puncture is free of tape.

Central Venous Catheters

Long-term infusion therapy has brought about many innovations in the central venous catheter (see also Part VI).

The *Arrow-Howes Multi-Lumen Catheter** is the first multilumen central venous catheter that, through one puncture site, provides for central venous pressure (CVP) monitoring and multiple infusions. This polyurethane radiopaque catheter contains three internal lumens with separate ports. The design allows for sampling of blood upstream from the ports used for infusions. The *Arrow Two-Lumen Central Venous Catheter* is ideal when only 2 lines are required.

Intrasil† is a silicone central venous catheter that permits peripheral access to the central venous system through a slotted needle, virtually eliminating the likelihood of shearing or damage to the catheter. The catheter with stylet is enclosed within a rotary introducer; the catheter is advanced by rotating the introducer top.

The *Corcath*‡ *Vascular Catheter* is a silicone elastomer catheter designed

---

*Arrow International, Inc., Reading, Pa.

†Vicra Division of Travenol Laboratories, Inc., Dallas, Tex.

‡Cormed Inc., Medina, N.Y.

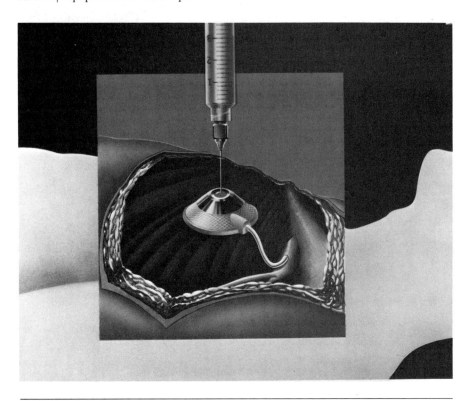

FIGURE 11.27
MediPort. The injection needle is inserted into the easily located needle insertion port. Its use provides introduction of fluids or medications into the body. Courtesy of CORMED,™ Inc., Medina, N.Y.

for chemotherapy, hyperalimentation, and other long-term therapies (Figure 11.24). The Dacron cuff promotes tissue growth, providing stability and a barrier against infection. A color-coded female Luer lock connector is permanently attached to the exterior segment. The catheter enters the selected vein from a subcutaneous tunnel formed on the anterior chest wall and exits through the chest wall about 6–8 inches from the vein insertion (Figure 11.25).

Implantable Vascular Access Devices

Totally implantable vascular access devices are a new concept which is increasingly replacing the external central venous catheters. The three different devices currently approved for use are MediPort,* Port-A-Cath,† and Infuse-A-Port.‡

The MediPort-DL is the first double-lumen implantable vascular access port (Figure 11.26). It consists of a dual lumen radiopaque silicone rubber catheter, 20 inches in length with a priming capacity of approximately 2.0 cc

---

*Cormed Inc., Medina, N.Y.

†Pharmacia Laboratories, Division of Pharmacia Inc., Piscataway, N.J.

‡Infusaid Inc., Norwood, Mass.

each lumen. A pair of rigid reservoir bodies with an inlet septum in the center of each is connected to the dual outlet catheter. The reservoir closest to the outlet catheter is connected to the catheter with the largest lumen. The self-sealing rubber septum accepts multiple punctures from a 22 gauge special "non-coring" needle (Figure 11.27). This device provides an easily located needle insertion site.

Complete information on central venous catheters is to be found in Chapters 18 and 19.

REFERENCES

1. Adriani, J. Venipuncture. *Am. J. Nurs.* 62:70, 1962.

2. Application Report AR-11. *Low Volume-Sterilizing Filtration*. Bedford, Mass.: Multipore Corporation, 1969, p.3.

3. Boyan, C. P. Cold or warmed blood for massive transfusion. *Ann. Surg.* 160:282, 1964.

4. Center for Disease Control. Guidelines for prevention of intravascular infection. *J. NITA* 5(1):39–90, 1982.

5. National Intravenous Therapy Association. NITA standards — I.V. therapy. *J. NITA* 5(1):24–29, 1982.

6. Stoklosa, M. J. *Pharmaceutical Calculations* (6th ed.). Philadelphia: Lea & Febiger, 1974, pp. 236, 237.

7. Tarail, R. Practice of fluid therapy. *J.A.M.A.* 171:45–49, 1950.

8. Turco, S. J. Inaccuracies in I.V. flow rates and the use of pumps and controllers. *J. Parent. Drug Assoc.* 32(5):242, 1978.

9. Webb, J. W., and Monahan, J. J. Intravenous infusion pumps — an added dimension to parenteral therapy. *Am. J. Hosp. Pharm.* 29:54–59, 1972.

10. Webb, J. W. Contemporary comments on infusion pumps. *J. NITA* 4(1):9–14, 1981.

CHAPTER 12

Techniques of Intravenous Therapy

Ada Lawrence Plumer

APPROACH TO THE PATIENT

The manner with which the nurse approaches the patient may have a direct bearing on that patient's response to intravenous therapy. Because an undesirable response can affect the patient's ability to accept treatment, emphasis must be placed on the significance of the nurse's manner and approach.

Intravenous therapy, though routine to the nurse, may be a new and frightening experience to the patient who is unfamiliar with the procedure. Patients may have heard rumors of fatalities associated with infusions or may misinterpret the treatment. By explaining the procedure, the nurse will alleviate fears and help the patient to accept therapy.

The critically ill patient is particularly susceptible to fears which can at times become exaggerated, triggering an undesirable autonomic nervous system response usually known as a vasovagal reaction. Such a reaction may manifest itself in the form of syncope and can be prevented if the nurse appears confident and reassures the patient. Sympathetic reaction may follow syncope and result in vasoconstriction. Peripheral collapse then limits available veins, complicating the venipuncture. Repeated attempts at venipuncture can result in an experience so traumatic as to affect the further course of fluid therapy. Only a skilled person should perform a venipuncture on an anxious patient with limited and difficult veins.

Reactions to exaggerated fear may not only make therapy difficult, but may constitute a real threat to the patient with severe cardiac disease. Fear incites stimulation of the adrenal medulla to secrete the vasopressors, which help maintain blood pressure and increase the work of the heart. Increased adrenal cortical secretions result in (1) sodium and chloride retention, which causes water retention; and (2) loss of cellular potassium, which draws water with it into the intravascular system. Increased antidiuretic hormone secretions cause a decreased urinary output, which results in retention of fluids and an increase in blood volume [4]. Such an increase may be sufficient to send a patient with an overburdened vascular system into pulmonary edema.

SELECTING THE VEIN

The selection of the vein may be a deciding factor in the success of the infusion and in the preservation of veins for future therapy. The most prominent vein is not necessarily the most suitable for venipuncture: prominence may be due to a sclerosed condition which occludes the lumen and interferes with the flow of solution, or the prominent vein may be located in an area impractical for infusion purposes. Scrutiny of the veins in both arms is desirable before a choice is made. The prime factors to be considered in selecting a vein are (1) suitable location, (2) condition of the vein, (3) purpose of the infusion, and (4) duration of therapy.

Location

Most superficial veins are accessible for venipuncture, but some of these veins, because of their location, are not practical. The *antecubital veins* are such veins, located over an area of joint flexion where any motion could dislodge the cannula and cause infiltration or result in mechanical phlebitis. If these large veins are impaired or damaged, phlebothrombosis may occur, which can limit the many available hand veins. The antecubital veins offer excellent sources for withdrawing blood and may be used numerous times without damage to the vein, provided good technique and sharp needles are used. But one infusion of long duration may traumatize the vein, limiting these vessels which most readily provide ample quantities of blood when large samples are needed.

Because of the close proximity of the arteries to the veins in the antecubital fossa, special care must be observed to prevent intraarterial injection when medications are introduced. An artery can generally be detected by the thicker and tougher wall, the brighter red blood, and usually the presence of a pulse. *Aberrant arteries* in the antecubital area have been found to exist in 1 person out of 10. When a patient complains of severe pain in the hand or arm upon infusion, an arteriospasm due to an intraarterial injection is to be suspected, and the infusion must be stopped immediately.

Surgery often dictates which extremity is to be used. Veins should be avoided in the affected arm of an axillary dissection, such as a radical mastectomy; the circulation may be embarrassed, affecting the flow of the infusion and increasing the edema. When the patient is turned sideways during the operation the upper arm is used for the intravenous infusion; increased venous pressure in the lower arm may interfere with the free flow of the solution.

The use of the veins in the lower extremities is frequently challenged. As stated in Chapter 6, these objections arise from the danger of pulmonary embolism due to a thrombus extending into the deep veins. Complications may also arise from the stagnant blood in varicosities; pooling of infused medications can cause untoward reactions when a toxic concentration reaches the circulating blood. Varicosities, because of the stagnant blood, are susceptible to trauma. Phlebitis interferes with ambulation of the patient.

Center of Disease Control (CDC) guidelines strongly recommend that "In adults, the upper extremity (or if necessary, subclavian and jugular sites) should be used in preference to lower extremity sites for I.V. cannulation. All cannulas inserted into a lower extremity should be changed as soon as a satisfactory site can be established elsewhere."[2]

Condition of the Vein

Frequently the dorsal metacarpal veins provide points of entry that should be utilized first in order to preserve the proximal veins for further therapy. The use of these veins depends upon their condition. In some elderly patients, the dorsal metacarpal veins may be a poor choice; blood extravasation occurs more readily in small thin veins, and difficulty may be encountered in adequately securing the cannula because of thin skin and lack of supportive tissue. At times these veins do not dilate sufficiently to allow for successful venipuncture; when hypovolemia occurs the peripheral veins collapse more quickly than do the large ones.

Palpation of the vein is an important step in determining the condition of the vein and in differentiating it from a pulsating artery. A thrombosed vein may be detected by its lack of resilience, by its hard, cord-like feeling, and by the ease with which it rolls. Use of such traumatized veins can result only in repeated venipunctures, pain, and undue stress.

Occasionally when thrombosis from multiple infusions interferes with the flow of solution and limits available veins, the venipuncture may be performed with the cannula inserted in the direction of the distal end; lack of valves in these small peripheral veins permits rerouting of the solution and a bypassing of the involved vein.

Often large veins may be detected by palpation and offer advantage over the smaller but more readily discernible veins. Owing to the small blood volume, the more superficial veins may not be easily palpated and may not make a satisfactory choice for venipuncture.

Continual use by the nurse of the same fingers for palpation will increase their sensitivity. The thumb should never be used since it is not as sensitive as the fingers; also a pulse may be detected in the nurse's thumb, and this may be confused with an aberrant artery.

Although not apparent, edema may conceal an available vein; pressure for a few seconds with the fingers often helps to disperse the fluid and define the vein.

Purpose of the Infusion

The purpose of the infusion dictates the rate of flow and the solution to be infused — two factors which inherently affect the selection of the vein. When large quantities of fluid are to be rapidly infused, or when positive pressure is indicated, a large vein must be used. When fluids with a high viscosity such as packed cells are required, a vein with an adequate blood volume is necessary to ensure flow of the solution.

Large veins are used when hypertonic solutions or solutions containing irritating drugs are to be infused. Such solutions traumatize small veins; the supply of blood in these veins is not sufficient to dilute the infused fluid.

Duration of Therapy

A prolonged course of therapy requires multiple infusions, which makes preservation of the veins essential. Performing the venipuncture distally with each subsequent puncture proximal to the previous one and alternating arms will contribute to this preservation.

The patient's comfort is also a factor that should be considered when infusions are required over an extended period of time; avoiding areas over joint flexion and performing venipunctures on veins located on the dorsal surface of the extremities will provide more freedom and comfort to the patient.

SELECTING THE CANNULA

Infusion may be administered through a plastic cannula or steel cannula (see also Chapter 19).

Three types of cannulas are available:

1. ONC (over-the-needle) catheter. Once the venipuncture is made, the catheter is slipped off the needle into the vein and the steel needle removed. Obturators are available but are not recommended for use by NITA [5]. They are inserted into the catheter to maintain patency for intermittent infusion.

2. INC (inside-the-needle) catheter. The venipuncture is performed and the catheter is then pushed through the needle until the desired length is within the lumen of the vein; the cutting edge is then protected by a shield to prevent the catheter from being severed.

3. Cutdown catheter. This catheter is inserted by means of a minor surgical procedure (cutdown) performed by the physician. This procedure has been largely replaced by central venous catheterization (see Part VI).

The choice of catheter depends upon the purpose of the infusion and the condition and availability of the veins.

Over-the-needle catheters are used in the operating room to ensure a ready route for the administration of blood and fluid. In long-term therapy these catheters serve a purpose when difficulty arises in keeping the needle in the vein. There are two schools of thought regarding the choice of over-the-needle catheters for routine infusions. Both National Intravenous Therapy Association (NITA) and CDC Guidelines are considered national standards. NITA states that over-the-needle catheters should be used for routine peripheral intravenous infusions [5]. CDC only moderately recommends the use of these cannulas for routine peripheral intravenous infusions and only if the hospital can assure the replacement of these cannulas every 48–72 hours; otherwise it recommends the stainless steel cannula for routine peripheral I.V. infusions and the plastic cannula "reserved for those clinical settings when a secure route for vascular access is imperative [2]."

Inside-the-needle catheters are used when a longer catheter is desired. They afford less risk of infiltration than does the steel cannula, often being used for administering drugs or hypertonic solutions which may cause necrosis if extravasation occurs. NITA does not recommend these cannulas for routine peripheral use.

The cutdown catheter is required when (1) veins become exhausted from prolonged therapy, (2) obesity obscures the veins, and (3) peripheral veins have collapsed from shock.

Catheters are made of polyethylene, Teflon, and Silastic. For many years polyvinyl chloride was used almost exclusively. Ideally the catheter should be of a hemo-repellant material to reduce the risk of thrombi formation on the catheter. Silicone catheters are thought to be helpful in this respect. Most catheters are fully radiopaque for detection by x-ray in the event the catheter is severed and lost in the circulation.

Steel needles are of two types, the steel cannula and the small-vein needle, often referred to as a Butterfly,* scalp vein, Miniset,† or pediatric set. The *steel cannula*, once the traditional intravenous cannula, is made of a metal such as stainless steel that is noncorrosive and relatively inert in relation to the tissues. It is usually siliconized for ease of insertion and to minimize clot formation. It varies in length and gauge. The gauge refers to both the inside and the outside diameters of the lumen — the smaller the gauge, the larger the lumen. Steel needles may be designed as *thin wall*. Because the wall of the needle is thinner than that of the standard needle, a larger lumen is obtained for the same external diameter, offering the advantage of higher flow rates. Today, the steel needle is most commonly used for drawing blood samples.

In the past it was common hospital practice to infuse intravenous fluids once or twice a day over a 3- or 4-hour period. Because of this short duration, the incidence of phlebitis and infiltration was kept to a minimum. The steel needle provided a practical means of administering intravenous fluids with a minimum of complications. With the advent of intravenous antibiotics and other drugs, hospital practice changed, and intravenous fluids are often administered on a keep-open or intermittent basis. The standard steel needle has given way to the small-vein needle. NITA does not recommend the use of the small-vein needle for routine vascular access because of the tendency of this cannula to dislodge. The steel cannula is useful only for short-term or one-dose peripheral I.V. therapy.

The *small-vein needle* is similar to the steel cannula, with the hub replaced with 2 flexible wings. Originally designed for pediatric and geriatric use, it has been used in prolonged therapy for all ages. Two types of small-vein needles are available, one with a short length of plastic tubing and a permanently attached resealable injection site, the other with a variable length of plastic tubing permanently attached to a female Luer adapter which accommodates an administration set. The small-vein needle with the resealable injection site offers a method for the intermittent administration of medications or fluids. A dilute solution of heparin maintains patency of the needle when it is not in use (see Chapter 20).

The small-vein needle is approximately ¾ inch long and ranges in size from a 27-gauge bore to a 16-gauge bore. It has definite advantages: the short bevel reduces the risk of infiltration from puncture to the wall of the vein, and the plastic wings provide a firm grip for inserting the needle and better control in performing the venipuncture. The wings fold flat against the skin, affording better anchoring power than the straight steel needle with a bulky hub.

The factors to be considered in selecting a steel needle are length of bevel, gauge, and length of the needle.

---

*Trade name, Deseret Co., Sandy, Utah.
†Trade name, Travenol Laboratories, Inc., Deerfield, Ill.

A short *bevel* reduces the risk of (1) trauma to the endothelial wall, (2) infiltration from a puncture to the posterior wall, and (3) hematoma or extravasation occurring when the steel needle enters the vein. When a steel needle with a long bevel is inserted into the vessel, blood may leak into the tissues before the entire bevel is within the lumen of the vein.

Whenever possible the *gauge* of the needle should be appreciably smaller than the lumen of the vein to be entered; when the gauge of the needle approaches the size of the vein, trauma may occur. When a large needle occludes the flow of blood, irritating solutions flowing through the vein, with no dilution of blood, may cause chemical phlebitis. Mechanical phlebitis may result from motion and pressure exerted by the needle on the endothelial wall of the vein.

When large amounts of fluid are required, a needle of adequate size must be used; a small lumen interferes with the flow of solution. As Adriani [1] stated,

> The flow of blood varies inversely as the fourth power of the radius of the lumen of the needle. Thus, a needle with an internal radius of 1 mm. delivering 1 cc. of blood with a fixed pressure on the plunger or in the infusion bottle delivers only $1/16$ of a cc. when the radius is reduced to $1/2$ mm.

A large needle is also required with fluids of high viscosity. The rate of flow of the solution decreases in proportion to the viscosity of the fluid.

The flow of the solution varies inversely with the *length of the needle shaft*. If the length of the needle is increased, other conditions being equal, the volume flowing will be reduced [1]. Use of a short needle for infusions reduces the risk of infiltration. Because a short needle affords more play than a long needle, more motion is needed to puncture the vessel wall.

SECURING PROPER LIGHTING

The importance of proper lighting should not be overlooked. A few extra seconds spent in obtaining adequate light may actually save time and free the patient from unnecessary venipunctures. The ideal light is either an ample amount of daylight or a spotlight which does not shine directly on the vein, but which leaves enough shadow for clearly defining the vessel.

APPLYING THE TOURNIQUET

Special care must be taken to distend the vein adequately. To achieve this, a soft rubber tourniquet is applied with enough pressure to impede the venous flow while the arterial flow is maintained; if the radial pulse cannot be felt, the tourniquet is too tight. In order to fill the veins to capacity, pressure is applied until radial pulsation ceases, and then released until pulsation begins. A blood pressure cuff may be used; inflate the cuff and then release it until the pressure drops to just below the diastolic pressure.

The tourniquet is applied to the mid-forearm if the selected vein is in the dorsum of the hand. If the selected vein is in the forearm, the tourniquet is applied to the upper arm.

Very little pressure is applied when performing venipunctures on patients with sclerosed veins. If the pressure is too great or the tourniquet is left on for an extended length of time the vein will become hard and tortuous, causing added difficulty when the cannula is introduced. For some sclerosed veins a tourniquet is unnecessary and only makes the phlebotomy more difficult.

If pressure exerted by the tourniquet does not fill the veins sufficiently, the patient may be asked to open and close his or her fist. The action of the muscles will force the blood into the veins, causing them to distend considerably more. Frequently a light tapping will help fill the vein. It may be helpful, before applying the tourniquet, to lower the extremity below the heart level to increase the blood supply to the veins. Occasionally these methods are inadequate to fill the vein sufficiently. In such cases application of heat is helpful. To be effective the heat must be applied to the entire extremity for 10 to 20 minutes and retained until the venipuncture is performed.

PREPARATION FOR VENIPUNCTURE

Check Solution and Container

Careful inspection must be made to ensure that the fluid is clear and free of particulate matter and that the container is intact — that there are no cracks in the glass bottle or holes in the plastic bag (see Chapter 17). The label must be checked to verify that the correct solution is being used and that the container is not outdated. Indicate the time and the date the bottle is opened; after 24 hours the fluid is outdated and should not be used.

Attach Administration Set to Fluid Container

The set is attached to the container by squeezing the drip chamber and entering the bottle with a thrust, not a twisting motion. The chamber is released, causing immediate function of the air vent and filling of the drip chamber on the suspension of the bottle. This prevents leakage of fluid through the air vent and expedites clearing the infusion set of air, thus preventing bubbles from entering the tubing. In systems that do not require air venting — plastic bags and semirigid bottles — squeezing the drip chamber before insertion avoids the introduction of air into the container.

Height of the Fluid Container

The fluid container is suspended at approximately 3 feet above the injection site. At this height adequate pressure is provided to achieve a maximum flow rate. The greater the height of the container, the greater the force with which the fluid will flow into the vein should the adjusting clamp release, and the greater the risk of speed shock.

Preparing the Patient and Provision of Privacy

Visitors should be asked to leave the room during procedure and curtains closed if a roommate is present. The patient should be in a comfortable position with his or her arm on a flat surface. If necessary a strip of tape is used to secure the arm to an armboard and prevent an uncooperative or disoriented patient from jerking the arm while the cannula is being inserted.

If the area selected for venipuncture is hairy, clipping the hair will permit better cleansing of the skin and make removal of the cannula less painful when the infusion is terminated. Shaving is not recommended (see Chapter 17).

TECHNIQUES IN VENIPUNCTURE

Direct Method or One-Step Entry

This method is performed with a thrust of the cannula through the skin and into the vein with one quick motion. The cannula enters the skin directly over the vein. This technique is excellent as long as large veins are available. However, owing to the many times one must resort to the use of small veins, this is not the preferred technique. Such an attempt at entry into the small veins will result in hematomas. A nurse who chooses to use this technique will never be adept at phlebotomies on tiny venules when the situation arises.

Indirect Method

This method consists of two complete motions:

1. Insertion of the cannula through the skin. The cannula enters the skin below the point where the vein is visible; entering the skin above the vein tends to depress the vein, obscuring its position.
2. Relocation of the vein and entry into the vein.

Recommended Skin Preparation [2]

The injection site should be scrubbed with an antiseptic and allowed to remain in contact for at least 30 seconds prior to venipuncture.

1. Tincture of iodine 1–2% is preferred.
2. Isopropyl 70% alcohol is recommended if the patient is sensitive to iodine.

BASIC VENIPUNCTURE

The basic venipuncture is performed as follows (Figure 12.1):

1. Put on gloves.
2. Apply tourniquet and select vein.
3. Prepare skin according to recommendations.
4. After establishing a minimum rate of flow by adjusting the clamp, kink the infusion tubing between the third and little fingers of the right hand. When the kinked tubing is released, the minimum rate of flow will prevent a rapid infusion of fluid and drugs with the potential danger of speed shock. Obstructing the flow of solution manually expedites the procedure and leaves the hands free for anchoring the steel cannula and caring for any collected blood samples.
5. Hold the patient's hand or arm with the left hand, using the thumb to keep the skin taut and to anchor the vein to prevent rolling.
6. Place the steel cannula in line with the vein, about ½ inch below the proposed site of entry. The bevel-up position of the cannula facilitates

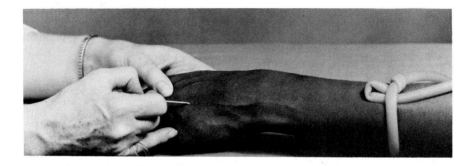

FIGURE 12.1
Basic venipuncture. Infusion tubing is kinked between third and little fingers. Left thumb keeps skin taut and anchors vein. The needle is held in line with the vein at 45-degree angle.

venipuncture and produces less trauma to the skin and the vein on puncture.

In small veins it is often necessary to enter the vein with the bevel down to prevent extravasation; any readjustment of the cannula should be made before releasing the tourniquet to prevent puncturing the vein and producing a hematoma [4].

7. Insert the cannula through skin and tissue at a 45-degree angle.
8. Relocate the vein and decrease the cannula angle slightly.
9. Slowly, with downward motion followed at once by raising point, pick up vein, leveling cannula until almost flush with skin.
10. On entering the vein there may be a backflow of blood, which indicates successful entry. There may be no blood return if the vein is small. Usually pinching the rubber tube just above the cannula adapter and then releasing it will back the blood into the plastic tubing. If doubtful of the cannula's position in the vein, check by this method. With experience the fingers will become sensitive to the cannula's entering the vein — the resistance encountered as the cannula meets the wall of the vein and the snap felt at the loss of resistance as the cannula enters the lumen. This is more difficult to discern on thin-walled veins with small blood volume. To prevent a through puncture, move the cannula slowly, checking at each movement for a backflow of blood.
11. Once the vein is entered, move the cannula cautiously up the lumen for about ¾ inch.
12. Release the tourniquet.
13. Release the pressure exerted by the little finger, unkinking the tube and allowing the solution to flow.
14. Check carefully for any signs of swelling.
15. Remove gloves. Wash hands.

Chapter 12 | Techniques of Intravenous Therapy

If the vein has sustained a through puncture (evidenced by a developing hematoma) and the venipuncture is unsuccessful, the cannula should be immediately removed and pressure applied to the site. Never reapply a tourniquet to the extremity immediately after a venipuncture; a hematoma will occur, limiting veins and providing an excellent culture medium for bacteria.

ANCHORING THE STEEL CANNULA AND SECURING THE ARMBOARD

The Cannula

1. Use 1-inch wide tape over the hub. Tape the cannula flush with the skin; no elevation of the hub is necessary, and it would only increase the risk of a through puncture from the point of the cannula.
2. Place a ½-inch strip of tape — adhesive up — under the hub of the cannula. Place one end tightly and diagonally over the cannula. Repeat with the other end, crossing the first. This secures the cannula firmly and prevents any sideward movement. Avoid placing tape directly over the actual injection site.
3. Loop the tubing and secure it with tape independently of the cannula. This eliminates dislodging the cannula by an accidental pull on the tubing.
4. Apply sterile, transparent, semi-permeable membrane adhesive dressing, over the cannula entrance site to allow for regular, standardized inspection.
5. Indicate type, gauge, insertion date, and initials near the dressing and in the medical record.

The Armboard

The use of an armboard is helpful in immobilizing the extremity when undue motion can result in infiltration or phlebitis. It is a valuable aid in restraining the arm when infusions are initiated on uncooperative, disoriented, or elderly patients or children, or when the cannula is inserted on the dorsum of the hand or in an area of joint flexion. When the metacarpal veins are used the fingers should be immobilized to prevent any movement of the cannula that could result in phlebitis.

The function of the hand may be endangered and even permanently impaired by the widespread hospital practice of flattening the hand on an armboard during intravenous therapy. This complication results from failure to recognize that the hand has both transverse and longitudinal arches and that if the knuckle joints (metacarpophalangeal) are immobilized in a straight position, they will develop contracture that will prevent motion (Figure 12.2). Patients on long-term therapy with edema or muscular weakness are particularly vulnerable. Intensive physical therapy, splinting, and even surgery may be required to restore mobility.

To preserve maximal function, the hand should be immobilized in a functional position on the armboard. Robert Leffert[*] recommends 20 degrees of

---

[*]Chief of the Surgical Upper Extremity Rehabilitation Unit and Department of Rehabilitation Medicine, Massachusetts General Hospital, Boston, Mass.

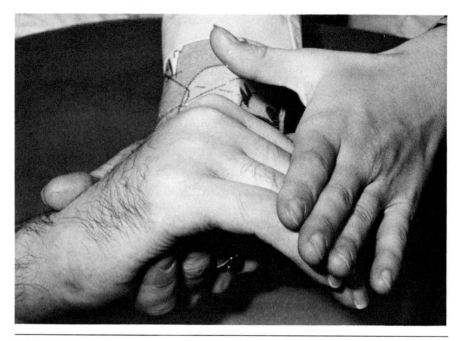

FIGURE 12.2
Maximal flexion of the hand of a patient who has developed a contracture from positioning the hand in a flat position. The patient cannot make a fist.

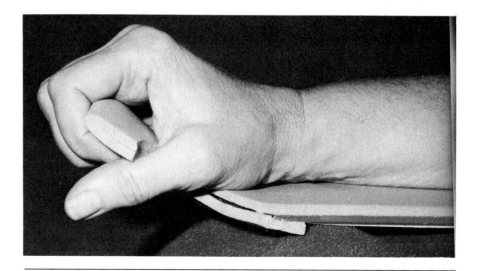

FIGURE 12.3
The hand is immobilized in a functional position on the armboard to prevent contracture, which may endanger or permanently impair the function of the hand.

dorsiflexion of the wrist, 45–60 degrees of flexion of the metacarpophalangeal joints, with the palm slightly cupped and the flexion increasing from index to little finger. The thumb should be in opposition so that it is away from the palm in the posture it would assume in pinch (Figure 12.3).

If a plastic armboard is used, cover it with absorbent paper or bandage to prevent the arm from perspiring and sticking to the board. Make certain that any tape placed on the cannula is independent of the board so that a motion of the arm on the board will not cause a pull on the cannula. If restraint of the arm is necessary, the restraint is secured to the board, not to the patient's arm above the puncture area; such restraint might act as a tourniquet, causing a backflow of blood into the cannula, resulting in clotting and obstruction of the flow.

THE "INSIDE-THE-NEEDLE" CATHETER AND ASSOCIATED RISKS

Because this type of catheter is associated with a higher incidence of serious complications, only the experienced therapist, alert to the risks involved, should attempt venipuncture by this method. The inherent danger of infection from bacteria invading the vein through the cutaneous opening and being carried along the plastic cannula makes thorough skin preparation necessary. Trauma caused by the insertion of a large catheter is increased when performed by an inexperienced operator.

A catheter severed by the cutting edge of the needle can result in a serious complication when lost in the bloodstream. A catheter introduced into a vein over a joint flexion increases the risk of complication if the extremity is not immobilized.

An inside-the-needle catheter facilitates prolonged therapy but increases the risk of thrombophlebitis. Limiting the length of time the catheter is in use reduces the incidence of phlebitis; a time limit is sometimes difficult to enforce, however, since veins may be exhausted in a critically ill patient whose life depends upon infusion therapy.

Insertion of the Inside-the-Needle Catheter

1. Put on gloves.
2. Apply a tourniquet and select the vein.
3. Prepare the injection site area according to recommendations.
4. Make the venipuncture.
5. Gently thread the catheter through the lumen of the needle into the vein until the desired length has been introduced.
6. Apply digital pressure on the vein to hold the catheter in place; withdraw the needle.
7. Apply pressure with a sterile sponge for 30 seconds to minimize bleeding through the puncture site.
8. Attach the needle to the infusion set, and regulate the flow rate. NEVER WITHDRAW THE CATHETER BACK THROUGH THE NEEDLE. If the

venipuncture is unsuccessful, the needle and catheter must be removed together; to pull the catheter back through the needle may sever the catheter and result in its loss in the circulation.

9. Slip the shield from the base of the needle over the bevel and tape; the shield must be kept in place to protect the cutting edge of the needle and prevent its severing the catheter. A tongue depressor is frequently used to secure the needle and catheter to further guard against kinking and breaking of the catheter at the junction of the needle.
10. Tape the catheter to prevent motion.
11. Ascertain the patency and position of the catheter in the vein.
12. Topical antibiotic or antiseptic ointment should be applied to the injection site.
13. Apply a sterile dressing; the puncture made by the needle is larger than the inlying catheter, and seepage of fluid and infection can occur.
14. Indicate length, gauge, and type of catheter, initials of operator, and date of insertion on tape near dressing and in medical record.
15. Use an armboard if the catheter lies over a point of flexion — motion contributes to phlebitis. The arm must not be fastened tightly to the armboard; vascular occlusion results in a plugged catheter, and stasis edema may occur.
16. Remove gloves. Wash hands.

THE "OVER-THE-NEEDLE" CATHETER

Venipuncture and Installation

1. Put on gloves.
2. Apply a tourniquet and select the vein.
3. Prepare the injection site according to recommendations. If palpation of the vein is necessary, prepare the finger tip in the same manner. Do not touch the proposed insertion site.
4. Perform the venipuncture in the usual manner. When the needle has punctured the venous wall, introduce it ½ inch farther to ensure entry of the catheter into the lumen of the vein.
5. Hold the needle in place and slowly slide the catheter hub until the desired length is in the vein (Figure 12.4). IF THE VENIPUNCTURE IS UNSUCCESSFUL, DO NOT REINSERT THE NEEDLE INTO THE CATHETER. To do so can sever the catheter.
6. Remove the needle by holding the catheter hub in place. To minimize leakage of blood while removing the needle and connecting the infusion set, apply pressure on the vein beyond the catheter with the little finger (Figure 12.5).
7. Attach the administration set, which has been previously cleared of air, and regulate the rate of flow.

Chapter 12 | Techniques of Intravenous Therapy

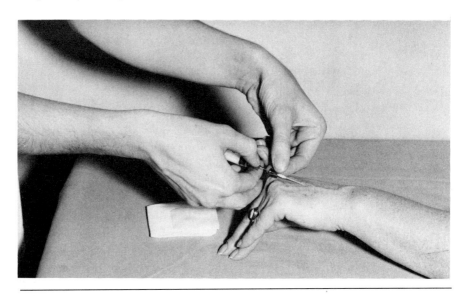

FIGURE 12.4
The hub of the needle is held in place while catheter (Jelco I.V.) is slipped off the shaft until the desired length is in the vein; CDC revised recommendations require gloves to be worn. Courtesy of Critikon Company, Division of Johnson & Johnson, Tampa, Fla.

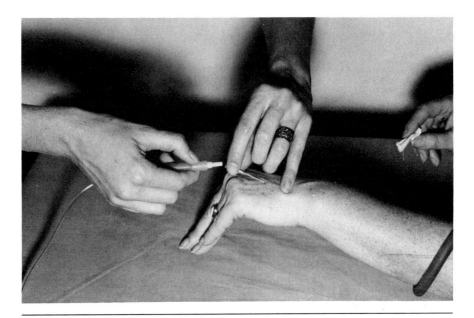

FIGURE 12.5
Pressure on vein reduces leakage of blood when needle is withdrawn from catheter (Jelco) and catheter is connected to infusion set; gloves must be worn. Courtesy of Critikon Company, Division of Johnson & Johnson, Tampa, Fla.

8. Topical antiseptic iodophor ointment should be considered or a broad spectrum antiseptic ointment for patients sensitive to iodine.
9. Tape catheter securely to prevent motion that could contribute to phlebitis. Avoid taping over injection site; cover site with sterile sponge.
10. Loop the tubing and tape independent of the catheter to prevent an accidental pull from withdrawing the catheter.
11. Indicate the length, gauge, and type of catheter, the date of insertion, and the initials of the operator on the tape, close to the dressing, and again in the medical record.
12. Remove gloves and wash hands after contact with patient.

THE CUTDOWN CATHETER

When lack of superficial veins prevents venipuncture, a surgical procedure for exposure and cannulation of the vein is performed by the physician. The commonest technique is insertion of the cannula or catheter into the exposed vein through the incision. This makes skin approximation difficult and may lead to a delay in healing and an increased risk of bacterial invasion in the vein through the incision.

Dudley [3] described a modified technique in which the incision is made in the usual manner to expose the vein. The cannula is then inserted slightly distal to the incision through a nick in the skin made by a small scalpel. The cannula is then introduced into the exposed vein in the usual manner. Later removal of the cannula does not disturb the incision.

Insertion and Care [2]

1. Hospital personnel should wash their hands with soap and water followed with an antiseptic before performing the cutdown.
2. Aseptic technique requires the use of sterile gloves, drapes, and equipment.
3. A topical antibiotic or antiseptic ointment should be applied to the cutdown site immediately after the catheter is inserted; follow with a sterile dressing.
4. The date of insertion should be recorded in the medical record and, if feasable, on the tape or dressing.
5. Cannulas should be replaced every 48–72 hours provided no complication has required earlier removal. The cannula may need to be used longer than the 48–72 hours if no other site is available. Cannulas inserted without proper asepsis, such as those inserted in an emergency, should be replaced as soon as a site is available.

Intravenous catheterization by surgical procedure is being replaced by subclavian insertion (see Chapter 18).

REFERENCES

1. Adriani, J. Venipuncture. *Am. J. Nurs.* 62:66, 1962.
2. Center for Disease Control. Guidelines for prevention of intravascular infection. *J. NITA* 5(1):39–50, 1982.
3. Center for Disease Control. Recommendations for prevention of HIV transmission in health-care settings. *J.A.M.A.* 258:1293–1305, 1987.
4. Dudley, H. A. F. Modified technique for intravenous cannulation. *Surg. Gynecol. Obstet.* 111:513, 1960.
5. Metheny, N. M., and Snively, W. D., Jr. *Nurses' Handbook of Fluid Balance* (4th ed.). Philadelphia: Lippincott, 1983, pp. 135, 185.
6. National Intravenous Therapy Association. NITA standards — I.V. therapy. *J. NITA* 5(1):24–29, 1982.

REVIEW QUESTIONS

1. Define the term *vasovagal reaction*.
2. Why is a vasovagal reaction a threat to a severely ill cardiac patient?
3. How can a nurse about to perform a venipuncture prevent a vasovagal reaction?
4. Why is the most prominent vein not necessarily a vein suitable for venipuncture?
5. Why are the antecubital veins impractical for intravenous infusions?
6. a. What hazards exist when veins of the lower extremity are used for intravenous infusions?
   b. What predisposes these veins to the related hazards?
7. What veins should be utilized first so that others may be preserved?
8. What prime factors are to be considered in selecting a vein for infusion purposes?
9. What method may be used to reroute the infusion should thrombosis limit available veins?
10. What precautions must be observed to prevent inadvertent intraarterial injection when medications are introduced into the veins located in the antecubital fossa?
11. How is a vein concealed by edema defined?
12. a. Why is there risk of a hematoma when a needle with a long bevel is introduced into a small vein?
    b. What technique may be used to prevent this occurrence?
13. a. How tightly is a tourniquet applied?
    b. How tightly is the blood pressure cuff applied when it is used as a tourniquet?
14. What effect does a tourniquet too tightly applied or left on for too long a period of time have on the vein?
15. At what rate do you adjust the flow of the solution before manually clamping the tubing and inserting the needle?
16. If a venipuncture is unsuccessful and the vein has sustained a puncture, what precaution is taken for the traumatized vein when attempting a second puncture?

17. What does the label placed on the needle after the infusion is started indicate?
18. What precautions are taken to prevent severing the catheter
    a. With an over-the-needle catheter?
    b. With an inside-the-needle catheter?

PART IV

Blood and Intravenous Therapy

CHAPTER 13

Transfusion Therapy

Ada Lawrence Plumer

With the increasing use of blood and its components, transfusion therapy has become an integral part of the daily treatment of patients. Administration of blood should be performed by competent, experienced, well-qualified personnel. Serious problems and complications that can lead to death and can result in litigation are associated with the administration of blood and its components. The intravenous nurse shares with the blood bank a responsibility for safe transfusion therapy and must recognize and understand the symptoms of untoward reactions.

Proper handling of the blood is vital. Contamination must be avoided; hemolysis must be prevented. The therapist must be familiar with the large variety of available blood products — their advantages and disadvantages, and the proper procedures for their safe administration. Knowledge of the fundamental principles of immunohematology provides the nurse with a better understanding of the problems associated with blood administration. Recognition of the factors that govern red cell destruction contributes to safe transfusion therapy. This information instills in the therapist an awareness of the possibility that patients may become sensitized to the many blood factors, and of the danger which this incurs. These facts bring out clearly the necessity for screening patients for antibodies that may develop from infused blood. Through an understanding of why bloods react unfavorably with other bloods, the therapist is keenly alert to the early symptoms of transfusion reactions.

BASIC IMMUNOHEMATOLOGY

Immunohematology is the science that deals with antigens of the blood and their antibodies. An *antigen* (or *agglutinogen*) is a substance capable of stimulating the production of an *antibody* and then reacting with that antibody in a specific way. The most important antigens in the blood transfusion are situated on the surface of the red cells. They are the A antigen and the B antigen in the ABO system. They are genetically inherited and determine the blood

TABLE 13.1
ABO Classification of Human Blood

Group	Cell Antigens		Plasma Antibodies		% U.S. Population
	A	B	A	B	
O	−	−	+	+	45
A	+	−	−	+	40
B	−	+	+	−	10
AB	+	+	−	−	5

group (Table 13.1). Individuals possessing red cells bearing the A antigen are classified as group A; B antigens, group B; A and B antigens, group AB; and neither A nor B antigens, group O.

The second most important antigens in the transfusion are those of the Rh system: D, (the strongest factor) C, E, c and e. These are located on the red cells in conjunction with the A and B antigens, and they are inherited.

Many antigens exist together on the red cells and some can, under favorable conditions and without proper precautions, stimulate the production of antibodies.

The antigens in the plasma are classified as human leukocyte antigens (HLA). Patients who have received numerous transfusions have been found to have a relatively high incidence of leukocyte antibodies. The use of leukocyte-depleted blood can substantially diminish the incidence of sensitization to leukocyte antigens following transfusion.

An important factor to bear in mind regarding antigens: if cells containing an antigen that is foreign to the recipient are injected into the bloodstream, the immune system, under favorable conditions, may produce an antibody to destroy the antigen.

An *antibody* (or *agglutinin*) is a protein in the plasma that reacts with a specific *antigen*. Antibodies may occur naturally or may be the result of immunization against their corresponding antigens (agglutinogens). The naturally occurring antibodies, anti-A and anti-B, are produced spontaneously without known antigenic stimulation. An antibody bears the same designation as the antigen with which it reacts. For instance, anti-A reacts with antigen A. A red cell antigen and its corresponding antibody are not produced in the same individual; that is, anti-A antibody is not produced by an individual whose red cells bear the A antigen (see Chapter 15). Immune antibodies (immunoglobulins) are produced by antigenic stimulation following either a transfusion or a pregnancy.

Antibodies may be classified according to their serological behavior. Naturally occurring antibodies are blood group antibodies that agglutinate erythrocytes containing the corresponding antigens in a saline solution; they are called *saline antibodies* or *complete antibodies*. Immune antibodies that will not agglutinate corresponding antigens in a saline solution but require additional reagents are classified as *incomplete* antibodies or *albumin antibodies*.

In vitro (in a test tube, or experimental) antibodies first react with their antigens by being adsorbed onto the red cells (coating). The reaction may stop there or may proceed to their agglutination, in which the red cells are stuck together in clumps, or hemolysis, in which the cells burst, releasing their hemoglobin. Which of these processes occurs depends upon the particular antibody involved: saline antibodies or albumin antibodies. Coating or agglutination in the test tube is associated in vivo (in the body) with sequestration of the affected cells in the liver or spleen prior to destruction (extravascular destruction). Hemolysis in the test tube is associated with in vivo destruction of red cells in the circulation (intravascular hemolysis).

Antibodies are also classified according to their physiochemical properties. The naturally occurring blood group antibodies are classified as IgM antibodies. They are the first class of immunoglobulins produced as the fetal system matures [3]. Most of the immune antibodies are structurally different and are classified as IgG.

THE PROCESS OF IMMUNE RESPONSE

Macrophages, B lymphocytes, and T lymphocytes are the cells principally involved in the immune response. Macrophages develop from monocytes, which are produced by the bone marrow, and migrate to the tissues. They are cells of the reticuloendothelial system that have the ability to absorb the foreign antigen, process (degrade) it, and present it to the antibody-forming cells, the T cells and the B cells. The T cells arise from the bone marrow and migrate to the thymus, where they mature. The B cells are derived from the bone marrow. In most cases the action of T cells affects the activity of B cells, B cells differentiate into plasma cells that produce the antibodies [3]. T cells include helper cells, which promote effector activity of both T and B cells; suppressor cells, which inhibit B and T cell activity; and cytoxic effector cells, which can destroy or alter foreign cells.

Primary immune response is a response in one who has never been exposed to the antigen. It occurs when the foreign antigen is injected, setting off a complex series of reactions which eventually leads to the production of a circulating antibody. The major antibody predominantly produced is IgM.

Secondary (or anamnestic) response occurs after the first injection of an antigen results in antibody-producing cells which develop a memory. This response occurs after a second injection of the same antigen and when the antibody production rapidly reaches a high titre. IgG is the major class of antibody produced [3].

BLOOD GROUP SYSTEMS

The best-known blood group system is the ABO system, discovered by Karl Landsteiner in 1901. Landsteiner demonstrated a classification of human blood based on antigens on the red cells and antibodies in the serum (see Table 13.1).

In 1940 Landsteiner and Wiener discovered the Rhesus (Rh) system, so called because of its relationship to the substance in the red cells of the rhesus monkey. The antigens belonging to the Rh system are C, D, E, c, and e. Because of the ease with which antibody D is built up, typing is done to ensure that D-negative recipients receive D-negative blood. A person whose blood contains a D antigen is classified as Rh-positive; lacking the D, Rh-negative. "Rh-negative recipients should receive Rh-negative Whole Blood or Red Blood Cell Components except for reasonable qualifying circumstances. Rh-positive recipients may receive either Rh-positive or Rh-negative Whole Blood or Red Blood Cell Components" [2]. (See Chapter 15.)

Occasionally, weak variants of the $Rh_o(D)$ factor exist and are identified by means of an indirect Coombs' test. These individuals, called D^u variants, are considered Rh-positive.

The serum of an Rh-negative individual differs from the main groups in that the anti-Rh antibodies usually are not present in significant quantities until the individual is exposed to an Rh-positive factor, through either transfusion or pregnancy.

Nine main blood group systems have been defined on the basis of reaction of cells with antibodies: ABO, Rh, Kell, Duffy, Kidd, Lewis, MNS, P, and Lutheran. Others are under investigation. Corresponding antibodies to the blood group antigens in most of these systems are found so infrequently that they do not cause an everyday problem. When present, these antibodies may produce hemolytic reactions; once discovered, precautions must be taken to ensure that the patient receives compatible blood. When difficulty arises in cross-matching, or when a transfusion reaction occurs, these systems take on a special significance. The American Association of Blood Banks (AABB) requires that a patient once transfused must be screened for irregular antibodies in the 48 hours preceding any further transfusions.

The term *hemolytic transfusion reaction* denotes the clinical symptoms caused when the red cells of either the recipient or the donor are destroyed in the recipient during a transfusion. Of prime importance in transfusion therapy is the assurance of ABO compatibility between donor and recipient. "Recipients shall receive ABO type-specific Whole Blood or ABO type-compatible Red Blood Cell Components" [2]. In situations in which delay in provision of blood may jeopardize life, blood may be issued before completion of routine tests according to AABB standards [2]:

> Recipients whose ABO type is not known may receive type O Red Blood Cells.
>
> Recipients whose ABO type has been determined by the transfusing facility without reliance on previous records, may receive ABO type-specific Whole Blood or Red Blood Cell Components before other tests for compatibility have been completed.

Physicians must indicate in the record that the clinical condition is sufficiently urgent to release blood before compatibility testing is completed; the tag or label must conspicuously indicate that compatibility testing is not completed; and standard compatibility tests should be completed promptly.

Chapter 13 | Transfusion Therapy

OBJECTIVES OF TRANSFUSION THERAPY

There are three main objectives of transfusion therapy:

1. Maintenance of blood volume
2. Maintenance of oxygen-carrying capacity of the blood by supplying red cells
3. Maintenance of coagulation properties by supplying the clotting factors found in platelets and plasma

Transfusion therapy is also vital when blood exchange is imperative, as in the treatment of newborn infants with hemolytic anemia. In cardiac surgery, blood is needed to prime the oxygenating pump and maintain circulation.

WHOLE BLOOD

Acid-citrate-dextrose (ACD) solution was for years the common anticoagulant used to preserve and store whole blood safely at a controlled temperature of 1–6°C for a period of 21 days. This time duration was based on the standard that 70 percent of the red cells of such blood (21 days old) must be present in the bloodstream of the recipient 24 hours after transfusion [3].

Today, citrate-phosphate-dextrose (CPD) and citrate-phosphate-dextrose-adenine (CPDA-1) are replacing ACD and have increased the storage of whole blood from 21 days in CPD to 35 days in CPDA-1. The phosphate acts as a buffer, allowing cells to be collected and stored at a higher pH and resulting in slower cellular breakdown. The capacity of the red cells to transport and release oxygen depends upon an organic phosphate in red cells called 2,3-DPG (2,3-diphosphoglycerate). Red blood cells stored in CPD retain adequate DPG levels for at least 10 days, while after one week, red cells stored in ACD are DPG-deficient. With the decrease in the concentration of 2,3-DPG, oxygen becomes more strongly bound to hemoglobin and the release of oxygen to the tissues is temporarily impaired. Once infused, DPG is quickly resynthesized, but if oxygen profusion is vital the delay could be hazardous [3, 5]. Although red blood cells prepared from CPDA-1 blood are approved officially, there is some question about the viability of the red cells in older blood units.

All the preservatives contain sodium citrate and dextrose. Sodium citrate, by combining with ionized calcium, inhibits clotting thus serving as an anticoagulant.

Dextrose prolongs the life of red cells. Large amounts of dextrose in preservatives provide adequate amounts of glucose for conversion to ATP (adenosine triphosphate). The red cell is dependent upon ATP for an energy source and any conditions that cause interference with this conversion are deleterious to red cell survival. Adenine in combination with CPD helps to maintain red cell ATP, but at the expense of red cell 2,3-DPG.

A new anticoagulant-preservative, CPD-AS, utilizes an additive solution (AS) in addition to the CPD. Two systems are available. One system uses 100 ml additive solution consisting of saline, dextrose, mannitol, and adenine with CPD. This system permits a 49-day expiration period from the date of collection for packed red cells. The second system uses 100 ml additive solution consisting of saline, dextrose, and adenine with CP2D and permits a 35-day dating period for red cell storage [3].

Whole blood transfusion is indicated when an acute blood loss has occurred, as in a massive hemorrhage. It is often used in cardiac surgery. It is also used for an exchange transfusion in an infant, child, or adult. The volume expanders — plasma, dextran, hydroxyethyl starch, and albumin — are useful only as a temporary measure. They lack the oxygen-carrying red cells necessary in treating hypoxia associated with hypovolemic shock. Frequently, acute blood loss requires massive transfusion.

In massive transfusion, the anticoagulant can present problems. Rapid administration of large quantities of citrated blood to a recipient with a severely damaged liver can cause a calcium deficit. A damaged liver may be unable to keep up with rapid administration of sodium-citrated blood and unable to metabolize the citrate ions. The citrate ions combine with ionized calcium in the bloodstream, causing a calcium deficit [8]. A low calcium sufficient to cause impairment of normal blood coagulation is incompatible with life. Citrate-induced ionized calcium deficit may interfere with the normal force of contraction of the heart.

Definite changes take place in stored blood which make age a consideration when a large quantity of blood (over 6 pints) is infused in a short period of time. With the continuous metabolic changes of red cells occurring during blood storage, the potassium leaks from the cells into the plasma. This potassium, plus that released from the intact cells, causes the plasma potassium level to rise from 7 mEq per liter on day 1 to 23 mEq per liter by day 21 [8]. This is an important factor in the event of massive transfusions and in blood exchange of the newborn infant.

During major surgery, when rapid transfusions of large quantities of blood are indicated, the freshest possible blood is used. When the patient's potassium level reaches 8 mEq per liter, cardiac manifestations are common, and when the level reaches 10 to 15 mEq per liter, cardiac arrest and death may occur [8].

Coagulation factors of the plasma and platelets are also affected by the age of the blood. In hemorrhage, when viable platelets are a consideration, fresh blood must be used. Fresh blood is also used in blood exchange in the newborn infant.

In conjunction with cardiac surgery, massive amounts of whole blood were formerly required to prime the oxygenating pumps, maintain circulation, and replace blood loss. The general use of bubble oxygenators has greatly reduced the amount of blood required for each cardiac surgical patient. Blood (preferably less than 5 days old) is used for the cardiac patients to provide optimum oxygen-carrying ability. Freshly collected blood may be needed if the patient is bleeding after operation.

Blood stored for transfusion is known to contain increasing amounts of cellular degradation debris such as microaggregates of leukocytes, platelets, and other amorphous material [11]. Studies suggest that the pulmonary insufficiency following massive transfusion may be due to this debris. Since the standard 170 micron filter has been found inadequate, several blood filters

Chapter 13 | Transfusion Therapy

with small pore size (40 microns and under) have been designed to protect the lung against this particulate matter when several units of stored blood are infused (see Chapter 17).

PACKED RED CELLS

Packed red cells are prepared by the removal of approximately 200–225 ml plasma from 1 pint whole blood, either by centrifuge or by sedimentation. Packed cells with a hematocrit of about 80 percent are readily transfusable. With the removal of greater amounts of plasma, difficulty is encountered upon infusion owing to the dense packing of the cells.

There are definite advantages in the use of packed red cells: reduced volume, reduced chemical content, and reduced agglutinins.

Reduced Volume

Because of its reduced volume, a unit of packed cells can supply red cells without overloading the circulation — a definite advantage in patients with normal or increased blood volume and those with heart disease. Packed red cells are used for patients not in need of plasma. One unit of packed cells, provides the same amount of oxygen-carrying red cells as one unit of whole blood.

Reduced Chemical Content

The excess plasma potassium content in stored blood is reduced by the removal of plasma. Red cells can be provided for a patient with kidney or heart disease without adding to the patient's hyperkalemia.

For patients on sodium restriction, sodium excess in the plasma (increased by the anticoagulant sodium citrate) is avoided. Packed cells also reduce hazards associated with sodium citrate, such as citrate intoxication caused by the inability of the liver to metabolize citrate.

Reduced Agglutinins

Packed cells provide relatively safe, low-titer type O blood. Most of the plasma is removed, thereby reducing the amount of anti-A and anti-B agglutinins.

FROZEN BLOOD

The storage time for donated blood has been increased to 3 years or more by the process of freezing blood. This processing is accomplished through a machine, the Cytoglomerator,* invented by Charles E. Huggins. Early attempts at freezing blood proved unsuccessful because of the ice crystals which damaged the red cells. Several techniques have been developed in the past 25 to 31 years, but Huggin's method has proved the simplest and quickest.

Plasma is extracted from the whole blood. The red cells are then coated with glycerol to prevent damage from freezing and packed in disposable plastic bags. They are then frozen at $-85°C$, labeled, and stored until used.

Just prior to use, the plastic bag with the frozen cells is thawed in a water bath of about 40°C. The thawing time is about 3 minutes. The bag is then inserted into the Cytoglomerator for a glycerol washout of about 20 minutes.

---

*International Equipment Co., Needham Heights, Mass.

Sugar solutions are used to cause a rapid sediment of the red cells. The machine takes its name from *cyto* (cell) and *glomerator* (cluster). Three dilutions are necessary. Five pints of blood can be processed every 20 minutes by one machine.

Frozen blood offers advantages other than the long storage period: (1) It is believed that the possibility of transmitting hepatitis by transfusion of frozen blood is negligible. (2) Owing to the selection of donors, frozen blood may be given to patients sensitized from previous transfusions. Type O frozen blood can safely be used as a universal donor because anti-A and anti-B antibodies are removed during washings. (3) Some surgeons believe that frozen blood plays a big part in improving results in kidney transplantations; fewer of the white blood cell antigens remain to trigger the body's rejection of foreign tissue [7].

The hematocrit of frozen blood is approximately 80 percent. Because of the lack of any plasma, the viscosity is less than that of packed cells, making frozen blood easily transfusable. It may be administered rapidly to most patients.

PLASMA

Plasma is the liquid content remaining after the red cells have been removed from whole blood by centrifuge. The storage of plasma presents less of a problem than does that of blood. When stored according to AABB standards [2] the shelf life of single-donor plasma in a liquid state stored at temperatures between 1°C and 6°C is no more than 26 days for blood collected into CPD and 42 days for blood collected into CPDA-1; the shelf life of a single-donor plasma frozen at −18°C or lower is no more than 5 years, and fresh-frozen single-donor plasma (human) may be stored at −18°C or lower for no longer than 1 year. After 1 year, fresh-frozen single-donor plasma may be frozen for 4 more years at temperatures of −18°C or lower, provided it is redesignated as single-donor plasma [3].

Liquid Stored Plasma

Liquid stored plasma is prepared from ACD and CPD blood. Special precaution must be taken to avoid contamination in the preparation of plasma. A closed system under sterile conditions is used to separate plasma from red cells. Further precautions include culture of the plasma plus visual inspection.

Plasma is prepared as single-donor plasma, and labeled with the specific blood group. Because plasma is a vehicle for transmitting hepatitis, the single-donor plasma carries fewer risks.

Plasma plays an important role in the treatment of burns. It supplies plasma protein and prevents shock without overloading the circulation with red cells. It may be used in an emergency to correct hypovolemia. Most of the clotting factors are lost during storage, making it of little use in patients with coagulation problems.

Under ordinary circumstances when single-donor plasma is used, it should be compatible with the recipient's red cells. AB plasma, because it lacks anti-A and anti-B agglutinins, may be used for all ABO groups. The group O

Chapter 13 | Transfusion Therapy

patient may receive plasma of any group. For the group A patient, only plasma taken from blood group A or AB may be used. For the group B patient, only plasma taken from blood group B or AB may be used. For the group AB patient, plasma from group AB blood only is used. In an emergency when the patient's blood group has not been determined, AB plasma is used.

Fresh-Frozen Plasma

Fresh-frozen plasma is beneficial to patients with inherited or acquired disorders of coagulation. Special donors with blood high in certain clotting factors are desirable. The plasma is separated from the cells and frozen within 6 hours of collection from the donor. Freezing preserves the various clotting factors, in particular factors V and VIII, to control hemorrhage in the presurgical hemophiliac.

Fresh-frozen plasma must be stored at −18° to −30°C and kept frozen until transfusion time. It is thawed in a water bath of 37°C. The fresh-frozen plasma must be administered within 6 hours after thawing; a delay causing a rise in the temperature of the plasma results in loss of factor VIII (antihemophiliac factor, AHF).

Plasma Components

Cryoprecipitate

Cryoprecipitate is a concentrate containing factor VIII (AHF) extracted from cold-thawed plasma. It was discovered by Judith G. Pool, Stanford University Medical Center, who began work on it in 1959. Since 1965 it has been used for treatment of hemophilia, this being the only coagulation deficiency for which it is therapeutically valuable [10].

The potency of AHF in cryoprecipitate far exceeds that in fresh-frozen plasma. Pool [10] stated that approximately 6 units, or 1,600 ml, of plasma would be necessary to raise the patient's AHF level from less than 1 percent of normal to 50 percent of normal, whereas only 55 ml or less of the concentrate produces the same results. It would take 2 hours or more to infuse the plasma but only 5 minutes to infuse the precipitate. This small volume avoids the risk of overloading circulation in patients who are not able to tolerate an increase in blood volume.

The blood from which the precipitate is taken can be reconstituted and used as whole blood or separated into components for patients other than the hemophiliac.

In the preparation of AHF, the plasma goes through a quick-freeze process. When frozen solid it is thawed at 4°C, which takes about 24 hours. The precipitate is then removed from the cold-thawed plasma.

Cryoprecipitate that contains 75 percent of the antihemophilic factor and 25 percent of the fibrinogen from the donor's original 250 ml plasma may be stored in the frozen state for no more than 12 months, from the time of donation, at temperatures of −30 to −18°C. Single-donor cryoprecipitate, once thawed, should be maintained at room temperature and administered within 6 hours; it should not be refrozen [2].

In the past, *fibrinogen,* a concentrate of the fibrinogen factor, was useful in the treatment of hemorrhage resulting from a deficiency of this protein. This deficiency is most frequently seen in the obstetrical patient and at times in patients with fibrinolysin undergoing major surgery. Because the hepatitis virus and fibrinogen combine during fractionation, there was increased risk of hepatitis to the patient infused with this product. Because of this risk, cryoprecipitate is now used in replacement therapy. Each bag of cryoprecipitate from a single blood donation should contain a minimum of 80 international units of factor VIII activity per bag.

Platelets

Platelets (thrombocytes) are cells in the plasma, the normal range in adults being between 150,000 and 350,000 per mm^3. Fresh whole blood provides the greatest number of platelets per donation but does not provide adequate treatment of platelet deficiency because more platelets are usually required than can be provided by a single unit of blood; large volumes of blood would be necessary.

Platelet transfusions are used primarily for the treatment of the bleeding thrombocytopenic patient and are usually administered when the count drops below 10,000 per cu mm of blood. Platelet Concentrates, prepared by centrifuging whole blood, should contain at least 5.5×10^{10} platelets per unit at maximum storage time; when prepared by cytapheresis the unit should contain 3×10^{11} platelets [2]. They must be suspended in sufficient plasma to maintain a pH of 6.0 or greater. Continuous gentle agitation is essential when stored at room temperature (20–24°C). They may be stored for 72 hours according to FDA requirements. Platelets, prepared in a closed system, may be stored at 1–6°C without agitation for 48 hours. The type of plastic bag used for storing platelets affects the preservation of platelet function. The newer plastics, such as polyolefin without plastizer, allow platelets to be stored at 20–24°C for up to 7 days before transfusing [3]. Gentle agitation is required; the type of agitation depends on the type of plastic used for the storage bag. Platelets stored at room temperature maintain function and viability better than do refrigerated platelets [3]. For maximum benefit, they should be infused within 6 hours of donation.

Platelet concentrate may be administered without a compatibility test although it is preferable for the donor plasma and the recipient's red cells to be ABO-compatible, especially when administered to the newborn infant [2]. Rh matching is preferable; when Rh-negative patients receive Rh-positive platelet concentrate, Rh (D) immune globulin should be considered to prevent Rh sensitization from the small amount of red cells in platelet concentrate. Rh-positive concentrate should not be used for female Rh-negative patients under 45 years of age if platelets from Rh-negative donors are available.

Platelets carry the risk of stimulating antibodies since they contain HLA antigens and additional antigens unique to platelets. They are ineffective in controlling hemorrhage when infused into patients who have developed antibodies to these antigens. In such cases, the patient's family members are used as donors since they provide a likely source of HLA-compatible platelets.

Platelet administration is preferably made by bolus through a standard Y-type blood component set (see Figure 11.8, p. 151). Administration may also be made by drip through a platelet set containing a small filter. Use of the large-size standard blood filter or the microaggregate filters may reduce the number of transfusable platelets as platelets tend to adhere to plastic.

Granulocytes

Leukocytes are white blood corpuscles consisting of 60 percent granulocytes, 35 percent lymphocytes, and 5 percent monocytes. There are 5,000–10,000 leukocytes per microliter of blood in the normal person; of these, 60 percent are granulocytes, found in the bone marrow and consisting of 58 percent neutrophils and 2 percent eosinophils. The neutrophils are the specific white cells that are infused as leukocyte or granulocyte transfusions. Their function is to engulf and kill bacteria by means of a chemical released from their granules [6].

Granulocytes are administered when serious bacterial infection occurs in a patient with severe granulocytopenia from marrow depletion due to chemotherapy, leukemia, or toxic drugs.

Because of the exposure, the severe reactions, and possible risk to the patient, granulocyte transfusions are used only after all other means of treatment have been exhausted. Transfusions are indicated only when the patient's absolute granulocyte count is less than 100 per µliter when there is definite evidence of infection, and after the patient has received antibiotic therapy for 2 days without response.

Leukopheresis is the procedure by which granulocytes are collected from a healthy donor for transfusion. *Centrifugation* is the method used, a method in which the donor's blood is continuously pumped into a machine which separates the blood elements by centrifugation and returns the other elements of the blood to the donor. The centrifugal techniques for granulocyte apheresis have replaced the nylon filtration technique formerly used.

The granulocytes may be stored at room temperature (20–24°C) no more than 24 hours and preferably less than 6 hours. Because granulocytes are contaminated with donor red cells, donor and recipient must have compatible blood types and a crossmatch must be performed.

Granulocyte transfusions are usually administered daily for 3 to 5 days or until there is increase in the granulocyte count (greater than 500/µliter the morning after transfusion) showing that the bone marrow is functioning, infection is reduced, or the patient cannot tolerate the transfusion.

The granulocytes are administered through a set containing the standard blood filter (170 microns) over a 4-hour period, depending upon the tolerance of the patient. Microaggregate filters should not be used in the administration set [2].

The common side-effects are febrile reactions to the granulocytes and occur when pyrogens are released from the granulocytes. They may cause discomfort but are usually not considered a serious threat to the patient. It is important to establish as soon as possible the cause of the reaction. Premedication 15 minutes before transfusion, with drugs such as hydrocortisone and morphine sulfate, may minimize severity of the reaction. Physicians may order the medication to be repeated if severe reaction occurs despite premedication. The infusion is slowed but is not usually discontinued unless chest pain and shortness of breath occur.

Human Serum Albumin

This albumin is available in two concentrations: a 5% solution in saline and a 25% solution.

Albumin-saline 5% is isotonic, being osmotically equivalent to an approximately equal volume of citrated plasma, and may be used as a substitute for plasma. It provides volume and colloid in the treatment of shock and burns without the risk of transmitting serum hepatitis; processing by heating destroys the hepatitis virus.

Albumin 25% is a hypertonic solution depending upon additional fluids, either drawn from the tissues or administered separately, for its maximal osmotic effect. Fifty ml is osmotically equivalent to 250 ml citrated plasma and produces a plasma volume increase of about 225 ml. It must be administered with caution since rapid infusion can result in circulatory overload or cardiopulmonary embarrassment. When administered to severely dehydrated patients, adequate amounts of supplemental fluid must be administered to prevent cellular dehydration. It is used primarily for protein replacement in severe hypoalbuminemia and infused at a slow rate of 2–3 ml per minute, adjusted to the patient's condition. It may be used in cerebral edema as a dehydrating agent.

Administration calls for strict aseptic and antiseptic handling. Once the container is entered with a needle or set, it must be used immediately or discarded, as there is no preservative in albumin. Drugs should not be added to albumin since many drugs contain phenol, a reducing agent which is incompatible with albumin. The product should be carefully examined and should not be administered if it is found to be turbid. The injection site of the 25% albumin must be scrubbed with an antiseptic. Compressing the drip chamber before its introduction into the vial will exert a negative pressure in the bottle and prevent albumin from leaking out the air vent, wetting and occluding the filter.

If albumin is piggybacked into an infusion, the primary infusion should be clamped off as there is danger of air entering the line once the albumin container runs dry. If it is essential that both run simultaneously, vigilance is necessary so that the line may be clamped off before the container empties.

Febrile reactions call for immediate termination of the infusion. The lot number should be noted and the blood bank notified. It may be necessary to recall and investigate all albumin of that lot number. If contamination during manufacture is suspected, the Food and Drug Administration is notified.

Plasma Protein Fraction (Human)

This type of plasma is plasma from which the fibrinogen and much of the globulin have been removed. It provides a substitute for plasma with minimal risk of viral hepatitis; processing by heating to 60°C for 10 hours inactivates the virus. It provides volume expansion.

PLASMA SUBSTITUTE: DEXTRAN

Dextran* is a plasma volume expander used for the treatment of hypovolemic shock. When introduced into the bloodstream, dextran increases the osmotic pressure, draws interstitial fluid into the vessels, and increases the blood volume. It is a synthetic product with two advantages: (1) no storage problem and (2) no danger of hepatitis.

It is available as dextran 6% in normal saline solution or dextran 5% in water for patients requiring low sodium intake. The usual dose is 500 ml.

Allergic reactions to dextran frequently occur, and precautions should be taken. The first few milliliters of dextran should be administered slowly and the patient observed for possible reactions. These may include mild urticaria, tightness of the chest, and hypotension [8]. If any such symptoms occur, the dextran must be discontinued.

The rate of flow should be ordered by the physician. Caution must be observed when dextran is administered to patients with heart or kidney disease; a rapid rate may cause congestive heart failure and pulmonary edema.

$RH_o(D)$ IMMUNE GLOBULIN†

The successful prevention of maternal sensitization to the Rh factor by an anti-Rh immunoglobulin was first announced by Freda, Gorman, and Pollack in 1965, and RhoGAM was approved for distribution to physicians in 1968 [9].

The $Rh_o(D)$ antibody produced by the Rh-negative mother after delivery of an Rh-positive infant is the cause of Rh hemolytic disease of the newborn in subsequent pregnancies. $Rh_o(D)$ immune globulin administered within 72 hours after delivery suppresses the development of this antibody in the mother.

To be considered a candidate for $Rh_o(D)$ immune globulin the postpartum mother must (1) be $Rh_o(D)$-negative, D^u-negative, (2) not be already immunized to the $Rh_o(D)$ factor, and (3) have delivered a baby who is either $Rh_o(D)$-positive or D^u-positive [9]. The same conditions apply in an abortion or miscarriage. Since the fetal blood type may be unknown, the mother should receive $Rh_o(D)$ immune globulin if the father is $Rh_o(D)$-positive or D^u-positive. Rh immunoglobulin is also used to protect the Rh-negative patient not already sensitized to the $Rh_o(D)$ factor against immunization from infused Rh-positive blood components.

One vial of RhoGAM will completely suppress immunity to 15 ml Rh-positive red blood cells and is sufficient to suppress immunity to the Rh antigen in the usual full-term delivery. The volume of Rh-positive blood that enters the bloodstream determines the dose of RhoGAM, which is administered intramuscularly. Reactions to Rh immunoglobulin are infrequent and mild and usually confined to the area of injection.

---

*Pharmacia Laboratories, Piscataway, N.J.; Division of Pharmacia, Inc.

†Gamulin Rh (Dow Pharmaceuticals, Indianapolis, Ind.); Hypo-Rho-D (Cutter Biological Division, MilesLabs, Inc., Emeryville, Calif.); RhoGAM (Ortho Diagnostics, Inc., Raritan, N.J.); Rho-Immune (Lederle Laboratories, Pearl River, N.Y.).

BLOOD ADMINISTRATION

With the rapid advancement in transfusion therapy, responsibility for administering this vital fluid increases. Only those well versed in every phase of therapy should hold this responsibility. The patient's safety depends upon adherence to specific rules regarding safe administration. The therapist is responsible for the following:

1. Patient-blood identification. The avoidance of mistaken identity is imperative.
2. Inspection of blood prior to administration to avoid infusing the patient with hemolyzed, clotted, or contaminated blood.
3. Proper technique.
4. Close observation of the patient. Early detection of symptoms of a reaction is important.

Issue and Transfer

Patient-blood identification is of paramount importance in preventing reactions from incompatible blood. The risk of identification errors occurring from copying information onto requisitions has been reduced by photocopying. The use of triplicate requisitions also reduces the danger of identification errors. Such requisitions, identifying the patient and indicating the amount and kind of blood and time needed, are sent to the blood bank with the blood sample. One copy is retained at dispatch or on the ward for demand of the processed blood. The upper portion is returned with the crossmatched blood to the floor.

The mode of transfer of blood components to the ward depends upon hospital policy. It may involve a messenger service, hospital personnel, or the individual who will administer the blood. One of the most common causes of hemolytic reaction is the accidental administration of incompatible blood, from the wrong container to the patient. To prevent administration of incompatible blood, only 1 unit should be transported by a person at a time.

Patient-Blood Identification

Absolute and positive identification of the donor blood and the patient must be made. All personnel handling the blood should be responsible for checking patient-blood identification. The intravenous nurse makes the final check and must decide whether to administer the blood or question it. *ABO-and Rh-compatibility identification* is made by comparing: (1) the patient's previous ABO and Rh determination with patient's and donor's ABO and Rh on the compatibility tag, and (2) the blood identification number on the blood container with the identification number on the blood tag and the blood unit itself.

Patient identification is made by checking the name and unit number on the blood tag with the face sheet in the patient's chart. The patient then must identify him- or herself by complete name. Identity should never be made by addressing the patient by name and awaiting a response. Errors can occur from faulty response of medicated patients. Hospital numbers on the identification bracelet must match hospital numbers on the tag to prevent errors in cases of similar names. Any discrepancy must be investigated and corrected before the blood is administered.

Chapter 13 | Transfusion Therapy

Blood must *never* be administered to a patient who has no identification bracelet.

Handling Blood

To prevent excessive warming, blood should be administered within 30 minutes of the time it leaves the bank. If blood is not maintained at 1–10°C while outside the control of the blood bank, it cannot be reissued. Blood-bank blood stored at FDA requirements of 1–6°C will exceed 10°C in approximately 30 minutes at room temperature; blood that cannot be administered immediately should be returned to the blood bank within this time.

Blood should never be placed in ward refrigerators; ward refrigerators are not controlled and contain no alarms to warn of temperature fluctuation.

If warm blood is ordered, special blood-warming devices (see Figure 11.7) that maintain a controlled temperature of between 32 and 37°C should be used to warm the blood in the tubing during administration; hot water must never be used to heat blood.

Before administering the blood component, the expiration date should be noted to avoid infusing an outdated product.

Sodium chloride injection, U.S.P. (normal saline) should be used to initiate the infusion of red blood cells, whole blood, platelets, or leukocytes. These components should not be hooked up with 5% dextrose in water, or run simultaneously with 5% dextrose in water through a Y tube. Hypotonic or hypertonic solutions should not be used to dilute blood. Extreme hypotonicity causes water to invade the red cells until they burst, resulting in hemolysis. Hypertonic solutions diluting blood result in reversal of this process with shrinkage of the red cells.

Medication should never be added to blood or administered simultaneously through the same set (normal saline is not considered a medication) for the following reasons:

1. Bacterial contamination is a real concern and potential hazard since blood hanging in a warm room is a good culture medium.
2. There is a possibility of pharmacological incompatibility between the drug and the blood or the anticoagulant.
3. Drugs may be administered too slowly to achieve therapeutic levels. For example, if an antihistamine is added to blood to prevent allergic reactions, the small amount given during the early administration may be inadequate to prevent a reaction. If a reaction occurs the drug is still in the container.

Blood Filters

A sterile pyrogen-free filter of 170 microns should be used for administration of all blood components. It is compressed and then inserted into the blood bag; squeezing the filter after insertion can introduce air into the bag. If the filter is not completely covered with blood, slight compression of the bag will fill it; utilizing the entire filter results in a much-improved flow rate. A single filter may be used to infuse 2–4 units of whole blood. Once the blood filter contains blood and debris it should be discarded; use of such filters allows bacterial contamination and hemolysis of the blood at room temperature.

The microaggregate filter (see Figure 11.9, p. 152) is often ordered for patients with compromised pulmonary function, for total replacement (in 24 hours), and for patients with a history of febrile reactions. The standard clot filter does not adequately trap microaggregates in stored blood-bank blood. It is suggested that 5–10 units of whole blood can be administered through a microaggregate filter under positive pressure, up to 300 mm Hg to maintain an adequate flow rate.

Venipuncture

A large vein with an adequate diameter should be used to ensure the flow of viscous components. The lower extremities and areas of joint flexion should be avoided.

Red blood cells and whole blood can usually be administered through a 19-gauge thin-walled cannula although smaller cannulas may be used for other components. Often, a 23-gauge thin-walled small-vein needle is used for pediatric patients.

Rate of Transfusion

The rate of the infusion is governed by the clinical condition of the patient and the component being infused. Infusion should be done at a slow rate for the first 15 minutes to avoid infusion of a large quantity of blood in case of an immediate reaction. Most patients can tolerate infusion of 1 unit red cells in 1½–2 hours; patients in congestive failure or in danger of fluid overload require infusions given over a much longer period of time. Whenever possible, blood should be infused within 4 hours; there is danger of bacterial proliferation and red cell hemolysis in blood kept at room temperature. When a unit is ordered to infuse over longer than 4 hours, the blood may be separated into aliquots and part of it stored in the blood bank while the first portion is transfused.

Whenever blood is needed with such rapidity that positive pressure is necessary, infusing it should be the physician's responsibility. *Caution is crucial.* Certain risks may be involved when the blood is infused rapidly: circulatory overloading with pulmonary edema, citrate toxicity, cardiac arrest, and air embolism.

Nursing Care

After the transfusion is initiated, the therapist should observe the patient for the initial 5 to 15 minutes of the infusion. Many of the fatal incompatible transfusion reactions produce symptoms early in the course of the infusion. The therapist and the attending nurse share a responsibility for safe transfusion administration. They must be familiar with the various transfusion reactions, recognize adverse reactions, and know what procedures to follow.

If venous spasm occurs from the cold blood being infused, a warm pack applied to the vein through which the blood is being infused will relieve the spasm and increase the rate of flow.

TRANSFUSION REACTIONS

Vast improvements in methods of collection and storage, together with growing knowledge in the field of immunohematology, have increased the safety of transfusion therapy. However, there is still an inherent risk with every unit of transfused blood. Both the therapist and the attending nurse should be aware of this fact and be alert to symptoms of untoward reactions. Reactions to administered blood can not all be eliminated by ABO- and Rh-compatibility testing. The most common causes of adverse reactions are leukocytes, platelets, and plasma proteins in which compatibility testing is not performed.

Whenever a transfusion reaction is suspected, manifested in more than hives, the transfusion should be terminated and the line kept open for possible therapeutic treatment. Vital signs should be taken and the physician and the blood bank should be notified. A blood sample of 10 ml should be sent to the blood bank with the blood container and the transfusion reaction report. When a hemolytic reaction occurs, urine is sent to the laboratory for hemoglobin analysis; urinary output should be monitored and all urine saved and observed for hemoglobin or bilirubin.

Transfusion reactions may be divided into three main classes: endogenous, exogenous, and delayed.

Endogenous Reactions

Endogenous reactions are those caused by antigen-antibody reactions in the recipient and are brought about by the body's response to foreign protein.

Hemolytic Transfusion Reactions

Hemolytic transfusion reactions occur when there is an antigen-antibody reaction in the recipient due to an incompatibility between red cell antigens and antibodies; the antibody combines with red cells possessing the corresponding antigen. The most serious, and major, incompatibility occurs between the recipient's antibodies and the donor's red cells. The recipient's entire antibody load reacts with the donor's red cells. Minor incompatibility occurs when the antibody is passively transfused from the donor's plasma and reacts with the recipient's red cells; severe reactions are less likely. The antibody may also react with other donor cells.

There are two types of red cell destruction: (1) *intravascular hemolysis,* in which the sensitized red cells are destroyed with hemolysis directly in the bloodstream (usually seen with ABO-incompatible red blood cells); and (2) *extravascular hemolysis,* in which the cells are coated with the antibody and subsequently removed by the reticuloendothelial system (as in Rh incompatibility).

Intravascular hemolysis is usually the more serious complication. Virtually all fatal blood-transfusion reactions are due to incompatibilities within the ABO blood group system. Investigation of such ABO errors shows that the most common cause is an improperly identified recipient sample sent to the blood bank for typing and crossmatching, an improperly identified blood unit, or an improperly identified blood recipient.

Serious reactions are characterized by chills, fever, flushing of face, burning sensation along the vein in which the blood is being infused, lumbar and flank pain, chest pain, frequent oozing of blood at the injection site and surgical areas, and shock. Hemoglobinemia may occur, followed by hemoglobinuria. If the free hemoglobin released from the destruction of the red cells is greater than the quantity that can combine with the haptoglobin in the plasma, the excess hemoglobin filters through the glomerular membrane into the kidney tubules and hemoglobinuria occurs.

When reactions occur, the transfusion must be stopped at once and the vein kept open with normal saline. When a Y blood tubing is used, a new set-up (container of fluid and a new administration set) should be connected directly to the cannula. DO NOT OPEN THE FLOW TO THE NORMAL SALINE HANGING WITH THE Y BLOOD TUBING. To do so could result in the patient receiving additional blood cells contained in the Y tubing.

Vigorous treatment of hypotension and promotion of adequate renal blood flow are imperative. Vasopressors such as levophed and adamine are usually reserved for life-threatening situations, because they may intensify existing renal vasoconstriction. Dopamine dilates the renal vasculature while increasing cardiac output and may be useful in low doses. Its administration requires careful monitoring of the patient's urinary flow, cardiac output, and blood pressure.

Fluid therapy may consist of rapidly infusing dilute intravenous fluids to cause diuresis and to help prevent renal damage; the patient's cardiac and renal disease may complicate therapy. Urinary flow rates in adults should be maintained at or over 100/ml per hour for at least 18–24 hours [3]. There are two schools of thought regarding the use of the osmotic diuretic, mannitol; some advocate its use while others feel that it should not be used for treatment of acute hemolytic transfusion reactions. Mannitol increases blood volume and may not increase renal blood flow. Furosemide, administered intravenously, improves renal blood flow and produces diuresis [3]. Peritoneal dialysis or hemodialysis may be initiated if kidney failure occurs.

Extravascular hemolysis is manifested by symptoms similar to, but usually less severe than, those for acute intravascular hemolysis.

Febrile Reactions

Febrile reactions are usually the result of antileukocyte antibodies in the recipient directed against the donor's white cells. Patients who have been sensitized to platelet and plasma proteins by numerous transfusions may also have febrile reactions.

Febrile symptoms may mimic those of a hemolytic reaction but are usually less severe. They tend to occur later in the transfusion or may occur even after the blood has been infused. The reaction is characterized by flushing of the face, palpitation, cough, tightness in chest, increased pulse rate followed by chills and fever of up to 104°F and not lasting more than 8 hours.

The treatment is usually symptomatic. If the patient requires subsequent transfusions, frozen red cells are usually administered because the white cells are largely destroyed and removed during their preparation.

Microaggregate filtration, when used for citrated blood stored longer

Chapter 13 | Transfusion Therapy

than 5 days, may prevent febrile reactions due to removal of unwanted leukocyte and platelet debris. This technique provides appreciable savings of cost and time over the more expensive automated cell washing systems used when frozen cells are not available [3].

Allergic Reactions

Allergic reactions are manifested by urticaria or hives and occasionally are accompanied by chills and fever. Severe reactions may occur with asthmatic symptoms, fever, and anaphylactic shock. The appearance of any of these symptoms is an indication for interruption of the transfusion.

Donors with allergies or hypersensitivity to certain drugs may be responsible for some of these reactions. A donor hypersensitive to a drug may develop antibodies against the drug; blood from the donor infused into a patient who is receiving the drug may cause allergic reactions [5].

Elimination of donors with allergies and hypersensitivity to drugs reduces, but does not eliminate, the incidence of allergic reactions. Treatment consists of administration of antihistamines. Epinephrine or steroids are used in the most severe cases.

Exogenous Reactions

Exogenous reactions are those caused by external factors in the administration of blood; antigen-antibody reactions are absent.

Circulatory Overload

Circulatory overload may occur when whole blood is infused too rapidly or given to a recipient who has an increased plasma volume. If the blood is infused too rapidly, a rise in the venous pressure may result. This is especially true in the aged and in patients on the verge of cardiac failure. Pulmonary edema, congestive failure, or hemorrhage into the lungs and the gastrointestinal tract may occur.

Monitoring the venous pressure guards against overtransfusion. The use of packed cells to infuse patients with normal blood volume may prevent overloading of the circulation.

The patient may complain of pounding headache, constriction of the chest, flushed feeling, back pain, chills, or fever. The nurse should stop the transfusion, elevate the head, and notify the physician.

Air Embolism

Air embolism may occur when large amounts of air enter the bloodstream, causing tenacious bubbles in the blood to become lodged in the pulmonary capillaries [1].

The risk of air embolism has been reduced by the closed infusion system using the plastic container. It may result from faulty technique in changing equipment or plastic bags, careless use of Y-type administration sets, and the use of air pressure for rapid blood infusion.

Symptoms are the same as those for circulatory collapse: cyanosis, dyspnea, shock, and sometimes, cardiac arrest.

The infusion should be clamped immediately, and the patient turned on the left side, head down. This position traps air in the right atrium, preventing it from entering the pulmonary artery; the pulmonic valve is kept clear until the air can escape gradually. The physician is notified.

Hypothermia
Hypothermia may occur from the rapid, massive replacement of cold blood. Such an infusion can result in chills, hypothermia, peripheral vasoconstriction, and cardiac arrest. Warming blood to 35°C with automatic blood warmers during rapid massive replacement prevents hypothermia.

Citrate Toxicity
Citrate toxicity may result from the rapid infusion of large quantities of citrated blood to patients with severely impaired liver function. The liver, unable to keep up with the rapid administration, is not able to metabolize the citrate ions; the citrate ions combine with calcium in the bloodstream, causing a calcium deficit.

Symptoms of excess citrate include tingling of fingers, muscular cramps, convulsions, hypotension, and cardiac arrest. Most of these symptoms are absent in the anesthetized patient, making detection of toxicity difficult.

Treatment consists of slow administration *by a physician* of ionized calcium such as calcium chloride.

Delayed Reactions

Delayed reactions may occur up to 160 days after the infusion and are the result of transmitted disease or isoimmunization.

Hepatitis
Transfusion-associated hepatitis, due to hepatitis A virus, is extremely rare as its presence in the blood is of a very short duration. The transmission of hepatitis type B to recipients has been greatly reduced by methods involved in screening donors for the hepatitis B surface antigen (HBsAg) and conversion from paid to voluntary donor systems; some risk still remains, however. The average incubation period is 90 days with a range of 15–180 days, the length of incubation period depending on the amount of hepatitis B virus (HBV) the patient is exposed to and the route of exposure [3].

If transfused recipients are carefully followed and tested, some degree of liver damage is found to occur in 7–10% of these recipients. Because no known viruses can be identified in 90 percent of these cases, the term non-A, non-B (NANB) hepatitis has been applied. About half of these have been thought to have chronic active hepatitis which may in some cases progress to cirrhosis. Incubation time for NANB hepatitis is approximately 50 days with a range of 15–180 days. Transfusion of any blood component or product with the exception of immune globulin preparations, heat-treated albumin, and plasma protein solutions can result in hepatitis B and NANB hepatitis [3].

AIDS
Acquired Immune Deficiency Syndrome (AIDS) is a disease caused by type III retrovirus called HTLV-III for Human T-Cell Lymphotropic Virus. It destroys the body's immune system and renders the individual vulnerable to infection

and cancers. "AIDS has occurred in hemophiliacs (1 percent of AIDS cases) who have been treated with large quantities of commercial Factor VIII concentrates" [3]. About 1 percent of AIDS cases are associated with blood transfusions [3].

In March 1985 a test for HTLV-III antibody became available to blood banks as a way to screen donors and to protect the nation's blood supply. The test gives information on exposure to the virus but does not diagnose AIDS. If a person has been exposed to AIDS and is still in an inactive period, the test may be negative. "The incubation period appears to be 6 to 24 months; in cases of suspected transfusion-associated AIDS, transfusion within the preceding 5 years should be considered relevant" [3].

Blood Specimens. Special caution must be observed in the care of blood specimens and blood-contaminated articles because blood from all patients should be considered infective. Blood specimens should not be allowed to spill on the outside of containers. Hospital policies for disposal of infectious materials must be observed. Cannulas should not be recapped or broken but disposed of intact in needle-proof containers. All personnel handling blood should wear gloves.

Syphilis
Serologic testing for syphilis required by the FDA and refrigerated blood storage have nearly eradicated the transmission of syphilis by blood transfusion; refrigeration has a spirocheticidal effect, eliminating treponemas after 72 hours at 4°C [3]. Fresh blood products carry the greatest risk of transmission of syphilis.

Malaria
Deferral of donors who have been in a malaria unit within the last 6 months or donors who have had malaria or have taken antimalarial prophylaxis within the last 3 years is the only factor in preventing transmission of malaria. There is no practical screening method to detect plasmodia in the donor's blood.

Delayed Hemolytic Reaction
Delayed hemolytic reaction is another endogenous reaction. The immune antibody, produced by the body's response to a foreign antigen in a previous transfusion, reacts with the corresponding antigen on the donor's red cells in subsequent transfusions. When the donor's red cells possessing the corresponding antigen are infused, they provoke an immune response in which rapid increase in antibodies is followed by increased destruction of the transfused cells. The incompatible red cells survive until there is ample antibody to initiate a rejection response. This reaction may be clinically severe with hemolysis; mild anemia and an increase in bilirubin occurring 2–11 days after transfusion. A direct Coombs' test may detect the antibody, but in very rapidly progressing delayed hemolytic reaction this test may be negative.

REFERENCES

1. Adriani, J. Venipuncture. *Am. J. Nurs.* 62:66, 1962.
2. American Association of Blood Banks. *Standards for Blood Banks and Transfusion Services* (11th ed.). Chicago: Twentieth Century Press, 1984, pp. 11, 18, 26, 29, 32.
3. American Association of Blood Banks. *Technical Manual* (9th ed.). Philadelphia: Lippincott, 1985, pp. 36, 44, 48, 73, 75, 77–78, 269, 277, 332, 339, 340, 345.
4. Grove-Rasmussen, M., Lesses, M. F., and Anstall, H. B. Medical progress: Transfusion therapy. *N. Engl. J. Med.* 264:1034–1044, 1088–1095, 1961.
5. Huestis, D. W., Bove, J. R., and Busch, S. *Practical Blood Transfusion* (2nd ed.). Boston: Little, Brown, 1976, pp. 60, 271.
6. Kumar, J. R. Leukapheresis and granulocyte transfusion. *J. NITA* 3(4): 115, 116, 1980.
7. Machine Extends Blood Storage Time. *Hospital Formulary Management.* Chicago: Clissold Publishing, 1966, p. 44.
8. Metheny, N. M., and Snively, W. D., Jr. *Nurse's Handbook of Fluid Balance* (4th ed.). Philadelphia: Lippincott, 1983, pp. 176, 181.
9. Ortho Diagnostics. *RhoGAM One Year Later* (Proceedings of Symposium on RhoGAM, Rh$_o$[D] Immune Globulin [Human], New York, April 17, 1969). Raritan, N.J., 1969, pp. 11, 14, 59.
10. Pool, J. G. Precipitate from cold thawed plasma potent in therapy for hemophiliacs. *J.A.M.A.* 193:27, 1965.
11. Solis, R. T., and Gibbs, M. B. Filtration of the microaggregates in stored blood. *Transfusion* 12:245, 1972.

REVIEW QUESTIONS

1. Where are antigens in blood transfusion therapy found?
2. Which are genetically inherited — antigens or antibodies?
3. What determines an individual's blood group — antigens or antibodies?
4. An antigen has the ability to evoke an immune response when infused into an individual who lacks this substance. True or false?
5. An individual's serum usually contains antibodies that are specific to the antigens on his or her red cells. True or false?
6. Immune antibodies can be produced only by active immunization following a blood transfusion or a pregnancy. True or false?
7. An antibody bears the same designation as the antigen with which it reacts. True or false?
8. Rh factors are antigens C, D, E, c, e, located on the surface of the red cells. True or false?
9. Which positive antigens are likely to evoke an immune response when introduced into Rh-negative recipients — CDE antigens or cde antigens?
10. In administering plasma the _____ in the donor plasma must be compatible with the _____ in the recipient's blood.
11. What blood type is the universal donor for plasma, and why?
12. Name the group plasma that can be administered to the following recipients: (a) AB, (b) A, (c) B, and (d) O.
13. Which packed cells — group O, A, or B — are considered preferable for administration to AB recipients in life-threatening situations, and why?

Chapter 13 | Transfusion Therapy

14. When Rh-positive blood components are administered to Rh-negative recipients, consideration should be given to the administration of _____ .
15. Albumin 25% is _hypertonic_ ; if rapidly infused, _circulatory overload_ may occur.
16. Granulocytes must be ABO- and Rh-matched. <u>True</u> or false?
17. Severe reactions usually accompany the administration of granulocytes, making medication necessary. <u>True</u> or false?
18. Major hemolytic reactions occur when the _antibodies_ in the recipient's blood reacts with the _antigens_ in the donor blood.
19. Intravascular hemolysis usually involves the naturally occurring antibodies, such as antibody A and B, with hemolysis of the sensitized red cells taking place in the bloodstream. True or false?

CHAPTER 14

Therapeutic Phlebotomy

Ada Lawrence Plumer

The purpose of this chapter is to acquaint the physician or nurse who may be called upon to perform a phlebotomy outside the confines of the blood bank with the equipment, the procedure, and the technique recommended for the protection of both the donor and the recipient. The phlebotomy, a bleeding of usually 400–500 ml blood, is performed for transfusion purposes and therapeutically for acute pulmonary congestion, polycythemia vera, hemochromatosis, and porphyria cutanea tarda.

BLOOD FOR TRANSFUSION PURPOSES

Routine Blood Bank Blood When the bleeding is performed for routine bank blood, donor selection is based on the medical history and the physical examination (weight, temperature, pulse, blood pressure, and hemoglobin). The technique is according to the standards of the American Association of Blood Banks (AABB) [1].

Autotransfusion Autotransfusion is used to return the patient's own blood to the circulation. The phlebotomy may be a:

1. *Blood bank procedure.* When the phlebotomy is performed in the blood bank, the usual blood bank procedure is followed. The blood can be stored at 4°C or the red cells can be frozen.

2. *Non-blood bank procedure.* When the bleeding is performed outside the confines of the blood bank, the same technique (according to the standards of the AABB) is used. However, the donor criteria can be modified; for example, a person with a history of cancer cannot make a routine donation but may donate for himself. Blood which is suitable only for the donor must be labeled with his name, hospital number, or social security number, and segregated from other donor bloods. The ABO type is confirmed just prior to transfusion.

Chapter 14 | Therapeutic Phlebotomy

An important fact to bear in mind is the possibility of sepsis; clinically undetected bacteremia may exist in the patient with a catheter, a tracheostomy, or a disease process.

BLOOD FOR THERAPEUTIC PURPOSES

The therapeutic phlebotomy is a valuable means by which a quantity of blood is removed to promote the health of the donor. It requires a written order by the physician specifying the date, the amount of blood to be drawn, the frequency of bleeding, and/or the hemoglobin or hematocrit at which the patient should be bled. If the recipient's physician approves and if the label conspicuously indicates the diagnosis and a therapeutic bleeding, the blood may be used for transfusion.

Acute Pulmonary Congestion (Inpatient)

The phlebotomy is performed to reduce venous pressure and to relieve the work load on the heart of a patient suffering from acute pulmonary edema of cardiac failure or overtransfusion. Overtransfusion is much less likely to occur today since central venous pressure monitoring provides a valuable guide for fluid administration; also, drugs are available to increase cardiac output and lower the central venous pressure. Since the patient with acute pulmonary congestion is critically ill, the phlebotomy should probably be done by, or in the presence of, the patient's physician.

Polycythemia Vera (Inpatient or Outpatient)

The therapeutic phlebotomy is most frequently performed on the hospital patient for the production of remissions in the treatment of polycythemia vera, a disease characterized by a striking absolute increase in the number of circulating red blood corpuscles. It is used to reduce the red cell mass, either alone or in combination with radioactive phosphorus (^{32}P), lowering the blood volume, reducing blood viscosity, and improving circulatory efficiency. The number of and interval between phlebotomies should be specified by the physician and the hematocrit value determined after the blood donation.

Hemochromatosis (Usually Outpatient)

Hemochromatosis is characterized by excessive body stores of iron. The phlebotomy is performed to reduce the total body iron. Because these patients usually have a hematocrit value in the normal range, periodic checks on the hematocrit value are desirable.

Porphyria Cutanea Tarda (Usually Outpatient)

The mechanism of relief of these skin lesions by phlebotomy is not clear. Because these patients have a normal hematocrit reading they are most likely to be bled too much; periodic hematocrit checks are desirable.

PROCEDURE FOR BLEEDING

To allay apprehension and to avoid a vasovagal reaction (an undesirable autonomic nervous system response), the procedure should be explained, and the patient reassured and put at ease.

Identification	1. Identify donor with the record and the order for the phlebotomy.
2. Make sure that identically numbered labels to donor record are attached to the blood collection container and to test tubes for donor blood samples.
3. Make sure that the processing tubes are correctly numbered and kept with the container during the collection of blood.
Donor Arm Preparation	Adequate preparation of the skin is vital in providing an aseptic site for venipuncture which will protect both the donor and the recipient. In preparing the area always start at the venipuncture site and move outward in concentric spirals for at least 1½ inches; use sterile materials and instruments.
1. Using a 15% aqueous (not alcoholic) soap or detergent solution, scrub vigorously for at least 30 seconds with gauze, or 60 seconds with cotton balls.
2. Apply 10% acetone in 70% isopropyl alcohol to remove the soap; let dry.
3. Apply tincture of iodine (3% in 70% ethyl alcohol) and allow to dry.
4. Use 10% acetone in 70% isopropyl alcohol to remove the iodine; allow to dry.
5. Place a dry sterile gauze over the site until ready to perform the venipuncture.

Alternative procedure:
1. Use 0.7% aqueous scrub solution of iodophor compound (povidone-iodine or poloxamer iodine complex), scrubbing the area for 30 seconds. Remove the foam; it is not necessary to dry the arm.
2. Prepare with iodophor complex solution (e.g., 10% povidone-iodine); allow to stand 30 seconds. The solution need not be removed.
3. Place a dry sterile gauze sponge over the site until ready to perform the venipuncture. Do not repalpate vein. |
| **Collection of Blood** | The following procedure for the collection of blood (see Figure 14.1) using the plastic bag is reproduced from the AABB's *Technical Methods and Procedures* [1]. Modification to this procedure may be made when the blood is to be discarded.
1. Inspect bag for any defects. Apply pressure to check for leaks. The anticoagulant solution must be clear.
2. Position bag carefully, being sure it is below the level of the donor's arm.
    a. If balance system is used, be sure counterbalance is level and adjusted for the amount of blood to be drawn. Unless metal clips and a hand sealer are used, make a very loose overhand knot in tubing. Hang the bag and route tubing through the pinch clamp. |

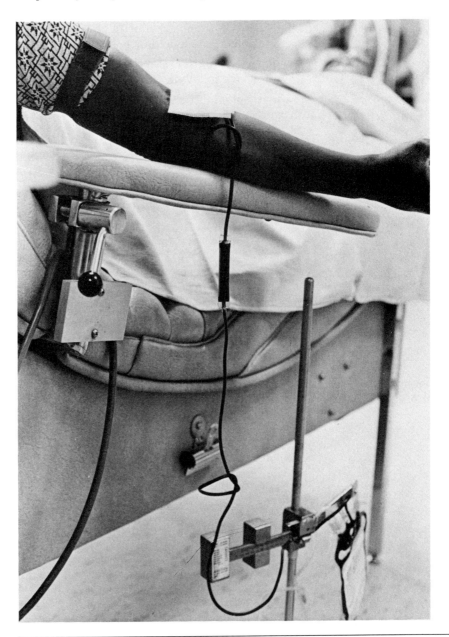

FIGURE 14.1
A phlebotomy. Note the sterile sponge placed over the venipuncture site during bleeding.

b. If balance system is not used, be sure there is some way to monitor the volume of blood drawn.

c. If a vacuum-assist device is used, the manufacturer's instructions should be followed.

3. Reapply tourniquet or blood pressure cuff. Have donor open and close hand until previously selected vein is again prominent.

4. Put on gloves. Uncover sterile needle and do venipuncture immediately. A clean, skillful venipuncture is essential for collection of a full, clot-free unit. Tape the tubing to hold needle in place and cover site with sterile gauze.

5. Open the temporary closure between the interior of the bag and the tubing, if present.

6. Have donor open and close hand, squeezing a rubber ball or other resilient object slowly every 10–12 seconds during collection. Keep the donor under observation throughout phlebotomy. The donor should never be left unattended during or immediately after donation.

7. Mix the blood and anticoagulant gently and periodically (approximately every 30 seconds) during collection. Mixing may be done by hand, by placing bag on a mechanical agitator, or by using a rocking vacuum-assist device.

8. Be sure blood flow remains fairly brisk, so that coagulation activity is not triggered. Rigid time limits are not warranted if there is continuous agitation, although units requiring more than 8 minutes to draw may not be suitable for preparation of platelet concentrates, fresh frozen plasma or cryoprecipitate.

9. Monitor volume of blood being drawn. If a balance or vacuum-assist device is used, blood flow will stop after the proper amount has been collected. One ml of blood weighs 1.053 gm, the minimum allowable specific gravity for female donors. A convenient figure to use is 1.06 gm; a unit containing 405–495 ml should weigh 425–520 gm plus the weight of the container with its anticoagulant.

10. Clamp tubing temporarily using a hemostat, metal clip, or other temporary clamp. Next, collect blood processing sample by a method that precludes contamination of the donor unit. There are several ways in which this may be accomplished.

    a. If the blood collection bag contains an in-line needle ("sid connector"), make an additional seal with a hemostat, metal clip, hand sealer, or a tight knot made from previously prepared loose knot just distal to the in-line needle. Open the connector by separating the needles. Insert the proximal needle into a processing test tube, remove the hemostat, allow the tube to fill, and reclamp tubing. Carefully reattach "sid connector." Donor needle is now ready for removal.

Chapter 14 | Therapeutic Phlebotomy

    b. If the blood collection bag contains an in-line processing tube, be certain that the processing tube, or pouch, is full when the collection is complete and the original clamp is placed near the donor needle. Entire assembly may now be removed from donor.

    c. If a straight-tubing assembly set is used there are two alternative procedures. In the first method, remove the needle from the donor's arm as soon as the tubing is clamped. Take bag and assembly to sealer area or collect processing tube at the donor chair by placing a hemostat close to where donor tubing enters the bag, leaving the tubing full of blood. Remove the clamp next to donor needle, empty contents of donor tubing into the processing test tube, reapply clamp or permanently seal next to donor needle, remove hemostat next to donor bag, and allow the donor tubing to refill with blood, well-mixed, from donor bag. In the second method, place two hemostats or temporary seals on the tubing. Cut tubing between seals, put cut end of tubing into processing test tube, remove proximal hemostat, allow tube to fill, and reclamp tubing.

11. Deflate and remove tourniquet. Remove needle from arm. Apply pressure over gauze and have donor raise arm (elbow straight) and hold gauze firmly over phlebotomy site with the other hand.

12. Discard needle assembly into special container designed to prevent accidental injury to and contamination of personnel.

13. Strip donor tubing as completely as possible into the bag, starting at seal. Work quickly, to avoid allowing the blood to clot in the tubing. Invert bag several times to mix thoroughly, then allow tubing to refill with anticoagulated blood from the bag. Repeat this procedure a second time.

14. Seal the tubing left attached to the bags into segments on which the segment number is clearly and completely readable. Knots, metal clips, or a dielectric sealer may be used to make segments suitable for crossmatching. It must be possible to separate segments from the container without breaking sterility of the container.

15. Reinspect container for defects.

16. Recheck numbers on container, processing tubes, and donation record. Be sure the expiration date of the unit is on the container label.

17. Place blood at appropriate temperature. Unless platelets are to be removed, whole blood should be placed at 1–6°C immediately after collection. If platelets are to be harvested, blood should not be chilled but should be maintained at room temperature (about 20–24°C) until platelets are separated. Platelets should be separated within 6 hours after collection of the unit of whole blood.

18. Remove gloves and wash hands.

Treatment of Adverse Donor Reactions

Stop the phlebotomy at the first sign of reaction and call the physician.

1. *Fainting*

   Elevate the donor's feet above head level.

   Loosen tight clothing.

   Ascertain that the donor has adequate airway.

   Apply cold compresses to forehead and back of neck.

   Check and record blood pressure, pulse, and respiration periodically.

2. *Nausea and vomiting*

   Instruct the donor to breathe slowly.

3. *Muscular twitching* or tetanic spasms of hands or face

   Instruct donor to rebreathe into a paper bag. DO NOT GIVE OXYGEN.

4. *Convulsions* (rare)

   Call for help.

   Prevent the donor from injuring himself or herself.

   Place tongue blades well-wrapped between donor's teeth.

5. *For more serious reactions* or if donor does not respond

   Call for medical aid.

Record the nature and treatment of all reactions on the donor's record; include opinion as to the future use of the donor for blood donations.

SUGGESTED PROCEDURE FOR THERAPEUTIC PHLEBOTOMY

The blood must be discarded. This procedure is not adequate for recipient protection.

Equipment

Phlebotomy pack (obtained from blood bank); if only double pack is available, ignore the satellite pack.

Counterbalance stand (obtained from blood bank) or small spring scale.

Blood pressure cuff or tourniquet.

Tincture of iodine (3% in 70% ethyl alcohol) or iodophor complex solution (10% povidone-iodine).

10% acetone in 70% isopropyl alcohol for use with tincture of iodine. Sterile sponges.

Technique

Preparation

1. Select the most suitable vein. Apply a tourniquet or a blood pressure cuff inflated to 50–60 mm of mercury. Opening and closing the fist will make the vein more prominent. Remove the tourniquet.

2. Prepare the venipuncture site. Always start at the puncture site and move out in concentric spirals for 1½ inches.
   a. Apply tincture of iodine; allow to dry. *Question patient before applying; some patients may be allergic to iodine.*
   b. Apply 10% acetone in 70% isopropyl alcohol to remove iodine. Allow to dry. Iodophor complex (10% povidone-iodine) may be substituted for iodine. It does not cause skin reactions even in iodine-sensitive individuals. Do not wash off iodophor complex. Cover the site with dry sterile gauze to prevent contamination until the phlebotomy is begun.

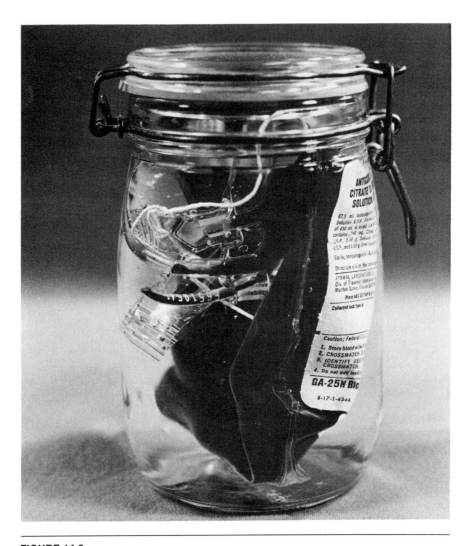

FIGURE 14.2
During autoclaving to decontaminate a unit of blood, bag is protected by a water bath in a sealed glass container. Specimen bottle, Wheaton Scientific, Millville, N.J.

Collection of Blood

1. Suspend bag from donor scale as far below donor's arm as possible.
2. If counterbalance scales are used, adjust the balance for amount of blood to be drawn.
3. Make loose overhand knot in donor tube near needle.
4. Apply tourniquet (do not impair arterial circulation).
5. *Do not touch or repalpate vein.*
6. Perform phlebotomy.
7. Tape needle in place and cover with sterile sponge.
8. Pinch bead into bag from junction of donor tube and bag to open lumen and allow blood to flow.
9. Instruct patient to open and close fist slowly.
10. Collect blood until bag falls on scale. If spring scales are used, collect until prescribed amount has been withdrawn.
11. Pull knot tight.
12. Release tourniquet, withdraw needle, and apply pressure with gauze pad until bleeding has stopped. *Do not flex arm.* The arm may be elevated while applying pressure.
13. Dispose of blood and equipment as directed by hospital procedure. *Caution:* Blood infected with the hepatitis virus should be decontaminated before disposal. The bag of blood, protected by a water bath in a sealed glass container (Figure 14.2), is autoclaved at 120°C at 15 pounds of pressure per square inch for 60 minutes.
14. Record procedure in patient's record.

REFERENCE

1. American Association of Blood Banks. *Technical Manual* (9th ed.). Washington, D.C., 1985, pp. 11–15.

REVIEW QUESTIONS

1. Define the term *autotransfusion*.
2. Define the term *therapeutic phlebotomy*.
3. A therapeutic phlebotomy requires a written order by the physician specifying the date and _____ .
4. Give three reasons for performing a therapeutic phlebotomy.
5. Negligence in reassuring the patient, explaining the procedure, and allaying apprehension can result in a _____ reaction.
6. The following preparation of the venipuncture site provides adequate recipient protection. True or false?
   ☐ Apply tincture of iodine; allow to dry.
   ☐ Apply 10% acetone in 70% alcohol.

Chapter 14 | Therapeutic Phlebotomy

7. When a blood pressure cuff is used as a tourniquet it is inflated to how many mmHg?
8. What treatment is suggested if the donor becomes faint?
9. What procedure is used if a faint muscular twitching or tetanic spasm of the hands or face resulting from hyperventilation occurs?
10. What method is used to dispose of blood infected with the hepatitis virus?

CHAPTER 15

Laboratory Tests

Ada Lawrence Plumer

In the past, intravenous departments included the collection of venous blood samples as one of their functions. Since intravenous therapy has become highly specialized and thus requires more of the nurse's time, the collection of venous blood now is often allocated to a team of technicians. There are still many instances in which the intravenous nurse will be involved: for example, in critical care units, when veins have become exhausted, when the patient is to receive an intravenous infusion and when the specimen is to be obtained from a central venous cannula that is to be removed, from a multilumen central venous cannula, from a Hickman/Broviac cannula, or from an implanted vascular access device. Definite advantages are gained when this nurse is involved in collecting venous blood [1]. The nurse, understanding the importance of the preservation of veins for infusion therapy, is cautious when choosing veins and in applying blood-drawing techniques [2]. Frequently one venipuncture permits both the withdrawal of blood and the initiation of the infusion, thereby preserving veins, reducing discomfort, and avoiding undue distress of the patient [3]. The patient-blood identification is of paramount importance in preventing the error of infusing incompatible blood. Because the department assumes responsibility in patient-blood identification in administering bloods and is aware of existing hazards, its personnel are well qualified and trained in the collection of samples for typing and crossmatching.

The nurse is often faced with the problem of collecting blood with little or no knowledge of the tests other than the amount of blood needed and the type of tube required. This chapter is intended primarily to provide the nurse with information concerning the most commonly performed laboratory tests — their purpose and normal values, and the collection and proper handling of the specimens. No attempt is made to explain laboratory procedures.

COLLECTION OF VENOUS BLOOD SAMPLES

The collection of blood samples for certain tests must meet special requirements. Some tests call for whole blood, while others require components such as plasma, serum, or cells. The proper requirement must be met to prevent erroneous or misleading laboratory analysis.

Serum consists of plasma minus fibrinogen and is obtained by drawing blood in a dry tube and allowing it to coagulate. Serum is required by the majority of laboratory tests in common use.

Plasma consists of the stable components of blood minus the cells and is obtained by using an anticoagulant to prevent the blood from clotting. Several anticoagulants are available in color-coded tubes. Choice of the anticoagulant depends upon the test to be performed. Most of the anticoagulants, including sodium or potassium oxalate, citrate, and ethylenediaminetetraacetic acid (EDTA), prevent coagulation by binding the serum calcium. Other anticoagulants, such as heparin, are valuable in specific tests but are not commonly used. Heparin prevents coagulation for only limited periods of time.

Whole blood is required for many tests, including blood counts and bleeding time. Potassium oxalate is commonly used to preserve whole blood.

Hemoconcentration through venous stasis should be avoided or inaccurate results will occur in some tests. Hemoconcentration increases proportionally with the length of time the tourniquet is applied. Once the venipuncture has been made, the tourniquet should be removed. This is a simple but important precaution, ignored by many. Carbon dioxide and pH are examples of tests affected by hemoconcentration. If the tourniquet is required to withdraw the blood, it should be noted on the requisition that the blood was drawn with stasis.

Hemolysis causes serious errors in many tests in which lysis of the red cells permits the substance being measured to escape into the serum. When red cells rich in potassium rupture, the serum potassium level rises, giving a false measurement. To avoid hemolysis, the following special precautions should be observed:

1. Dry syringes and dry tubes must be used.
2. Excess pressure on the plunger of the syringe should be avoided; such pressure collapses the vein and may cause air bubbles to be sucked from around the hub of the needle into the blood.
3. Clotted blood specimens should not be shaken unnecessarily.
4. Force should be avoided in transferring blood to a container or tube; force of the blood against the tube results in rupture of the cells. In transferring blood to a vacuum tube, no needle larger than 20 gauge should be used.

Intravenous Solutions

Intravenous solutions may contribute to misleading laboratory interpretations. Blood samples should never be drawn proximal to an infusion but preferably from the contralateral extremity. If the solution contains a substance which may affect the analysis, an indication of its presence should be made on the requisition — for example, potassium determination during an infusion of electrolyte solution.

Special Handling

Special handling is required with some samples when a delay is unavoidable. Some determinations, such as the pH, must be done within 10 minutes after the blood is drawn. When a delay is inevitable, the sample is placed in ice, which partially inhibits *glycolysis,* the production of lactic acid by the glycolytic enzymes of the blood cells, resulting in a rapid lowering of pH on standing.

Blood gases also require special handling and must be analyzed as soon as collected. When the carbon dioxide content of serum is to be determined, the blood must completely fill the tube or carbon dioxide will escape. There are several procedures currently in use; in each the escape of carbon dioxide must be prevented.

Fasting
As absorption of food may alter the blood, some tests depend upon the patient's fasting. Blood glucose and serum lipid levels are increased by ingestion of food. Serum inorganic phosphorous values are depressed after meals.

Promptness of Examination
Immediate dispatch of blood samples to the laboratory is vital to the accurate determination of some blood tests; promptness in examining blood samples is necessary in the analysis of labile constituents of blood. In certain tests, such as potassium, the substance being measured diffuses out of the cells into the serum being examined and gives a false measurement. To prevent this rise in serum concentration, the cells must be separated from the serum promptly.

Infected Samples
Special caution must be observed in the care of all blood specimens, because blood from all patients is to be considered infective. Specimens should not be allowed to spill on the outside of the containers. Contaminated material should be placed in bags and treated in accordance with institutional policies for disposal of infectious material. Cannulas should not be recapped or broken but disposed of intact in cannula-proof containers. All personnel handling blood should wear gloves.

Emergency Tests
Blood tests ordered as emergency must be sent directly to the laboratory. Red cellophane tape or other alert-type stickers, according to facility preference, may be used to indicate a state of emergency. Tests most likely to be designated as emergencies include amylase, blood urea nitrogen (BUN), carbon dioxide, potassium, prothrombin, sodium, sugar, and blood typing.

VENIPUNCTURE FOR WITHDRAWING BLOOD

A venipuncture, when skillfully executed, subjects the patient to little discomfort. The numerous blood determinations necessary for diagnosis and treatment make good technique imperative.

The one-step entry technique should be avoided as it too often results in through-and-through punctures, contributing to hematoma formation. The needle should be inserted under the skin and then, after relocation of the vein, into the vessel.

The veins most commonly used are those in the antecubital fossa. The median antecubital vein, though not always visible, is usually large and palpable. Since it is well supported by subcutaneous tissue and least likely to roll, it is often the best choice for venipuncture. Second choice is the cephalic vein. The basilic vein, though oftentimes the most prominent, is likely to be the least desirable. This vein rolls easily, making the venipuncture difficult, and a hematoma may readily occur if the patient is allowed to flex his or her arm; flexing the arm squeezes the blood from the engorged vein into the tissues.

Sufficient time should be spent in locating the vein before attempting venipuncture. Whenever the veins are difficult to see or palpate, the patient should lie down. If the patient is seated the arm should be well supported on a pillow.

Complications

Hematomas

Hematomas are the most common complication of routine venipuncture for withdrawing blood, and they contribute more to the limitation of available veins than any other complication. They may result from through-and-through puncture to the vein or from incomplete insertion of the needle into the lumen of the vein, which allows the blood to leak into the tissues by way of the bevel of the needle. In the latter case, correction may be made by advancing the needle into the vein. At the first sign of uncontrolled bleeding, the tourniquet should be released and the needle withdrawn.

Hematomas also result from the application of the tourniquet after an unsuccessful attempt has been made to draw blood. The tourniquet should never be applied to the extremity immediately after a venipuncture.

Hematomas most frequently result from insufficient time spent in applying pressure and from the bad habit of flexing the arm to stop the bleeding. Once the venipuncture is completed, the patient should be instructed to elevate the arm; elevation causes a negative pressure in the vein, collapsing it and facilitating clotting. With cardiac patients, elevation of the arm should be avoided. Constant pressure is maintained until the bleeding has stopped. Pressure is applied with a dry sterile sponge; a wet sponge encourages bleeding. Band-Aids do not take the place of pressure and, if ordered, are not applied until the bleeding has stopped. Ecchymoses on the arm indicate poor technique or haphazard manner.

Hepatitis
Special caution must be exercised in the care of needles used to draw blood from patients suspected of harboring microorganisms. Contaminated needles should be placed immediately in a separate container for disposal. A vacuum tube with stopper provides adequate protection against accidental puncture from the contaminated needle until proper disposal can be made. Any needle puncture should be reported at once.

Other complications of venipuncture include syncope, continued bleeding, and thrombosis of the vein. Serum hepatitis may occur if the same syringes or needle holders are used for multiple punctures.

Syncope is rarely encountered when the therapist is confident, skillful, and reassures the patient.

Continued bleeding is a complication that may affect the patient receiving anticoagulants, the patient with a blood dyscrasia or the oncology patient undergoing chemotherapy. To prevent bleeding and to preserve the vein, pressure to the site may be required for an extended period of time. The therapist should remain with the patient until the bleeding has stopped.

Thrombosis in routine venipuncture occurs from injury to the endothelial lining of the vein during the venipuncture. Antecubital veins may be used indefinitely if the therapist has skillful technique.

THE VACUUM SYSTEM

The vacuum system, which is replacing the syringe for withdrawing blood, has done much to increase the efficiency of the program. It consists of a plastic holder into which screws a sterile disposable double-ended needle. A rubber-stoppered vacuum tube slips into the barrel. The barrel has a measured line denoting the distance the tube is inserted into the barrel; at this point the needle becomes embedded in the stopper. The stopper is not punctured until the needle has been introduced into the vein.

After entry into the vein, the rubber-stoppered tube is pushed the remaining distance into the barrel. As the needle is pushed into the vacuum tube, a rubber sheath covering the shaft is forced back, allowing the blood to flow. The tourniquet is released and several specimens may be obtained by simply removing the tube containing the sample and replacing it with another tube. As the tube is removed, the rubber sheath slips back over the needle, preventing blood from dripping into the holder.

If there is failure in locating the vein, removal of the tube before the needle is withdrawn will preserve the vacuum in the tube.

At times it becomes necessary to draw blood from small veins. If suction from the vacuum tube collapses the vein, difficulty will be encountered in drawing the blood. By pressing the finger against the vein beyond the point of the needle or by placing the bevel of the needle lightly against the wall of the vein, suction is reduced and the vein allowed to fill. In the latter process, particular caution should be exercised to prevent injury to the endothelial lining of the vein. The pressure is intermittently applied and released, filling and emptying the vein. A 22-gauge needle is available and often used successfully when

Chapter 15 | Laboratory Tests

small amounts of blood are needed; the smaller needle reduces the amount of suction and may prevent collapse of the vein. A syringe is often used to draw blood from small veins as the amount of suction can be more easily controlled.

DRAWING BLOOD VIA THE CENTRAL VENOUS CATHETER

Occasionally it becomes desirable to draw blood samples via the central venous catheter (see also Part VI). Such occasions include difficulty in obtaining an adequate vein, cases in which the avoidance of stress is imperative, and situations in which blood tests are ordered frequently and repeatedly.

Aseptic technique is vital in preventing the introduction of bacteria into the catheter. A sterile I.V. Catheter Plug,* placed in the stopcock outlet at the time the catheter is inserted, reduces the risk of bacterial invasion.

Procedure Follow this procedure in drawing blood by way of the central venous catheter from a patient not on drug therapy:

1. Put on gloves. Clamp off the infusion.
2. Remove catheter plug, protecting stopcock outlet, and with a sterile syringe withdraw 4 ml of blood; discard it.
3. Using a sterile syringe, withdraw the required amount of blood. If difficulty is encountered in drawing blood samples, raise patient's arm to shoulder level or higher to reduce axillary pressure on catheter.
4. Recap stopcock with a sterile plug.
5. Open clamp and flush catheter with about 5 ml of infusion fluid to maintain patency of catheter.
6. Adjust flow to prescribed flow rate. After contact with patient, remove gloves and wash hands.

If the patient is receiving drug therapy, follow the same procedure, except *use a hemostat* to stop the infusion temporarily; after the blood is drawn, the control clamp maintains the prescribed rate of flow without readjustment.

Precaution Patients receiving vasopressors may not tolerate an interruption of medication. Check with the charge nurse before stopping the infusion; extra caution may be required, with a standby nurse to watch the monitor.

WITHDRAWING BLOOD AND INITIATING AN INFUSION

Drawing blood samples and initiating an infusion can be efficiently accomplished by a single venipuncture in the following way:

1. Put on gloves. Fill intravenous set with solution.
2. Regulate the flow to a minimum rate.

---

*American McGaw Laboratories, Inc., Irvine, Calif.; Division of American Hospital Supply Corporation.

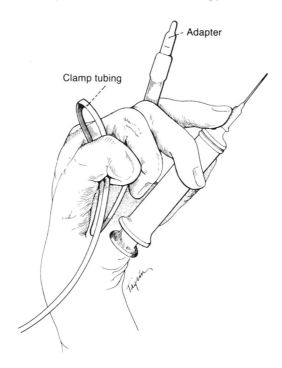

FIGURE 15.1
Infusion tubing is kinked and held by the little finger; adapter is held between the forefinger and second finger, leaving the hand free for drawing blood sample; a small-vein needle or over-the-needle catheter is replacing the metal needle. New CDC revisions call for gloves to be worn.

3. Clamp tubing manually by kinking between third and little fingers (Figure 15.1).
4. Hold adapter between the forefinger and second finger, leaving the hand free for holding the syringe and cannula and collecting blood.
5. Draw blood.
6. Remove syringe; attach the infusion set to the cannula, releasing little finger; solution will flow at the previously adjusted rate.
7. Secure cannula with a piece of tape.
8. Attach syringe to needle, previously imbedded in stopper of vacuum tube, and transfer blood. Vacuum will cause tube to fill — never apply force. Use no larger needle than 20 gauge; lysis of cells can occur.
9. Remove gloves and wash hands.

COMMONLY USED LABORATORY TESTS

Laboratory tests are performed (1) routinely, because they point out disorders which are relatively common; (2) for diagnostic purposes; (3) for following the course of a disease; and (4) in regulating therapy (Table 15.1, pp. 242–265).

Blood Cultures — In cases of suspected bacteremia, blood cultures are performed to identify the causative microorganisms. Isolation of the organism is necessary to enable the physician to direct proper antimicrobial therapy. Blood cultures are performed during febrile illnesses or when the patient is having chills with spiking fever. Intermittent bacteremia accompanies such infections as pyelonephritis, brucellosis, cholangitis, and other infections. In such cases repeated blood cultures are usually ordered to be performed when the fever spikes. In other infections, such as subacute bacterial endocarditis, the bacteremia is more constant during the 4–5 febrile days. Usually 4 or 5 cultures are obtained over a span of 1–2 days, and antimicrobial therapy is initiated with the realization that the majority of cultures will be found to harbor the offending microorganism. If antimicrobial therapy is administered prior to the blood culture or prior to the patient's admittance to the hospital, the bacteremia may be suppressed, rendering isolation difficult.

Penicillinase is often ordered to be added to the blood culture medium to neutralize the existing penicillinemia and to recover the organism. Usually antimicrobial therapy must be withheld to await report of culture in order to make a precise diagnosis. The penicillinase is added to the culture medium before or immediately after the blood sample is drawn.

Some bacteriology laboratories routinely culture blood under both aerobic and anaerobic conditions. If this is not done routinely and bacteremia with strict anaerobes is suspected, the laboratory should be notified, as a special culture broth is necessary.

Extreme care must be observed in preparing the area for venipuncture as the skin affords a fertile field for bacterial growth. *Staphylococcus albus*, diphtheroids, and yeast (common skin or environment contaminants) usually indicate contamination, whereas *S. aureus* presents a greater problem by indicating either a contaminant or the presence of a serious pathogen.

Procedure

Several procedures are currently in use. Newer methods, for collecting the blood sample, use special vacuum tubes containing prepared culture media. The amount of blood required depends on laboratory and procedure used. All require thorough preparation of the puncture area with an effective antiseptic. An iodine preparation followed by 70% isopropanol is a highly recommended preparation; question the patient about iodine sensitivity. Gloves should be worn by all personnel performing venipuncture.

MEASUREMENTS OF ELECTROLYTE CONCENTRATION

Electrolyte imbalances are serious complications in the critically ill. Such imbalances must be recognized and corrected at once. Frequently electrolyte determinations are ordered on an emergency basis. Accurate measurement is essential and to a large degree depends upon the proper collection and handling of blood specimens.

Potassium

Potassium is an electrolyte essential to body function. Approximately 98 percent of all body potassium is found in the cells; only small amounts are contained in the serum.

The kidneys normally do not conserve potassium. When large quantities of body fluid are lost without potassium replacement, a severe deficiency occurs. Chronic kidney disease and the use of diuretics may cause a potassium deficit. Adrenal steroids play a major role in controlling the concentration of potassium: hyperadrenalism causes increased potassium loss, with deficiency resulting; steroid therapy promotes potassium excretion.

An elevated potassium level results from potassium retention in renal failure or in adrenal cortical deficiency. Hypoventilation and cellular damage also result in an elevated potassium level.

Because intracellular ions are not accessible for measurement, determination must be made on the serum. As the concentration of potassium in the cells is roughly 15 times greater than that in the serum, the blood for potassium determination must be carefully drawn to prevent hemolysis.

Blood Collection. Blood (2 ml) is drawn in a dry tube and allowed to clot or, preferably, placed under oil; oil minimizes friction and hemolysis of the red blood cells. The blood should be sent to the laboratory immediately as potassium diffuses out of the cells and gives a falsely high reading.

Normal serum range is 3.6 to 5.5 mEq per liter [2].

Sodium

The main role of sodium is the control of the distribution of water throughout the body and the maintenance of a normal fluid balance.

The excretion of sodium is regulated to a large degree by the adrenocortical hormone aldosterone. The regulation of water excretion is regulated by ADH (antidiuretic hormone), and as long as these two systems are in harmony, the sodium and water remain in isosmotic proportion. Any change in the normal sodium concentration indicates that the loss or gain of water and sodium are in other than isosmotic proportion. Increased sodium levels may be caused by excessive infusions of sodium, insufficient water intake, or excess loss of fluid without a sodium loss, as in tracheobronchitis. Decreased sodium levels may be caused by excessive sweating accompanied by intake of large amounts of water by mouth, adrenal insufficiency, excessive infusions of nonelectrolyte fluids, or gastrointestinal suction accompanied with water by mouth.

Blood Collection. Blood (3 ml) is drawn carefully to prevent hemolysis and placed in a dry tube or a tube with oil.

Normal serum range is 135 to 145 mEq per liter [1].

Chlorides

Chlorides are usually measured along with other blood electrolytes. The measurement of chlorides is helpful in diagnosing disorders of acid–base balance and water balance of the body. Chloride has a reciprocal power of increasing or decreasing in concentration whenever changes in concentration of other anions occur. In metabolic acidosis there is a reciprocal rise in chloride concentration when the bicarbonate concentration drops.

Elevation in blood chlorides occurs in such conditions as Cushing's syndrome, hyperventilation, and some kidney disorders. A decrease in blood chlorides may occur in diabetic acidosis, heat exhaustion, and following vomiting and diarrhea.

Blood Collection. Venous blood (5 ml) is withdrawn and placed in a dry tube to clot.

Normal serum range is 100 to 106 mEq per liter.

Calcium

Calcium, an essential electrolyte of the body, is required for blood clotting, muscular contraction, and nerve transmission. Only ionized calcium is useful but, since it cannot be satisfactorily measured, the total amount of body calcium is determined; 50 percent of the total is believed to be ionized [2]. In acidosis there is a higher level of ionized calcium; in alkalosis, a lower level.

Hypocalcemia (decrease in normal blood calcium) occurs whenever impairment of the gastrointestinal tract, such as sprue or celiac disease, prevents absorption. Deficiency also occurs in hypoparathyroidism and in some kidney diseases and is characterized by muscular twitching and tetanic convulsions.

Hypercalcemia (excess of calcium in the blood) occurs in hyperparathyroidism and in respiratory disturbance where carbon dioxide blood content is increased, such as in respiratory acidosis.

Blood Collection. Venous blood (5 ml) is placed in a dry tube and allowed to clot. Analysis is performed on the serum.

Normal serum range in adults is 8.5 to 10.5 mg per 100 ml [1]. The range is slightly higher in children.

Phosphorus

Phosphorus metabolism is related to calcium metabolism and the serum level varies inversely with calcium.

Increased concentration of phosphorus may occur in such conditions as hypoparathyroidism, kidney disease, or excessive intake of vitamin D. Decreased concentrations may occur in hyperparathyroidism, rickets, and some kidney diseases.

Blood Collection. Since red cells are rich in phosphorus, hemolysis of the blood must be avoided. Analysis is performed on the serum; 4 ml of blood is placed in a dry tube to clot.

Normal serum range is 3.0 to 4.5 mg per 100 ml [1]. In infants in the first year, the range is up to 6.0 mg per 100 ml.

VENOUS BLOOD MEASUREMENTS OF ACID–BASE BALANCE

Acid–base balance is maintained by the buffer system, carbonic acid–base bicarbonate at a 1–20 ratio. When deviations occur in the normal ratio, a change in pH results and is accompanied by a change in bicarbonate concentration.

Carbon Dioxide Content

Carbon dioxide content is the measurement of the free carbon dioxide and the bicarbonate content of the serum, which provides a general measure of acidity or alkalinity. An increase in carbon dioxide content usually indicates alkalosis; a decrease indicates acidosis. This test, along with clinical findings, is helpful in surmising the severity and nature of the disorder. Measurement of pH is necessary for accuracy — a change in carbon dioxide does not always signify a change in pH, as pH depends on the ratio and not the carbon dioxide content. When the carbon dioxide and pH are known, the buffer ratio can be determined.

An elevated carbon dioxide content is present in metabolic alkalosis, hypoventilation, loss of acid secretions such as occurs in persistent vomiting or drainage of the stomach, and excessive administration of ACTH or cortisone. A low carbon dioxide content usually occurs in loss of alkaline secretions such as in severe diarrhea, certain kidney diseases, diabetic acidosis, and hyperventilation.

Blood Collection. There are several procedures now in use: collection in a heparinized syringe with immediate placement on ice, collection in a heparinized vacuum tube, or collection in a dry tube without an anticoagulant. The procedure used depends upon the laboratory's routine. The containers must always be filled with blood to prevent carbon dioxide from escaping. In all methods it is important that the patient avoid clenching the fist; excess muscular activity of the arm can increase the carbon dioxide level in the blood.

Normal serum range is 24 to 30 mEq per liter [1].

Acidity (pH) Content

pH, a symbol for acidity, indicates the serum concentration of hydrogen ions. The pH becomes lower in acid conditions such as hypoventilation, diarrhea, and diabetic acidosis. The pH rises in alkaline conditions such as hyperventilation and excessive vomiting.

Blood Collection. The blood is collected *without stasis* in a heparinized 2-cc syringe; the syringe is then capped. The blood may be drawn with a small-vein needle, the needle discarded, and the tubing tied off. The specimen is left in the syringe and packed in ice. Loss of carbon dioxide from contact with the air is thus avoided and excess production of lactic acid by enzymic reaction reduced. Five ml blood may also be collected in a green-stoppered vacuum tube containing heparin.

Normal blood range is 7.35–7.45.

ENZYMES

Amylase

Amylase determination is helpful in the diagnosis of acute pancreatitis or the acute recurrence of chronic pancreatitis. Amylase is secreted by the pancreas; a rise in the serum level occurs when outflow of pancreatic juice is restricted. This test is usually performed on patients with acute abdominal pain, or on surgical patients in whom questionable injury may have occurred to the pancreas. Amylase levels usually remain elevated for only a short time — 3–6 days.

Blood Collection. Venous blood (6 ml) is allowed to clot in a dry tube.

Normal serum range is 4–25 units per milliliter. The range may depend upon the normal values established by clinical laboratories, as the method may be modified.

Lipase

Lipase determination is used for detecting damage to the pancreas and is valuable when too much time has elapsed for the amylase level to remain elevated. When secretions of the pancreas are blocked, the serum lipase level rises.

Blood Collection. The test is performed on serum from 6 ml clotted blood.
Normal serum range is 2 units per milliliter or less.

Phosphatase, Acid

Acid phosphatase is useful in determining metastasizing tumors of the prostate. The prostate gland and carcinoma of the gland are rich in phosphatase but do not normally release the enzyme into the serum. Once the carcinoma has spread, it starts to release acid phosphatase, increasing the serum concentration [2]. In addition to carcinoma of the prostate, other conditions that produce increased serum acid phosphatase levels are Paget's disease, hyperparathyroidism, metastatic mammary carcinoma, renal insufficiency, multiple myeloma, some liver disease, arterial embolism, myocardial infarction, and sickle-cell crisis [2].

Blood Collection. Blood (5 ml) is allowed to clot in a dry tube. Hemolysis should be avoided. Analysis should be done immediately or the serum frozen.
Normal serum range. (1) Male: Total, 0.13–0.63 Sigma unit per milliliter. (2) Female: Total, 0.01–0.56 Sigma unit per milliliter. (3) Prostatic: 0–0.5 Fishman-Lerner unit per 100 ml [1].

Phosphatase, Alkaline

Alkaline phosphatase is a useful test in diagnosing bone diseases and obstructive jaundice. In bone diseases the small amount of alkaline usually present in the serum rises in proportion to the new-bone cells. When excretion of alkaline phosphatase is impaired as in some disorders of the liver and biliary tract, the serum level rises and may give some evidence of the degree of blockage in the biliary tract [2].

Blood Collection. Blood (5 ml) is drawn and the test is performed on the serum. Sodium sulfobromophthalein dye should be avoided.
Normal serum range is 13 to 39 units per liter [1].

TRANSAMINASE

The transaminases are enzymes found in large quantities in the heart, liver, muscle, kidney, and pancreas cells. Any disease that causes damage to these cells will result in an elevated serum transaminase level; clinical signs and other tests are used in diagnosis.

SGOT (Serum Glutamic Oxaloacetic Transaminase)

SGOT is used to distinguish between myocardial infarction and acute coronary insufficiency without infarction. It is also useful as a liver function test in following the progression of liver damage or in ascertaining when the liver has recovered.

Blood Collection. The test is performed on serum from 5 ml clotted blood.
Normal serum range is 10–40 units per milliliter. In myocardial infarction, the level is increased 4–10 times, whereas in liver involvement a high of 10–100 times normal may occur. The serum level remains elevated for about 5 days.

SGPT (Serum Glutamic Pyruvate Transaminase)

SGPT is another transaminase that is more specific for hepatic malfunction than SGOT.

Blood Collection. The test is performed on serum from 5 ml blood.
Normal serum range is 6–36 Karmen units per milliliter [2].

SLD (Serum Lactic Dehydrogenase)

The transaminase SLD is present in all tissues and in large quantities in the kidney, heart, and skeletal muscles. Elevated serum levels usually parallel the SGOT levels. Elevation occurs in myocardial infarction and may continue through the sixth day. Elevations have been found in lymphoma, disseminated carcinoma, and some cases of leukemia.

Blood Collection. Blood (3 ml) is collected and allowed to coagulate. Care must be taken to avoid hemolysis, as only a slight degree may give an incorrect reading.
Normal serum range is 60–120 units per milliliter [1].

LIVER FUNCTION TESTS

Albumin, Globulin, Total Protein, and A/G Ratio

These tests may be useful in diagnosing kidney and liver disease or in judging the effectiveness of treatment. The chief role of serum albumin is to maintain osmotic pressure of the blood; globulin assists. The globulin molecule, being larger than the albumin, is less efficient in maintaining osmotic pressure and does not leak out of the blood. With the loss of albumin through the capillary wall, the body compensates by producing more globulin. The osmotic pressure is reduced and may result in some edema. Certain conditions, such as chronic nephritis, lipoid nephrosis, liver disease, and malnutrition result in a lowered albumin concentration [2].

Blood Collection. The test is performed on serum from 6 ml clotted blood.
Normal serum range. (1) Total protein, 6.0–8.0 gm per 100 ml. (2) Albumin, 3.2–5.6 gm per 100 ml. (3) Globulin, 1.3–3.5 gm per 100 ml.

Bilirubin (Direct and Indirect)

The bilirubin test, which is becoming less common, differentiates between impairment of the liver by obstruction and hemolysis. Bilirubin arises from the hemoglobin liberated from broken-down red cells. It is the chief pigment of the bile, excreted by the liver. If the excretory power of the liver is impaired by obstruction, there is an excess of circulatory bilirubin and it is free of any attached protein. Measurement of free bilirubin (direct) usually indicates obstruction.

When increased red cell destruction (hemolysis) occurs, the increased bilirubin is believed to be bound to protein (indirect).

A *total bilirubin* determination detects increased concentration of bilirubin before jaundice is seen.

Blood Collection. The test is performed on serum from 5 ml clotted blood.
Normal serum range is 0.1–1.0 mg per 100 ml [2].

Cephalin Flocculation

This test, commonly used in diagnosing liver damage, is being replaced in many hospitals by more specific tests. In diagnosing liver damage, it frequently detects damage before jaundice becomes evident. It is also useful in following the course of liver disease such as cirrhosis. The serum of patients with damaged liver cells flocculates a colloidal suspension of cephalin and cholesterol, while the serum of normal patients does not clump the suspension. Abscesses and neoplasms do not damage liver cells and therefore give negative results [2].

Blood Collection. The test is performed on serum from 5 ml of clotted blood.
Normal serum range is either negative or 1+. Reports are delayed 24–48 hours.

Cholesterol

Cholesterol, a normal constituent of the blood, is present in all body cells. In various disease states the cholesterol concentration in the serum may be raised or lowered. Elevation of the cholesterol level may be helpful in indicating certain liver diseases, hypothyroidism, and xanthomatosis [2].

Blood Collection. The test is performed on serum from 5 ml clotted blood.
Normal serum range is 120–260 mg per 100 ml.

Prothrombin Time

The prothrombin time, considered one of the most important screening tests in coagulation studies, indirectly measures the ability of the blood to clot. During the clotting process, prothrombin is converted to thrombin. It is thought that when the prothrombin level is reduced to below normal, the tendency for the blood to clot in the blood vessel is reduced. It is an important guide in controlling drug therapy and is commonly used when anticoagulants are prescribed. The prothrombin content is reduced in liver diseases.

Blood Collection. Venous blood (4 ml) is collected, added to the coagulant, and quickly mixed. It is important to avoid clot formation and hemolysis. The blood should be examined as soon as possible.
    The *normal value* is between 11–18 seconds, depending on the type of thromboplastin used.

Thymol Turbidity

Thymol turbidity detects damaged liver cells and differentiates between liver disease and biliary obstruction. Turbidity is usually increased when the serum of patients with liver damage is mixed with a saturated solution of thymol. Turbidity is usually normal in biliary obstruction without liver damage.

Blood Collection. The test is performed on serum from 5 ml clotted blood.
Normal serum range is 0–4 units [1].

KIDNEY FUNCTION TESTS

Creatinine

The creatinine test measures kidney function. Creatinine, the result of a breakdown of muscle creatine phosphate, is produced daily in a constant amount in each individual. A disorder of kidney function prevents excretion and an elevated creatinine value gives a reliable indication of impaired kidney function. A normal serum creatinine value does not indicate unimpaired renal function, however.

Blood Collection. The test is performed on serum from 6 ml of clotted blood.
Normal serum range is 0.6–1.3 mg per 100 ml.

BUN (Blood Urea Nitrogen)

The BUN is a measure of kidney function. Urea, the end product of protein metabolism, is excreted by the kidneys. Impairment in kidney function results in an elevated concentration of urea nitrogen in the blood. Rapid protein catabolism may also increase the urea nitrogen above normal limits. The *nonprotein nitrogen* is a similar test for measuring kidney function.

Blood Collection. The test is performed on blood or serum. Blood (5 ml) is added to an oxalate tube and shaken or placed in a dry tube to clot.
Normal ranges are 9–20 mg per 100 ml.

BLOOD SUGAR TESTS

The test for blood sugar is used to detect a disorder of glucose metabolism, which may be the result of any one of several factors, including (1) inability of pancreas islet cells to produce insulin, (2) inability of intestines to absorb glucose, and (3) inability of liver to accumulate and break down glycogen.

An elevated blood sugar level may indicate diabetes, chronic liver disease, or overactivity of the endocrine glands. A decrease in blood sugar may result from an overdose of insulin, tumors of the pancreas, or insufficiency of various endocrine glands.

FBS (Fasting Blood Sugar)

A fasting blood sugar test requires that the patient fast for 8 hours.

Blood Collection. Venous blood (3–5 ml) is collected in an oxalate tube and shaken to prevent microscopic clots.
Normal serum range is 70–100 mg per 100 ml (true blood sugar method). The normal value depends upon the method of determination. Values over 120 mg per 100 ml on several occasions may indicate diabetes mellitus.

Postprandial Blood Sugar Determinations

The postprandial sugar test is helpful in diagnosing diabetes mellitus. Blood is drawn 2 hours after the patient has begun to eat. If the blood sugar value is above the upper limits of normal for fasting, a glucose tolerance test is performed.

Glucose Tolerance

The glucose tolerance test is indicated

1. When the patient shows glycosuria.
2. When fasting or 2-hour blood sugar concentration is only slightly elevated.

3. When Cushing's syndrome or acromegaly is a questionable diagnosis.
4. To establish cause of hypoglycemia.

Blood Collection. A fasting blood sugar sample is drawn. The patient drinks 100 gm glucose in lemon-flavored water (some laboratories use 1.75 gm glucose per kilogram of ideal body weight). Blood and urine samples are collected at 30, 60, 90, 120, and 180 minutes after ingestion of glucose.

Normal (true blood sugar) values are (1) FBS below 100 mg per 100 ml. (2) Peak below 160 mg per 100 ml in 30 or 60 minutes. (3) Two-hour value returning to fasting level. The values depend upon the standards used.

BLOOD TYPING

Blood typing is one of the commonest tests performed on blood, being required by all donors and by all patients who may need blood. The ABO system denotes four main groups: O, A, B, and AB. The designations refer to the particular antigen present on the red cells: group A contains red cells with the A antigen, B with B antigen, AB with A and B antigens, and O red cells contain neither A nor B antigens.

When red cells containing antigens are placed with serum containing corresponding antibodies under favorable conditions, agglutination (clumping) occurs. Therefore an antigen is known as an agglutinogen, and an antibody as an agglutinin.

An individual's serum contains antibodies that will react to corresponding antigens not usually found on the individual's own cells. For instance, serum of group O contains antibodies A and B, which will react with the corresponding antigens A and B found on the red cells of group AB.

Although agglutination occurs in antigen–antibody reaction in the laboratory, hemolysis occurs in vivo; antibody attacks red cells, causing rupture with liberation of hemoglobin. Hemolysis results from infusing incompatible blood and may lead to fatal consequences.

Rh Factor

The antigens belonging to the Rh system are D, C, E, c, and e; they are found in conjunction with the ABO group. The strongest of these factors is the $Rh_o(D)$ factor, found in about 85 percent of the white population. Therefore the $Rh_o(D)$ factor is often the only factor identified in Rh typing. When not present, further typing may be done to identify any of the less common Rh factors.

Blood Collection

Venous blood is collected and allowed to clot. Usually one tube (10 ml) will set up 4–5 units of blood. Positive patient identification must be made before the blood is drawn; the name and number on the identification bracelet must correspond to that on the requisition and label. Identity should never be made by addressing the patient by name and awaiting the response. The label is placed on the blood tube at the patient's bedside.

Blood Grouping

Various methods are used in typing blood, but all involve the same general principle: The patient's cells are mixed in standard saline serum samples of anti-A and of anti-B. The type of serum, A or B, which agglutinates the patient's cells indicates the blood group. As a double check, the patient's serum is mixed with saline suspensions of A and of B red cells. The ABO group is determined on the basis of agglutination or absence of agglutination of A and of B cells.

Coombs' Test

Not all antibodies cause agglutination in saline; some merely coat the red cells by combining with the antigen, which is not a visible reaction. The Coombs' test is performed to detect antibodies that cannot cause agglutination in saline; these are known as *incomplete antibodies*. Antihuman globulin serum is used. This serum is obtained by the immunization of various animals, usually rabbits, against human gamma globulin by the injection of human serum, plasma, or isolated globulin. This antiserum, when added to sensitized red cells (red cells coated with incomplete antibody), causes visible agglutination (Figure 15.2).

The Coombs' test is performed in two ways. The *direct Coombs' test* is performed when the patient's red cells have become coated in vivo. This test is a valuable procedure in

1. Diagnosis of erythroblastosis fetalis. The red cells of the baby are tested for sensitization.

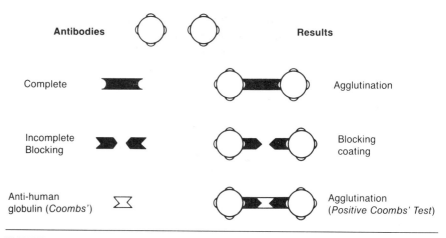

FIGURE 15.2
Red cell agglutination is produced either by complete antibodies or indirectly by coating of the red cell antigens by incomplete (blocking) antibodies followed by exposure to antihuman globulin (Coombs') antibodies, which form the final bridge between the red cells. (Reprinted with permission from the *New England Journal of Medicine* 264:1089, 1961 [3]).

2. Acquired hemolytic anemia. The patient may have produced an antibody that coats his or her own cells.
3. Investigation of reactions. The patient may have received incompatible blood that has sensitized his red cells.

The *indirect Coombs' test* detects incomplete antibodies in the serum of patients sensitized to blood antigens. It involves use of the patient's serum, in contrast to the use of the patient's red cells in the direct Coombs' test. When pooled, normal red cells containing the most important antigens are exposed in a test tube to the patient's serum and to Coombs serum, agglutination of the red cells occurs and indicates the incomplete antibody present. This test is valuable in

1. Detecting incompatibilities not found by other methods.
2. Detecting weak or variant antigens.
3. Typing with certain antiserums, such as anti-Duffy or anti-Kidd, which require Coombs' serum to produce agglutination.
4. Detecting antiagglutinins produced by exposure during pregnancy.

REFERENCES

1. Castleman, B., and McNeely, B. Case records of the Massachusetts General Hospital: Normal laboratory values. *N. Engl. J. Med.* 314:39–49 (January 2), 1986.
2. Garb, S. *Laboratory Tests in Common Use* (6th ed.). New York: Springer, 1976. pp. 23–123.
3. Grove-Rasmussen, M., Lesses, M. F., and Anstall, H. B. Transfusion therapy. *N. Engl. J. Med.* 264:1089, 1961.

REVIEW QUESTIONS

1. Serum consists of plasma minus _____ .
2. Plasma consists of all the stable components of blood minus _____ .
3. Serum is obtained by drawing blood in a dry tube and allowing it to coagulate. True or false?
4. How is plasma obtained?
5. What special handling of blood samples is required when a delay in getting them to the laboratory is unavoidable, such as in samples collected for pH analysis?
6. Define the term *glycolysis*.
7. Why is it important to fill the tube completely when drawing blood for carbon dioxide analysis?
8. What does "without stasis" imply?
9. What tests are required to be performed "without stasis"?
10. Define the term *hemolysis*.

TABLE 15.1
Normal Reference Laboratory Values

Blood, Plasma or Serum Values

Determination	Reference Range Conventional	SI
Acetoacetate plus acetone	Negative	
Aldolase	1.3–8.2 U/liter	22–137 nmol · sec^{-1}/liter
Ammonia	12–55 μmol/liter	12–55 μmol/liter
Amylase	4–25 units/ml	4–25 arb. unit
Ascorbic acid	0.4–1.5 mg/100 ml	23–85 μmol/liter
Bilirubin	Direct: up to 0.4 mg/100 ml	Up to 7 μmol/liter
	Total: up to 1.0 mg/100 ml	Up to 17 μmol/liter
Blood volume	8.5–9.0% of body weight in kg	80–85 ml/kg
Calcium	8.5–10.5 mg/100 ml (slightly higher in children)	2.1–2.6 mmol/liter
Carbon dioxide content	24–30 meq/liter	24–30 mmol/liter
Carbamazepine	4.0–12.0 μg/ml	17–51 μmol/liter
Carbon monoxide	Less than 5% of total hemoglobin	
Carotenoids	0.8–4.0 μg/ml	1.5–7.4 μmol/liter
Ceruloplasmin	27–37 mg/100 ml	1.8–2.5 μmol/liter
Chloramphenicol	10–20 μg/ml	31–62 μmol/liter
Chloride	100–106 meq/liter	100–106 mmol/liter
CK isoenzymes	5% MB or less	
Copper	Total: 100–200 μg/100 ml	16–31 μmol/liter
Creatine kinase (CK)	Female: 10–79 U/liter	167–1317 nmol · sec^{-1}/liter
	Male: 17–148 U/liter	283–2467 nmol · sec^{-1}/liter
Creatinine	0.6–1.5 mg/100 ml	53–133 μmol/liter
Ethanol	0 mg/100 ml	0 mmol/liter
Glucose	Fasting: 70–110 mg/100 ml	3.9–5.6 mmol/liter
Iron	50–150 μg/100 ml (higher in males)	9.0–26.9 μmol/liter
Iron-binding capacity	250–410 μg/100 ml	44.8–73.4 μmol/liter
Lactic acid	0.6–1.8 meq/liter	0.6–1.8 mmol/liter

Chapter 15 | Laboratory Tests   243

Minimal Ml Required	Note	Method
1-B		Behre: J Lab Clin Med 13:770, 1928 (modified)
2-S	Use unhemolyzed serum	Beisenherz et al.: Z Naturforsch 86:555, 1963
2-B	Collect in heparinized tube; deliver *immediately* packed in ice	Da Fonseca-Wolheim: J Clin Chem Clin Biochem 11:421, 1973
1-S		Zinterhofer et al.: Clin Chim Acta 43:5, 1973
7-B	Collect in heparinized tube before any food is given	Roe, Kuether: J Biol Chem 147:399, 1943
1-S		Gambino: Standard Methods Clin Chem 5:55, 1965
		Isotope dilution technique with ^{131}I albumin
1-S		Spectrophotometry using cresolphthalein complexone
1-S	Fill tube to top	By CO_2 electrode
		Liquid chromatography
3-B	Fill tube to top	Multi-wavelength spectrophotometry
3-S	Vitamin A may be done on same specimen	Natelson: Microtechniques of Clinical Chemistry, 2nd ed., 1961, p. 454
2-S		Ravin: J Lab Clin Med 58:161, 1961
0.2-S		Liquid chromatography
1-S		Cotlove: Standard Methods Clin Chem 3:81, 1961
0.2-S		Electrophoresis
1-S		Atomic-absorption spectrophotometry
1-S		Szasz: Clin Chem 22:650, 1976
1-S		Fabiny, Ertingshausen: Clin Chem 17:696, 1971
2-B	Collect in oxalate and refrigerate	Gas-liquid chromatography
1-P	Collect with oxalate-fluoride mixture	Bergmeyer: Methods of Enzymatic Analysis, 1965, p. 117
1-S		Spectrophotometry using Ferrozine
1-S		Spectrophotometry using Ferrozine
2-B	Collect with oxalate-fluoride; deliver immediately packed in ice	Hadjivassiliou, Rieder: Clin Chim Acta 19:357, 1968

TABLE 15.1 (continued)

Blood, Plasma or Serum Values

Determination	Reference Range	
	Conventional	SI
Lactic dehydrogenase	45–90 U/liter	750–1500 nmol · sec^{-1}/liter
Lead	50 μg/100 ml or less	Up to 2.4 μmol/liter
Lipase	2 units/ml or less	Up to 2 arb. unit
Lipids		
Cholesterol	120–220 mg/100 ml	3.10–5.69 mmol/liter
Triglycerides	40–150 mg/100 ml	0.4–1.5 g/liter
Lipoprotein electrophoresis (LEP)		
Lithium	0.5–1.5 meq/liter	0.5–1.5 mmol/liter
Magnesium	1.5–2.0 meq/liter	0.8–1.3 mmol/liter
5′ Nucleotidase	1–11 U/liter	17–183 nmol · sec^{-1}/liter
Osmolality	280–296 mOsm/kg water	280–296 mmol/kg
Oxygen saturation (arterial)	96–100%	0.96–1.00
PCO$_2$	35–45 mm Hg	4.7–6.0 kPa
pH	7.35–7.45	Same
PO$_2$	75–100 mm Hg (dependent on age) while breathing room air Above 500 mm Hg while on 100% O$_2$	10.0–13.3 kPa
Phenobarbital	15–50 μg/ml	65–215 μmol/liter
Phenytoin (Dilantin)	5–20 μg/ml	20–80 μmol/liter
Phosphatase (acid)	Male — Total: 0.13–0.63 sigma U/ml	36–175 nmol · sec^{-1}/liter
	Female — Total: 0.01–0.56 sigma U/ml	2.8–156 nmol · sec^{-1}/liter
	Prostatic: 0–0.5 Fishman-Lerner U/100 ml	
Phosphatase (alkaline)	13–39 U/liter; infants and adolescents up to 104 U/liter	217–650 nmol · sec^{-1}/liter; up to 1.26 μmol · sec^{-1}/liter
Phosphorus (inorganic)	3.0–4.5 mg/100 ml (infants in first year up to 6.0 mg/100 ml)	1.0–1.5 mmol/liter

Chapter 15 | Laboratory Tests 245

Minimal Ml Required	Note	Method
1-S	Unsuitable if hemolyzed	Gay, McComb, Bowers: Clin Chem 14:740, 1968
2-B	Collect with oxalate-fluoride mixture	Berman: Atom Absorp Newslett 3:9, 1964 (modified)
1-S		Zinterhofer: Clin Chim Acta 44:173, 1973
1-S	Fasting	Siedel: J Clin Chem Clin Biochem 19:838, 1981
1-S	Fasting	Ziegenhorn: Clin Chem 21:1627, 1975
2-S	Fasting, do not freeze serum	Less, Hatch: J Lab Clin Med 61:518, 1963
1-S		Pybus, Bowers: Clin Chem 16:139, 1970
1-S		Willis: Clin Chem 11:251, 1965 (modified)
1-S		Arkesteijn: J Clin Chem Clin Biochem 14:155, 1976
1-S		Osmometry using freezing-point depression
3-B	Deliver in sealed heparinized syringe packed in ice	Gordy, Drabkin: J Biol Chem 227:285, 1957
2-B	Collect and deliver in sealed heparinized syringe	By CO_2 electrode
2-B	Collect without stasis in sealed heparinized syringe; deliver packed in ice	Glass electrode
2-B		Oxygen electrode
1-S		Liquid chromatography
1-S		Liquid chromatography
1-S	Must always be drawn just before analysis or stored as frozen serum; avoid hemolysis	Bessey et al.: J Biol Chem 164:321, 1946 Babson et al.: Clin Chim Acta 13:264, 1966
1-S		Stevens, Thomas: Clin Chim Acta 37:541, 1972
1-S		Daly, Ertingshausen: Clin Chem 18:263, 1972

TABLE 15.1 (continued)

Blood, Plasma or Serum Values

Determination	Reference Range	
	Conventional	SI
Potassium	3.5–5.0 meq/liter	3.5–5.0 mmol/liter
Primidone (Mysoline)	4–12 µg/ml	18–55 µmol/liter
Procainamide	4–10 µg/ml	17–42 µmol/liter
Protein: Total	6.0–8.4 g/100 ml	60–84 g/liter
Albumin	3.5–5.0 g/100 ml	35–50 g/liter
Globulin	2.3–3.5 g/100 ml	23–35 g/liter
Electrophoresis	(% of total protein)	
Albumin	52–68	
Globulin:		
$Alpha_1$	4.2–7.2	
$Alpha_2$	6.8–12	
Beta	9.3–15	
Gamma	13–23	
Pyruvic acid	0–0.11 meq/liter	0–0.11 mmol/liter
Quinidine	1.2–4.0 µg/ml	3.7–12.3 µmol/liter
Salicylate:	0	
Therapeutic	20–25 mg/100 ml; 25–30 mg/100 ml to age 10 yr 3 hr post dose	1.4–1.8 mmol/liter 1.8–2.2 mmol/liter
Sodium	135–145 meq/liter	135–145 mmol/liter
Sulfonamide	5–15 mg/100 ml	
Transaminase, SGOT (aspartate aminotransferase)	7–27 U/liter	117–450 nmol · sec^{-1}/liter
Transaminase, SGPT (alanine aminotransferase)	1–21 U/liter	17–350 nmol · sec^{-1}/liter
Urea nitrogen (BUN)	8–25 mg/100 ml	2.9–8.9 mmol/liter
Uric acid	3.0–7.0 mg/100 ml	0.18–0.42 mmol/liter
Vitamin A	0.15–0.6 µg/ml	0.5–2.1 µmol/liter

Minimal Ml Required	Note	Method
1-S	Serum must be separated promptly from cells	Ion-selective electrode
1-S		Enzyme immunoassay
1-S		Liquid chromatography
1-S		Weichselbaum: Am J Clin Pathol 16:40, 1946
1-S		Doumas et al.: Clin Chim Acta 31:87, 1971
	Globulin equals total protein minus albumin	
1-S	Quantitation by densitometry	Kunkel, Tiselius: J Gen Physiol 35:89, 1951
		Durrum: J Am Chem Soc 72:2943, 1950
2-B	Collect with oxalate fluoride. Deliver immediately packed in ice	Hadjivassiliou, Rieder: Clin Chim Acta 19:357, 1968
1-S		Liquid chromatography
2-P		Keller: Am J Clin Pathol 17:415, 1947
1-S		Ion-selective electrode
2-P		Bratton, Marshall: J Biol Chem 128:537, 1939
1-S		Karmen et al.: J Clin Invest 34:126, 1955
1-S		Henry et al.: Am J Clin Pathol 34:381, 1960
1-S		Paulson et al.: Clin Chem 17:644, 1971
1-S		Spectrophotometry using uricase
3-S		Natelson: Microtechniques of Clinical Chemistry, 2nd ed. 1961, p. 451

TABLE 15.1 (continued)

Special Endocrine Tests
Steroid Hormones

Determination	Reference Range	
	Conventional	SI
Aldosterone	Excretion: 5–19 μg/24 hr	14–53 nmol/day
	Supine: 48 ± 29 pg/ml	133 ± 80 pmol/liter
	Upright (2 hr): 65 ± 23 pg/ml	180 ± 64 pmol/liter
	Supine: 107 ± 45 pg/ml	279 ± 125 pmol/liter
	Upright (2 hr): 239 ± 123 pg/ml	663 ± 341 pmol/liter
	Supine: 175 ± 75 pg/ml	485 ± 208 pmol/liter
	Upright (2 hr): 532 ± 228 pg/ml	1476 ± 632 pmol/liter
Cortisol	8 a.m.: 5–25 μg/100 ml	0.14–0.69 μmol/liter
	8 p.m.: Below 10 μg/100 ml	0–0.28 μmol/liter
	4-hr ACTH test: 30–45 μg/100 ml	0.83–1.24 μmol/liter
	Overnight suppression test: Below 5 μg/100 ml	0.14 nmol/liter
	Excretion: 20–70 μg/24 hr	55–193 nmol/day
Dehydroepiandrosterone (DHEA)	Male: 0.5–5.5 ng/ml	1.7–19 nmol/liter
	Female:	
	1.4–8.0 ng/ml	4.9–28 nmol/liter
	0.3–4.5 ng/ml	1.0–15.6 nmol/liter
Dehydroepiandrosterone sulfate (DHEA-S)	Male: 151–446 μg/100 ml	3.9–11.4 μmol/liter
	Female:	
	84–433 μg/100 ml	2.2–11.1 μmol/liter
	1.7–177 μg/100 ml	0.04–4.5 μmol/liter
11-Deoxycortisol	Responsive: Over 7.5 μg/100 ml	> 0.22 μmol/liter
Estradiol	Male: < 50 pg/ml	< 184 pmol/liter
	Female: 23–361 pg/ml	84–1325 pmol/liter
	< 30 pg/ml	< 110 pmol/liter
	< 20 pg/ml	< 73 pmol/liter
Progesterone	Male: < 1.0 ng/ml	< 3.2 nmol/liter
	Female: 0.2–0.6 ng/ml	0.6–1.9 nmol/liter
	0.3–3.5 ng/ml	0.95–11 nmol/liter
	6.5–32.2 ng/ml	21–102 nmol/liter

Minimal Ml Required	Note	Method
5/day	Keep specimen cold	Bayard et al.: J Clin Endocrinol Metab 31:507, 1970
3-S, P	Fasting, at rest, 210-meq sodium diet	Poulson et al.: Clin Immunol Immunopathol 2:373, 1974
	Upright, 2 hr, 210/meq sodium diet	
	Fasting, at rest, 110-meq sodium diet	
	Upright, 2 hr, 110-meq sodium diet	
	Fasting, at rest, 10-meq sodium diet	
	Upright, 2 hr, 10-meq sodium diet	
1-P	Fasting	Catt, Tregear: Science 158:1670, 1967
1-P	At rest	
1-P	20 U ACTH, IV per 4 hr	
1-P	8 a.m. sample after 0.5 mg dexamethasone by mouth at midnight	
2/day	Keep specimen cold	
2-S, P		Sekihara, Ohsawa: Steroids 24:317, 1974
	Adult	
	Post-menopausal	
2-S, P		Buster, Abraham: Anal Lett 5:543, 1972
	Adult	
	Post-menopausal	
1-P	8 a.m. sample, preceded by 4.5 g of metyrapone by mouth per 24 hr or by single dose of 2.5 g by mouth at midnight	Mahajan et al.: Steroids 20:609, 1972
5-S, P		Mikhail et al.: Steroids 15:333, 1970
	Adult	
	Post-menopausal	
	Pre-pubertal	
5-S, P		Furuyama, Nugent: Steroids 17:663, 1971
	Follicular phase	
	Midcycle peak	
	Post-ovulatory	

TABLE 15.1 (continued)

Special Endocrine Tests
Steroid Hormones

Determination	Reference Range	
	Conventional	SI
Testosterone	Adult male: 300–1100 ng/100 ml	10.4–38.1 nmol/liter
	Adolescent male: Over 100 ng/100 ml	> 3.5 nmol/liter
	Female: 25–90 ng/100 ml	0.87–3.12 nmol/liter
Unbound testosterone	Adult male: 3.06–24.0 ng/100 ml	106–832 pmol/liter
	Adult female: 0.09–1.28 ng/100 ml	3.1–44.4 pmol/liter

Polypeptide Hormones

Determination	Reference Range	
	Conventional	SI
Adrenocorticotropin (ACTH)	15–70 pg/ml	3.3–15.4 pmol/liter
Alpha subunit	< 0.5–2.5 mg/ml	< 0.4–2.0 nmol/liter
	< 0.5–5.0 ng/ml	< 0.4–4.0 nmol/liter
Calcitonin	Male: 0–14 pg/ml	0–4.1 pmol/liter
	Female: 0–28 pg/ml	0–8.2 pmol/liter
	> 100 pg/ml in medullary carcinoma	> 29.3 pmol/liter
Follicle-stimulating hormone (FSH)	Male: 3–18 mU/ml	3–18 arb. unit
	Female: 4.6–22.4 mU/ml	4.6–22.4 arb. unit
	13–41 mU/ml	13–41 arb. unit
	30–170 mU/ml	30–170 arb. unit
Growth hormone	Below 5 ng/ml	< 233 pmol/liter
	Children: Over 10 ng/ml	> 465 pmol/liter
	Male: Below 5 ng/ml	< 233 pmol/liter
	Female: Up to 30 ng/ml	0–1395 pmol/liter
	Male: Below 5 ng/ml	< 233 pmol/liter
	Female: Below 5 ng/ml	< 233 pmol/liter
Insulin	6–26 μU/ml	43–187 pmol/liter
	Below 20 μU/ml	< 144 pmol/liter
	Up to 150 μU/ml	0–1078 pmol/liter
Luteinizing hormone (LH)	Male: 3–18 mU/ml	3–18 arb. unit
	Female: 2.4–34.5 mU/ml	2.4–34.5 arb. unit
	43–187 mU/ml	43–187 arb. unit
	30–150 mU/ml	30–150 arb. unit

Minimal Ml Required	Note	Method
1-P	a.m. sample	Catt, Tregear: Science 158:1670, 1967
2-P	a.m. sample	Forest et al.: Steroids 12:323, 1968

Minimal Ml Required	Note	Method
5-P	Place specimen on ice and send promptly to laboratory. Use EDTA tube only	Gonzales: Clin Chem 26:1228, 1980
2-S	Adult male or female Postmenopausal female	Kourides et al.: Endocrinology 94:1411, 1974
5-S	Test done only on known or suspected cases of medullary carcinoma of the thyroid	Deftos et al.: Metabolism 20:1129, 1971 Deftos et al.: Metabolism 20:428, 1971
5-S, P	Same sample may be used for LH Pre- or post-ovulatory Mid-cycle peak Post-menopausal	Midgley: J Clin Endocrinol Metab 27:295, 1967
1-S	Fasting, at rest After exercise After glucose load	Glick et al.: Nature 199:784, 1963
1-S	Fasting During hypoglycemia After glucose load	Morgan, Lazarow: Proc Soc Exp Biol Med 110:29, 1962
5-S, P	Same sample may be used for FSH Pre- or post-ovulatory Mid-cycle peak Post-menopausal	Odell et al.: J Clin Invest 46:248, 1967

TABLE 15.1 (continued)

Polypeptide Hormones

Determination	Reference Range	
	Conventional	SI
Parathyroid hormone	< 25 pg/ml	< 2.94 pmol/liter
Prolactin	2–15 ng/ml	0.08–6.0 nmol/liter
Renin activity	Supine: 1.1 ± 0.8 ng/ml/hr	0.9 ± 0.6 nmol/liter/hr
	Upright: 1.9 ± 1.7 ng/ml/hr	1.5 ± 1.3 nmol/liter/hr
	Supine: 2.7 ± 1.8 ng/ml/hr	2.1 ± 1.4 nmol/liter/hr
	Upright: 6.6 ± 2.5 ng/ml/hr	5.1 ± 1.9 nmol/liter/hr
	Diuretics: 10.0 ± 3.7 ng/ml/hr	7.7 ± 2.9 nmol/liter/hr
Somatomedin C (Sm-C, IGF-1)	0.08–2.8 U/ml	0.08–2.8 arb. unit
	0.9–5.9 U/ml	0.9–5.9 arb. unit
	0.34–1.9 U/ml	0.34–1.9 arb. unit
	0.45–2.2 U/ml	0.45–2.2 arb. unit

Thyroid Hormones

Determination	Reference Range	
	Conventional	SI
Thyroid-stimulating hormone (TSH)	0.5–5.0 µU/ml	0.5–5.0 arb. unit
Thyroxine-binding globulin capacity	15–25 µg T_4/100 ml	193–322 nmol/liter
Total triiodothyronine (T_3)	75–195 ng/100 ml	1.16–3.00 nmol/liter
Reverse triiodothyronine (rT3)	13–53 ng/ml	0.2–0.8 nmol/liter
Total thyroxine by RIA (T_4)	4–12 µg/100 ml	52–154 nmol/liter
T_3 resin uptake	25–35%	0.25–0.35
Free thyroxine index (FT_4I)	1–4	

Vitamin D Derivatives

Determination	Reference Range	
	Conventional	SI
1,25-Dihydroxyvitamin D	26–65 pg/ml	62–155 pmol/liter
25-Hydroxyvitamin D	8–55 ng/ml	19.4–137 nmol/liter

Minimal Ml Required	Note	Method
5-P	Keep blood on ice, or plasma must be frozen if it is to be sent any distance; a.m. sample	Stewart et al.: N Engl J Med 306: 1982
2-S		Sinha et al.: J Clin Endocrinol Metab 36:509, 1973
4-P	EDTA tubes, on ice, normal diet Low-sodium diet	Haber et al.: J Clin Endocrinol Metab 29:1349, 1969
2-P	Low-sodium diet EDTA plasma Prepubertal During puberty Adult males Adult females	Furlanetto et al.: J Clin Invest 60:648, 1977

Minimal Ml Required	Note	Method
2-S		Ridgway et al.: J Clin Invest 52:2785, 1973
2-S		Levy et al.: J Clin Endocrinol Metab 32:372, 1971
2-S		Larsen et al.: J Clin Invest 51:1939, 1972
2-S		Cooper et al.: J Clin Endocrinol Metab 54:101, 1982
1-S		Chopra: J Clin Endocrinol Metab 34:938, 1972
2-S		Taybearn et al.: J Nucl Med 8:739, 1967
2-S		Sarin, Anderson: Arch Intern Med 126:631, 1970

Minimal Ml Required	Note	Method
1-S		Reinhardt et al.: J Clin Endocrinol Metab 58:91, 1984
1-S		Preece et al.: Clin Chim Acta 54:235, 1974

		SI
		4.0–10.0 μmol/liter
		0.60–1.40
		0.60–1.40
		0.70–1.30
		0.70–1.30
		0.50–2.0
		0.60–1.40
(... cofactor)		
Factor XI (plasma thromboplastic antecedent)	60–140%	0.60–1.40
Factor XII (Hageman factor)	60–140%	0.60–1.40
Coagulation Screening tests:		
Bleeding time (Simplate)	3–9.5 min	180–570 sec
Prothrombin time	Less than 2-sec deviation from control	Less than 2-sec deviation from control
Partial thromboplastin time (activated)	25–38 sec	25–38 sec
Whole-blood clot lysis	No clot lysis in 24 hr	0/day
Fibrinolytic studies:		
Euglobin lysis	No lysis in 2 hr	0/2 hr
Fibrinogen split products	Negative reaction at > 1:4 dilution	0 (at 1:4 dilution)
Thrombin time	Control ± 5 sec	Control ± 5 sec

Minimal Ml Required	Note	Method
4.5-P	Collect in Vacutainer containing sodium citrate	Ratnoff, Menzies: J Lab Clin Med 37:316, 1951
4.5-P	Collect in plastic tubes with 3.8% sodium citrate	Owren, Aas: Scand J Clin Lab Invest 3:201, 1951
4.5-P	Collect as in factor II determination	Lewis, Ware: Proc Soc Exp Biol Med 84:640, 1953
4.5-P	Collect as in factor II determination	Same as factor II
4.5-P	Collect as in factor II determination	Bachman et al.: Thromb Diath Haemorrh 2:29, 1958
4.5-P	Collect as in factor II determination	Tocantins, Kazal: Blood Coagulation, Hemorrhage and Thrombosis, 2nd ed., 1964
4.5-P	Collect as in factor II determination	*Idem*
4.5-P	Collect as in factor II determination	*Idem*
4.5-P	Collect as in factor II determination	*Idem*
		Simplate Bleeding Time Device (General Diagnostics)
4.5-P	Collect in Vacutainer containing 3.8% sodium citrate	Colman et al.: Am J Clin Pathol 64:108, 1975
4.5-P	Collect in Vacutainer containing 3.8% sodium citrate	Babson, Babson: Am J Clin Pathol 62:856, 1974
2.0-whole blood	Collect in sterile tube and incubate at 37°C	Page, Culver: Syllabus, Laboratory Examination and Clinical Diagnosis, 1960, p. 207
4.5-P	Collect as in factor II determination	Sherry et al.: J Clin Invest 38:810, 1959
4.5-S	Collect in special tube containing thrombin and epsilon aminocaproic acid	Carvalho: Am J Clin Pathol 62:107, 1974
4.5-P	Collect as in factor II determination	Stefanini, Dameshek: Hemorrhagic Disorders, 1962, p. 492

Part IV | Blood and Intravenous Therapy

TABLE 15.1 (continued)

Hematologic Values

Determination	Reference Range	
	Conventional	SI
"Complete" blood count:		
Hematocrit	Male: 45–52%	Male: 0.45–0.52
	Female: 37–48%	Female: 0.37–0.48
Hemoglobin	Male: 13–18 g/100 ml	Male: 8.1–11.2 mmol/liter
	Female: 12–16 g/100 ml	Female: 7.4–9.9 mmol/liter
Leukocyte count	4300—10,800/mm^3	4.3–10.8 × 10^9/liter
Erythrocyte count	4.2–5.9 million/mm^3	4.2–5.9 × 10^{12}/liter
Mean corpuscular volume (MCV)	86–98 μm^3/cell	86–98 fl
Mean corpuscular hemoglobin (MCH)	27–32 pg/RBC	1.7–2.0 pg/cell
Mean corpuscular hemoglobin concentration (MCHC)	32–36%	0.32–0.36
Erythrocyte sedimentation rate	Male: 1–13 mm/hr	Male: 1–13 mm/hr
	Female: 1–20 mm/hr	Female: 1–20 mm/hr
Erythrocyte enzymes:		
Glucose-6-phosphate dehydrogenase	5–15 U/g Hb	5–15 U/g
Pyruvate kinase	13–17 U/g Hb	13–17 U/g
Ferritin (serum)		
Iron deficiency	0–12 ng/ml	0–4.8 nmol/liter
	13–20 Borderline	5.2–8 nmol/liter Borderline
Iron excess	> 400 ng/liter	> 160 nmol/liter
Folic acid		
Normal	> 3.3 ng/ml	> 7.3 nmol/liter
Borderline	2.5–3.2 ng/ml	5.75–7.39 nmol/liter
Haptoglobin	40–336 mg/100 ml	0.4–3.36 g/liter
Hemoglobin studies:		
Electrophoresis for abnormal hemoglobin		
Electrophoresis for A$_2$ hemoglobin	3.0%	0.015–0.035
Borderline	0.3–3.5%	0.03–0.035
Hemoglobin F (fetal hemoglobin)	Less than 2%	< 0.02
Hemoglobin, met- and sulf-	0	0
Serum hemoglobin	2–3 mg/100 ml	1.2–1.9 μmol/liter

Chapter 15 | Laboratory Tests 257

Minimal Ml Required	Note	Method
1-B	Use EDTA as anticoagulant; the seven listed tests are performed automatically on the Ortho ELT 800, which directly determines cell counts, hemoglobin (as the cyanmethemoglobin derivative), and MCV and computes hematocrit, MCH, and MCHC	
5-B	Use EDTA as anticoagulant	Modified Westergren method. Gambino et al.: Am J Clin Pathol 35:173, 1965
9-B	Use special anticoagulant (ACD solution)	Beck: J Biol Chem 232:251, 1958
8-B	Use special anticoagulant (ACD solution)	Beutler: Red Cell Metabolism, 2nd ed., 1975, p. 60
		Addison et al.: J Clin Pathol 25:326, 1972
1-S		Waxman, Schreiber: Blood 42:281, 1973
1-S		
1-S		Behring Diagnostic Reagent Kit
5-B	Collect with anticoagulant	Singer: Am J Med 18:633, 1955
5-B	Use oxalate as anticoagulant	Abraham: Hemoglobin 1:27, 1976
5-B	Collect with anticoagulant	Maile: Laboratory Medicine—Hematology, 2nd ed., 1962, p. 845
5-B	Use heparin as anticoagulant	Michel, Harris: J Lab Clin Med 29:445, 1940
2-S		Hunter et al.: Am J Clin Pathol 20:429, 1950

TABLE 15.1 (continued)

Hematologic Values

Determination	Reference Range	
	Conventional	SI
Thermolabile hemoglobin	0	0
Lupus anticoagulant	0	0
LE (lupus erythematosus) preparation:		
Method I	0	0
Method II	0	0
Leukocyte alkaline phosphatase:		
Qualitative method	Males: 33–188 U	33–188 U
	Females (off contraceptive pill): 30–160 U	30–160 U
Muramidase	Serum, 3–7 µg/ml	3–7 mg/liter
	Urine, 0–2 µg/ml	0–2 mg/liter
Osmotic fragility of erythrocytes	Increased if hemolysis occurs in over 0.5% NaCl; decreased if hemolysis is incomplete in 0.3% NaCl	
Peroxide hemolysis	Less than 10%	0.10
Platelet count	150,000–350,000/mm^3	150–350 × 10^9/liter
Platelet function tests:		
Clot retraction	50–100%/2 hr	0.50–1.00/2 hr
Platelet aggregation	Full response to ADP, epinephrine, and collagen	1.0
Platelet factor 3	33–57 sec	33–57 sec
Reticulocyte count	0.5–2.5% red cells	0.005–0.025
Vitamin B$_{12}$	205–876 pg/ml	150–674 pmol/liter
Borderline	140–204 pg/ml	102.6–149 pmol/liter

Minimal Ml Required	Note	Method
1-B	Any anticoagulant	Dacie et al.: Br J Haematol 10:388, 1964
4.5-P	Collect as in factor II determination	Boxer et al.: Arthritis Rheum 19:1244, 1976
5-B	Use heparin as anticoagulant	Hargraves et al.: Proc Staff Meet Mayo Clin 24:234, 1949
5-B	Use defibrinated blood	Barnes et al.: J Invest Dermatol 14:397, 1950
20-Isolated blood leukocytes	Special handling of blood necessary	Valentine, Beck: J Lab Clin Med 38:39, 1951
Smear-B		Kaplow: Am J Clin Pathol 39:439, 1963
1-S		Osserman, Lawlor: J Exp Med 124:921, 1966
1-U		
5-B	Use heparin as anticoagulant	Beutler. In: Williams et al., eds. Hematology, McGraw-Hill, 1972, p. 1375
6-B	Use EDTA as anticoagulant	Gordon et al.: Am J Dis Child 90:669, 1955
0.5-B	Use EDTA as anticoagulant; counts are performed on Clay Adams Ultraflow; when counts are low, results are confirmed by hand counting	(Hand count): Brecher et al.: Am J Clin Pathol 23:15, 1955
4.5-P	Collect as in factor II determination	Benthaus: Thromb Diath Haemorrh 3:311, 1959
18-P	Collect as in factor II determination	Born: Nature 194:927, 1962
4.5-P	Collect as in factor II determination	Rabiner, Hrodek: J Clin Invest 47:901, 1968
0.1-B		Brecher: Am J Clin Pathol 19:895, 1949
12-S		Difco Manual, 9th ed., 1953, p. 221 (modified)

TABLE 15.1 (continued)

Miscellaneous Values

Determination	Reference Range Conventional	SI
Carcinoembryonic antigen (CEA)	0–2.5 ng/ml	0–2.5 µg/liter
Chylous fluid		
Digitoxin	17 ± 6 ng/ml	22 ± 7.8 nmol/liter
Digoxin	1.2 ± 0.4 ng/ml	1.54 ± 0.5 nmol/liter
	1.5 ± 0.4 ng/ml	1.92 ± 0.5 nmol/liter
Duodenal drainage		
pH (urine)	5–7	5–7
Gastric analysis	Basal: Females: 2.0 ± 1.8 meq/hr Males: 3.0 ± 2.0 meq/hr Maximal (after histalog or gastrin): Females: 16 ± 5 meq/hr Males: 23 ± 5 meq/hr	0.6 ± 0.5 µmol/sec 0.8 ± 0.6 µmol/sec 4.4 ± 1.4 µmol/sec 6.4 ± 1.4 µmol/sec
Gastrin-I	0–200 pg/ml	0–95 pmol/liter
Immunologic tests:		
Alpha-fetoprotein	Undetectable in normal adults	
Alpha-1-antitrypsin	85–213 mg/100 ml	0.85–2.13 g/liter
Rheumatoid factor	< 60 IU/ml	
Antinuclear antibodies	Negative at a 1:8 dilution of serum	
Anti-DNA antibodies	Negative at a 1:10 dilution of serum	
Antibodies to Sm and RNP (ENA)	None detected	
Antibodies to SS-A (Ro) and SS-B (La)	None detected	
Autoantibodies to:		
Thyroid colloid and microsomal antigens	Negative at a 1:10 dilution of serum	
Gastric parietal cells	Negative at a 1:20 dilution of serum	
Smooth muscle	Negative at a 1:20 dilution of serum	

Minimal Ml Required	Note	Method
20-P	Must be sent on ice	Hansen et al.: J Clin Res 19:143, 1971
	Use fresh specimen	Todd et al.: Clinical Diagnosis, 12th ed., 1953, p. 624
1-S	Medication with digitoxin or digitalis	Smith, Butler, Haber: N Engl J Med 281:1212, 1969
1-S	Medication with digoxin 0.25 mg per day	Smith, Haber: J Clin Invest 49:2377, 1970
1-S	Medication with digoxin 0.5 mg per day	
	pH should be in proper range with minimal amount of gastric juice	
		Marks: Gastroenterology 41:599, 1961
4-P	Heparinized sample	Dent et al.: Ann Surg 176:360, 1972
2-S		
10-B		Nephelometric assay
10 ml clotted blood	Fasting sample preferred	Nephelometric assay
2-S	Send to laboratory promptly	Immunofluorescence assay
2-S		*Crithidia lucilliae* assay
10 ml clotted blood		Double diffusion
10 ml clotted blood		Double diffusion
2-S	Low titers in some elderly normal women	Doniach, Bottazzo, Drexhage: The autoimmune endocrinopathies. In: Lachmann, Peters, eds. Clinical Aspects of Immunology, Vol. 2, Oxford: Blackwell Scientific, 1982, p. 903
2-S		
2-S		

TABLE 15.1 (continued)

Miscellaneous Values

Determination	Reference Range	
	Conventional	SI
Mitochondria	Negative at a 1:20 dilution of serum	
Interstitial cells of the testes	Negative at a 1:10 dilution of serum	
Skeletal muscle	Negative at a 1:60 dilution of serum	
Adrenal gland	Negative at a 1:10 dilution of serum	
Bence Jones protein	No Bence Jones protein detected in a 50-fold concentrate of urine	
Complement, total hemolytic	150–250 U/ml	
Cryoprecipitable proteins	None detected	0 arb. unit
C3	Range, 83–177 mg/100 ml	0.83–1.77 g/liter
C4	Range, 15–45 mg/100 ml	0.15–0.45 g/liter
Factor B	12–30 mg/100 ml	
C1 esterase inhibitor	13.2–24 mg/100 ml	
Hemoglobin A_{1c}	3.8–6.4%	0.038–0.064
Hypersensitivity pneumonitis screen	No antibodies to those antigens assayed	
Immunoglobulins:		
IgG	639–1349 mg/100 ml	6.39–13.49 g/liter
IgA	70–312 mg/100 ml	0.7–3.12 g/liter
IgM	86–352 mg/100 ml	0.86–3.52 g/liter
Viscosity	1.4–1.8 relative viscosity units	
Iontophoresis	Children: 0–40 meq sodium/liter	0–40 mmol/liter
	Adults: 0–60 meq sodium/liter	0–60 mmol/liter
Propranolol (includes bioactive 4-OH metabolite)	100–300 ng/ml	386–1158 mmol/liter
Stool fat	Less than 5 g in 24 hr or less than 4% of measured fat intake in 3-day period	< 5 g/day

Chapter 15 | Laboratory Tests   263

Minimal Ml Required	Note	Method
2-S		
2-S		
50-U		Doniach et al.: Protocol of Autoimmunity Laboratories. London: Middlesex Medical School
10-B	Must be sent on ice	Hook, Muschel: Proc Soc Exp Biol Med 117:292, 1964
10-S	Collect and transport at 37°C	Barr et al.: Ann Intern Med 32:6, 1950 (modified)
2-S		Nephelometric assay
2-S		Nephelometric assay
5 ml clotted blood		Nephelometric assay
5 ml clotted blood		Nephelometric assay
5-P	Send EDTA tube on ice promptly to laboratory	Nathan et al.: Clin Chem 28:512, 1982
5 ml clotted blood		Double diffusion
2-S		
2-S		
2-S		
10-B	Expressed as the relative viscosity of serum compared with water	Barth: Viscosimetry of serum in relation to the serum globulins. In: Sunderman, Sunderman, eds. Serum Proteins and the Dysproteinemias, 1964, p. 102
	Value given in terms of sodium	Gibson, Cooke: Pediatrics 23:545, 1959
1-S	Obtain blood sample 4 hr after last dose of beta-blocking agent	M.G.H. method of Rockson, Homcy, Haber: by radioimmunoassay
24-hr or 3-day specimen		Jover et al.: J Lab Clin Med 59:878, 1962

TABLE 15.1 (continued)

Miscellaneous Values

Determination	Reference Range	
	Conventional	SI
Stool nitrogen	Less than 2 g/day or 10% of urinary nitrogen	< 2 g/day
Synovial fluid: Glucose	Not less than 20 mg/100 ml lower than simultaneously drawn blood sugar	See Blood Glucose
D-Xylose absorption	5–8 g/5 hr in urine; 40 mg per 100 ml in blood 2 hr after ingestion of 25 g of D-xylose	33–53 mmol/day 2.7 mmol/liter

Note: To update the normal reference values* of laboratory procedures recorded in the Case Records of the Massachusetts General Hospital and to give the methods used, the tabular summaries previously published have been revised. Both the conventional values and SI units are listed.†‡

*Normal Laboratory Values, N Engl J Med 234:24–28, 1946; 243:748–753, 1950; 254:29–35, 1956; 262:84–91, 1960; 268:1462–1469, 1963; 276:167–174, 1967; 283:1276–1285, 1970; 290:39–49, 1974; and 198:34–45, 1978, and 302:37–48, 1980. These values are in common use in the laboratories at the Massachusetts General Hospital and were compiled with the aid of James G. Flood, Ph.D., the Chemistry Laboratory; Leonard Ellman, M.D., the Clinical Laboratories; Bernard Kliman, M.D., the Endocrine Clinical Laboratories; and Kurt J. Bloch, M.D., the Clinical Immunology Laboratory.

11. What special considerations should be taken when drawing blood from a patient who is receiving an intravenous infusion?
12. What methods may be used to obtain blood when suction from a vacuum tube collapses the vein?
13. What precautions should be taken to prevent a hematoma when a successive venipuncture is necessary?
14. After drawing blood from an antecubital vein, such as the basilic, the arm should be flexed to stop the bleeding. True or false?
15. How long is pressure applied to the puncture site?
16. What special cautions are taken when a specimen is suspected of harboring microorganisms that cause infectious disease?
17. The most important factor in drawing blood for blood grouping and typing is _____ .

Chapter 15 | Laboratory Tests

Minimal Ml Required	Note	Method
24-hr or 3-day specimen		Peters, Van Slyke: Quantitative Clinical Chemistry, Vol. 2 (Methods), 1932, p. 353
1 ml of fresh fluid	Collect with oxalate-fluoride mixture	See Blood Glucose
5-U 5-B	For directions see Benson et al.: N Engl J Med 256:335, 1957	Roe, Rice: J Biol Chem 173:507, 1948

†The SI for the Health Professions. World Health Organization, Office of Publications, Geneva, Switzerland, 1977.

‡Abbreviations used: SI, Système international d'Unités; d, 24 hours; P, plasma; S, serum; B, blood; U, urine; l, liter; h, hour; and s, second.

Source: Reprinted by permission of the *New England Journal of Medicine* 314:39–49 (January 2), 1986. © Copyright, 1986, by the Massachusetts Medical Society.

PART V
Hazards and Complications

CHAPTER 16

Hazards and Complications of Intravenous Therapy

Ada Lawrence Plumer

Intravenous therapy subjects the patient to numerous hazards, many of which can be avoided if the nurse understands the risks involved and uses all available measures to prevent their occurrence. Local complications occur frequently but are rarely of serious nature. Systemic complications, though rarer, are most serious and are frequently life-threatening, requiring immediate recognition and medical attention.

LOCAL COMPLICATIONS

Occasionally local complications are not recognized until considerable damage is done. Early recognition may prevent (1) extensive edema depriving the patient of urgently needed fluid and medications, (2) necrosis, and (3) thrombophlebitis with the subsequent danger of emobolism. The local complications occur as the result of trauma to the wall of the vein.

THROMBOSIS

Any injury that roughens the endothelial cells of the venous wall allows platelets to adhere and a thrombus to form. Because the point of the cannula traumatizes the wall of the vein where it touches, thrombi form on the vein and at the tip of the cannula. Thrombosis occurs when a local thrombus obstructs the circulation of blood. It must be remembered that thrombi form an excellent trap for bacteria, whether carried by the bloodstream from an infection in a remote part of the body or introduced through the subcutaneous orifice [2].

THROMBOPHLEBITIS

Thrombophlebitis is the term used to denote a twofold injury: thrombosis plus inflammation. The development of thrombophlebitis is easily recognized. A painful inflammation develops along the length of the vein. If the infusion is allowed to continue, the vein progressively thromboses, becoming hard, tortuous, tender, and painful [6]. Early detection may prevent an obstructive thrombophlebitis which causes the infusion to slow and finally stop. This condition is most painful, persisting indefinitely, incapacitating the patient, and limiting valuable veins for future therapy.

Usually a sterile inflammation develops from a chemical or mechanical irritation. When the inflammation is the result of sepsis it is much more serious and carries with it the potential danger of septicemia and acute bacterial endocarditis.

There is always the inherent danger of embolism when thrombosis occurs. The more pronounced the inflammation and the more intense the pain, the more organized the thrombus is likely to become. It has been frequently stated that embolism is less likely to occur from the well-attached clot of thrombophlebitis than from phlebothrombosis [5].

PHLEBOTHROMBOSIS

Phlebothrombosis denotes thrombosis and usually indicates that the inflammation is relatively inconspicuous. It is thought to give rise to embolism since the thrombus is poorly attached to the wall of the vein [5]. Both thrombophlebitis and phlebothrombosis have a degree of inflammation and are associated with potential embolism.

Contributing Factors

Any irritation involving the wall of the vein predisposes the patient to thrombophlebitis. Inflammation to the vein will occur from any foreign body and is mediated by the following: (1) duration of the infusion, (2) composition of the solution, (3) site of the infusion, (4) technique, and (5) method employed.

Duration of the infusion is a significant factor in the development of thrombophlebitis. As the duration of time is lengthened, the incidence and degree of inflammation increase.

The *composition of the solution* may play a role. Venous irritation and inflammation may result from the infusion of hypertonic glucose solutions, certain drug additives, or solutions with a pH significantly different from that of the plasma. Solutions of dextrose are known to be irritating to the vein [3, 4]. The United States Pharmacopeia specifications for pH of dextrose solutions range from 3.5 to 6.5; acidity is necessary to prevent "caramelization" of the dextrose during autoclaving and to preserve the stability of the solution during storage. Studies have been performed which show a significant reduction in thrombophlebitis when buffered glucose solutions have been infused [4]. Abbott Laboratories, recognizing this problem, identifies the pH of each solution and provides Neut, a sodium bicarbonate 1% additive solution, to increase the pH of acid intravenous solutions. This additive, however, poses a problem of incompatibility when added to solutions containing drugs. Abbott's circular on Neut calls attention to the precaution that "When Neut is added to solutions, the compatibility of these solutions with other drugs may be altered." The largest number of incompatibilities may be produced by changes in pH [8]. As an example, tetracycline hydrochloride, with a pH of 2.5–3.0, is unstable in an alkaline environment.

The *site of infusion* can be a factor contributing to thrombophlebitis. The veins in areas over joint flexion undergo injury when motion of the cannula irritates the venous wall. The veins in the lower extremities are especially susceptible to trauma, enhanced by the stagnant blood in varicosities and the stasis in the peripheral venous circulation.

Small veins are subject to inflammation when used to infuse an irritating solution. The infusion cannula may occlude the entire lumen of the vein, obstructing the flow of circulating blood; the solution then flows undiluted, irritating the wall of the vein.

Technique can mean the difference between a successful infusion and the complication of thrombophlebitis. Only minimal trauma results from a skillfully executed venipuncture, whereas a carelessly performed venipuncture may seriously traumatize the venous wall.

Phlebitis associated with sepsis may be related to the technique of the operator. There is always the risk of infection if sterile technique is not zealously observed. Thorough cleansing of the skin is important in preventing infections. Maintenance of asepsis is essential during long-term therapy, particularly in the use of the through-the-needle cannula [9].

Methods employed to infuse parenteral solutions may foster septic thrombophlebitis. This complication is most often associated with the through-the-needle cannula. The cannula threaded through the needle remains sterile, does not come in contact with the skin, but provides a large subcutaneous orifice facilitating entry of bacteria around the catheter and seepage of fluid.

The over-the-needle cannula is not without fault as it comes in direct contact with the skin before being introduced into the vein. However, the tight fit through the skin may bar further bacterial entry.

Preventive Measures

In performing venipunctures, the therapist should exercise every caution to avoid injuring the wall of the vein needlessly. Multiple punctures, through-and-through punctures, and damage to the posterior wall of the vein with the point of the cannula can cause thrombosis. The risk of phlebitis may be minimized if the nurse:

1. Refrains from using veins in the lower extremities.
2. Selects veins with ample blood volume when infusing irritating substances.
3. Avoids veins in areas over joint flexion; utilize an armboard if the vein must be located in an area of flexion.
4. Anchors cannulas securely to prevent motion.

To prevent septic phlebitis, thorough preparation of the skin, together with aseptic technique and maintenance of asepsis during infusion, is imperative.

Periodic inspection of the injection site will detect developing complications before serious damage occurs. Complaints of a painful infusion make it necessary to differentiate between early phlebitis and venospasm from an irritating solution. If the latter is present, slowing the solution and applying heat to the vein will dilate the vessel and increase the blood flow, diluting the solution and relieving the pain. Following hypertonic solutions with isotonic fluids will flush the vein of irritating substances.

If inflammation accompanies the pain, a change in the injection site should be considered. To continue the infusion will only bring progressive trauma and limit available veins. An enforced time limit for removal of the cannula reduces the incidence of phlebitis [3].

During removal of the infusion cannula, care must be taken to prevent injury to the wall of the vein; the cannula should be removed at an angle nearly flush with the skin. Pressure should be applied for a reasonable length of time to prevent extravasation of blood.

INFILTRATION

Dislodgment of the cannula with consequent infiltration of fluid is not uncommon and is too frequently considered of minor significance. With the increasing numbers of irritating solutions and the frequency with which potent drugs are infused via intravenous solutions, serious problems may occur when the fluid invades the surrounding tissues. Hypertonic, acid, and alkaline solutions are contraindicated for hypodermoclysis and are not intended for other than venous infusions. If they are allowed to infiltrate, necrosis may occur (Figures 16.1, 16.2).

If necrosis is avoided, edema may nevertheless:

1. Deprive the patient of fluid and drug absorption at the rate essential for successful therapy.
2. Limit veins available for venipuncture, complicating therapy.
3. Predispose the patient to infection.

Extravasation can easily be recognized by the increasing edema at the site of the infusion. A comparison of the infusion area with the identical area in the opposite extremity assists in determining whether there is a swelling.

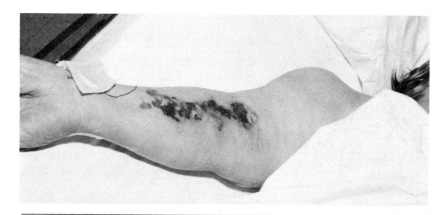

FIGURE 16.1
Necrosis of tissues resulting from infiltration of concentrated solution of potassium chloride.

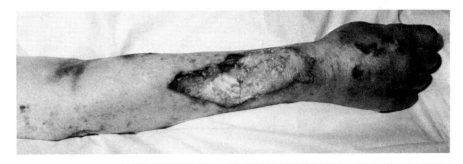

FIGURE 16.2
Necrosis from infiltration of hypertonic solution.

Frequently the edema is allowed to increase to great proportions because of a misconception that a backflow of blood into the adapter is significant proof that the infusion is entering the vein. This is not a reliable method for checking a possible infiltration. The point of the cannula may puncture the posterior wall of the vein, leaving the greater portion of the bevel within the lumen of the vein. Blood return will be obtained on negative pressure, but if the infusion is allowed to continue fluid will seep into the tissues at the point of the cannula, increasing the edema.

Occasionally, a blood return is not obtained on negative pressure. This may occur when the needle occludes the lumen of a small vein, obstructing the flow of blood.

To confirm an infiltration, apply a tourniquet proximal to the injection site tightly enough to restrict the venous flow. If the infusion continues regardless of this venous obstruction, extravasation is evident.

Once an infiltration has occurred, the cannula should be removed immediately.

SYSTEMIC COMPLICATIONS

Septicemia

Septicemia occurs when pathogenic bacteria invade the bloodstream. Early symptoms usually include chills, fever, general malaise, and headache. Immediate recognition and treatment must begin before organisms are allowed to multiply and cause overwhelming infection leading to vascular collapse, shock, and death. Adhering to established infection control procedures will minimize the occurrence of this serious complication.

Early symptoms must be reported to the physician immediately. If infection develops from an unknown source the entire infusion system should be suspected, removed, and cultured (see Chapter 17). The 0.22 micron air-eliminating filter, which is both bacteria and endotoxin retentive, provides a method of reducing the occurrence of septicemia related to infusion systems.

Use of Sterile Solutions

The solution should be carefully inspected for abnormal cloudiness or for the presence of extraneous particulate matter which may represent fungi. Fungal septicemia develops from the infusion of pathogenic fungi (see Chapter 17).

Methods of sterilization of parenteral fluids vary with manufacturing companies. If the method used produces a vacuum in solution bottles, presence of a vacuum should be noted; lack of vacuum indicates possible loss of sterility and contamination.

Use of Freshly Opened Solutions
Protein solutions, such as albumin and protein hydrolysates, must be used as soon as the seal is broken. To refrigerate these opened solutions for future use can result in serious consequence.

Other solutions should be used within 24 hours. The wise practice of indicating on the container the time and date that the seal is broken safeguards patients from possible contaminated infusions, especially patients on keep-open infusions for intermittent drug therapy.

Protection of Solution From Contamination
In the drug-additive program, sterile technique is essential to prevent organisms from being introduced into the solution. All drugs must be reconstituted with a sterile diluent. Once opened, any unused diluent should be discarded.

Keep-open solutions, terminated temporarily for blood infusion or drug therapy, must be protected from contamination. Sterile caps are available for some containers; sterile sponges may provide protection.

Pulmonary Embolism

Pulmonary embolism occurs when a substance, usually a blood clot, becomes free floating and is propelled by the venous circulation to the right side of the heart and on into the pulmonary artery [5]. Emboli may obstruct the main pulmonary artery or the arteries to the lobes, occluding arterial apertures at major bifurcations [5]. Obstruction of the main artery results in circulatory and cardiac disturbances. Recurrent small emboli may eventually result in pulmonary hypertension and right heart failure [7].

Preventive Measures
Certain precautions must be taken to prevent this serious complication from occurring.

1. Blood or plasma must be infused through an adequate filter to remove any particulate matter which could result in small emboli.
2. Veins on the lower extremities should be avoided when venipunctures are performed. These veins are particularly susceptible to trauma, predisposing the patient to thrombophlebitis. Although superficial veins rarely seem to be the source of emboli consequence [5], a thrombus may extend into the deep veins, resulting in a potentially viable clot; superficial and deep veins unite freely in the lower extremities.
3. Positive pressure should not be employed to relieve clot formation. To check for patency of the lumen of the cannula, kink the infusion tubing about 8 inches from the cannula. Then kink and release the tubing between the cannula and the pinched tubing — if the tubing becomes hard and meets with resistance, obstruction is evident, necessitating removal and reinstatement of the infusion.

4. Special precautions should be observed in the drug-additive program. Reconstituted drugs must be completely dissolved before being added to parenteral solutions; it is the inherent nature of red cells to adhere to particles, adding to the danger of clot formation.

5. Solutions should be examined to detect any particulate matter.

Air Embolism

Although air embolism is a significant possible complication with air-dependent containers, it is much more frequently associated with central venous lines. There is a potential risk for air embolism on the insertion of a central venous catheter, on inadequate sealing of the tract subsequent to disconnection of a central venous catheter, with disconnection of central lines, and with bypassing the "pump housing" of an electronic volumetric pump with an intravenous piggy back connection. Fatal embolism may occur when small bubbles accumulate dangerously and form tenacious bubbles that block the pulmonary capillaries [1]. Recognition of the circumstances which contribute to this hazard and measures taken to prevent their occurrence are imperative for safe fluid therapy.

Infusions run by gravity. If a vented container is allowed to run dry, air enters the tubing and the fluid level drops to the proximity of the patient's chest. The pressure exerted by the blood on the walls of the veins controls the level to which the air drops in the tubing. A negative pressure in the vein may allow air to enter the bloodstream. A negative pressure occurs when the extremity receiving the infusion is elevated above the heart [8]. Infusions flowing through a central venous catheter carry an even greater risk of air embolism when the container empties than those flowing through a peripheral vein; since the central venous pressure is less than the peripheral venous pressure, there is more apt to be a negative pressure which could suck air into the circulation. Precautions should be taken by the nurse while changing the administration set of a central venous infusion. The patient should be lying flat in bed and should be instructed to perform the Valsalva maneuver (forced expiration with the mouth closed) immediately before and during the time that the catheter is open to the air.

If the fluid container on a continuous infusion should empty, fresh solution will force the trapped air into the circulation. To remove the air from the administration set (Figure 16.3):

1. Place a hemostat close to the infusion cannula.
2. Hang the fresh solution.
3. With an antiseptic, clean the rubber section of the tubing proximal to the hemostat and below the air level in the tubing.
4. Insert a sterile needle to allow the air to escape.
5. Remove clamp and readjust flow.

The Y-type infusion set used with vented containers (Figure 16.4) is a less obvious source but one by which great quantities of air can be drawn into the bloodstream. Running solutions simultaneously is the contributing factor. If one vented container empties, it becomes the source of air for the flowing

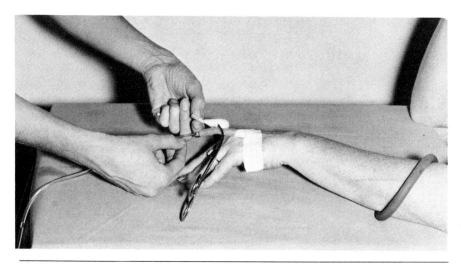

FIGURE 16.3
Removing air from the infusion set. The hemostat prevents air from entering the vein while a sterile needle allows air to escape from the administration set.

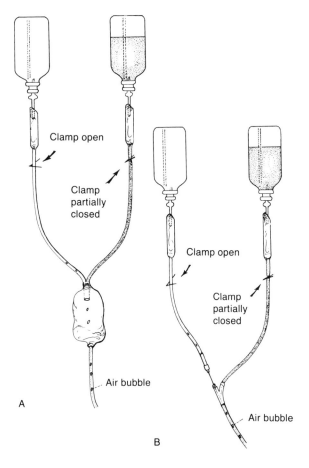

FIGURE 16.4
(A) The container runs dry during simultaneous infusion of fluids through Y-type administration set. Pressure below the partially constricted clamp is less than atmospheric, allowing air from the empty container (atmospheric) to enter infusion. (B) A secondary infusion "piggybacked" through the injection site of a primary intravenous set. Lacking an automatic shut-off valve, air from the empty container will enter the circulation. The same principle is involved as in the Y-type set.

solution. This is explained by the fact that the atmospheric pressure is greater in the open tubing to the empty container than below the partially restricted caamp on the infusion side. Recurrent small air bubbles are constantly aspirated into the flowing solution and on into the venous system. The introduction of air may be prevented by running one solution at a time. Vigilance is imperative if vented solutions are ordered to run simultaneously. The tubing must be clamped completely off before the solution container is allowed to empty [10].

This same principle is involved in the piggyback setup for secondary infusions. The potential danger of air embolism exists whenever solutions from two vented sets run simultaneously through a common cannula.

All connections of an infusion set must be tight. Any faulty opening or defective hole in the set allows air to be emitted into the flowing solution. If a stopcock is used, the outlets not in use must be completely shut off.

The regulating clamp on the infusion set should be located no higher than the chest level of the patient. Since the pressure exerted by the blood on the venous wall will normally raise a column of water from 4 to 11 cm above the heart, a restricting clamp placed above this point will result in a negative pressure in the tubing [8]. If great enough, the pressure can suck air into the flowing solution should a loose connection or a faulty opening exist between the clamp and the cannula [8]. The lower the clamp, the greater is the chance of any defects occurring above the clamp, where positive pressure can force the solution to leak out [10].

An infusion set long enough to drop below the extremity gives added protection against air's being drawn into the vein should the infusion bottle empty. Inlying pressure chambers on administration sets should be kept filled at all times. Manual compression of an empty chamber will force air into the bloodstream.

Occurrence of an Air Embolism

The nurse should be familiar with the symptoms associated with air embolism which arise from sudden vascular collapse: cyanosis, drop in blood pressure, weak rapid pulse, rise in venous pressure, and loss of consciousness. If air embolism occurs, the source of air entry must be immediately rectified. The patient should be turned on his left side with his head down [8]. This causes the air to rise in the right atrium, preventing it from entering the pulmonary artery. Oxygen is then administered and the physician notified.

Catheter Embolism Catheter embolism may occur during the insertion of a through-the-needle catheter if strict adherence to the proper procedure is not followed. The catheter should never be pulled back through the needle. If it becomes necessary to remove the catheter, the entire unit should be removed and a new catheter inserted. Catheter embolism may also occur during the insertion of an over-the-needle catheter if the needle is either partially or totally withdrawn and then reinserted. If the catheter is sheared off and embolized, the intervention of cardiac catheterization with shearing the catheter under the fluoroscope may be necessary.

Pulmonary Edema

Overloading the circulation is a real hazard to the elderly patient and to patients with impaired renal and cardiac function. Fluids too rapidly infused increase the venous pressure, with the possibility of cardiac dilatation and subsequent pulmonary edema.

Preventive Measures
These measures should be taken to prevent pulmonary edema:

1. Infusions should be maintained at the flow rate prescribed.
2. Positive pressure, using the pressure-chamber administration sets, should never be applied by the nurse to infuse solutions. If the patient requires fluids at such rapidity that positive pressure is required, infusion then becomes the physician's responsibility.
3. Controlled-volume infusion sets give added protection by preventing large quantities of fluid from being accidentally infused. These sets control the volume from 10 to 150 ml.
4. Solutions not infused within the 24-hour period ordered should be discarded and not infused with the following day's solutions; fluids administered in excess of the quantity ordered can overtax the homeostatic controls, increasing the danger of pulmonary edema.

The attending nurse must be alert to any signs or symptoms suggestive of circulatory overloading. Venous dilatation, with engorged neck veins, increased blood pressure, and a rise in venous pressure, should alert the nurse to the danger of pulmonary edema. Rapid respiration and shortness of breath may occur. The infusion should be slowed to a minimal rate and the physician notified. Raising the patient to a sitting position may facilitate breathing.

Speed Shock

Speed shock is the term used to denote the systemic reaction which occurs when a substance foreign to the body is rapidly introduced into the circulation. Caution must be observed in the administration of I.V. push injections. Rapid injection permits the concentration of a medication in the plasma to reach toxic proportions, flooding the organs rich in blood — the heart and the brain. As a result syncope, shock, and cardiac arrest may occur [1].

Preventive Measures
Certain precautions can minimize the potential danger of speed shock.

1. By reducing the size of the drop, pediatric-type infusion sets provide greater accuracy, thereby reducing the risk of rapid administration. These sets are valuable when solutions containing potent drugs must be maintained at a minimal rate of flow.
2. Electronic flow-control devices control the rate of infusion, an asset imperative to the administration of I.V. medications.
3. Upon initiating the infusion, ascertain that the solution is flowing freely before adjusting the rate. Movement of a cannula in which the aperature is partially obstructed by the wall of the vein can cause an increase in the flow, contributing to the danger of speed shock.

REFERENCES

1. Adriani, J. Venipuncture. *Am. J. Nurs.* 62:66–70, 1962.
2. Druskin, M. S., and Siegel, P. D. Bacterial contamination of indwelling intravenous polyethylene catheters. *J.A.M.A.* 185:966–968, 1963.
3. Editorial. Thrombophlebitis following intravenous infusions. *Lancet* 1:907–909, 1960.
4. Fonkalsrud, E. W., Pederson, B. M., Murphy, J., and Beckerman, J. H. Reduction of infusion thrombophlebitis with buffered glucose solutions. *Surgery* 63:280–284, 1968.
5. Hickan, J. B., and Sieker, H. O. Pulmonary embolism and infarction. *Disease-A-Month*, January 1959.
6. McNair, T. J., and Dudley, H. A. F. The local complications of intravenous therapy. *Lancet* 2:365–368, 1959.
7. Mavor, G. E., and Galloway, J. M. D. The ileofemoral venous segment as a source of pulmonary emboli. *Lancet* 1:873, 1967.
8. Metheny, N. M., and Snively, W. D., Jr. *Nurses' Handbook of Fluid Balance* 4th ed. Philadelphia: Lippincott, 1983, pp. 164, 174, 175.
9. Moran, J. M., Atwood, R. P., and Rowe, M. I. A clinical and bacteriologic study of infections associated with venous cutdown. *N. Engl. J. Med.* 272:554–556, 1965.
10. Tarail, R. Practice of fluid therapy. *J.A.M.A.* 171:45–49, 1950.

REVIEW QUESTIONS

1. Thrombophlebitis consists of what two injuries to the vein?
2. A sterile thrombophlebitis develops from a _____ or a _____ irritation.
3. Differentiate between thrombophlebitis and phlebothrombosis.
4. Septic thrombophlebitis carries the potential danger of _____ and _____.
5. Both thrombophlebitis and phlebothrombosis are associated with potential embolism. Which is considered more likely to give rise to embolism?
6. Name factors that may contribute to thrombophlebitis.
7. Name four preventive measures that may be taken by the nurse to minimize the risk of phlebitis.
8. What serious problems arise as the result of an infiltration?
9. What two precautions must be taken to prevent septicemia?
10. List three precautions that must be taken to prevent the occurrence of pulmonary embolism.
11. What precautions must be taken to prevent an air embolism?
12. Cyanosis, drop in blood pressure, weak rapid pulse, rise in venous pressure, and loss of consciousness are the symptoms of a sudden vascular collapse resulting from a(n) _____.
13. What three emergency measures can be taken in the event of an air embolism?
14. What would symptoms such as venous dilatation, engorged neck veins, increased blood pressure, and a rise in venous pressure suggest?
15. What three measures should be taken to prevent pulmonary edema?
16. What does the term *speed shock* denote?
17. What can be done to minimize the potential danger of speed shock?

CHAPTER 17

Bacterial, Fungal, and Particulate Contamination

Ada Lawrence Plumer

COMPLICATIONS OF INTRAVENOUS THERAPY

Scientific, technological, and medical advances have extended the lifesaving capabilities of intravenous therapy. However, in spite of these advances, intravenous-associated morbidity and mortality continue to increase.

The literature is full of warnings citing intravenous fluids and administration sets as potential vehicles for transmission of infection in hospitals. Cases of septicemia and fungemia have been directly traced to contamination of in-use intravenous apparatus and solutions [8, 11]. In 1969, 33 patients with fungal septicemia had been seen over an 18-month period in one university hospital. This complication was the primary cause of death in 13 patients. A correlation with prolonged intravenous catheterization was found [8].

From 1970 to 1971, 150 cases of bacteremia associated with intravenous therapy occurred in 8 United States hospitals. These were associated with the intravenous fluids of a major manufacturer; gram-negative bacteria were found contaminating sterile equipment. As a result, the Center for Disease Control (CDC) performed a study of all commercial intravenous systems in use in hospitals. The study showed a minimum of 6 percent prevalence of contamination within tubing and bottles after infusion equipment had been in use [4]. Conditions were shown to exist that potentially contributed to contamination: the characteristics of the apparatus itself and the manipulation of sets and solutions by hospital personnel. Hospital staffs were found to lack an understanding of asepsis, and therefore to practice poor antiseptic technique.

Much has been published concerning the alarming escalation of intravenous therapy complications, but owing to a lack of communication hospital personnel remain ignorant of the potential dangers. In hospitals utilizing intravenous teams, communication is better and personnel are more cognizant of complications and their warning symptoms. Infusion-associated infections "can be minimized if physicians, nurses, and other hospital personnel adhere to established infection control procedures when administering intravenous fluids" [16]. As long as intravenous therapy is taken for granted and the staff remain uninformed, intravenous-associated infection will continue to plague the recovery of the ill patient. Sixty to seventy percent of people hospitalized in the United States receive intravenous therapy each year [28]. These patients must be protected from the hazards complicating intravenous infusions.

To this end, official organizations have developed improvements in their requirements, guidelines, and standards for hospital practice. Learning the technical maneuvers of venipuncture is often accomplished by trial and error; the trauma resulting from such an approach contributes to complications. To overcome this and other problems, hospitals do now require periodic reassessment of therapeutic measures and training procedures. The principles of asepsis relevant to intravenous therapy are taught to all personnel involved in the preparation, administration, and maintenance of intravenous infusions.

A background knowledge of the epidemiology of nosocomial infections helps to instill in the therapist a greater awareness of the importance of aseptic and antiseptic technique in the prevention of infection. Epidemiology has been defined as "the division of medical science concerned with defining and explaining the interrelationship of the host, the agent and environment in causing disease" [39]. The host is the organism or patient from which a parasite obtains its nourishment. Bacteria which cause disease are said to be agents of the specific disease they cause [39].

SOURCES OF BACTERIA

There are three main sources of bacteria responsible for intravenous-associated infection: the air, the skin, and the blood. Microorganisms (flora and fauna) characteristic of a given location are referred to accordingly, thus the terms *skin flora, intestinal flora,* and so on.

The Air

The number of microbes per cubic foot of air varies, depending upon the particular area involved. Where infection is present, bacteria escape in body discharges, contaminating clothing, bedding, and dressings. Activity, such as bed making, sends bacteria flying into the air on particles of lint, pus, and dried epithelium [20]. Increased activity causes a rise in the number of airborne particles and provides an environment that interferes with aseptic technique and potentially contributes to contamination. Patient areas and utility rooms are places where airborne microorganisms may be plentiful. These contaminants find easy access to unprotected intravenous fluids.

The Skin

The skin is the main source of bacteria responsible for intravenous-associated infection. The bacteria found on the skin are referred to as *resident* or *transient*. Resident bacteria are those normally present, and they are relatively constant in a given individual. They adhere tightly to the skin, and usually include *Staphylococcus albus* as well as diphtheroids and *Bacillus* species [20]. Since not all bacteria are removed by scrubbing, meticulous care must be observed to avoid touching sterile equipment.

"The 'transient' flora is loosely attached to the skin and is composed of bacteria which have been picked up by the individual from his environment, and it varies from day to day in quality and quantity.... It is scant on clean protected skin, and profuse on dirty, greasy, exposed areas of the body" [20]. The transient bacteria are responsible for infection carried from one person to another. Touch contamination is a potential hazard of infection since hospital personnel move about frequently, touching patients and objects. Frequent hand washing is imperative.

The skin of the patient offers fertile soil for bacteria growth. "It has been estimated that a minimum of 10,000 organisms are present per square centimeter of normal skin" [44]. A square centimeter is equal to 0.155 square inches. Organisms such as *S. epidermidis, S. aureus,* gram-negative bacilli (especially *Klebsiella, Enterobacter,* and *Serratia*), and enterococci are ubiquitous on the skin of hospital patients [27].

The Blood

The blood may harbor potentially dangerous microorganisms. Therefore care must be taken to prevent bacterial contamination from blood spills when drawing samples and performing venipuncture. However, more likely to be a problem in blood is the hepatitis virus and the AIDS retrovirus. Hepatitis is transmitted by blood containing the hepatitis B virus and unidentified viruses non-A, non-B. Screening blood donors became a reality in 1970 when a test for HBsAG became available, reducing the occurrence of post-transfusion hepatitis. As no test is as yet available for non-A, non-B variety, post-transfusion hepatitis is still occurring in about 7 percent of all patients receiving blood or blood components (see Chapter 13). The hepatitis virus is easily transmitted and can be destroyed only by heat or gas sterilization. Proper care of cannulas, syringes, and intravenous sets is imperative. Adequate precaution and warning on blood samples that may possibly be contaminated with hepatitis virus are necessary to prevent the spread of any infection among hospital employees.

AIDS (acquired immune deficiency syndrome) is caused by the retrovirus HTLV-111, which destroys the body's immune system leaving the patient vulnerable to infection and other diseases. The epidemic of acquired immune deficiency syndrome, first recognized in 1981, seriously affected the nation's blood supply and complicated transfusion therapy [21]. In the spring of 1985 the AIDS test, to detect the presence of antibodies to the virus HTLV-111 in potential donors, became available.

Precautions must be taken to prevent the spread of the AIDS virus. Blood from all patients should be considered infective. Hand washing and wearing gloves are a must when handling blood and body fluid specimens. Hands must be washed after removing gloves, and always after becoming contaminated with blood. If contamination of the outside of the container has occurred, it should be cleaned with a disinfectant, such as 1:10 dilution of 5.25% sodium hypochlorite, household bleach, with water [22]. The blood specimen should be placed in a second container for transport. Hospital policies for disposable of infectious wastes must be observed. Needles should not be bent or reinserted into their sheaths because this action potentiates the risk of an inadvertent skin puncture. They should be placed in a puncture-resistant container.

Chapter 17 | Bacterial, Fungal, and Particulate Contamination 283

FACTORS INFLUENCING THE SURVIVAL OF BACTERIA

Infection depends upon the ability of bacteria to survive and proliferate. The factors that influence their survival are: (1) the specific organisms present, (2) the number of such organisms, (3) the resistance of the host, and (4) the environmental conditions [31].

The Specific Organisms

Bacteria are referred to as *pathogenic* or *nonpathogenic*. Pathogenic bacteria are capable of producing disease. All bacteria should be considered pathogenic. Reports show that bacteria previously considered nonpathogenic may produce infection. In one study, *Serratia* was implicated in 35 percent of cases of gram-negative septicemia resulting from intravenous therapy [1]. "Evidence is piling up that we can no longer ignore culture reports showing that patients or equipment are positive for organisms supposedly 'non-pathogenic for man'"[30].

Bacteria are classified as *gram-positive* and *gram-negative*. In recent years gram-negative bacteria have replaced gram-positive bacteria as the leading cause of death from septicemia [34]. "The single most important reason for the seriousness of the problem is probably the increased usage of antibiotics highly effective against gram-positive organisms but only selectively effective against gram-negative organisms. With the competitive inhibition of gram-positive bacteria eliminated, the more resistant gram-negative organisms have proliferated in the hospital environment" [26].

Number of Organisms

The number of contaminants present influences the probability of production of an infection. The power of bacteria to proliferate must not be underestimated. It is simply *not true* that a small amount of bacteria from touch contamination is harmless. Contamination of intravenous fluids and bottles with even a few organisms is extremely dangerous since some fungi and many bacteria can proliferate at room temperature in a variety of intravenous solutions to more than 10^5 organisms per milliliter within 24 hours [13].

Host Resistance

The resistance of the host influences the development and course of septicemia. Underlying conditions such as diabetes mellitus, chronic uremia, cirrhosis, cancer, and leukemia may adversely affect the patient's capacity to resist infection. Various forms of treatment such as immunosuppressive drugs, corticosteroids, anticancer agents, and extensive radiation therapy may depress immunological response and permit the invasion of infection. Therapy may mask infection so that septicemia may be unrecognized until autopsy [1].

Environmental Factors

Environmental factors that affect the survival and propagation of bacteria in intravenous fluids are (1) the pH, (2) the temperature, and (3) the presence of essential nutrients in the infusion.

Some organisms grow rapidly in a neutral solution and are less likely to grow in an acid medium. Buffering of acidic dextrose solutions has been recommended for prevention of phlebitis [14], but at the same time, the neutral environment provided by the buffer may enhance the survival and proliferation of bacteria.

The temperature of the fluid may affect the ability of bacteria to multiply. At room temperatures, strains of *E. cloacae, E. agglomerans,* and other members of the tribe Klebsiellae have been found to proliferate rapidly in commercial solutions of 5% dextrose in water [4, 27]. Total parenteral nutrition fluids should be used as soon as possible after preparation, and when it becomes necessary to store them temporarily they should be refrigerated at 4°C; at this temperature growth of *Candida albicans* is suppressed [27].

The presence of certain nutrients is essential to the growth of bacteria. Blood and crystalloid solutions provide nutrients that broaden the spectrum of pathogens capable of proliferation. Maki and associates [27] stated that the administration of blood or reflux of blood into the infusion system may provide sufficient nutrients to broaden this spectrum. The American Association of Blood Banks requires blood to be stored at a constant controlled refrigeration of 1–6°C.

It has been reported [32] that saline solutions are likely to contain enough biologically available carbon, nitrogen, sulphur, and phosphate together with traces of other material to support, under favorable conditions, the survival and multiplication of any gram-negative bacillus introduced to as many as a million organisms per milliliter.

FACTORS CONTRIBUTING TO CONTAMINATION AND INFECTION

Local complications of phlebitis and infection, as well as systemic complications and septicemias, are hazards of prolonged intravenous therapy which complicate recovery. Extrinsic contamination (introduced from without) may occur via the administration sets, the medication sites, and supplementary apparatus such as extension tubes, containers of fluid, and cannulas. Each time a medication is added, a container is changed, or supplementary equipment is added, the likelihood of contamination increases. Dudrick [12] pointed out that "each violation of the system's integrity geometrically increases the chances for contamination of the tubing, the bottle, or the catheter."

Breaks in aseptic technique contribute to contamination. Too much reliance on antibiotics has fostered a decline in aseptic technique. "Instead of overcoming contamination, antibiotic therapy has simply changed the spectrum of organisms from gram-positive to gram-negative" [30]. "Experience has suggested that antibiotic therapy, particularly with large and prolonged dosage, may have contributed to the development and increasing incidence of gram-negative septicemia. In some instances, toxemia and shock seemed to be temporarily intensified, presumably by the sudden destruction and lysis of gram-negative bacteria and the liberation of endotoxin" [1].

Faulty Handling   Faulty handling and procedures contribute to contamination. Containers of parenteral fluid are accepted as being sterile and nonpyrogenic on arrival from the manufacturer. The potential risk of contamination occurring in transit or in use is frequently overlooked by hospital personnel. However, through faulty handling or carelessness, glass containers may become cracked or damaged and plastic bags punctured. Bacteria and fungi may penetrate a hairline crack in an intravenous container, even though the crack is so fine that fluid is not lost from the container (Figure 17.1). Robertson [37] reported two cases in which fluid contaminated with fungi was inadvertently administered; the containers were cracked. These two patients were treated with an effective drug (amphotericin B), and recovery was complete.

Intravenous solutions of dextrose, as well as providing carbon and an energy source, include the extra nutrients needed to support the growth of 10 million organisms per milliliter. If the fluid is not examined closely, its opalescence may be overlooked, and subsequent infusion of a few hundred milliliters of such contaminated fluid will result in deep shock or possibly death [32].

Prior to use, containers of fluid should be examined, preferably against a light and dark background, for cracks, defects, turbidity, and particulate matter; plastic containers should be squeezed to detect any puncture hole.

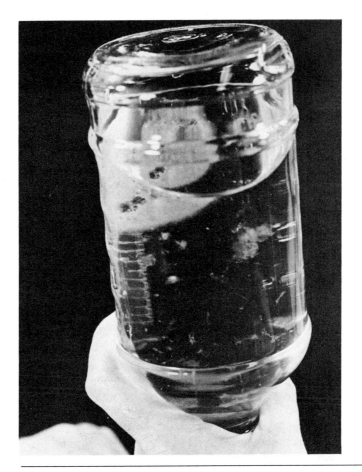

FIGURE 17.1
Intravenous fluid contaminated with fungi, which penetrated a hairline crack in the container.

Accidental puncture may occur without being evident and provide a point of entry for microorganisms [27, 43]. Any container with a crack or defect must be regarded as suspect and not used. Any glass container lacking a vacuum when opened should not be used.

Airborne Contamination

Studies by Hansen and Hepler [19] showed that intravenous fluids in an open intravenous stream (without an air filter) may become contaminated by airborne microbes when the container vacuum is replaced by unsterile air. When a 1-liter glass container is opened, approximately 100 ml air rushes in to replace the vacuum. In areas with a high concentration of airborne particles, contamination of unprotected fluids is a potential risk. Many hospitals, recognizing this risk, are having intravenous containers opened and the appropriate set added in the pharmacy under the sterile environment of a laminar flow hood. An alternative to this method is the use of the filter cannula to break the vacuum and allow particulate-free air to enter the container.

Discarding Outdated Intravenous Solutions

Several studies [4, 8, 11] have demonstrated that intravenous fluids and sets often become contaminated while in use. The longer the container is in use, the greater the proliferation of bacteria and the greater the infection should contamination inadvertently occur. The risk of infusing outdated fluids can be avoided by the utilization of special 24-hour limit labels, supported by a strong monitoring policy. Every container should be labeled with the time it is opened. The CDC recommends that all parenteral fluids should be completely used or discarded within 24 hours, and that lipid emulsions should be completely used within 12 hours of starting [5].

The CDC previously recommended also that intravenous administration sets be changed at least every 24 hours [5]. This recommendation was based on studies carried out during an epidemic period [5, 27]. To evaluate this recommendation, controlled studies have been performed. These studies "suggest that changing IV fluid administration sets daily has no important effect on the frequency of fluid contamination or phlebitis when exogenous contamination occurs infrequently and when the contaminants are not able to proliferate in dextrose-containing solutions" [3]. Study results implied that any benefits derived from a daily changing of intravenous administration sets were offset by the more frequent violation of the integrity of the system and the risk of introducing contaminants.

Today, CDC guidelines advocate that I.V. administration tubing, including "piggyback" tubing, be routinely changed every 48 hours and that tubing used for hyperalimentation be routinely changed every 24–48 hours. The set should be changed after administering blood, blood products, or lipid emulsions. Blood samples should not be withdrawn through I.V. tubing except in an emergency and just before discontinuation of the set and cannula. The administration set should not be flushed or irrigated to improve flow [5]. Strict asepsis must be maintained during bottle and tubing changes.

Should the spike or the adapter of the set become contaminated by inadvertent contact with unsterile objects, the set must be discarded. A sterile sponge placed under the hub of the cannula during the attachment of a sterile set will reduce the risk of touch contamination.

Admixtures

Allowing untrained hospital personnel to add drugs to intravenous containers potentially contributes to the risk of contamination. This risk is reduced when admixtures are prepared under laminar flow hoods by trained personnel adhering to strict aseptic technique such as is regulated by a pharmacy additive program. Such a program may not be practical or possible in all hospitals, and even where it exists, the necessity for nurses and physicians to prepare admixtures in an emergency does arise. All personnel involved in the preparation and administration of intravenous drugs should receive special training in the preparation of admixtures and the handling of intravenous fluids and equipment. Adherence to strict aseptic methods is vital. It must be understood that touch contamination is the primary source of infection and that although laminar flow hoods prevent airborne contamination, they do not ensure sterility when a break in aseptic technique occurs.

Manipulation of In-Use Intravenous Equipment

Intravenous fluids can be inadvertently contaminated by faulty techniques in the manipulation of equipment. In open systems, where solutions are not protected by air filters, the simple procedure of hanging the container may be taken for granted and the risk of contamination overlooked. When an administration set is inserted into the container and the container is inverted, the fluid tends to leak out the vent onto the unsterile surface of the container. Regurgitation of the contaminated fluid into the container occurs when the container vents. Instructions in the use of the equipment often go unread and unheeded. Squeezing the drip chamber of the administration set before inserting it into the container and releasing it when the container is inverted will prevent regurgitation of fluid and minimize the risk of contamination.

Injection Ports

Meticulous care, both aseptic and antiseptic, must be observed in the use of injection ports since they are a potential source of contamination when used to "piggyback" infusions. Its location, at the distal end of the tubing, exposes the injection port to patient excreta and drainage which enhance the growth of microorganisms and contribute to contamination. The injection port must be *scrubbed* over at least one minute with an accepted antiseptic; 70% isopropyl alcohol is commonly used. Scrubbing the injection cap for 30 seconds with an antimicrobial (povidone-iodine) solution provides very good protection. The needle should be firmly engaged up to the hub in the injection site and securely taped to prevent an in-and-out motion of the needle from introducing bacteria into the infusion.

Three-Way Stopcocks

Three-way stopcocks are potential mechanisms for transmission of bacteria to the host since their ports, unprotected by sterile covering, are open to moisture and contaminants. Connected to central venous catheters and arterial lines, they are frequently used for drawing blood samples. Aseptic practices are vital in preventing the introduction of bacteria into the line. A sterile catheter plug attached at the time the stopcock is added and changed after each use will reduce the risk of contamination.

Whenever fluid leakage is discovered at injection sites, connections, or vents, the intravenous set should be replaced. McDonough [30] stated that "many of the gram-negative organisms, including *Serratia,* have been found contaminating intravenous solutions and equipment. Their entry from 'standing water' about loose or defective caps or other ports is simple and swift; and their resultant sepsis in the patient is equally swift."

Small-Vein Needles

Small-vein needles have been recommended for parenteral infusions because most studies show that the use of these devices results in very low rates of infection or serious local reactions [40]. Because the insertion of a small-vein needle is relatively atraumatic and phlebitis is not a common complication, the same vein may be used repeatedly. CDC recommends the use of small-vein needles for routine peripheral I.V. infusions in hospitals that cannot assure replacement of plastic cannulas every 48–72 hours. NITA does not recommend the small-vein needles for routine use.

Plastic Cannulas

In the past plastic cannulas have been associated with a high incidence of complications in comparison with steel cannulas. "Venous complications from plastic catheters were found to be approximately 2½ times more prevalent than with steel needles." [40]

The traumatic insertion of a plastic cannula can result in the formation of local thrombi which can support bacterial or fungal proliferation. The trauma is increased when a large cannula is used or when the venipuncture is performed by inexperienced personnel.

Characteristics inherent with the plastic cannula encourage the introduction of bacteria through the cutaneous opening. In the over-the-needle catheter, the catheter is larger than the cutaneous puncture wound made by the inlying needle. The result is a definite drag through the skin as the catheter is slipped off the needle, with the potential risk of transporting cutaneous bacteria into the puncture wound. Skin flora has been implicated as an important source of organisms responsible for catheter-associated infection. In the through-the-needle catheter, the sterility of the catheter is maintained by its sterile protective sleeve and the sterile needle through which the catheter is slipped into the vein. Once the catheter is within the lumen of the vein, the needle is withdrawn, leaving a puncture wound larger than the catheter and one through which fluid can seep and bacteria can gain entrance. CDC guidelines, today, moderately recommend: [5]

a. Plastic cannulas are acceptable for routine peripheral infusions if and only if the hospital can be sure that cannulas are replaced every 48–72 hours, such as can be done by an I.V. team.
b. Otherwise, stainless steel cannulas should be used for routine peripheral I.V. infusion, and plastic cannulas should be reserved for those clinical settings when a secure route for vascular access is imperative.

Today national standards and guidelines, through their recommendations, are providing added protection and increased safety in the use of plastic cannulas.

Skin Preparation

Microbes on the hands of hospital personnel contribute to hospital-associated infection. Too often breaks in sterile technique occur from failure to wash the hands before changing containers or sets or preparing admixtures. Besides the usual skin flora, antibiotic-resistant gram-negative organisms frequently contaminate the hands of hospital personnel [27].

To maintain asepsis, the CDC recommends that the hands be thoroughly washed for insertion of central venous catheters and that sterile gloves be worn for cannulas requiring cutdowns [5].

Adequate and reliable preparation of the patient's skin and maintenance of asepsis is imperative when a catheter is used for intravenous therapy. The skin, the first defense barrier of the body, is broken, providing a vulnerable port for the migration of bacteria. Skin flora has been implicated as a source of contamination of catheters. In a study made of 118 patients receiving intravenous therapy via an indwelling polyvinyl catheter, 53 catheters were found to be contaminated with bacteria; in 28 of these the organisms were comparable to those cultured from the skin of the patient before the skin was cleaned with iodine [2].

Frequently the question arises of whether or not to shave the skin. The need to remove the hair is not substantiated by scientific evidence; antiseptics used to clean the skin also clean the hair. Shaving facilitates removal of the tape, but may produce microabrasions which enhance the proliferation of bacteria [27]. Clipping excess hair with scissors will facilitate the removal of tape.

Alcohol 70% is frequently used to prepare the skin site for venipuncture. How reliable is alcohol? Studies show that ethyl alcohol, 70% by weight, is an effective germicide for the skin when *applied with friction for 1 minute*. It is as effective as 12 minutes of scrubbing and reduces the bacterial count by 75 percent [44]. Since a minimum of 10,000 organisms per square centimeter are present on normal skin, the count would be reduced to 2,500. Too frequently the use of alcohol consists of a quick wipe which fails to reduce the bacterial count significantly.

Iodine and iodine-containing disinfectants are still the most reliable agents for preparing the skin for venipuncture since they provide bactericidal, fungicidal, and sporicidal activity. Because of occasional patient allergy to iodine, the possibility of sensitivity should be investigated before its use. Tincture of iodine (2% iodine in 70% alcohol) is inexpensive and well tolerated. "Solution should be liberally applied, allowed to dry for at least 30 seconds, and washed off with 70% alcohol. Both agents should be applied with friction, working from the center of the field to periphery" [27]. Iodophor preparations, when used for patients with sensitive skin, should not be washed off since the sustained release of free iodine may be necessary for germicidal action. Iodophor preparations require 30 second contact time.

Quaternary ammonium compounds such as aqueous benzalkonium chloride are inactivated by organic debris and are ineffective against gram-negative organisms, and so should not be used for skin disinfection [27].

The tourniquet itself may very well provide a source of cross-infection and contamination since it is used repeatedly from patient to patient and handled just prior to venipuncture. This possibility should be kept in mind and the tourniquet disinfected periodically.

Once the venipuncture is completed and it is within the lumen of the vein, the cannula must be securely anchored; to-and-fro motions of the catheter in the puncture wound may irritate the intima of the vein and introduce cutaneous bacteria. Thought should be given to the possible contamination of the adhesive tape that is used to secure the cannula. Rolls of tape last indefinitely and may be a source of contamination; they are transported from room to room, placed on patients' beds and tables, and frequently roll to the floor. Furthermore, before venipuncture, strips of tape often are torn off the roll and placed in convenient locations on the bed, table, and uniform. These facts should be borne in mind. Adhesive tape should not be applied over the puncture wound. The puncture wound must be considered an open wound and asepsis must be maintained.

CARE OF THE CATHETER

The CDC recommends: "a topical antibiotic or antiseptic ointment should be applied at the I.V. site immediately after cannula insertion, especially for insertion by cutdown." The wound should be protected by a sterile dressing. The dressing should be changed every 48–72 hours using aseptic technique and the ointment reapplied. Occlusive dressings create a moist, warm environment which may alter the cutaneous flora and enhance the proliferation of bacteria [27].

Recommendations [5] require that indwelling cannulas be left in place no longer than 72 hours and preferably for only 48 hours. The date and time of insertion written on a piece of tape and placed in the vicinity of the dressing will alert the nurse and assist in ensuring removal within a safe period of time.

Frequent observations should be made for signs of malfunction of the cannula; infiltration; and phlebitis characterized by erythema, induration, or tenderness. Such signs require immediate removal of the cannula. Fuchs [15] has noted that the major factor influencing the frequency of catheter colonization is the presence of other catheter complications such as subcutaneous infiltration and phlebitis. He defined *colonization* as positive culture of the catheter tip without evidence of local or systemic infection.

Irrigation of a plugged catheter may embolize small catheter thrombi, some of which are infected. Contamination of the catheter may result from a break in aseptic technique, from contaminated fluid or set, from bacterial invasion of the puncture wound, or from clinically undetected bacteremia arising from an infection in a remote area of the body, such as a tracheostomy, the urinary tract, or a surgical wound. The clot around or in the catheter serves as an excellent trap for circulatory microorganisms and as a nutrient for bacterial proliferation.

INTRAVENOUS-ASSOCIATED INFECTIONS

Intravenous-associated sepsis is not always accompanied by phlebitis. Symptoms of infection consist of chills and fever, gastric symptoms, headache, hyperventilation, and shock. Should infection develop from an unknown source in a patient receiving intravenous therapy, the intravenous system should be suspected and the entire system, including the cannula, removed. The catheter and the infusion fluid should be cultured.

The following procedure should be used for culturing the catheter [16].

1. Cleanse the skin about the cannula site with alcohol, allowing the alcohol to dry before removing the cannula.
2. Maintaining asepsis, remove the catheter and with sterile scissors snip 1 cm of the catheter tip into blood culture or other appropriate culture medium.

The following procedure should be used for culturing the infusion fluid [16].

1. Aseptically withdraw 20 ml fluid from the intravenous line: 1 ml is used to prepare a pour plate; the remaining fluid is used to inoculate two blood culture containers.
2. Add to the remaining intravenous fluid in the container an equal volume of brain-heart infusion broth enriched with 0.5% beef extract. Inoculate at 37°C; this is a more sensitive culture for detecting low-level contamination.

All containers of fluid previously administered to the patient should be suspected and, if possible, retained and cultured. All information and identification, including the lot number of the suspected solution, should be recorded on the culture requisition and the patient chart. The U.S. Food and Drug Administration, the CDC, and the local health authorities should be notified if contamination during manufacturing is suspected; fluids bearing implicated lot numbers should be stored for investigation.

PARTICULATE MATTER

The literature concerning particulate matter in infusions and its clinical significance is increasing. Many articles indicate that intravenously administered particles can cause pathogenic states [42]. Particulate matter is defined as the mobile, undissolved substances unintentionally present in parenteral fluids [24]. Such foreign matter may consist of rubber, glass, cotton fibers, drug particles, molds, metal, or paper fibers.

Vascular Route of Infused Particles

The pulmonary vascular bed acts as a filter for infused particles. Particles introduced into the vein travel to the right atrium of the heart, down through the tricuspid valve, and into the right ventricle. From there they are pumped into the pulmonary artery and on through branches of arteries which decrease in size until the particles are trapped in the massive capillary bed in the lungs, where the capillaries measure 7 to 12 microns in diameter.

Five microns, the size of an erythrocyte suspended in fluid, has been suggested as the largest allowable size for a particle in the pulmonary capillary bed [17]. Particles larger than 5 microns are recognized as potentially dangerous since they are likely to become lodged. Particles as large as 300 microns can pass through an 18-gauge cannula, and much larger particles may pass through an indwelling catheter with a larger lumen. See Table 17.1 for particle size comparisons. If occlusion of a small arteriole inhibits oxygenation or normal metabolic activities, cellular damage or tissue death may result. Where there is ample collateral circulation, the occlusion would have no appreciable

TABLE 17.1
Particle Size Comparisons

Microns		Inches
175	=	.007
150	=	.006
125	=	.005
100	=	.004
75	=	.003
50	=	.002
25	=	.001

Source: Contamination Control Laboratories. *Particle Size Comparisons* (information circular). Livonia, Mich., 1970.

Note: One micron equals 40 millionths of an inch (approx.). A human hair is approximately 125 microns in thickness. Bacteria range in size from 0.3 to 0.5 micron. We cannot see a particle or hole smaller than 20 microns. A hole 25 microns in diameter in a HEPA filter is over 75 times larger than the contaminants and bacteria passing through.

biological effect. However, a particle that is not biologically inert may incite an inflammatory reaction, a neoplastic response, or an antigenic, sensitizing response [23].

Particles may gain access to the systemic circulation, where occlusion of a small arteriole in the brain, kidney, or eye can be serious, in one of the following ways:

1. The pulmonary vascular bed does not filter out all particles. Prinzmetal and associates [36] demonstrated that glass beads up to 390 microns may pass through the pulmonary capillary bed and reach the systemic circulation.
2. Large arteriovenous shunts have been demonstrated to exist in the human lung [18, 25]. Particles bypass the pulmonary capillary bed and enter the systemic circulation, where a systemic occlusion could be serious.
3. Particles larger than 5 microns may reach the systemic circulation by interarterial injection or infusion.

Sources of Contamination

Studies [10] have shown that particulate contamination is present in all intravenous fluids and administration sets. The U.S.P. has established an acceptable limit of particles for single-dose infusion as not more than 50 particles per milliliter that are equal to or larger than 10.0 μm, and not more than 5 particles per milliliter that are equal to or larger than 25.0 μm in effective linear dimension (see Chapter 9). Great efforts are being made by manufacturers to produce high-quality intravenous injections. Their efforts are being defeated by numerous manipulations before final infusion.

Medication Additives
Drugs constitute a major source of contamination. Improper technique in the preparation of drugs results in the formation of insoluble particles. When personnel with no pharmaceutical knowledge add drugs to intravenous fluids, they contribute to incompatibilities which substantially increase the particle

count. Rubber closures also have been implicated as a major source of contamination.

Glass Ampules

Glass ampules may be responsible for the injection of thousands of glass particles into the circulation. Turco and Davis [41], in a study prompted by the frequency of high-dose administration of furosemide, showed that a dose of 400 mg, which at that time required the breaking of 20 ampules, could add to the injection 1,085 glass particles larger than 5 microns. A dose of 600 mg, requiring 30 ampules, could result in 2,387 particles larger than 5 microns.

Antibiotic Injectables

Studies have been performed in relation to particulate matter in commercial antibiotic injectable products [29]. They showed particulate contamination levels of bulk-filled antibiotics to be 2 to 10 times greater than those of stable antibiotic solutions and lyophilized antibiotics. Filtration is impossible since packaging by the sterile bulk-fill method involves extracting and processing the antibiotic in sterile bulk powder form and then aseptically placing the bulk antibiotic into dry presterilized vials. In the lyophilized and the stable liquid packaging processes the particulate matter can be terminally removed by filtration directly into presterilized vials. The majority of the antibiotics are packed by the bulk-fill method.

Particulate matter in intravenous injections may be responsible for much of the phlebitis that so often occurs with the infusion of these drugs. Russell [38] listed the major pathological conditions caused by particulate matter as (1) direct blockage of vessels, (2) platelet agglutination leading to formation of emboli, (3) local inflammation caused by impaction of particles, and (4) antigenic reactions with subsequent allergic consequence.

Intravenous Fluids

Walter [45] noted that critically ill patients who had received large amounts of intravenous fluid died of pulmonary insufficiency characterized by increased venous pressure and pulmonary hypertension. He observed that the lungs looked like leather and speculated that the cause of death might be the result of accumulated matter from the many liters of infused fluids.

Massive Infusions of Old Banked Blood

Deaths caused by pulmonary emboli following massive transfusions have been reported [33]. Cellular debris in stored blood has been implicated; the standard blood filter of 170 microns has been found inadequate to remove the microaggregates that accumulate in stored bank blood. Commercially available blood filters (see Figure 11.9) of small micropore size (40 microns or lower) are available and trap degenerating platelets, white cells, and fibrin strands that form in blood after 5 or more days of storage.

Reducing the Level of Contamination

Since particulate matter infused via intravenous fluids may produce pathological changes which can have an adverse effect on critically ill patients, every effort must be made to reduce the particulate count in intravenous injections.

Nurses and doctors in general have been unaware of the potential dangers that exist and have unknowingly added to the contamination. Official agencies have developed standards for an acceptable limit for particles in intravenous fluids. Industry has provided the medical profession with filters to limit direct access of bacteria, fungi, and particulate matter to the bloodstream.

Filters

A filter aspiration needle* specially designed to remove particulate matter from intravenous medicaments is available. With this device attached to a syringe the medication is drawn from the vial or glass ampule filtering out the particles. The filter needle must then be discarded to prevent the particles trapped on the filter from being injected when the medication is added to the intravenous fluid.

Final Filters

The National Coordinating Committee on Large Volume Parenterals† has recommended the in-line filter that is both particulate and microbe retentive for the following: hyperalimentation patients and immune-deficient or immune-compromised patients. The intravenous filter that is particulate retentive is generally recommended for patients receiving intravenous infusions with many additives, when drugs requiring constitution are known to be heavily particulated, or to minimize particulate matter in infusions to which additives have been introduced. In-line filters should be used when drugs are administered in minute doses (less than 5 µg per milliliter or total amount of less than 5 mg over a 24-hour period) but only after studies confirm that the specific drug being administered is not absorbed to the filter and I.V. device.

There are two schools of thought regarding the routine use of filters. CDC does not recommend the in-line filter as a routine infection control measure. Some experts feel that these filters are not cost effective in the prevention of infections, which today occur infrequently.

NITA policy advocates the routine use of 0.22 micron air-eliminating filters in delivering routine intravenous therapy since these filters remove particulates, bacteria, and air, and some remove endotoxins as well [35].

Filters are manufactured in a variety of forms, sizes, and materials. Some — not all — when wet block the passage of air under normal pressure. Used in conjunction with infusion pumps, they play an important role in preventing air from being pumped into the bloodstream should the fluid container become empty.

A knowledge of filter characteristics, use, and proper handling is important to the safety of the patient. Faulty handling can cause plugging of the filter, resulting in the patient not receiving prescribed fluids and the necessity of performing a venipuncture to insert a new line. A ruptured filter may go

---

*Monoject Filter Aspiration Needle, Sherwood Medical Industries, St. Louis, Mo.

†National Coordinating Committee on Large Volume Parenterals, cosponsored by the United Pharmacopeial Convention and the Food and Drug Administration under FDA contract with U.S.P.C. Ref. No.:79–01, Nov. 30, 1979.

undetected and introduce filter fragments, bacteria, and air into the infusion line. (See Chapter 11.)

Handling of Filters

Although they provide added protection for the patient, filters are not a substitute for sterile technique. The manual addition or frequent changes of the filter increase the likelihood of contamination. In-line membrane filters with a self-venting air filter reduce the risk of contamination by eliminating the need for (1) manual addition of the filter and (2) frequent changes due to obstruction of the filter by air block.

Some administration sets contain air vent filters which allow only sterile air to enter the container. Such sets are also available for the administration of salt-poor albumin. Misuse occasionally occurs, contributing to contamination. The drip chamber of the set *must be compressed* before it is introduced into the fluid bottle. This creates a vacuum which immediately causes the air vent to function, avoiding regurgitation of fluid and a wet filter which may cease to function. Occasionally a staff member inserts a needle into the air vent to provide a patent vent; however, this ruptures the filter and contributes to particulate contamination.

Final filters complicate a system by which viscous fluids, such as blood, and some drugs, such as amphotericin B, are infused. An injection site distal to the filter provides a means of infusion. A clamp located between the filter and the injection site plays an important role; if, through ignorance or carelessness, the injection is made without clamping off the tubing, the filter may become blocked by viscous fluid or back pressure from the injection may rupture the membrane and allow particulate matter and bacteria to enter the bloodstream.

In-line filters limit the access of bacteria, fungi, particulate matter, air, and — one filter — endotoxins into the bloodstream; but their safety depends upon the knowledge of the individuals involved in their use.

REFERENCES

1. Altemeier, W. A., Todd, J. C., and Inge, W. W. Gram-negative septicemia: A growing threat. *Ann. Surg.* 166:530–542, 1967.

2. Banks, D. C., Cawdreys, H. M., Yates, D. B., and Harries, M. G. *Lancet* 1:443, 1970.

3. Buxton, A. E., Highsmith, A. K., Garner, J. S., West, C. M., Stamm, W. E., Dixon, R. E., and McGowan, J. E. Contamination of intravenous infusion fluid; Effects of changing administration sets. *Ann. Intern. Med.* 90:764–768, 1979.

4. Center for Disease Control. *Nosocomical Bacteremias Associated with Intravenous Fluid Therapy* (U.S.A. Morbidity and Mortality Weekly Report 20). (Special Suppl.) Vol. 20, no. 9, 1971.

5. Center for Disease Control. Guidelines for prevention of intravascular infection. *J. NITA* 5(1):39–50, 1982.

6. Contamination Control Laboratories. *Particle Size Comparisons* (information circular). Livonia, Mich., 1970.

7. Crossley, K., and Matsen, J. M. The scalp-vein needle: A prospective study of complications. *J.A.M.A.* 220:985, 1972.

8. Curry, C. R., and Quie, P. G. Fungal septicemia in patients receiving parenteral hyperalimentation. *N. Engl. J. Med.* 285:1221, 1971.

9. Davis, N. M., and Turco, S. A study of particulate matter in I.V. infusion fluids — phase 2. *Am. J. Hosp. Pharm.* 28:620–623, 1971.

10. Davis, N. M., Turco, S., and Sivielly, E. A study of particulate matter in I.V. infusion fluids. *Am. J. Hosp. Pharm.* 27:822–826, 1970.

11. Deeb, E. N., and Natsios, G. A. Contamination of intravenous fluids by bacteria and fungi during preparation and administration. *Am. J. Hosp. Pharm.* 28:764, 1971.

12. Dudrick, S. J. Article in *Hospital Tribune* (University and Hospital Edition of *Medical Tribune and Medical News*)8(3):1, 1974.

13. Felts, S. K., Shaffner, W., Melly, M. A., and Koenig, M. G. Sepsis caused by contaminated intravenous fluids: Epidemiological clinical and laboratory investigation of an outbreak in one hospital. *Ann. Intern. Med.* 77:881, 1972.

14. Fonkalsrud, E. W., Murphy, J., and Smith, F. G., Jr. Effect of pH in glucose infusions on development of thrombophlebitis. *J. Surg. Res.* 8:539, 1968.

15. Fuchs, P. C. Indwelling intravenous polyethylene catheters: Factors influencing the risk of microbial colonization and sepsis. *J.A.M.A.* 216:1447–1450, 1971.

16. Goldmann, D. A., Maki, G. D., Rhame, F. S., and Kaiser, A. B. Guidelines for infection control in intravenous therapy. *Ann. Intern. Med.* 79:849, 1973.

17. Groves, M. J. Particles in intravenous fluids (letter). *Lancet* 2:344, 1965.

18. Hales, M. R. Multiple small arteriovenous fistulae of the lungs. *Am. J. Pathol.* 32:927, 1956.

19. Hansen, J. S., and Hepler, C. D. Contamination of intravenous solutions by airborne microbes. *Am. J. Hosp. Pharm.* 30:326–331, 1973.

20. Hirshfield, J. W. Bacterial contamination of wounds from the air, from the skin of the operator, and from the skin of the patient. *Surg. Gynecol. Obstet.* 73:72–78, 1941.

21. Inderlied, C. B., and Young, L. S. Clinical microbiology of acquired immune deficiency syndrome (AIDS). *J. Med. Technicians* 2(3):167, 169, March 1985.

22. Jemison-Smith, P. Understanding the acquired immune deficiency syndrome, *J. NITA* 7(2):115, 1984.

23. Jonas, A. M. Potentially Hazardous Effects of Introducing Particulate Matter into the Vascular System of Man and Animals. In *Safety of Large Volume Parenteral Solutions* (Proceedings of National Symposium of the U.S. Food and Drug Administration, Washington, D.C., 1966). Washington, D.C.: Government Printing Office, 1967.

24. Kruger, E. O., and Riggs, T. H. Objectives: Pharmaceutical Manufacturers Association Parenteral Particulate Matter Committee. *Bull. Parent. Drug Assoc.* 22:99–103, 1968.

25. Liebow, A. A., Hales, M. R., and Lindskog, G. B. Enlargement of the bronchial arteries and their anastomoses with the pulmonary arteries in bronchiectasis. *Am. J. Pathol.* 25:211–231, 1949.

26. Lillehei, R. C., Dietzman, R., Moras, S., and Block, J. H. Treatment of septic shock. *Modern Treatment* 4(2):32–346, 1967.

27. Maki, D. G., Goldman, D. A., and Rhama, F. S. Infection control in intravenous therapy. *Ann. Intern. Med.* 79:869, 870, 872, 875, 876, 878, 880, 1973.

28. Maki, D. G. Preventing infection in intravenous therapy. *Hosp. Prac.* 11(4):1976.

29. Masuda, J. V., and Beckerman, J. H. Particulate matter in commercial antibiotic injectable products. *Am. J. Hosp. Pharm.* 30:72–76, 1973.

30. McDonough, J. J. Preventing contamination in I.V. therapy. *Hosp. Phys.* Nov. 1971, p. 70.

31. McGaw Laboratories. *McGaw Technical Information Bulletin #16.* Glendale, Calif., 1969.

32. Microbiological hazards of intravenous infusions. *Lancet* 1:43, 1974.

33. Moseley, R. V., and Doty, D. B. Death associated with multiple pulmonary emboli soon after battle. *Ann. Surg.* 171:336, 1970.

34. Motsay, G. J., Dietzman, R. H., Ersek, R. A., and Lillehei, R. C. Hemodynamic alterations and results of treatment in patients with Gram-negative septic shock. *Surgery* 67:577–583, 1970.

35. National Intravenous Therapy Association. NITA standards — I.V. therapy. *J. NITA* 5(1):24–29, 1982.

36. Prinzmetal, M., Ornitz, E. M., Jr., Simkin, B., and Bergman, H. C. Arteriovenous anastomoses in liver, spleen, and lungs. *Am. J. Physiol.* 152:48–52, 1948.

37. Robertson, M. H. Fungi in fluids — A hazard of intravenous therapy. *J. Med. Microbiol.* 3:99, 1970.

38. Russell, J. H. Pharmaceutical application of filtration, part 2. *Am. J. Hosp. Pharm.* 28:125–126, 1970.

39. Taber's *Cyclopedic Medical Dictionary*. Revised and edited by C. L. Thomas, Philadelphia: Davis, 1973.

40. Thomas, E. T., Evers, W., and Racz, C. B. Post infusion phlebitis. *Anesth. Analg.* 49:150–159, 1970.

41. Turco, S., and Davis, N. M. Glass particles in intravenous injections. *N. Engl. J. Med.* 287:1264–1265, 1972.

42. Turco, S., and Davis, N. M. Clinical significance of particulate matter — A review of literature. *Lippincott's Hospital Pharmacy* 8:137, 1973.

43. Viaflex containers. *Med. Lett. Drugs Ther.* 14:69–71, 1972.

44. Walter, C. W. *The Aseptic Treatment of Wounds*. New York: Macmillan, 1956.

45. Walter, C. W. *FDA Symposium on Safety of Large Volume Parenteral Solutions*. Washington, D.C.: U.S. Government Printing Office, 1967.

BIBLIOGRAPHY

Bivins, B. A., Rapp, R. P., Deluca, P. P., McKean, H., and Ward, O. G., Jr. Fluid inline filtration: A means of decreasing the incidence of infusion phlebitis. *Surgery* 85(4):388–394, 1979.

National Coordinating Committee on Large Volume Parenterals. Recommendations to pharmacists for solving problems with large volume parenterals. *Am. J. Hosp. Pharm.* 33:231–236, Mar., 1976.

REVIEW QUESTIONS

1. The three main sources of bacteria responsible for intravenous-associated infections are the _____, the _____, and the _____.

2. Of the three sources of bacteria, the _____ is the major one.

3. Will the use of laminar flow in the preparation of admixtures reduce the risk of intravenous infections associated with skin flora?

4. Define the term *resident flora*.

5. Define the term *transient flora*.

6. *Staphylococcus albus* and *Bacillus* species are usually considered to be transient flora. True or false?

7. Blood may harbor potentially dangerous microorganisms. Name the virus that is easily transmitted and can be destroyed only by heat or gas sterilization.

8. Differentiate between pathogenic and nonpathogenic.

9. Is *Serratia* pathogenic or nonpathogenic?

10. Gram-negative bacteria have replaced gram-positive bacteria as the leading cause of death from septicemia. Why?

11. Is a small amount of bacteria from touch contamination considered harmless?

12. What five underlying conditions adversely affect the patient's capacity to resist infection?

13. What four forms of treatment may depress immunological response and permit the invasion of infection?
14. Give three factors that affect the survival and propagation of bacteria in intravenous fluids.
15. Name five areas where extrinsic contamination may occur.
16. The CDC recommends that intravenous fluid containers be changed at least every _____ hours.
17. The CDC recommends that intravenous administration sets be changed at least every _____ hours.
18. Laminar flow hoods prevent airborne contamination and ensure sterility when a break in aseptic technique occurs. True or false?
19. What precautions must be taken when injection sites are used for fluid or drug administration?
20. Whenever fluid leakage is discovered at injection sites, connections, or vents, the intravenous set should be replaced. Many of the gram-negative organisms, including _____, may enter the system from standing water.
21. How must ethyl alcohol, 70% by weight, be applied to be an effective germicide for the skin?
22. Iodine and iodine-containing disinfectants are the most reliable agents for preparing the skin because they provide _____, _____, and _____ activity.
23. Why should iodophor preparations not be washed off the skin with alcohol?
24. Why does the tourniquet provide a potential source of cross-infection and contamination?
25. What complications may result from improper taping of the catheter?
26. How often should the catheter site be inspected and the dressing changed?
27. Is it beneficial to shave the skin in preparation for cannula insertion?
28. What potential hazards may arise from irrigating a plugged catheter?
29. Name three sources which contribute to particulate contamination.
30. What devices are available to remove particulate matter?

PART VI

Specific Applications

CHAPTER 18

Central Venous Catheterization

Faye Cosentino

In the past, when a successful venipuncture could not be obtained a cutdown (surgical venesection) was performed by the physician. Cutdowns are rarely done today because of the high risk of infection. According to Center for Disease Control (CDC) guidelines, all cutdowns must be treated with the same recommendations as given for peripheral cannula insertion. They must be replaced every 48–72 hours [1]. Percutaneously inserted central venous catheters have replaced cutdowns.

The advantages of central venous catheterization include (1) placement usually by percutaneous puncture, avoiding minor surgery which could result in the loss of the vein for future use; (2) a lower risk of infection; and (3) catheter tip placement in the superior vena cava.

The tip placement allows for rapid dilution of the infusate, thus reducing the risk of phlebitis and vein sclerosis. The tip placement also allows for monitoring central venous pressure (CVP).

VASCULAR ANATOMY

To apply the principles relating to the use of central venous catheters, it is necessary to review a section of the vascular system.

Vessels involved include the cephalic, basilic, axillary, jugular, subclavian, and innominate veins as well as the superior vena cava (Figures 18.1, 18.2).

The Cephalic Vein The cephalic vein ascends along the outer border of the biceps muscle to the upper third of the arm. It passes in the space between the pectoralis major and deltoid muscles. It terminates in the axillary vein, with a descending curve, just below the clavicle.

The cephalic vein is occasionally connected with the external jugular or subclavian vein by a branch which passes from it upward in front of the clavicle [2].

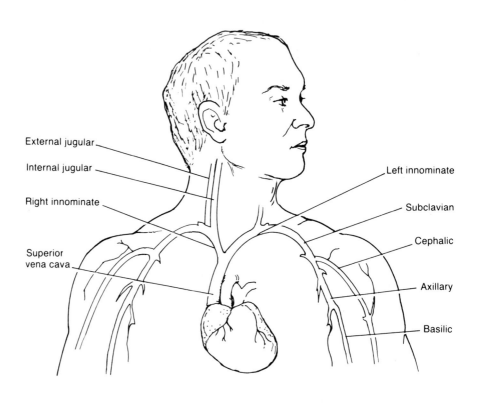

FIGURE 18.1
Central venous catheters are inserted via the subclavian and internal or external jugular veins.

The Basilic Vein	The basilic vein is larger than the cephalic. It passes upward in a smooth path along the inner side of the biceps muscle and terminates in the axillary vein [2].
The Axillary Vein	The axillary vein commences upward as a continuation of the basilic vein, increasing in size as it ascends. It receives the cephalic vein and terminates immediately beneath the clavicle, at the outer border of the first rib. At this point it becomes the subclavian vein [2].
The External Jugular Vein	The external jugular vein is easily recognized on the side of the neck. It follows a descending inward path to join the subclavian vein above the middle of the clavicle [2].
The Internal Jugular Vein	The internal jugular vein descends first behind and then to the outer side of the internal and common carotid arteries. The carotid plexus is situated on the outer side of the internal carotid artery. The internal jugular vein joins the

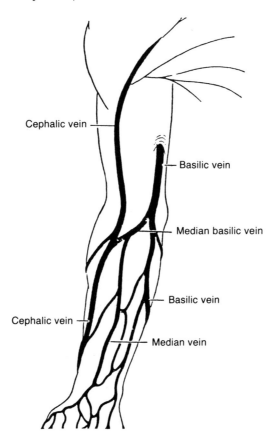

FIGURE 18.2
The cephalic and basilic veins are used for peripheral insertion of central venous catheters. From Gray, H. Anatomy, Descriptive and Surgical. New York: Crown, 1977.

subclavian vein at the root of the neck. At the angle of junction, the left subclavian receives the thoracic duct while the right subclavian receives the right lymphatic duct [2].

The Subclavian Vein

The subclavian vein, a continuation of the axillary, extends from the outer edge of the first rib to the inner end of the clavicle, where it unites with the internal jugular to form the innominate vein.

Valves are present in the venous system, until approximately one inch before the formation of the innominate vein [2].

The Right Innominate Vein

The right innominate vein is about an inch long. It passes almost vertically downward and joins the left innominate just below the cartilage of the first rib [2].

The Left Innominate Vein

The left innominate vein is about 2.5 inches in length and larger than the right. It passes from left to right across the upper front chest, in a downward slant. It joins the right innominate to form the superior vena cava [2].

The Superior Vena Cava	The superior vena cava receives all blood from the upper half of the body. It is comprised of a short trunk 2.5–3 inches in length. It begins below the first rib close to the sternum on the right side, descends vertically slightly to the right, and empties into the right atrium of the heart [2].

CENTRAL VENOUS PRESSURE

Peripheral insertions of central venous catheters were first used for monitoring central venous pressure (CVP). *Central venous pressure* denotes the pressure in the right atrium or vena cava of the venous blood as it returns from all parts of the body. The pressure varies among individuals, usually ranging between 4 and 11 cm H_2O in the vena cava while the pressure in the right atrium is usually 0–4 cm H_2O [3]. The normal range has little significance since the true value lies in the change or lack of change following attempts to alter the blood volume or to improve cardiac action. Because central venous pressure relates to a fully sufficient circulation, it facilitates assessment of both the blood volume and the ability of the heart to tolerate an increased volume, thereby providing a valuable guide for fluid administration. It requires no laboratory personnel and no expensive equipment; it is simple in technique; and, once set up, it may be monitored quickly and as often as required.

Because central venous pressure relates to an adequate circulatory blood volume it is dependent upon [3].

1. Volume of blood.
2. Status of the myocardium (heart muscle).
3. Tone of blood vessels.

Circulatory failure may result from deficiency in any one or combination of these essential factors.

Blood Volume	Changes in blood volume alter the tone of the blood vessels and the ability of the heart to circulate the blood. A reduced blood volume results in less pressure at the right atrium, indicated by a drop in central venous pressure; an increased blood volume produces more pressure at the atrium, with a rise in central venous pressure [3].

In managing an inadequate circulation, one must first establish a normal blood volume. If the inadequate circulation is due to deficiency in the blood volume, manipulation is made by administering expanders, or in the case of increased volume, phlebotomy.

If the circulation still remains insufficient, it becomes necessary to look at the remaining two essential components — status of the myocardium and tone of the blood vessels.

Status of the Myocardium	The status of the myocardium may be affected by disease, drugs, fluids, or anesthesia. Because the central venous pressure is a measure of the capacity of the myocardium as well as the blood volume, it is invaluable in monitoring the effects of anesthesia and surgery on elderly patients with arteriosclerosis or

patients with myocardial insufficiency. The central venous pressure rises if the heart muscle is impaired — the pressure of the volume of blood at the heart increases because the heart muscle is no longer able to pump an adequate flow of blood out of the right atrium [3]. A high central venous pressure may suggest cardiac failure [3]. This is one of the commonest causes of an elevated central venous pressure in shock.

Drugs or chemicals are administered to improve myocardial response, thus increasing cardiac output and lowering the central venous pressure.

Tone of the Blood Vessels

The third essential component, the tone of the blood vessels, is dependent upon the arterial pressure and upon external and internal pressures on the veins. The arterial pressure arises from the contractile force of the left ventricle and is transmitted through the capillaries to the veins.

The external pressures upon the vein result from (1) the muscular and fascial pumping action in the extremities, (2) the intraabdominal pressure from straining and distension, and (3) the intrathoracic pressure due to contraction of the diaphragm and chest wall. Central venous pressure of patients on positive pressure respirators is usually increased by 4 cm, while patients on negative pressure show a decreased central venous pressure [4].

The internal pressure on the veins is due to blood volume, myocardial response, and sympathomimetic amines (epinephrine, norepinephrine). Vasopressors, by stimulating contraction of the venous wall, decrease the capacity of the venous system and improve vascular tone.

Applications

Hypotension
The management of hypotension continues to be one of the most urgent problems facing the surgeon. The parameters used in evaluating a patient in shock consist of the following:

1. Blood pressure.
2. Rate and quality of pulse.
3. Skin temperature and color.
4. Urinary output.
5. Peripheral venous filling.
6. Blood pH.

Blood Volume
Maintenance of an optimal blood volume is essential for survival. Prolonged hypovolemia may cause poor tissue perfusion with the inherent risk of renal and myocardial complication; hypovolemia, uncorrected, can eventually lead to shock and death. Blood volume is not necessarily reflected by the blood pressure. In cardiogenic shock the blood volume is increased and the blood pressure is low. In septic shock, hypotension accompanies a normal blood volume.

Various methods have been employed to detect change in a patient's blood volume: hematocrit, change in patient's weight, and blood volume computations. Today the central venous pressure is the parameter frequently used to assess blood volume. It is an important guide during

1. *Surgery,* when there is a risk of overloading an anesthetized, traumatized patient who is continuously losing blood.
2. *Shock,* when origin is unknown.
3. *Massive fluid replacement* in open-heart surgery and in critical cases, such as the severely burned, where circulatory overload is a hazard.
4. *Anuria* or *oliguria,* when questionable cause is dehydration.

Total Parenteral Nutrition

Subclavian insertions were first used for administration of total parenteral nutrition (TPN). This subject is thoroughly discussed in Chapter 21.

Short-Term Infusion

As more physicians mastered subclavian techniques, central venous catheters were used for other purposes. A common use was for administration of short-term infusions of fluids, admixtures, and/or blood when a secure venous access was required for *very large volumes and/or fast rates* of administration. This was frequently seen during surgery, in intensive care units, and in trauma patients.

Cancer Therapy

With the advent of tunneling techniques, antithrombogenic catheter materials, new device designs, and lowered infection rates, central venous catheters became popular for many other uses. The administration of long-term chemotherapeutic agents, blood or blood components, and antibiotics, as well as blood sample drawing, is frequently done with a central catheter device in cancer patients; see Chapter 22.

Unsuccessful Peripheral Entry

In any hospital patient requiring a venous access whose peripheral veins cannot be cannulated, a central catheter is often the best solution.

Home I.V. Therapy

Many home patients have been taught to self-administer their continuous or intermittent medications through a central device; see Chapter 25.

Therapeutic Phlebotomy

This catheter has also been used for long-term therapeutic phlebotomies, when peripheral access is extremely difficult or impossible [5]; see Chapter 13.

Today, all types of central venous catheters are common on every patient care unit in acute care hospitals, and are used for all kinds of I.V. therapy in the home; see Chapter 19.

Chapter 18 | Central Venous Catheterization

CENTRAL VENOUS PRESSURE MONITORING

Central venous pressure monitoring is achieved by attaching an intravenous set to a three-way stopcock and to an extension tube with a radiopaque catheter of approximately 24 inches. A vertical length of infusion tubing that serves as the manometer is connected to the stopcock and attached to the intravenous stand against a marked centimeter tape. Central venous pressure sets are available with disposable water manometers, graduated in units. The zero mark on the tape is adjusted to the level of the patient's right atrium. The pressure is measured at either the superior vena cava by introducing the catheter via the antecubital, jugular, or subclavian vein, or at the inferior vena cava via the femoral vein.

The superior vena cava is most commonly used. Complications have been associated with inferior vena caval catheters. Use of the femoral vein and the long duration of time the catheter is in the vein enhance the risk of thrombotic complications. A second disadvantage is the fact that abdominal distension interferes with monitoring an accurate right atrial pressure.

Equipment

With a central venous catheter in site, the following equipment is needed for monitoring central venous pressure.

Intravenous pole
Solution as ordered
Intravenous or transfusion tubing
Central venous monometer set
Venous pressure level (optional)
Dye (methylene blue), if ordered
Vitamin B complex, if ordered
Heparin 1 : 1,000, if ordered
Armboard with cover
Adhesive tape

Procedure

Connecting pressure manometer to central venous catheter (Figure 18.3).

1. Wash hands thoroughly and dry.
2. Add dye (methylene blue) or vitamin B complex to the container, if ordered. This facilitates reading of the manometer.
3. Add heparin to the container, if ordered. This reduces thrombus formation and provides catheter patency.
4. Close three-way stopcock.
5. Hold and squeeze drip chamber while inserting tubing spike into upright bottle or hanging plastic bag. The use of a tubing with a Luer-lock connector will aid in the prevention of a connection separation, which could result in an air embolism.

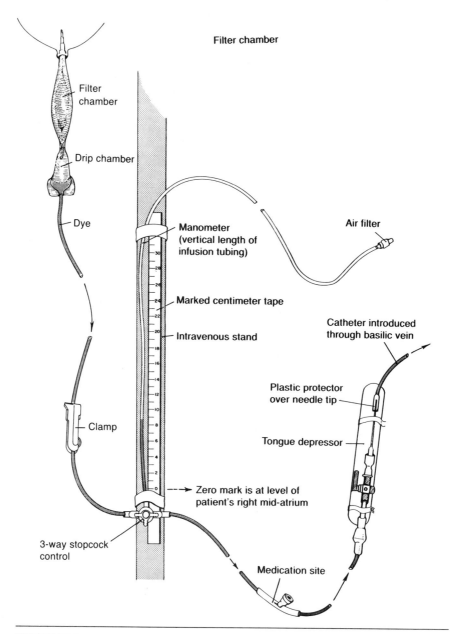

FIGURE 18.3
Equipment for monitoring central venous pressure. Zero mark on the tape is level with the right atrium. Notice precautions taken to prevent cutting edge of the needle from severing the catheter: the bevel shield is in place and the tongue depressor provides added protection.

Chapter 18 | Central Venous Catheterization

6. Release squeeze, allowing drip chamber to fill one-quarter to one-third full. Prefilling drip chamber prevents air bubbles from entering the system.
7. If the manometer is to be permanently attached to the I.V. pole, tape centimeter strip onto intravenous pole with zero point adjusted to the midatrial level. Patient should be in a supine position with the bed flat. Use venous pressure level for accuracy. Midatrial level is at a point approximately equidistant from the sternum and the back. Tape stopcock to pole at a level below patient's right atrium. Do not tape directly on the stopcock. Tape upper end of manometer taut to intravenous pole.

   If the manometer contains clips and will be removed for each reading, secure manometer to intravenous pole. When this type of manometer is used, placing a waterproof "X" on the side of the patient's chest at midatrial level will ensure that all readings are taken with zero point at the same level.
8. Adjust stopcock to allow solution to flow into manometer, filling it halfway.
9. Adjust stopcock to flush remainder of tubing.
10. Connect manometer system to central venous catheter.
    a. Use strict aseptic techniques while disconnecting present I.V. system and connecting manometer system.
    b. Be sure to use air embolism precautions when the catheter is open to air (see air embolism, under the complications section of this chapter).
    c. Secure catheter hub–tubing connection with tape to aid in prevention of connection separation.
    d. Secure arm to covered armboard. Motion of catheter upon flexion of the arm increases the potential risk of phlebitis. A kinked catheter results in unreliable readings and leads to clogging of the lumen.

Central Venous Pressure Measurement

The pressure is usually read at half-hour or hourly intervals. The patient must be quiet, not coughing or straining, and in a supine position with the zero point on the manometer at the midatrial level. The procedure is as follows:

1. Turn stopcock so solution flows from the container to the manometer.
2. When manometer level reaches 30 cm, turn stopcock to stop flow from the container and direct manometer flow to the patient.
3. The fluid level will drop rapidly, reaching the reading level in about 15 seconds. The central venous pressure is measured at the high point of the fluctuation.
4. Readjust the stopcock so the infusion resumes.
5. Record measurements on Vital Signs Record.

The catheter is presumed to be in the thoracic cavity when (1) manometer fluid fluctuates 3–5 cm during breathing, and (2) coughing and straining cause the column of water to rise. If the catheter is inserted too far and reaches the heart, higher pressure waves synchronous with the pulse will be seen [6].

PATIENT PREPARATION

To allay fears and to obtain patient cooperation, the reasons for the insertion and the procedure must be explained in detail to the patient. The nurse should make sure that the patient knows what to expect and what each step of the procedure accomplishes.

Position During Insertion

If a subclavian entry is to be used, explaining to the patient that he or she will be positioned flat in bed with the head lowered and knees bent, to increase the blood supply to the vein, and that a rolled towel will be placed under the back between the shoulder blades to make it easier for the physician to enter the vein, will obtain patient cooperation when the uncomfortable position must be maintained.

Gowns and Masks

Explaining that the nurse and the physician will both wear gowns and masks to keep normal bacteria away from the area will allay apprehension. If the patient will be required to wear a mask, having him or her wear one before the procedure will give reassurance that a mask does not really interfere with breathing.

The Valsalva Maneuver

Practicing the Valsalva maneuver prior to the insertion will obtain patient cooperation when he or she is asked to hold the breath and "bear down" at the time the catheter is open to the air.

Becoming Acquainted with the Device

If a tunneled catheter or implanted venous access or pump device is being inserted, seeing and touching the device which will remain in their bodies is reassuring to most patients. Any limitations of activity the device will create should be thoroughly discussed. If the patient will be required to give any self-care, this should be completely explained and agreed to by the patient before insertion.

Consent Form

A patient consent form must be signed before any central venous catheter or device insertion.

Blood Studies

Preinsertion blood studies include platelet count, prothrombin time (PT), and partial thromboplastin time (PTT). Any abnormal result may require correction with vitamin K, fresh frozen plasma, or platelet concentrates before insertion is attempted.

Premedication

Depending upon the type of device, insertion site, and individual patient needs, some form of sedation may be required prior to the procedure. This should be explained to the patient.

CENTRAL VENOUS CANNULATION

Any central venous catheter has its inherent risks. *If peripheral veins are obtainable and adequate for the desired treatment, a central venous catheter should not be inserted.*

Contraindications

Contraindications for any type of central venous catheter insertion may include:

1. Abnormal coagulation studies.
2. Septicemia.
3. Anomalies of the central venous vascular structures.
4. Thrombosis of the innominate or subclavian veins, or of the superior vena cava.
5. Superior vena cava syndrome.

Catheter Tip Placement

Even though tunneled catheters are often called "right atrium" catheters, the preferred tip placement is usually at the junction of the superior vena cava and the right atrium. If the tip lies in the right atrium, atrial arrhythmias may occur as a result of catheter irritation. For various reasons it is not always possible to advance the catheter far enough to achieve the desired tip location. Depending upon the specific purpose of the catheter, innominate or subclavian catheter tip placement may be adequate.

Infection Control

Except for emergency situations, all central catheters should be inserted with sterile technique. Sterile gloves, gowns, and masks are worn [17]. If the patient cannot be masked, the head should be turned away from the insertion area. If the site is very hairy the dressing may not adhere well. Because shaving can cause microabrasions which can increase the risk of infection, cutting the hair with scissors is recommended [17]. The skin is defatted with acetone and prepped with povidone-iodine solution or tincture of iodine followed by a complete removal with alcohol. A sterile field is provided by a fenestrated drape or sterile towels. During the procedure the nurse should be alert to the possibility of touch contamination of any sterile item. Having a central catheter insertion cart will provide a means of replacing any possibly contaminated items immediately. A repeat site prep with povidone-iodine solution is frequently done after catheter insertion. Povidone-iodine ointment is placed at the insertion site and the area covered with an occlusive dressing [18].

Air Embolism Precautions

There is always the risk of air embolism during catheter insertion because central venous pressure can be negative. Placing the patient in Trendelenburg's position will increase the pressure. If possible, the patient should perform the Valsalva maneuver whenever the catheter is opened to the air. If the catheter stylet has been removed, the hub should be occluded with either a syringe or the gloved finger to prevent air entry.

Patient Positioning During a central venous catheter insertion the patient is placed in Trendelenburg's position. This not only increases central venous pressure; it also distends the vein and facilitates entry. When the subclavian approach is used, a rolled towel is placed along the spinal cord to hyperextend the neck and elevate the clavicle. For the jugular approach, the head is turned to the opposite direction and extended. This stretches and stabilizes the vein and accentuates the muscular landmarks. During a cephalic or brachial insertion, abduction of the arm may be required to pass the catheter past the shoulder area.

INSERTION SITES

There are basically three approaches for central venous catheter insertions. The veins used for entry are the subclavian and the internal or external jugular veins for central insertion, and the cephalic or basilic vein for peripheral insertion.

CENTRAL INSERTION

The subclavian vein is frequently the entry of choice. It requires the shortest length catheter because it utilizes the most central veins, thus creating a high blood flow around a large portion of the catheter. This results in minimal catheter irritation or obstruction. All these factors lower the risks of complications, resulting in a longer catheter life.

Subclavian Vein A subclavian entry is always performed by a physician because major complications can occur during or from this insertion; see Complications section of this chapter, below.

The subclavian entry may be performed by the infraclavicular or the supraclavicular approach. In both approaches the cannula is inserted under the clavicle, aiming for the jugular notch. For the infraclavicular approach the cannula is inserted at approximately the midpoint of the clavicle. For the supraclavicular approach the cannula is frequently inserted at the base of the triangle formed by the sternal and clavicular heads of the sternocleidomastoid muscle.

Contraindications
Contraindications for the subclavian approach may include:

1. Radiation burns at intended insertion site.
2. Fractured clavicle.
3. Hyperinflated lungs.
4. Cancer growth at the base of the neck or apex of the lungs.

Internal Jugular Vein Because of the possibility of major insertion complications, the insertion of central venous catheters into the internal jugular vein should be left to physicians. Many physicians select the internal jugular vein as a first choice of site for the insertion of a central venous catheter.

The constant anatomical location of the internal jugular vein makes its cannulation easier than that of the subclavian vein. The right internal jugular vein is usually chosen because it forms a straighter, shorter line to the superior vena cava. It also avoids the higher left pleura and thoracic duct. This insertion is frequently performed by first locating the vein with a small-gauge needle. After making a small skin incision to facilitate entry, a larger gauge cannula is inserted, following the same direction as the locator needle, aiming for the ipsilateral nipple.

External Jugular Vein

The external jugular vein is observable and easily entered. Insertion complications are rare, so cannulation can be performed by specialty nurses.

The external jugular vein varies in size and its junction with the subclavian vein is acutely angulated. It contains two pairs of valves. The uppermost pair are 4 cm above the clavicle, the lower pair are located at the vein's entrance to the subclavian vein. Because of these factors central cannulation can be difficult. As a short cannula may be easily inserted, central cannulation may be achieved by the use of an introducer with a guide wire. Entry into the superficial vein is performed by directing the cannula toward the ipsilateral nipple.

Objections to Jugular Insertions

The main objections to any jugular cannulation are:

1. *Catheter occlusion* is a persistent problem as a result of head movement.
2. *Vein irritation* is created by the same movements. These factors result in a *shorter catheter life*.
3. It is *difficult to maintain an intact dressing* on the area.
4. The idea of having a catheter in the neck is *esthetically and psychologically disturbing* to many patients and families.

PERIPHERAL INSERTION

Because subclavian and internal jugular insertions usually have a longer life span, peripheral insertions are frequently performed when the subclavian or the jugular vein is either contraindicated or attempted unsuccessfully. Peripheral insertion of a central venous catheter via the cephalic or the basilic vein incurs minimal insertion complications. Therefore, cephalic or basilic vein insertion is frequently performed by specially trained nurses.

Cephalic Vein

The cephalic vein is usually superficial and easy to enter at the antecubital fossa. However, because of the abrupt angle with which the cephalic joins the axillary, difficulties are frequently encountered while attempting to thread a long catheter through this vein. Positioning the patient's arm at a right angle to the body may facilitate catheter passage. If the cephalic vein is connected to the external jugular or the subclavian veins by a branch, catheter passage may be impossible.

Basilic Vein

The basilic vein is usually the first choice of veins for the peripheral insertion of a central venous catheter. This larger vein, following a smooth path, will facilitate catheter passage into the axillary, subclavian, and innominate veins, and into the superior vena cava. However, the entry point is not as superficial as the cephalic and frequently requires entry by palpation. The basilic vein is in close proximity to the brachial artery and some of the branches of the internal cutaneous nerve. Care must be taken to prevent injury to either of these structures during venipuncture.

Objections to Peripheral Insertions

1. There is a high risk of *catheter malpositioning* with tip placement in the jugular vein. Having the patient lower the head toward the insertion site can help avoid this problem.
2. The extreme length of the peripherally inserted catheter creates a higher risk of catheter irritation with resultant *phlebitis*.
3. If the insertion site is directly at the antecubital fossa, mechanical irritation will occur with patient movement. This may require *immobilization of the joint* with an armboard. Selection of an entry site in the upper arm, above the antecubital fossa, can help avoid this problem.

Postinsertion Care

A chest x-ray is always done immediately after catheter insertion to rule out pneumothorax and to document tip placement. An isotonic solution is infused until tip placement is confirmed. The site should be observed for any signs of excess bleeding or swelling. The patient's breathing should be monitored for any signs of respiratory distress. Any unexpected observation should be reported to the physician immediately.

COMPLICATIONS

Arterial Puncture

Arterial puncture, one of the most frequently reported complications of subclavian insertions, is usually not a major problem if it is recognized early. The puncture of an artery requires the immediate application of digital pressure for at least 5 minutes. If the patient has a coagulation abnormality, digital pressure must be maintained until all bleeding stops. If the artery puncture is not recognized and treated early, a massive hematoma resulting in tracheal compression or respiratory distress can occur.

Pneumothorax

Pneumothorax, another common complication of subclavian insertion, occurs as a result of pleural puncture; the patient may experience difficult breathing or chest pain. It can be asymptomatic and discovered by radiography. A chest tube may be required to treat the symptoms.

Hemothorax

Hemothorax may result if the subclavian or adjacent veins have been traumatized or transected during the insertion. Symptoms and treatment are the same as for pneumothorax.

Hydrothorax

Hydrothorax results when the I.V. fluid infiltrates into the chest. The symptoms and treatment are identical to a pneumothorax.

Catheter Embolism

Catheter embolism is always a risk whenever an inside-the-needle (INC) device is inserted or left in situ. During insertion, care must be taken NEVER to withdraw the catheter back through the needle. While the INC is in place, care must be taken to ensure that the needle tip is always protected with a secured tip cover. A severed catheter may require cardiac catheterization to retrieve the embolism. The use of catheter designs which do not require sharp metal needles can almost eliminate this complication.

Air Embolism

Air embolism is always a potential danger whenever any central venous catheter is open to air. This can occur because it is always possible to have negative central venous pressure. During insertion, placing the patient in Trendelenburg's position will increase central venous pressure. Placing the sterile gloved finger over the catheter hub, between catheter stylet removal and I.V. system connection, can prevent air from entering the catheter.

If the patient can cooperate, performing the Valsalva maneuver will increase central venous pressure. However, be sure that the patient takes the deep breath and bears down *before* the disconnection. Performing the disconnection while the patient is inhaling can *increase* the risk of air embolism. During tubing changes the same precautions are necessary to prevent air embolism. Using taped Luer lock connections between the catheter and the air-eliminating filter can reduce the risk of tubing separations resulting in air embolism [9].

Air embolism precautions should also be taken during catheter removal. The Valsalva maneuver should also be performed at this time. Positioning the patient flat in bed and immediately upon catheter removal placing a sterile sponge with antimicrobial ointment directly over the puncture site will prevent air from entering the system. This dressing should be left intact for 24–48 hours to allow time for tissue healing.

Signs and symptoms of air embolism can include chest pain, dyspnea, hypoxia, apnea, tachycardia, hypotension, or a precordial murmur. Immediate treatment includes placing the patient in a supine position on the left side with the feet elevated. This position is used in an attempt to trap the air in the right atrium, where it can be aspirated with an intracardiac needle.

Catheter-Related Infection

Catheter-related infection is a serious complication of central venous catheters. The majority of steps taken in maintenance of the I.V. system and site are performed to prevent I.V.-related sepsis.

Whenever a patient with a central venous catheter has an unexpected fever spike, I.V.-related sepsis must be suspected. The insertion site should be carefully inspected for any signs of infection. A blood culture drawn through the catheter may be ordered. To rule out all sources of contamination, all tubings and containers should be changed immediately and sent promptly to bacteriology for culturing. A complete "fever work-up" must be done to rule out any other obvious source of infection. If the fever remains and no other possible source can be established, catheter removal may be necessary [10].

Some practitioners perform a catheter exchange with a guide wire. If the blood culture is positive or the semiquantitative culture of the catheter tip yields 15 or more colonies, the new catheter is removed and the patient is considered to have catheter sepsis. If both cultures are negative, then the catheter can be used despite the fever. If septic shock, shaking chills, recent positive blood cultures for staphylococcus or Candida, or if local infection of the catheter entry site is present, the catheter must be removed immediately [11].

Of primary importance in the prevention of I.V.-related infection is maintaining strict aseptic techniques during insertion, admixture, any line manipulations, and aseptically performing recommended site dressing and tubing changes.

Deep-Vein Thrombosis

Deep-vein thrombosis is not as common with the new catheter materials. The addition of 1,000 units of heparin per liter of infusate has been recommended as a preventive measure [11]. Thrombosis may be present without any symptoms. Arm and neck pain may suggest the diagnosis. A venogram may be necessary to establish the diagnosis. Signs and symptoms of pulmonary embolism in a patient with a central venous catheter strongly suggests deep-vein thrombosis. Treatment consists of thrombolytic therapy with streptokinase or urokinase [11].

Thrombus Catheter Occlusion

Thrombus catheter occlusion used to be a frequent cause for catheter removal. A fibrin sheath forms over the catheter tip. This may result in only a withdrawal occlusion. In this case it is impossible to withdraw a blood sample, but there is no difficulty with infusion. If there is little or no infusion flow, the patency of the catheter can be restored with the use of a thrombolytic agent. Small-dose vials are available for the declotting procedure.

Preparing the Solution
Urokinase 5,000 I.U. is packaged in a 2-chamber vial. The following steps are used to prepare the solution:

1. Remove protective cap and turn plunger-stopper a quarter turn, press to force diluent into lower chamber.
2. Roll and tilt to dissolve, avoid shaking solution.
3. Sterilize stopper top with alcohol.
4. Insert needle through the center of stopper until tip is barely visible. Invert vial and withdraw dose.

Declotting the Catheter
Catheter declotting, with urokinase, may be achieved by the following steps [12, 13]:

1. Using air embolism precautions, aseptically disconnect the I.V. tubing at the catheter hub and attach an empty 10 ml syringe.

2. Gently attempt to aspirate blood. If aspiration is not possible remove the syringe.
3. Attach 1 ml tuberculin syringe filled with prepared urokinase.
4. Slowly and gently inject amount equal to volume of catheter.
5. Remove syringe and connect empty 5 ml syringe.
6. Wait at least 5 minutes before attempting to aspirate drug and residual clot.
7. Repeat aspiration attempts every 5 minutes.
8. If the catheter cannot be opened within 30 minutes, cap the catheter and allow drug to remain for 30–60 minutes.
9. A second urokinase injection may be required.
10. When patency is restored, aspirate 4–5 ml blood to assure removal of all drug and clot residual.
11. Remove blood-filled syringe and connect 10 ml syringe with 0.9% sodium chloride and gently flush to assure patency.
12. Remove syringe and aseptically reconnect sterile I.V. tubing to catheter hub.

CARE AND MAINTENANCE OF CENTRAL VENOUS CATHETER LINES

The risks of postinsertion complications from a central venous catheter are directly related to the care and maintenance of the system. Established protocols primarily address the prevention of catheter clotting and 2 life-threatening complications, catheter-related sepsis and air embolism. To minimize these complications, in some institutions the I.V. therapy team is responsible for insertions of peripheral and external jugular central catheters, assisting the physician with internal jugular and subclavian catheter insertions, as well as performing all tubing and dressing changes, catheter flushing, and drawing blood specimens from central catheters. A small group of highly dedicated nurses can rigidly maintain aseptic technique and follow all protocols essential for minimizing complications.

Electronic Control Instruments

Consideration should be given to the use of an electronic control instrument to maintain flow accuracy and catheter patency. A clotted central catheter can result in delay of prescribed medications and the need for catheter replacement with all its inherent risks.

When a positive-pressure instrument is used the pressure must not be greater than that which is recommended for the particular catheter and/or any device being used.

Catheter Clamp

A smooth-blade catheter clamp is used with tunneled silicone catheters to prevent air embolism or an inadvertent bleed whenever the catheter is opened to the air. A grooved-blade clamp should never be used, for catheter damage could result. The clamp should be applied to the distal two-thirds portion of the external catheter. If clamp damage should occur, catheter repair is easier in this area. Clamp sites should be alternated to prevent a weakened area on the catheter.

There are many types and styles of clamp available. If the clamp is to be used by a patient, it is important that the patient can easily open and close it. Some clip-type clamps are difficult to work with because they require great hand strength and thus would not be appropriate for an elderly patient. The clamp should be with the patient at all times. If the catheter should break, the clamp should be immediately applied proximal to the rupture point. Immediate medical assistance is required to repair the catheter before occlusion occurs.

Catheter Repair

A sterile repair kit, specific to the individual type of catheter, should be readily available. Repairing the external portion of a tunneled catheter is a sterile procedure requiring surgical gloves, mask, and cap. It may be performed by the following steps [14].

Equipment

Sterile repair kit containing (1) replacement silicone rubber segment with Luer-lock connector, (2) silicone rubber splice sleeve, (3) splice segment, (4) Luer-lock cap, (5) tube of medical adhesive, and (6) blunt 18-gauge needle.

- Sterile drapes
- 3 cc syringe
- 4 × 4 inch sterile sponges
- Small beaker for alcohol
- Scalpel blades
- Iris scissors
- Guarded hemostat
- Tongue blade
- Povidone-iodine solution
- Alcohol
- Heparin flush
- Tape

Procedure

1. Surgically prep catheter and create sterile field.
2. Clean powder from gloves with 4 × 4 inch sponge and alcohol.
3. Load adhesive into syringe barrel, then insert plunger and attach blunted needle.
4. If catheter is not clamped, clamp with guarded hemostat near chest wall.
5. Cut off the existing damaged catheter 15–20 cm from chest wall (Figure 18.4A).

Chapter 18 | Central Venous Catheterization

6. Insert splice segment into lumen of catheter (lubricate with alcohol if necessary, but be sure all alcohol is removed or evaporated before proceeding).

7. Trim repair segment to desired length and slip onto the splice segment protruding from the implanted catheter. Do not remove the larger splice sleeve loose mounted on the repair segment.

8. Inject adhesive on the outside of the tubing in the area of the splice segment and slide the larger splice sleeve over the area of the splice segment. Inject adhesive underneath each end of splice sleeve (Figure 18.4B). Roll between fingers to extrude excess adhesive and wipe excess adhesive away.

9. A sterile field is no longer required. Splint the repaired joint by taping the area to a tongue blade (Figure 18.4C).

10. Remove clamp and *gently* flush with heparin. Excessive pressure may rupture joint.

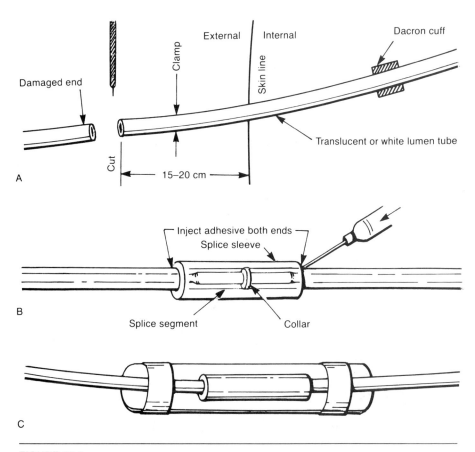

FIGURE 18.4
(A) The damaged catheter is cut off 15–20 cm from the chest wall. (B) Adhesive is injected underneath each end of splice sleeve. (C) The repaired joint is splinted by taping the area to a tongue blade. Courtesy Davol, Inc., Cranston, R.I.

320 Part VI | Specific Applications

The catheter may be used for infusion after a few hours. The splint may be removed after 48 hours, when the joint will have achieved full mechanical strength.

0.22 Micron Air-Eliminating Filter

Taping a Luer lock air-eliminating filter directly to the catheter hub will reduce the risk of connection separation and air infusion which could result in a fatal emobolism [18]. If a separation occurs distal to the filter, this device will prevent air infusion and an inadvertent bleed. The 0.22 micron filter can also prevent any particulate matter, fungi, bacteria, and endotoxins from entering the system through the filter.

I.V. Containers and Admixtures

All recommendations for peripheral containers or admixtures should be strictly adhered to for central catheter usage. To prevent risks of contamination, all manipulation for admixture and container changes must be performed with strict adherence to aseptic technique. All containers must be changed at least every 24 hours and fat emulsions should not hang longer than 12 hours [1, 17].

If an air-eliminating filter is not used, a closed non-air dependent container will reduce the risk of air embolism when the container totally empties.

Tubing Changes

All tubings should be aseptically changed every 24–48 hours [1, 7]. It is extremely important to remember that there is always the possibility of negative pressure with a central catheter. Therefore, the risk of an air embolism is always present when the catheter is open to the air. If the patient cannot perform the Valsalva maneuver, consideration should be given to the use of an extension tubing with a clamp which can be closed during the tubing change. Many practitioners use this system especially for critically ill patients. Care must be taken to maintain the sterility of the extension tubing during each I.V. tubing change. The extension tubing is changed at least weekly.

Between changes of components the system should be maintained as a

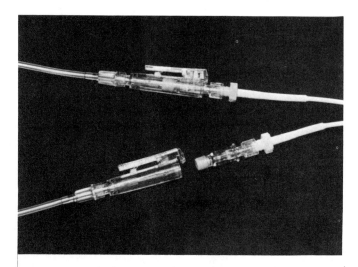

FIGURE 18.5
Needle-locking device, Click Lock®.
Courtesy ICU Medical, Inc., Huntington Beach, Calif.

closed system as much as possible. All entries into the system should be made through injection ports which have been disinfected just before entry [1].

Looping the tubing and taping it to the chest wall will prevent any relayed stress to the connection or insertion site when the tubing is pulled or stretched. To prevent separations of any additional lines, all secondary and piggyback connections should be Luer locked or locked with special needle-locking devices and taped (Figure 18.5).

REFERENCES

1. Center for Disease Control. *Guidelines for the Prevention and Control of Nosocomial Infections*. Atlanta, 1983.
2. Gray, H. *Anatomy, Descriptive and Surgical*. (Revised American edition from the 15th English edition). New York: Crown, 1977.
3. Metheny, N. M., and Snively, W. D., Jr. *Nurses' Handbook of Fluid Balance* (4th ed.). Philadelphia: Lippincott, 1983, pp. 182–184.
4. Russell, M. V., and Maier, W. P. The ABCs of C.V.P. measurement. *R.N.* 32:34, 1969.
5. Neave, L. C. The use of Intrasil catheters in long-term phlebotomy patients. *J. NITA* 6:423–425, 1983.
6. Ryan, G. M., and Howland, W. S. An evaluation of central venous pressure monitoring. *Anesth. Analg.* 45:754–759, 1966.
7. National Intravenous Therapy Association, Inc. Nursing standards of practice. *J. NITA* 5:19–34, 1982.
8. Maki, D. G., and Band, J. D. A comparative study of polyantibiotic and iodophor ointments in prevention of vascular-catheter-related infection. *Am. J. Med.* 70:739–744, 1981.
9. Coppa, G. F., Gouge, T. H., et al. Air embolism: A lethal but preventable complication of subclavian vein catheterization. *J.P.E.N.* 5:166–168, 1981.
10. Bower, R. H. A logical approach to catheter sepsis. Presented at the 9th Annual NITA Convention, Boston, March, 1981.
11. Ryan, J. A. Jr., and Gough, J. A. Complications of central venous catheterization for total parenteral nutrition: The role of the nurse. *J. NITA* 7:29–35, 1984.
12. Abbott Laboratories. *Abbokinase™ Open-Cath Instruction Booklet*. Chicago, 1984.
13. Lawson, M., Bottino, J. C., et al. The use of urokinase to restore the patency of occluded central venous catheters. *Am. J. I.V. Ther. Clin. Nutr.* 9:29–30, 32–43, 1982.
14. Evermed. *Repair Kit for Hickman Right Atrial Catheter Instruction Sheet*. Medina, Wash.

BIBLIOGRAPHY

Bradham, G. B., and Walsh, N. Silastic for intravenous intubation. *J.S.L. Med. Assoc.* 61:165, 1965.
Brendel, V. Current concepts in the care of central line catheters. *J. NITA* 6:272–274, 1983.
Gilligan, J. E., Phillips, P. J., et al. Streptokinase and blocked central venous catheter. *Lancet* 2:1189, 1979.
Hoshal, V. L. Jr., Ause, R. G., et al. Fibrin sleeve formation on indwelling subclavian central venous catheters. *Arch. Surg.* 102:353–358, 1971.
Hurtubise, M. R., Lawson, M., et al. Restoring patency of occluded central venous catheters. *Arch. Surg.* 115:212–213, 1980.

Lindblad, B. Thromboembolic complications and central venous catheters (letter). *Lancet* 2:936, 1982.

Maki, D. G., Weise, C. E., et al. A semiquantitative culture method for identifying intravenous-catheter-related infection. *N. Engl. J. Med.* 296:1305–1309, 1977.

Mansell, C. W. Peripherally inserted central venous catheterization by I.V. nurses: Establishing a precedent. *J. NITA* 6:355–356, 1983.

Nursing Photobook. *Managing I.V. Therapy.* Horsham, Pa.: Intermed Communications, Inc., 1980.

Ostrow, L. S. Air embolism and central venous lines. *Am. J. Nurs.* 81:2036, 1981.

Peters, W. R., Bush, W. H., et al. The development of fibrin sheath on indwelling venous catheters. *Surg. Gynecol. Obstet.* 137:43–47, 1973.

Rubin, R. N. Local installation of small doses of streptokinase for treatment of thrombotic occlusions of long-term access catheters. *J. Clin. Oncol.* 1:572, 1983.

Sriram, K., Kaminski, M. V., et al. A safe technique of central venous catheterization. *J.P.E.N.* 6:245–248, 1982.

Stephens, W., and Lawler, W. Thrombus formation and central venous catheters. *Lancet* 2:664, 1982.

REVIEW QUESTIONS

1. Where is the ideal location for the tip of a central venous catheter?
2. When measuring central venous pressure, zero point on the manometer is adjusted to the level of _____ .
3. During the insertion of a central venous catheter, the patient is placed in Trendelenburg's position to _____ and _____ .
4. Which vein is usually the first choice for peripheral insertion of a central venous catheter?
5. What test is always ordered after the insertion of a central venous catheter?
6. The Valsalva maneuver is used to minimize the risk of _____ .
7. What is the immediate treatment for an air embolism?
8. If the semiquantitative culture of a catheter tip yields _____ colonies, the patient is considered to have catheter-related sepsis.
9. What precaution should be taken when using a positive-pressure electronic instrument with a central venous catheter?
10. What complication will be reduced by taping a Luer locked air-eliminating filter to a central venous catheter?
11. A regular, standardized site inspection, disinfection, and dressing change should minimize _____ .

CHAPTER 19

Central Venous Catheters

Faye Cosentino

CATHETER MATERIALS

The ideal material for a central venous catheter would inhibit thrombus formation, be easily insertable, and be radiopaque.

Deep-Vein Thrombosis

Deep-vein thrombosis from central venous catheters has many contributing factors. Any foreign material in the bloodstream becomes coated with a protein and fibrin deposit. Internal coagulation is activated, causing platelet activation, and platelets adhere to the catheter. Damage to endothelial cells at the puncture site enhances platelet activation. Patients requiring central venous catheters often have activated coagulation systems due to trauma or severe disease; both conditions also promote the development of central venous catheter thrombosis. Thrombosis may be limited to a fibrin sheath formation or may be severe enough to cause vein occlusion. It may have no clinical significance or it may result in a fatal pulmonary embolism [1].

The majority of central venous catheters are made of polyvinyl chloride, Teflon,* polyurethane, or silicone.

Polyvinyl Chloride
Polyvinyl chloride was the first catheter material. High incidences of thrombosis have been associated with this material [2]. Today, most central venous catheters are made of less thrombogenic materials.

Teflon
Teflon catheters are easily inserted because they are relatively stiff. However, they are reported to have high incidences of thrombus formation [2].

---

*DuPont.

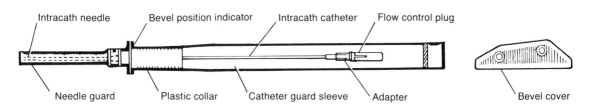

FIGURE 19.1
Components of an inside-the-needle catheter (INC). Intracath™. Courtesy Deseret Medical, Inc., Sandy, Utah.

Polyurethane
Polyurethane is only moderately firm, so it is not as easily inserted. Thrombus formation is reported to be less than with Teflon. *Hydromer-coated polyurethane* catheters have reports of low thrombus formation [3].

Silicone
Silicone catheters are very soft, much like a wet noodle, so they require special mechanisms for insertion. They are reported to have the lowest incidences of thrombus formation [14].

Radiopaque Catheters
Radiopaque catheters are available in all materials. This property is required to affirm catheter tip placement postinsertion.

CATHETER DESIGNS

The design of the device is frequently related to the properties of the catheter material. The design also dictates insertion methods.

Inside-the-Needle Catheter (INC)

The inside-the-needle catheter (INC), the first central catheter device, is often made of Vialon* (a polyurethane) or polyvinyl chloride (PVC).

Device Components
The unit consists of a stainless steel needle attached to a plastic sheath containing a catheter with or without a stylet, and needle tip cover (Figure 19.1).

Insertion Technique
The venipuncture is performed with the stainless steel needle (Figure 19.2A). The catheter is advanced through the needle (Figure 19.2B). The needle is drawn back over the catheter (Figure 19.2C), and its tip protected with a cover (Figure 19.2D).

---

*Deseret Medical, Inc.

Chapter 19 | Central Venous Catheters

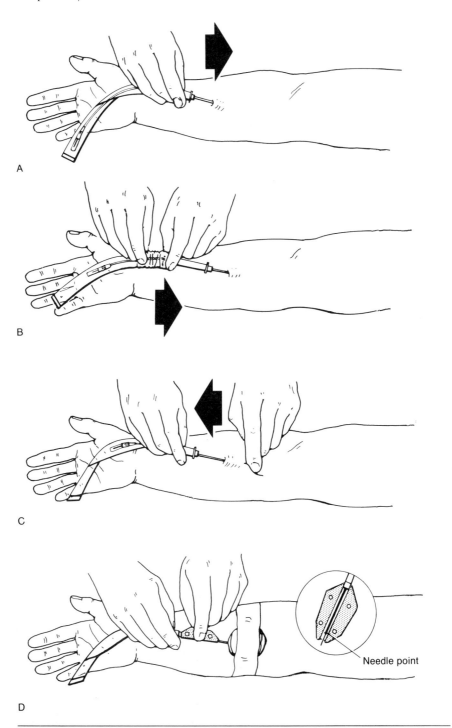

FIGURE 19.2
(A) Venipuncture is performed with the stainless steel needle. (B) The catheter is advanced through the needle. (C) The needle is withdrawn over the catheter. (D) The needle tip is protected with the cover. Courtesy Deseret Medical, Inc., Sandy, Utah.

Part VI | Specific Applications

Device Features

Because of its stiffness, the catheter is easy to insert a short distance into the vein. When attempting to thread a long catheter, difficulty may be encountered due to the stiffness. If this occurs, the stylet (if present) can be partially withdrawn to soften the catheter. A smooth insertion requires a vein without sharp twists or curves. The INC is always a single-lumen catheter. If not used according to manufacturer's instructions, this device has a high risk of catheter embolism. During insertion the catheter must NEVER be drawn back through the needle. The sharp needle can easily sever the catheter with a resultant embolism. Because the sharp needle must remain over the catheter, there is always the risk of catheter severance if manufacturer's instructions as to needle point protection are not followed. The catheter material, for the illustrated model, is polyurethane. This is less thrombogenic than either Teflon or PVC catheters of this design. The INC is an excellent *short-term* inpatient central venous catheter. It was not designed for long-term or home care usage.

Catheter with Removable Introducer

Catheters with removable introducers are frequently made of polyurethane.

Device Components

The unit consists of an introducer catheter or syringe and needle, and a catheter with stylet (Figure 19.3).

Insertion Technique

The venipuncture is performed with the needle and syringe (Figure 19.4A). The syringe is removed and the catheter threaded through the needle (Figure 19.4B). The needle is withdrawn from the vein and removed from the catheter by splitting into two parts (Figure 19.4C).

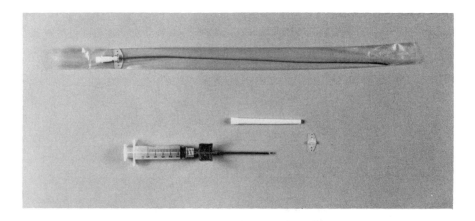

FIGURE 19.3
Components of an introducer cannula and catheter with stylet. L-Cath®. Courtesy Luther Medical Products, Inc., Santa Ana, Calif.

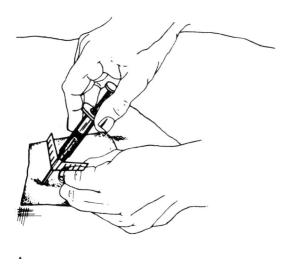
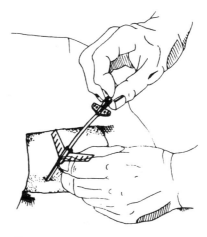
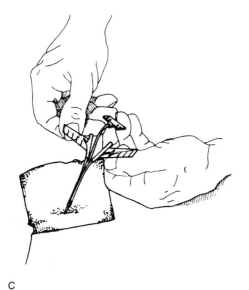

FIGURE 19.4
(A) Venipuncture is performed with the introducer needle and syringe. (B) The syringe is removed and the catheter threaded through the needle. (C) The needle is withdrawn from the vein and removed from the catheter by splitting into two parts. Courtesy Luther Medical Products, Inc., Santa, Ana, Calif.

Device Features

A catheter with a removable introducer is a single-lumen catheter with a fairly easy method of insertion. Because the device is usually made of polyurethane it is softer than Teflon and easier to thread through twists and curves. Removal of any sharp needle eliminates the risk of catheter embolism. Because thrombus formation can be a problem with polyurethane, this may not be the catheter of choice for long-term therapy. However, minimal thrombus formation has been reported with hydromer-coated polyurethane and long-term usage.

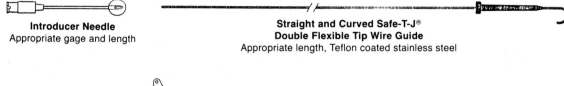

Introducer Needle
Appropriate gage and length

Straight and Curved Safe-T-J®
Double Flexible Tip Wire Guide
Appropriate length, Teflon coated stainless steel

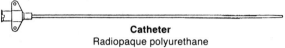

Catheter
Radiopaque polyurethane

FIGURE 19.5
Components of a catheter with introducer and guide wire. Courtesy Cook Critical Care, Bloomington, Ind.

Catheter with Introducer and Guide Wire

A catheter with an introducer and guide wire allows for the insertion of a multiple-lumen silicone catheter.

Device Components
The unit consists of a syringe and needle or an over-the-needle catheter (ONC), long central catheter, and a guide wire (Figure 19.5).

Insertion Technique
The venipuncture is performed with the syringe and needle or ONC. The syringe or stylet is removed. The guide wire is threaded through the short catheter or needle (Figure 19.6A), and the short catheter or needle is withdrawn (Figure 19.6B). The puncture site may be enlarged with a number 11 scalpel blade (Figure 19.6C). The long catheter is threaded over the guide wire (Figure 19.6D), and the guide wire withdrawn, leaving the long catheter in the vein (Figure 19.6E).

Device Features
The silicone catheter has the lowest reports of thrombus formation. The design of the device allows for multiple-lumen catheter placement. It requires a fairly complex method of insertion with a large amount of "in-and-out" manipulation in the vein. The silicone catheter is an excellent *long-term* central catheter for both inpatient and home care usage.

Catheter on a Spool

A catheter on a spool is made of silicone elastomer. It is a single-lumen catheter.

Device Components
The unit consists of a catheter coiled in a spool which has a slotted needle attachment (Figure 19.7).

Insertion Technique
After venipuncture with the slotted needle (Figure 19.8A), the spool is turned until the desired length of catheter has been threaded into the vein (Figure 19.8B). The spool is opened (Figure 19.8C) and the needle removed from the vein and the catheter (Figure 19.8D).

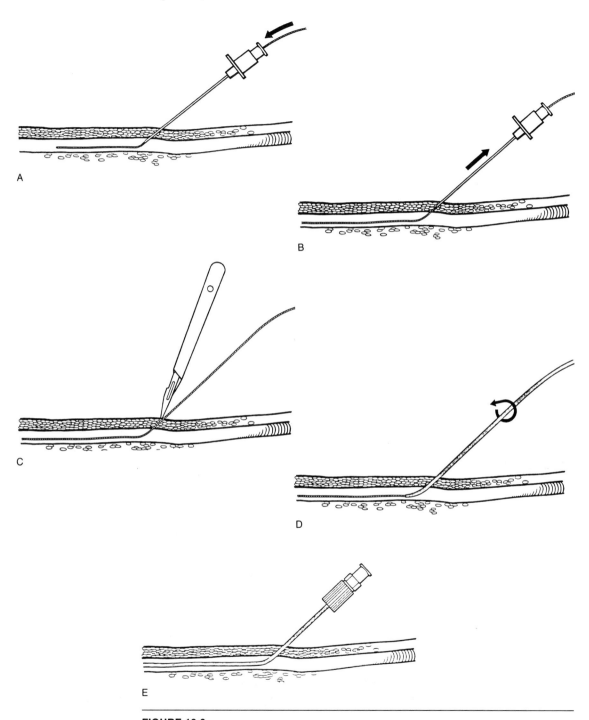

FIGURE 19.6
(A) The guide wire is threaded through the inserted needle. (B) The needle is withdrawn from the vein. (C) The puncture site may be enlarged with a no. 11 scalpel blade. (D) The catheter is threaded over the guide wire. (E) The guide wire is withdrawn, leaving the catheter in the vein. Courtesy Cook Critical Care, Bloomington, Ind.

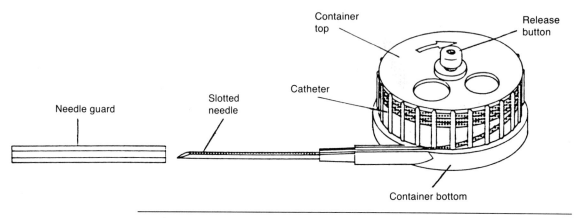

FIGURE 19.7
Components of a catheter on a spool. Intracil® © Copyright 1985 Travenol Laboratories, Inc. Reproduced with permission of Travenol Laboratories, Inc., Deerfield, Ill.

Device Features
The insertion is fairly complex but does not require a lot of "in-and-out" manipulation in the vein. Because this catheter is silicone elastomer, very low thrombus formation has been reported. Many nurse practitioners insert this device peripherally. It provides a long-term central venous catheter without the risks or costs of a subclavian insertion. This is an excellent *long-term* catheter for both inpatients and home patients.

Indwelling Tunneled Catheter

The indwelling tunneled catheter is made of polymeric silicone.

Device Components
This single- or double-lumen catheter contains a Dacron cuff. The external end has a "ring" with a threaded Luer lock adapter covered with a Luer lock cap. An integral clamp may be present (Figure 19.9). One version of this catheter has a closed tip and a lateral two-way valve. The valve opens outward for infusion and inward for blood sample drawing. This model does not require heparin flush to maintain catheter patency (Figure 19.10).

Insertion Technique
The insertion may be performed by cutdown or percutaneous puncture. This is performed under fluoroscopy, usually in a minor surgery operating room.
   Placement of the catheter is achieved by locating the subclavian vein, forming a tunnel from the vein to an area between the sternum and the nipple, pulling the catheter through the tunnel, inserting it into the vein and threading the catheter until the tip is in the superior vena cava (Figure 19.11).

Catheter Features
Fibrous tissue forms around the Dacron cuff. The cuff and tunnel anchor the catheter and help prevent infection. Because the material is polymeric silicone, this catheter has reports of low thrombus formation. It is a perfect central

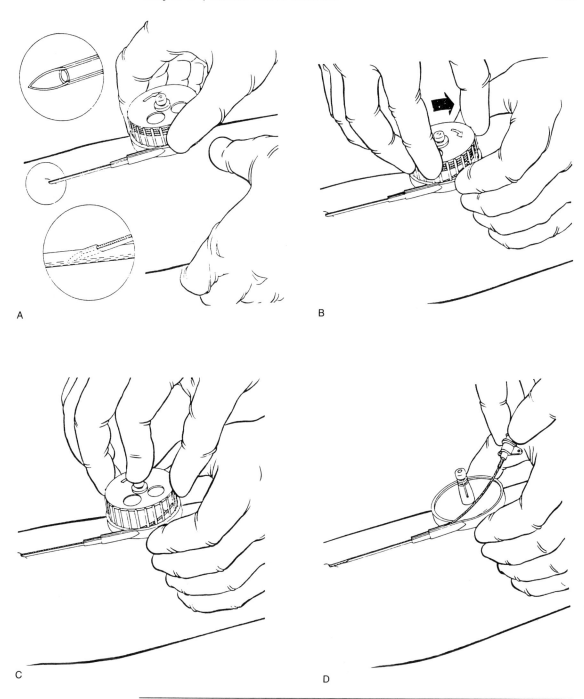

FIGURE 19.8
(A) Venipuncture is performed with the slotted needle. (B) The spool is turned until the desired length of catheter has been threaded into the vein. (C) The spool is opened by pushing the button on top of the device. (D) The needle and spool unit are removed from the vein and catheter. Reproduced with permission of Travenol Laboratories, Inc., Deerfield, Ill.

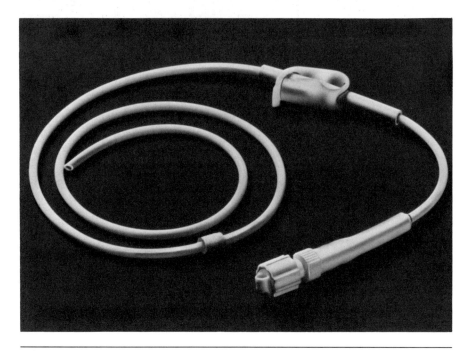

FIGURE 19.9
Indwelling tunneled catheter with integral clamp. CorCath™ Cormed, Inc., Medina, N.Y.

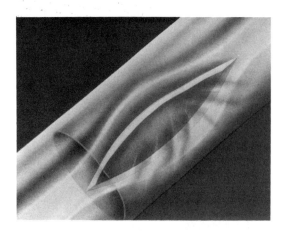 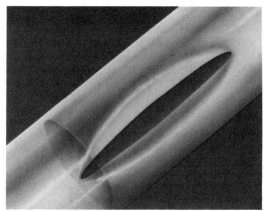

FIGURE 19.10
Indwelling tunneled catheter with a closed tip and two-way valve. Groshong™ Catheter Technology Corp., Salt Lake City, Utah.

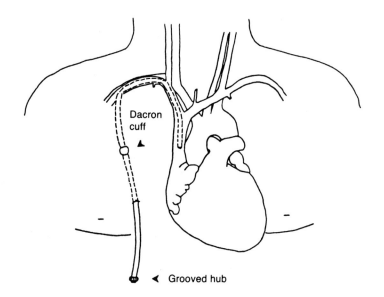

FIGURE 19.11
A tunnel is formed from the vein to an area between the sternum and the nipple. The catheter tip is placed in the superior vena cava.

venous catheter for home I.V. therapy. This catheter is also inserted for long-term inpatient use.

Totally Implanted Venous Access Device

Totally implanted devices for repeated venous access eliminate the need for frequent venipunctures.

Device Components
The unit consists of a silicone catheter attached to a reservoir with a self-sealing septum. At the present time there are four manufacturers of this device (Figures 19.12–19.15). Units are available with single or double lumens. Special noncoring needles are required to use these devices.

Insertion Technique
The unit is surgically placed under local or general anesthesia. The insertion technique is similar to that used for implanted tunneled catheters. The catheter is placed in the subclavian vein and threaded into the vein until the tip lies in the superior vena cava. This position is confirmed by fluoroscopy. A pocket is made for the reservoir (Figure 19.16A). The reservoir is sutured in the pocket. As the center of the port will be punctured repeatedly, when the pocket is closed the suture line is lateral, medial, superior, or inferior to the port septum (Figure 19.16B).

Device Features
This device has reports of low thrombus formation due to the silicone catheter. When not in use, the only care required is a monthly heparin flush. The fact that this is totally implanted, leaving no catheter exiting from the chest, makes it a favorite device with many patients. It is an "artificial vein" perfect for any

334 Part VI | Specific Applications

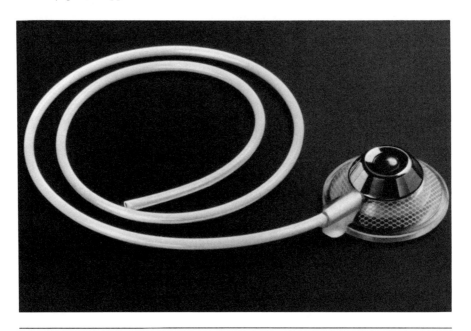

FIGURE 19.12
Med-I-Port™. Cormed, Inc., Medina, N.Y.

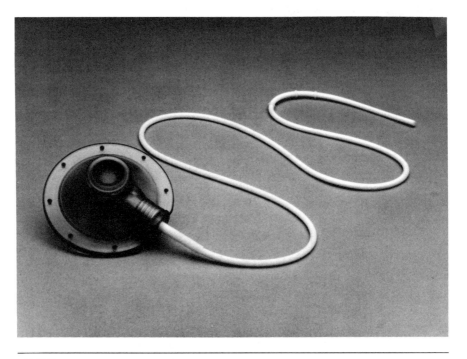

FIGURE 19.13
Infuse-A-Port™. Intermedics Infusaid, Inc., Norwood, Mass.

Chapter 19 | Central Venous Catheters

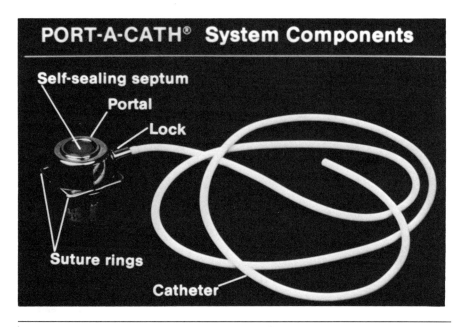

FIGURE 19.14
Port-A-Cath™. Pharmacia Laboratories, Piscataway, N.J.

patient receiving *long-term periodic* infusion therapy, in the home or in the hospital.

Totally Implanted Pump

Totally implanted pumps are designed for continuous, low-volume, long-term ambulatory therapy. It may be used for arterial or venous infusion and tissue perfusion.

Device Components
The device consists of two chambers separated by flexible metal bellows. One chamber is the drug reservoir, the other contains the charging fluid in a completely sealed compartment. The vapor pressure of the charging fluid exerts a constant pressure on the bellows, forcing the drug out of the reservoir through an outlet filter and flow restrictor into a silicone catheter (Figure 19.17). When the pump is refilled, the increasing pressure within the drug chamber exerts a pressure on the charging fluid, causing the fluid vapor to condense to its liquid state, thereby storing energy for the next pumping cycle.

Various models are available. The basic device has one catheter (Figure 19.18A). One model also has a direct access port that bypasses the reservoir for administering bolus injections. Another model has double catheters (Figure 19.18B). This can be used to administer a drug to more than one site.

Insertion Technique
The pump is implanted in the operating room under fluroscopy. To activate the charging fluid, the pump must be heated for 30 minutes at 30–40°C prior to implantation. This is done with a heating pad. The insertion technique is

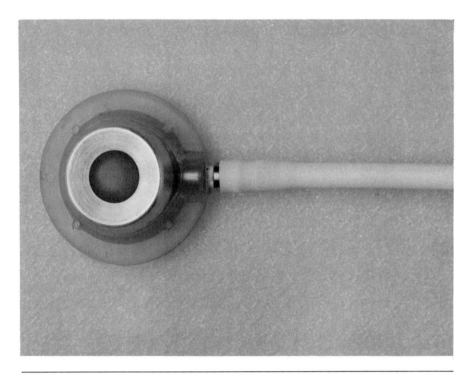

FIGURE 19.15
Chemo-Port®. HDC Corp., Mountain View, Calif.

the same as for the implanted venous access. The pocket is frequently located below the umbilicus on the abdomen.

Device Features
Several factors will influence the pump flow rate. If the catheter site is arterial and *arterial blood pressure increases significantly,* the flow rate can decrease by as much as 15 percent. *Hypotension* can increase the rate by as much as 6 percent. When the patient moves from one *altitude* to another, the rate can increase by as much as 38 percent. *Fever* can increase flow rate by as much as 13 percent. The *amount of drug in the reservoir* will affect the flow rate. The pump flow rate is established with the reservoir half full. At full volume the rate will be approximately 3 percent faster and at low volume 3 percent slower than the mean flow rate [5].

The silicone catheter results in low thrombus formation. This is an excellent method for *continuous long-term administration* of *low-volume* narcotics or chemotherapeutic agents on cancer patients. As there are no external parts, it requires no care between port refills.

Contraindications
Contraindications for the implanted pump include:

1. All but very small volumes of drugs.

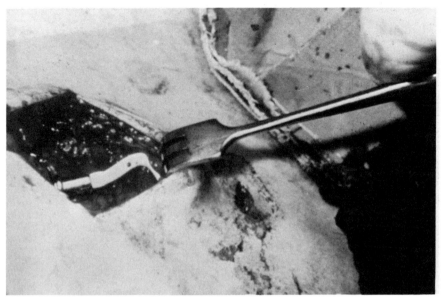

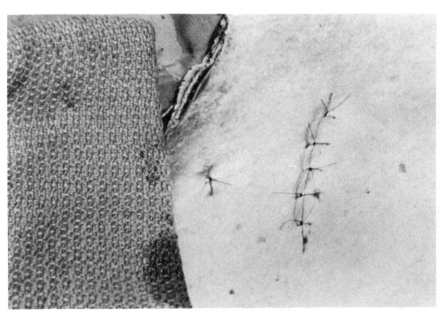

FIGURE 19.16
(A) A pocket is made for the reservoir. (B) All components are completely under the skin. The suture line is away from the entry point of the septum. Courtesy Pharmacia Laboratories, Piscataway, N.J.

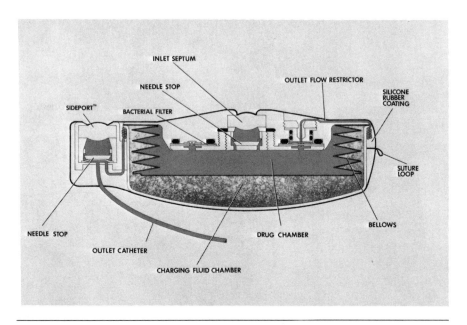

FIGURE 19.17
Components of the implanted pump. Infusaid™. Courtesy Intermedics Infusaid, Inc., Norwood, Mass.

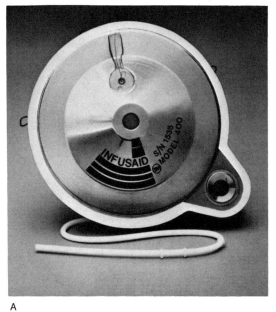
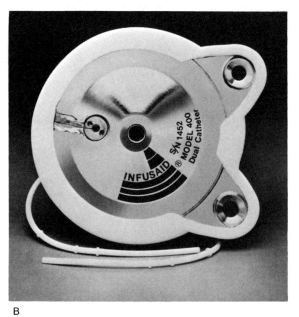

FIGURE 19.18
(A) Basic model Infusaid™ pump. (B) Infusaid™ pump with two catheters. Courtesy Intermedics Infusaid, Inc., Norwood, Mass.

Chapter 19 | Central Venous Catheters

2. A body size not large enough for the size and weight of the pump.
3. Patients with severe emotional, psychiatric, or neurological disturbances.
4. Patients who travel extensively or frequently and experience altitudinal changes [5].

CATHETER SITE CARE

A regular, standardized site inspection, disinfection, and dressing change should minimize catheter-related sepsis. Catheter site care and dressing change should be performed every 48–72 hours. If the dressing becomes wet, soiled, or loose, it should be changed immediately. Aseptic technique must be maintained during the procedure [16].

Nontunneled Catheter

There are many acceptable variations for performing site care and changing central venous catheter dressings. However, they are all based on the same principles. On a routine basis the old dressing must be removed; both site and catheter carefully inspected, cleaned, and disinfected; an antimicrobial ointment applied; and an occlusive dressing secured. The person performing the care thoroughly washes the hands and wears sterile gloves and a mask. If the patient cannot be masked, the face should be turned away from the dressing site.

Equipment
The use of a prepackaged dressing kit will assure the immediate availability of all required supplies. It will also help to assure that all persons performing the care are using a standard procedure.

Procedure

1. Prepare a clean table for a work area.
2. Prepare the patient in a comfortable position on the bed.
3. Put on the mask, wash hands thoroughly, and dry.
4. Carefully, remove old dressing. Removing the tape from the outside edges inward toward the center will prevent stress at the insertion site. The site should be carefully inspected for any signs of discharge or leakage. The catheter should be inspected to assure (a) that the sutures are intact; (b) that the length of the external portion has not increased, (c) that any needle protective cover is in place and locked, and (d) that the catheter and hub are intact.

    If the hands should become contaminated during the dressing removal, they must be rewashed. If the procedure is performed with two pairs of gloves, the first pair are worn to remove the old dressing.
5. Open kit. The overlay will provide a sterile field.
6. Put on the sterile gloves.

7. The site and the portion of the catheter close to the site should be cleansed of all debris. Polyurethane and silicone catheters should not come in contact with 100% acetone, which could weaken the material and cause possible leakage. Concentrated acetone may also cause skin irritation which can increase the risk of infection. Some practitioners use a combination of dilute acetone and alcohol for cleansing purposes. Hydrogen peroxide has become very popular for this step of the procedure. The cleansing is performed in a circular fashion, starting at the center and working outward. The cleansing agent must be allowed to dry before the disinfection is started.
8. Disinfection may be done with (a) 1% or 2% tincture of iodine followed by a complete removal with alcohol, or (b) povidone-iodine solution. Povidone-iodine must not be removed with alcohol. The skin prep is applied in the circular method as described for cleansing (Figure 19.19A). The nurse must not forget to disinfect the portion of the catheter that is close to the insertion site. Allow the agent to dry.
9. Apply antimicrobial ointment sparingly directly to the insertion site (Figure 19.19B). Povidone-iodine is recommended for central catheter sites [17].
10. Placing a sterile 2 × 2 inch sponge directly over the ointment will assure that the ointment stays at the site (Figure 19.19C). A sterile sponge may be placed under the catheter and hub for patient comfort.
11. If the tape used causes skin damage, tincture of benzoin may be used to protect the exposed skin. Be sure that it dries before applying the tape.
12. An adhesive cover is applied to maintain an occlusive dressing. There are several types available. Sterile elastic or foam adhesive bandage, or transparent tape are frequently used. The sterile tape is placed directly over the site with the catheter exiting from the bottom of the tape. This position is important to prevent stress at the catheter hub–tubing connection when the patient moves. Be sure this connection is outside the tape to facilitate tubing changes.
13. The catheter hub–tubing connection is inspected to assure that it is locked and taped. The tubing is looped and taped to the chest wall to prevent stress at the connection or insertion site when the tubing is pulled or stretched.
14. The dressing change label is signed, dated, and applied to the dressing (Figure 19.19D).

Tunneled Catheters

The dressing change procedure may be modified for the tunneled catheter. If the patient is immunosuppressed or if site healing is not complete, the same care given to the nontunneled catheter may be used for this catheter. If the patient is not immunosuppressed and site healing is complete, site care may be limited to daily inspection and cleansing with soap and water while bathing.

Totally Implanted Devices

Totally implanted devices do not require any site care as the entire device is under the skin.

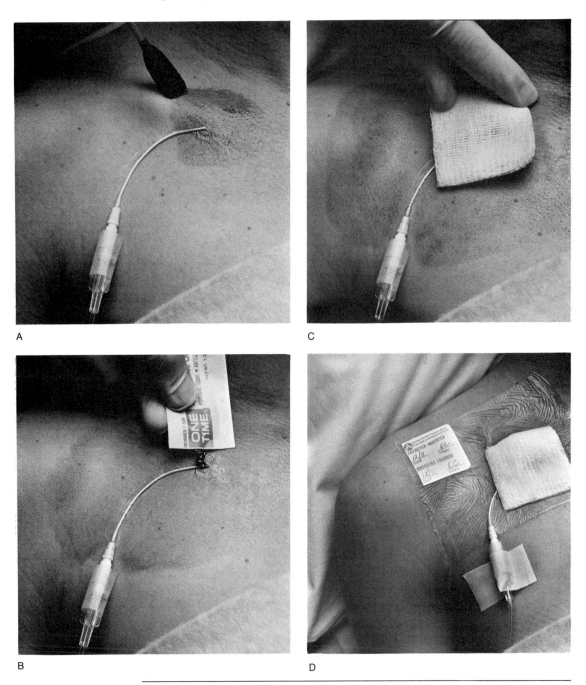

FIGURE 19.19
(A) The skin prep is applied in a circular fashion, starting at the site working outward. (B) Antimicrobial ointment may be applied to the site. (C) A sterile 2 × 2 inch sponge is placed over the ointment and site. (D) An adhesive cover is applied to maintain an occlusive dressing. The dressing change label is signed, dated and applied to the dressing. Courtesy Acme United Corp., Fairfield, Conn.

CATHETER MAINTENANCE AND OPERATION

Heparin Flush

After using the catheter and at routine intervals, flushing with heparin solution will maintain catheter patency. For tunneled or nontunneled catheters, the frequency and heparin strength varies considerably between institutions. Some authors believe too much is given too frequently [8–10]. The volume of heparin needs to be only slightly more than the volume of the catheter. Because the largest tunneled catheter contains less than 2 ml, 2.5–3 ml should be sufficient. Many practitioners have found that every-other-day flushes maintain catheter patency. The strength of heparin may depend upon the condition of the patient. Any patient with decreased coagulation factors may require only 100 units per milliliter. Patients with normal coagulation factors may require up to 1,000 units per milliliter. Both strengths are available in 2.5 ml or 3 ml prefilled syringes.

Prefilled Heparin Flush Syringe
Using a prefilled heparin syringe reduces the risk of touch contamination during preparation and ensures administration of the correct dosage of heparin.

Gauge and Length of Needles
Whenever injections are made into injection ports or intermittent injection caps, using a short-length needle prevents the risk of accidental puncture of the tubing or catheter. Small-gauge needles prevent large holes in the cap or injection port, which can result in fluid leakage or an entry point for air or bacteria.

Aids for Preventing Catheter Clotting
While injecting the heparin flush, the clamp is applied before the syringe is completely empty. The syringe and needle are removed while pressure is applied upon the plunger. This prevents reflux of blood into the lumen, which could result in catheter clotting.

When the catheter is not in use, taping the hub to the chest wall above heart level will minimize blood pressure at the catheter tip.

Discontinuing Infusion

When an infusion is completed, an injection cap and heparin flush are used to maintain catheter patency. A normal saline flush is given before the heparin to rinse the I.V. fluid from the catheter. If the catheter is of a material which cannot be clamped without possible damage and there is no extension tubing which can be clamped, the patient must perform the Valsalva maneuver at any time the catheter is open to the air.

The following steps may be used to discontinue the infusion, connect an injection cap, and flush with normal saline and heparin.

Equipment

Smooth blade catheter clamp (1)

Luer lock injection cap (1)

Chapter 19 | Central Venous Catheters

   10 cc syringe (1)
   22 gauge × 1 inch needle (1)
   Sodium chloride 0.9% 10 ml (1)
   Prefilled syringe with heparin flush (1)
   Povidone-iodine swab (3)
   Alcohol sponge (1)
   Sterile 2 × 2 inch sponge (1)
   Tape
   Sterile gloves 1 pr (optional)

Procedure

1. Wash hands thoroughly and dry.
2. Aseptically open all sterile supplies.
3. Prepare air-purged 10 ml 0.9% sodium chloride syringe with a 22G × 1 inch needle.
4. Prepare air-purged heparin flush.
5. Shut infusion off and clamp catheter.
6. Remove old tape from catheter filter–I.V. tubing connection.
7. Cleanse connection with povidone-iodine swab for 30 seconds.
8. Place connection on sterile 2 × 2 inch sponge and allow to dry.
9. If sterile gloves are worn, they may be used at this time. Pick up connection by holding catheter hub with the sterile sponge.
10. Aseptically disconnect and discard infusion tubing.
11. Aseptically connect and lock injection cap.
12. Remove clamp.
13. Cleanse rubber end of injection cap with povidone-iodine for 30 seconds. Allow to dry.
14. *Carefully* insert needle of syringe with normal saline flush into center of injection cap. Do not exert force. If an obstruction is felt, realign needle angle.
15. Inject normal saline flush (Figure 19.20).
16. While still holding catheter hub, remove empty syringe. Recleanse injection cap end with povidone-iodine for 30 seconds, allow to dry.
17. *Carefully* insert needle of heparin flush. Do not force insertion. If an obstruction is felt, realign needle angle.
18. Inject heparin flush. Before the syringe is completely empty, close catheter clamp.
19. Remove syringe and needle, applying pressure on plunger during withdrawal.
20. Remove clamp.

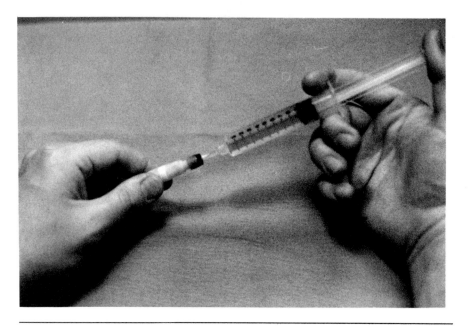

FIGURE 19.20
Injecting normal saline flush through intermittent injection cap.

21. Secure injection cap to catheter with a strip of tape.
22. Tape catheter hub on the chest wall above heart level.

Routine Heparin Flushing

Routine heparin flushing is required to maintain patency of unused catheters. If the catheter has more than one lumen, remember to flush each unused lumen.

The following steps may be used to perform heparin flush without changing the intermittent injection cap.

Equipment

Smooth-blade catheter clamp (1)
Prefilled syringe with heparin dosage (1)
Povidone-iodine swab (1)
Tape

Procedure

1. Wash hands thoroughly and dry.
2. Prepare air-purged heparin flush.
3. Remove tape holding end of catheter to chest wall.
4. Cleanse rubber end of injection cap with povidone-iodine for 30 seconds. Allow to dry.

Chapter 19 | Central Venous Catheters

5. While stabilizing the catheter hub, carefully insert needle of heparin flush syringe into center of cap. If an obstruction is felt, do not apply force but realign needle angle.
6. Gently inject heparin flush. Clamp the catheter before the syringe is completely empty.
7. Apply pressure on plunger while removing syringe and needle.
8. Remove clamp.
9. Tape catheter hub on chest wall above heart level.

Changing Intermittent Injection Cap

The injection cap must be changed at routine intervals. If the catheter is flushed every other day, cap changing may be coordinated with each third flushing (every 6 days). Using an intermittent injection cap which has a very small amount of dead space eliminates to need to preflush the cap. This minimizes the risk of touch contamination.

If the catheter contains more than one lumen, remember to change the caps on all unused lumens. If the catheter is made of a material which cannot be clamped without catheter damage, be sure that the patient is flat in bed and performs the Valsalva maneuver at any time the catheter is open to the air.

The following steps may be used to change the intermittent injection cap at the time of heparin flushing.

Equipment

Smooth-blade catheter clamp (1)
Prefilled syringe with heparin dosage (1)
Luer lock intermittent injection cap (1)
Sterile 2 × 2 inch sponge (1)
Povidone-iodine swabs (2)
Tape

Procedure

1. Wash hands thoroughly and dry.
2. Aseptically prepare sterile supplies.
3. Prepare air-purged heparin flush.
4. Remove tape holding catheter to chest wall. Remove tape securing cap to catheter.
5. Cleanse cap-catheter connection point with povidone-iodine for 30 seconds. Place on sterile sponge and allow to dry.
6. Close clamp.
7. Pick up catheter hub protected by sterile sponge. Be careful not to touch the cleansed connection.
8. *Carefully,* unlock, remove, and discard old cap.
9. Holding the new cap by the rubber injection end, connect and lock to catheter.

10. Secure connection with a strip of tape.
11. Remove clamp.
12. Cleanse rubber end of injection cap with povidone-iodine for 30 seconds. Allow to dry.
13. *Carefully* insert needle of heparin flush into center of rubber end. Do not force insertion. If an obstruction is felt, realign needle angle.
14. Gently inject heparin. Before the syringe is completely empty, close clamp.
15. Apply pressure on plunger while withdrawing syringe and needle.
16. Remove clamp.
17. Tape catheter hub on the chest wall above heart level.

Drawing Blood Specimens

Many central venous catheters are placed on patients without available peripheral veins, or on patients to minimize peripheral venipunctures. Therefore, drawing blood specimens through central catheters is common practice. There are basically 3 methods by which this can be done with tunneled and nontunneled catheters: (1) drawing specimens from continuous infusion line maintaining the closed system, (2) drawing specimens from continuous infusion line by opening the system, and (3) drawing specimens from catheter with in-place intermittent injection cap.

If the system does not have the possibility of catheter clamping, the patient must be placed flat in bed and perform the Valsalva maneuver whenever the catheter is open to the air. If this is not done, there always remains the possibility of air embolism.

PT and PTT Tests and Heparin

One must be aware that any blood specimen drawn through a central catheter that has been flushed with heparin, or that has heparin as a solution additive, should not be used for prothrombin time or partial prothrombin time testing. Heparin adheres to the catheter and can result in falsely elevated values for these tests.

Catheter Withdrawal Occlusion

The inability to withdraw blood through a central venous catheter even though infusion creates no difficulties is frequently encountered. It has been postulated that the formation of a fibrin sheath over the catheter tip allows infusion but inhibits blood withdrawal [11]. Having the patient cough, or move into various positions, may be helpful. Sometimes the problem will be intermittent; after an hour's wait blood specimens can be obtained without difficulty. At other times and on some patients it may continue to be impossible to withdraw blood through the central venous catheter. Flushing the catheter with normal saline prior to blood withdrawal appears to be helpful.

Patient Identification

Before drawing any blood specimens the patient must be accurately identified. This should be done by the patient's hospital identification band. Asking the patient to state his or her name may supplement but should never be substituted for some form of written identification on the patient.

Labeling Specimen Tubes
Before drawing the blood specimen, all tubes should be labeled with the patient's full name, room number, hospital identification number, and the initials of the person drawing the blood. This is done to prevent mislabeling which can result in inadequate or inappropriate treatment.

Drawing Blood Specimens from Continuous Infusion Line Maintaining a Closed System. This procedure requires an injection port between the filter and the catheter. It may be performed by the following steps.

Equipment

    Vacuum tube holder (1)

    Multiple draw needle 22G × 1 inch (1)

    Appropriate number and type vacuum tube(s) for tests

    0.9% sodium chloride 10 ml (2)

    10 cc syringe (2)

    Needles 22g × 1 inch (2)

    Povidone-iodine swab (3)

    Alcohol sponge (1)

Procedure

1. Put on gloves. Strict aseptic technique must be used throughout the entire procedure.
2. Prepare two air-purged 10 ml 0.9% sodium chloride syringes with 22G × 1 inch needles.
3. Prepare vacuum tube holder, needle and tube. Do not fully insert tube into needle as vacuum will be lost.
4. Shut off infusion for 1 minute before drawing blood specimens to prevent blood contamination with infusion fluid. This is especially important when total parenteral nutrition is infusing.
5. Close clamp distal to injection port (Figure 19.21A).
6. Cleanse injection port with povidone-iodine for 30 seconds. Allow to dry.
7. Hold injection port while performing all entries and withdrawals. Aseptically insert needle of first normal saline flush directly into center of port. Gently inject solution to flush extension tubing (if used) and catheter of infusate (Figure 19.21B).
8. Withdraw syringe full (10 ml) of blood and fluid mixture. Remove and discard syringe and needle.
9. Recleanse injection port with povidone-iodine for 30 seconds. Allow to dry.

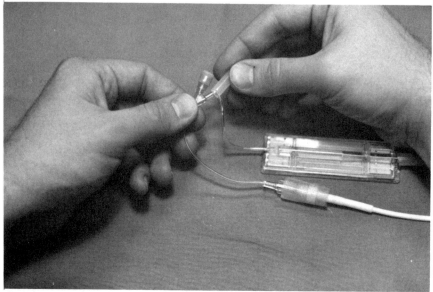

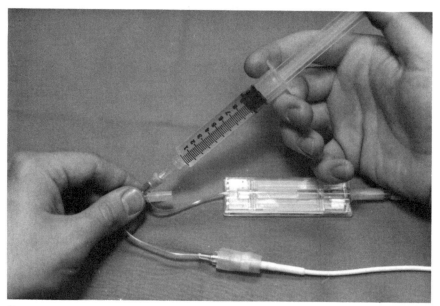

FIGURE 19.21
(A) The clamp distal to the injection port is closed. (B) Normal saline is injected to clear system of infusate. (C) Allow vacuum tube to fill with blood.

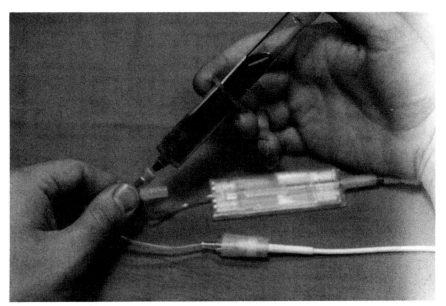

C

10. Aseptically insert needle of vacuum tube unit into center of injection port.
11. Fully insert tube into needle. Allow tube to fill with blood (Figure 19.21C).
12. Remove tube. Continue to insert, allow to fill, and remove required tube(s) for blood specimen(s). Be sure to mix, by gentle rotation, all specimens drawn in tubes with an anticoagulant.
13. Remove holder, tube, and needle.
14. Recleanse injection port with povidone-iodine for 30 seconds. Allow to dry.
15. Aseptically, insert needle of second syringe with 0.9% sodium chloride into center of injection port. Gently flush to rinse blood cells from the catheter.
16. Open clamp and regulate infusion drip rate.

Drawing Blood Specimens from Continuous Infusion Line by Opening the System. This procedure requires a catheter which can be clamped because the catheter will be opened to the air several times. An extension tubing which contains a clamp may be aseptically Luer locked and taped to the catheter hub as a substitute. Extreme care must be taken to maintain sterility when the extension tubing is used for this purpose. This procedure should be performed in correlation with the tubing change to avoid reconnecting a used tubing after the blood specimens are drawn.

The following steps may be used to perform the blood drawing procedure.

Equipment

    Catheter clamp or in-site extension tubing with clamp (1)
    Appropriate number and type vacuum tubes for tests
    Syringe large enough to hold required amount of blood (1)
    10 cc syringes (2)
    Needles 20G × 1 inch (3)
    0.9% sodium chloride 10 ml (2)
    Povidone-iodine swab (1)
    Alcohol sponge (1)
    Sterile 2 × 2 inch sponge (1)
    Appropriate infusion tubing (1)
    Luer lock 0.22 micron air-eliminating filter (1)

Procedure

1. Put on gloves. Strict aseptic technique must be maintained throughout the entire procedure.
2. Prepare fresh I.V. system, flush tubing and filter.
3. Prepare two air-purged syringes of 10 ml 0.9% sodium chloride.
4. Shut infusion off for 1 minute. Close clamp.
5. Remove old tape at catheter–tubing or filter connection.
6. Cleanse connection for 30 seconds with povidone-iodine swab. Place on sterile sponge to dry.
7. Pick up connection by protecting catheter hub with sterile sponge.
8. Disconnect and discard infusion system.
9. Continue to hold hub with sterile sponge during all connection and disconnection manipulations. Connect first air-purged syringe of 0.9% sodium chloride.
10. Open clamp. Gently inject flush to rinse catheter, and extension tubing, if used.
11. Withdraw 10 ml blood and fluid mixture. Close clamp.
12. Disconnect and discard syringe.
13. Connect large syringe, open clamp, and withdraw required amount of blood for all ordered tests (Figure 19.22).
14. Close clamp. Disconnect syringe filled with blood. A second person may be required to add needle and fill specimen tube(s). Be sure to mix by gentle rotation all tubes with an anticoagulant.
15. Connect second air-purged syringe with 0.9% sodium chloride. Open clamp and inject flush to rinse blood from catheter.

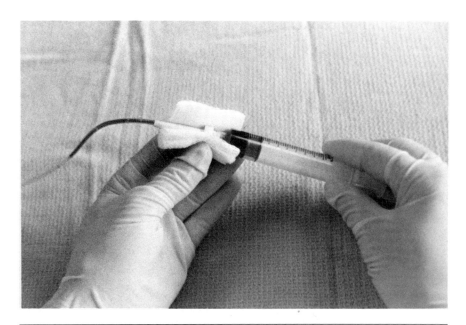

FIGURE 19.22
Withdraw required amount of blood for all ordered tests.

16. Close clamp, remove syringe. Connect, lock, and tape Luer-lock connection of I.V. tubing or filter to catheter. Open clamp. Reestablish infusion flow rate.
17. Tape tubing to chest wall to prevent relayed stress to the connection if the tubing is pulled or stretched.

Drawing Blood Specimens from Catheters with Injection Cap in Place. This procedure is frequently performed, especially with multiple-lumen catheters. The most proximal lumen is usually reserved for this purpose. By utilizing the distal lumen(s) for infusions, the fluid is downstream from the site where the blood will be drawn. This decreases the risk of blood contamination with the infusate if the solution cannot be turned off, or can be turned off only for a very short period of time.

When inserting needles into an intermittent injection cap, force should never be applied. If an obstruction is felt, realigning the angle of the needle will facilitate entry.

Blood may be drawn from a central catheter with an injection cap in place by following these steps.

Equipment

Vacuum tube holder (1)

Multiple sample needle 22G × 1 inch (1)

Appropriate number and type vacuum tubes for tests

0.9% sodium chloride 10 ml (2)

10 cc syringes (2)

Needles 22G × 1 inch (2)

Prefilled syringe with heparin dosage (1)

Povidone-iodine swabs (4)

Alcohol swab (1)

Tape

Procedure

1. Put on gloves. Aseptic technique must be maintained throughout the entire procedure.
2. Prepare two air-purged 10 ml 0.9% sodium chloride flushes. Prepare air-purged heparin flush.
3. Prepare vacuum tube holder and needle with first tube. Do not fully insert tube into needle as vacuum will be lost.
4. Cleanse rubber end of injection cap with povidone-iodine for 30 seconds. Allow to dry.
5. Hold catheter hub without touching end of injection cap during all needle entries and withdrawals. Insert needle of first air-purged syringe with normal saline flush into center of rubber cap.
6. Inject flush to rinse heparin from catheter.
7. Withdraw 10 ml blood and solution mixture. Remove and discard needle and syringe.
8. Recleanse rubber end of injection cap with povidone-iodine for 30 seconds. Allow to dry.
9. Insert needle of vacuum tube unit into center of injection cap. Fully insert tube into needle. Allow tube to fill with blood. Remove tube.
10. Insert, allow to fill, and remove required specimen tubes. Be sure to mix by gentle rotation all tubes with an anticoagulant.
11. Recleanse rubber end of injection cap with povidone-iodine for 30 seconds. Allow to dry.
12. Insert needle of second syringe with normal saline flush into center of injection cap.
13. Inject flush to rinse blood from catheter. Remove syringe and needle.
14. Recleanse rubber end of injection port with povidone-iodine for 30 seconds. Allow to dry.
15. Insert needle of heparin flush into center of injection cap.
16. Gently inject heparin. Before the syringe is completely empty, clamp tubing. Apply pressure on plunger while withdrawing needle and syringe.
17. Remove clamp and tape catheter hub on chest wall above heart level.
18. Remove gloves and wash hands.

TOTALLY IMPLANTED CATHETERS

Sterile Technique Because this device is placed for long-term usage, extreme care must be taken to maintain sterile technique while performing any manipulations. Therefore, the use of sterile gloves becomes an important part of all procedures.

Needles To prevent septum damage, only noncoring needles may be used for cannulation of the device. Straight needles are used for heparin flush, bolus injection, or blood drawing. Needles bent to a 90° angle are used for continuous or frequent intermittent infusions. The bent needle may also be used for heparin flush, bolus injection, or blood drawing. Noncoring needles are also available with a permanently attached extension tubing and clamp (Figure 19.23).

Needles are available, with metal or plastic hubs, in gauges 24 to 19, and in lengths from ½ inch to 2½ inches. The needle length required will depend upon how superficial or deep the septum is implanted. The gauge will depend upon the type and rate of infusate to be given. Packed red cells may require a 19 gauge needle, while a 24 gauge may be adequate for flushing.

The needle must be held securely against the needle stop during all procedures to avoid injecting the drug into the subcutaneous tissue. Do not use an angular motion or twist the needle once in the septum. This action will cut the septum and create a drug leakage path. If the heparin flush is given without an extension tubing, 3 ml heparin (100 units/per milliliter) is used. If an extension tubing is used, 5 ml heparin may be required.

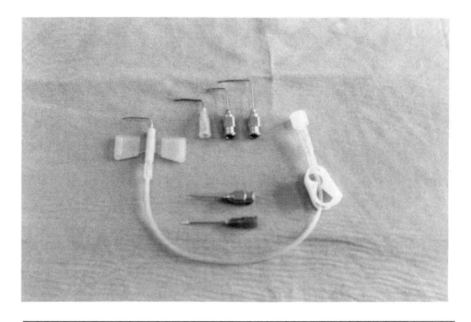

FIGURE 19.23
Straight and 90° bend noncoring needles.

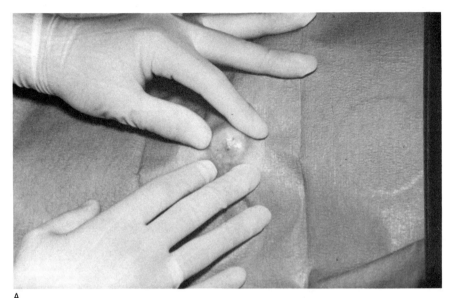

A

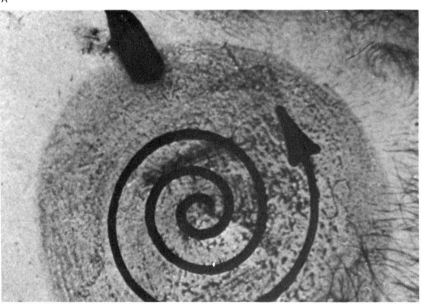

B

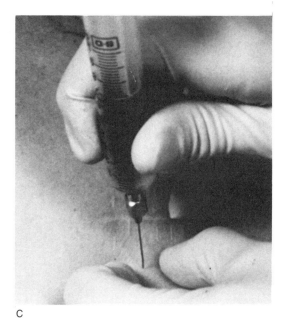

C

FIGURE 19.24
(A) The septum is located by palpating the outer perimeter of the port. (B) The skin prep is performed in a circular fashion, starting at the center of the septum and working outward toward the periphery of the port. (C) While stabilizing the port, using a perpendicular angle, insert the needle into the septum until the needle stop is felt. Courtesy Pharmacia Laboratories, Piscataway, N.J.

Heparin Flush

Implanted catheters require heparin flushing after each use and monthly when not in use. This is almost universally done with 3–5 ml of 100 units per milliliter heparin.

The heparin flush may be performed by the following steps.

Equipment

    Sterile noncoring needle (1)

    Sterile syringe with 3 ml heparin flush (100 units per milliliter)

    Sterile gloves (1 pr)

    Sterile towel (1)

    Sterile fenestrated drape (optional)

    Povidone-iodine swabs (3)

Procedure

1. Identify septum by palpating the outer perimeter of the port. Confirm septum location (Figure 19.24A).
2. Wash hands thoroughly and dry.
3. Aseptically prepare sterile supplies on opened sterile towel.
4. Put on sterile gloves. Observing sterile technique, perform *three* separate skin preps with povidone-iodine. Start at center of septum and work outward toward the periphery of the port (Figure 19.24B).
5. Place fenestrated drape over prepped area (optional). The availability of a sterile field at the insertion site will decrease risk of touch contamination during the procedure.

6. Attach syringe with heparin flush to noncoring needle and eliminate air from syringe and needle. A straight or 90° angled needle may be used for heparin flush.
7. *While stabilizing the port,* using a *perpendicular angle,* insert needle into septum until the needle stop is felt (Figure 19.24C).
8. Inject flush no faster than 5 ml per minute.
9. Withdraw needle while *maintaining stability of the port.*
10. Examine the site closely for any signs of infiltration or leakage. Apply sterile dressing if necessary.

Connecting Implanted Catheter to Continuous Infusion System

When a continuous infusion is to be started, the device is cannulated with an extension tubing connected between the needle and the infusion tubing. If frequent intermittent infusions are given, the needle and extension tubing are left in place and the extension tubing covered with an intermittent injection cap. This prevents the need for frequent septum punctures.

Equipment

Electronic infusion instrument (optional)
Appropriate infusion tubing
Luer lock air-eliminating 0.22 micron filter (1)
Luer lock extension tubing with clamp or stopcock (1)
Admixture or infusion solution
Noncoring 90° angled needle
Sterile towel (1)
Sterile fenestrated drape (optional)
Sterile 10 cc syringe with 0.9% sodium chloride
Sterile strip of tape (1)
Povidone-iodine swabs (3)
Povidone-iodine ointment (optional)
Sterile gloves (1 pr)
Sterile 2 × 2 inch sponges (2)
Sterile transparent tape dressing (1)

Procedure

1. Identify septum by palpating the outer perimeter of the port. Confirm septum location.
2. Wash hands thoroughly and dry.
3. Prepare solution container, tubing, and filter. Flush system. If infusion pump is used, be sure psi is <15 to prevent possibility of catheter rupture.

Chapter 19 | Central Venous Catheters

4. Aseptically prepare all sterile supplies on opened sterile towel.
5. Put on sterile gloves. Using sterile technique perform *three* separate site preps with povidone-iodine. Start at the center of the septum and work outward beyond the periphery of the port.
6. Place fenestrated drape over prepped area (optional).
7. Attach 10 cc syringe with 0.9% sodium chloride to extension tubing.
8. Firmly lock noncoring 90° angle needle to extension tubing.
9. Flush extension tubing and needle with the 0.9% sodium chloride. Close stopcock or clamp (Figure 19.25A).
10. *While stabilizing the port,* using a perpendicular angle, insert needle into septum until the needle stop is felt. Digital pressure on top of the needle at the bend point will facilitate septum entry (Figure 19.25B).
11. Open stopcock or clamp, stabilize port, and inject normal saline to affirm needle placement. Carefully observe site for any signs of infiltration. If desired, a small amount of blood may be withdrawn to affirm septum entry.
12. Close stopcock or clamp and remove syringe.
13. Securely connect and lock prepared infusion system to the extension tubing. The use of Luer locks and taping connections will reduce the risk of separation.
14. Open stopcock or clamp and start the infusion.
15. If the needle does not lie flush with the skin, place a sterile sponge under needle or needle hub.
16. If povidone-iodine ointment is to be used, apply to insertion site. The use of an ointment at this access point may create increased risk of needle movement with resultant dislodgement, and can prevent direct observation of the insertion site.
17. Placing a strip of sterile tape over the needle at the insertion site can help prevent needle dislodgement.
18. Using aseptic technique, apply sterile transparent tape dressing over site and a portion of the extension tubing. Using clear sterile tape allows for site inspection without removing the dressing (Figure 19.26).
19. Loop the tubing and tape on the skin to prevent stress at the needle site if the tubing is stretched or pulled.

Discontinuing Infusion

A continuous infusion may be discontinued by the following steps.

1. Shut infusion off. Close clamp on extension tubing or turn stopcock off.
2. Aseptically disconnect I.V. tubing from stopcock or extension tubing.
3. Aseptically connect air-purged syringe with 10 ml 0.9% sodium chloride. Open clamp or stopcock. Inject sodium chloride to flush system. Close clamp or stopcock.

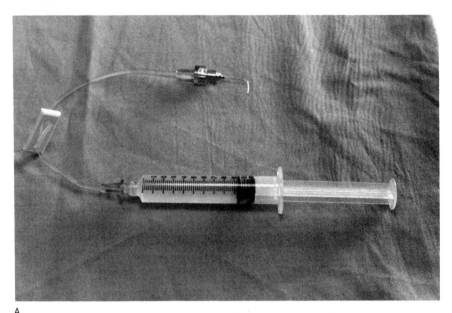

A

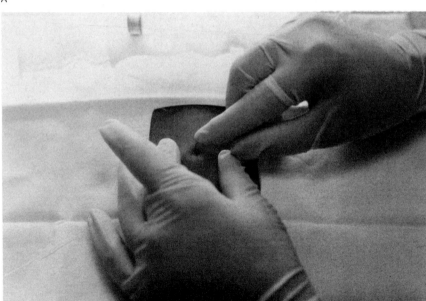

B

FIGURE 19.25
(A) The 90° angle needle is connected to the extension tubing and syringe. The entire unit is flushed. (B) Digital pressure on the bend point of the needle will facilitate septum entry.

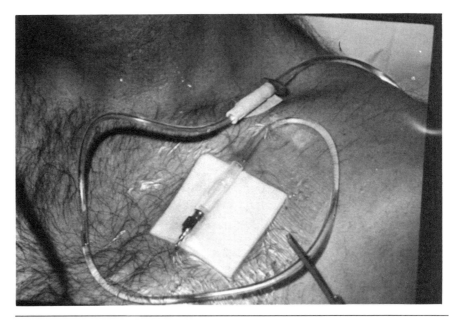

FIGURE 19.26
Completed access to an implanted catheter. Courtesy Pharmacia Laboratories, Piscataway, N.J.

4. Remove empty syringe. Connect air-purged syringe with 5 ml (100 units per milliliter) heparin. Open clamp or stopcock. Inject heparin flush.
5. Stabilize the needle while removing the clear tape and any sponges (Figure 19.27).
6. Remove the needle while *maintaining stability of the port*.
7. Examine injection site for any signs of swelling or fluid seepage.
8. Apply a sterile dressing if necessary.

Administering a Bolus Injection

A bolus injection may be given by the following steps.

Equipment

Sterile noncoring needle (1)
Sterile extension tubing with clamp or 2-way stopcock (1)
Sterile syringes 10 cc (2)
Sterile syringe 5 cc (1)
Sterile syringe appropriate size for drug (1)
Sterile needles 22G × 1 inch (4)

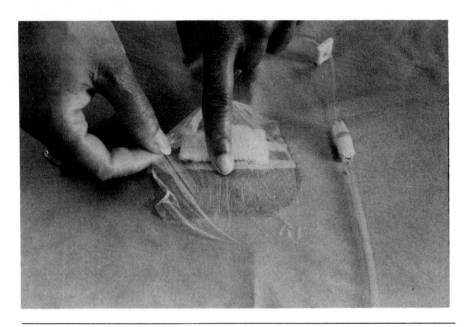

FIGURE 19.27
Stabilize the needle while removing the tape and sponges.

Sodium chloride 0.9% 20 ml
Heparin flush 5 ml (100 units per milliliter)
Drug to be injected
Sterile gloves (1 pr)
Sterile towel (1)
Sterile fenestrated drape (optional)
Povidone-iodine swabs (3)
Alcohol sponge (1)

Procedure

1. Identify septum by palpating the outer perimeter of the port. Confirm septum location.
2. Wash hands thoroughly and dry.
3. Open sterile towel and aseptically prepare all sterile supplies.
4. Put on sterile gloves. Observing sterile technique perform *three* separate skin preps with povidone-iodine. Start at center of septum and work outward toward the periphery of the port.
5. Place fenestrated drape over prepped area (optional). The availability of a sterile field at the needle insertion site will decrease risk of touch contamination during the procedure.
6. Using sterile technique, prepare two air-purged syringes with 10 ml

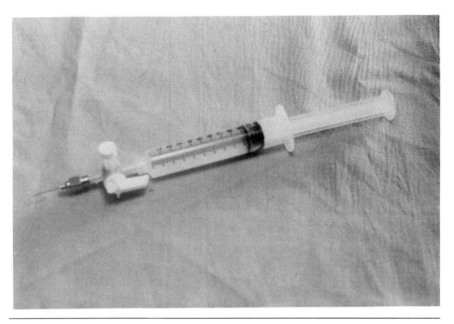

FIGURE 19.28
The needle, stopcock, and syringe are connected and flushed.

normal saline, one air-purged syringe with 5 ml heparin flush, and an air-purged syringe with drug to be injected.

7. Connect extension tubing or stopcock to first syringe with 0.9% sodium chloride and noncoring needle. Flush the system. Close clamp or turn stopcock off (Figure 19.28).
8. While stabilizing port, using a perpendicular angle insert needle into septum until needle stop is felt. Open clamp or turn stopcock on. Inject sodium chloride. To prevent needle dislodgement during any injection, the needle should be stabilized either digitally or, with a 90° angle needle by the use of a sterile strip of tape.
9. Turn stopcock off or clamp extension tubing, disconnect empty syringe, and connect air-purged syringe with drug. Turn stopcock on or open tubing clamp, inject drug at recommended rate but no faster than 5 ml per minute.
10. Turn stopcock off or clamp extension tubing, disconnect empty syringe, and connect second air-purged 10 cc syringe of 0.9% sodium chloride. Turn stopcock on or open tubing clamp, inject flush.
11. Turn stopcock off or clamp extension tubing, disconnect empty syringe, and connect air-purged syringe with heparin flush. Turn stopcock on or open tubing clamp, and inject heparin flush.
12. Remove needle while *maintaining stability of the port.*
13. Examine site closely for any signs of infiltration or leakage. Apply sterile dressing if necessary.

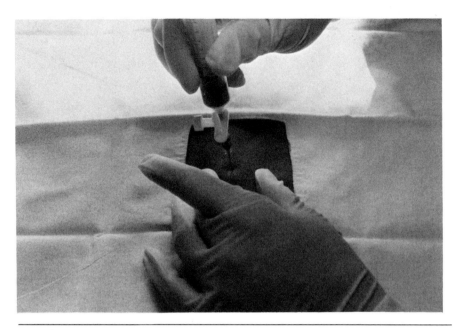

FIGURE 19.29
Drawing a blood specimen from an implanted catheter.

Drawing Blood Samples

Blood samples may be drawn as a separate procedure or at the time of a bolus injection or during continuous infusion. To draw a blood sample as a separate procedure or at the time of a bolus injection.

1. Follow all steps including the first flush with 0.9% sodium chloride given for a bolus injection (steps 1 through 7).
2. Using the empty syringe, draw back 10 ml blood and saline mixture. Close stopcock or clamp and remove and discard syringe with blood.
3. Attach fresh sterile syringe, open stopcock or clamp, withdraw required amount of blood for ordered specimen (Figure 19.29). Close stopcock or clamp and remove syringe.
4. Immediately attach second syringe with 10 ml 0.9% sodium chloride. Open stopcock or clamp and flush device. Close stopcock or clamp.
5. If bolus injection is to be given, proceed with bolus procedure after first 0.9% sodium chloride flush (steps 8 through 11).
6. If the catheter will not be used, perform heparin flush by the following steps.
    a. Remove empty syringe and connect air-purged heparin syringe.
    b. Inject flush at 5 ml per minute.
    c. Remove needle while *maintaining stability of the device*. Inspect site closely for any signs of infiltration of leakage. Sterile dressing may be applied to site if necessary.

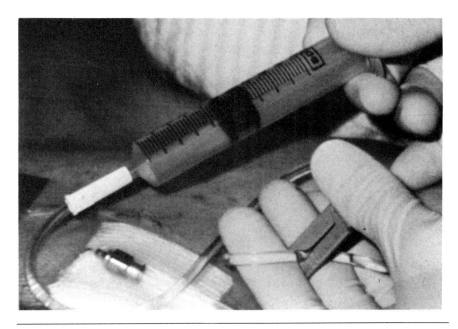

FIGURE 19.30
The catheter and extension tubing are flushed with normal saline. Courtesy Pharmacia Laboratories, Piscataway, N.J.

Drawing Blood Samples during Continuous Infusion

1. Shut off infusion.
2. Close clamp on extension tubing.
3. Aseptically disconnect system at extension tubing–I.V. system connection. Blood samples should be drawn in coordination with tubing and filter changes. This prevents unnecessary manipulation of the system and prevents the risk of contamination that is present if the same tubing is reconnected.
4. Aseptically connect air-purged syringe with 10 ml 0.9% sodium chloride. Open clamp. Inject normal saline to flush infusate from septum and catheter.
5. Using empty syringe, withdraw 10 ml blood and saline mixture. Close clamp.
6. Aseptically remove and discard syringe with blood and connect empty syringe. Make sure the syringe is large enough to collect all blood required for specimens.
7. Open clamp and withdraw required amount of blood. Close clamp.
8. Aseptically remove syringe with blood, attach air-purged syringe with 10 ml sodium chloride.
9. Open clamp and inject to flush blood from the catheter and septum (Figure 19.30).

10. Close clamp. Remove syringe. Reconnect sterile I.V. system and lock and tape connections.
11. Reestablish flow rate.

Tubing and Dressing Changes

Many centers are changing the tubing and filter down to the extension tubing or stopcock every 24–48 hours. The sterile clear tape dressing is changed when the needle and extension tubing or stopcock are changed, every 5–7 days. If this protocol is followed, extreme care must be taken to assure that a thorough handwashing precedes all line manipulations, that sterile gloves are worn for cannulation, that *three* sterile skin preps are performed, and that touch contamination does not occur.

IMPLANTABLE PUMPS

Patient Identification Card

When the pump is implanted the surgeon should fill out the Patient Registration and Implantation Record. The manufacturer will issue the patient a wallet-sized identification card containing information pertinent to the implanted pump. The physician should fill in the space provided for any medical emergency instructions. This card should be carried by the patient at all times.

Postimplantation Care

Patients should be monitored carefully postimplantation to confirm proper pump performance, wound healing, and favorable response to therapy. The pump should not be used for the administration of drugs for several days after implantation to allow for adequate wound healing [5].

Patient Instructions

The patient should be instructed to [5]:

1. Avoid traumatic physical activity to prevent tissue damage around the implant site.
2. Avoid long hot baths, saunas, and other activities which increase body temperature and result in increased drug flow.
3. Consult the physician during febrile illness to assess the effects of increased drug flow.
4. Consult the physician prior to air travel or change of residence to another geographic location. Adjustments in drug dosage may be required to compensate for an anticipated change in drug flow.
5. Avoid deep sea or scuba diving.
6. Report any unusual symptoms or complications relating to the specific drug therapy or the device.
7. Return at the prescribed time for pump refill.

Pump Refill Procedure

The pump will require refills at specific intervals of time. The intervals will depend upon the volume of the reservoir and the rate of administration.

The pump may be refilled by the following steps [5].

Equipment

    Sterile fenestrated drape (1)
    Sterile towel (1)
    50 cc syringe with drug solution (1)
    Sterile empty 50 cc syringe (1)
    Sterile noncoring needle (1)
    Sterile extension tubing with clamp (1)
    Sterile gloves (1 pair)
    Sterile 2 × 2 inch sponge (1)
    Povidone-iodine swabs (3)
    Heating pad (1)

Procedure

1. Warm 50 cc syringe with drug solution to 15–35°C with the heating pad.
2. Identify the outer perimeter of the pump by palpating the pump pocket. Locate pump septum.
3. Wash hands thoroughly and dry.
4. Using sterile technique, place all sterile items on opened sterile towel.
5. Put on sterile gloves.
6. Disinfect pump site with povidone-iodine. Use *three* separate preps. Start at the center of the pump and work outward beyond the periphery of the pump.
7. Place fenestrated drape over prepped pump site. Sterile template may be aligned over septum.
8. *Securely* connect *barrel* of empty 5 cc syringe and extension tubing to the noncoring needle. Close clamp.
9. Using a perpendicular angle, insert needle into center of septum.
10. Open clamp. Lower syringe barrel to below patient level and allow pump to empty (Figure 19.31A).
11. Close clamp. Record returned volume, adding 1 ml for amount of drug remaining in extension tubing. Disconnect and discard syringe barrel
12. *Securely* attach air-purged syringe with drug solution to extension tubing. Open clamp.
13. Using both hands, inject 5 ml solution into pump. Release pressure and allow drug to return to syringe. This test confirms proper needle placement. Continue to inject and check needle placement at 5 ml increments until syringe is emptied (Figure 19.31B).
14. Pull needle out quickly and apply digital pressure with sterile sponge. If necessary, apply a sterile adhesive bandage.

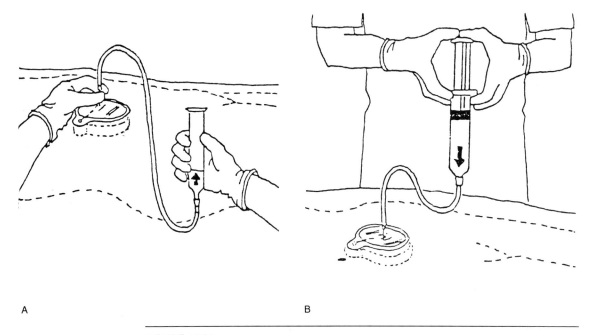

FIGURE 19.31
(A) The syringe barrel is lowered to allow the pump to empty. (B) Using both hands, 5 ml is injected into the pump. Courtesy Intermedics Infusaid, Inc., Norwood, Mass.

Important Considerations	Never attempt to aspirate fluid from the pump. This will cause blood to be drawn back into the catheter, resulting in occlusion. If no fluid is returned into the syringe barrel, either the septum has not been penetrated or the pump is completely empty of infusate. To test for septum penetration, remove the syringe barrel and connect 5 cc syringe with normal saline. Inject the solution and release the plunger to allow the fluid to return to the syringe. If the fluid does not return, again attempt to locate and penetrate the septum, using 5 ml normal saline to test penetration. If you are not successful the physician should be notified as pump failure may have occurred. Accurate fill and refill records are essential to ensure that the pump is refilled at the required intervals; these records also document appropriate pump functioning.
Bolus Injection Through the Sideport	A bolus injection may be given through the sideport of the implanted pump by the following steps [5].

Equipment

    Sterile 5 cc syringes (2)

    Sterile syringe appropriate size for drug to be injected (1)

Sterile needles 22G × 1 inch (3)
Noncoring needle (1)
Stopcock or extension tubing with clamp (1)
0.9% sodium chloride 10 ml (1)
Drug to be injected (1)
Sterile towel (1)
Sterile fenestrated drape (1)
Sterile gloves (1 pr)
Alcohol sponge (1)
Povidone-iodine swabs (3)

Procedure

1. Identify the outer perimeter of the pump by palpating the pump pocket. Locate the *sideport* septum.
2. Wash hands thoroughly and dry.
3. Using sterile technique, place all sterile items on opened sterile towel.
4. Put on sterile gloves.
5. Disinfect sideport septum with povidone iodine. Use *three* separate preps. Start at the center of the sideport and work outward beyond the periphery of the port.
6. Place fenestrated drape over prepped area.
7. Using sterile technique, prepare two syringes with 5 ml 0.9% sodium chloride. Prepare drug to be injected in separate syringe.
8. Connect first normal saline syringe to stopcock or extension tubing and noncoring needle. Secure all connections. Flush system with solution. Close clamp or stopcock.
9. While stabilizing port, insert noncoring needle into *sideport* septum at a perpendicular angle.
10. Open stopcock or clamp. Inject saline to flush catheter and confirm needle placement. Close stopcock or clamp.
11. Disconnect and discard syringe. Connect syringe with drug. Open stopcock or clamp. Inject drug at manufacturer's recommended rate, but do not exceed 10 ml per minute. Close stopcock or clamp. Disconnect and discard syringe.
12. Connect second syringe with normal saline flush. Open stopcock or clamp. Flush catheter. Close clamp.
13. Stabilize port while gently withdrawing needle.
14. Carefully check area for any signs of infiltration or leakage. A sterile dressing may be applied if necessary.

REFERENCES

1. Ryan, J. A., Jr., and Gough, J. A. Complications of central venous catheterization for total parenteral nutrition: The role of the nurse. *J. NITA* 7:29–35, 1984.
2. McIntyre, P. B., Laidlow, J. M., et al. Thromboembolic complications and central venous catheters (letter). *Lancet* 2:936, 1982.
3. Brendel, V. Catheters utilized in delivering total parenteral nutrition. *J. NITA* 7:488–490, 1984.
4. Welch, G. W., McKeel, D. W., et al. The role of catheter composition in the development of thrombophlebitis. *Surg. Gynecol. Obstet.* 138:421–424, 1974.
5. Intermedics Infusaid Corporation. *Implantable Drug Delivery System — Physician's Manual.* Norwood, Mass. 1983.
6. National Intravenous Therapy Association, Inc. Nursing standards of practice. *J. NITA* 5:19–34, 1982.
7. Maki, D. G., and Band, J. D. A comparative study of polyantibiotic and iodiphor ointments in prevention of vascular-catheter-related infection. *Am. J. Med.* 70:739–744, 1981.
8. Gillies, H., Rogers, H. J., Johnston, J., et al. Is repeated flushing of Hickman catheters necessary? *Br. Med. J.* 290:1708, 1985.
9. Pituk, T. L., DeYoung, J. L., and Levin, H. J. Volumes of selected central venous catheters: Implications for heparin flush use. *J. NITA* 6:98–100, 1983.
10. Newton, R., DeYoung, J. L., and Levin, H. J. Volumes of implantable vascular access devices and heparin flush requirements. *J. NITA* 8:137–140, 1985.
11. Lokick, J. J., Bothe, A., Jr., et al. Complications and management of implanted venous access catheters. *J. Clin. Oncol.* 3:710–717, 1985.

BIBLIOGRAPHY

Annest, L. S., and Ryan, J. A. Use of a split-sheath vein introducer for subclavian venipuncture in the placement of silicone catheters for chronic venous access. *Am. J. Surg.* 144:367–369, 1982.

Bjeletich, J., and Hickman, R. O. The Hickman indwelling catheter. *Am. J. Nurs.* 80:62–65, 1980.

Bjornson, H. S., Colley, R., et al. Association between the number of microorganisms present at the catheter insertion site and the colonization of the central venous catheter in patients receiving total parenteral nutrition. *Surgery* 94:720–727, 1982.

Carelli, R. M., and Herink, E. Hickman/Broviac catheters: Results of survey and patient care considerations. *J. NITA* 7:287–289, 1984.

Duval, A., and Hennessy, K. Care of the Broviac catheter. *J. NITA* 6:40–42, 1983.

Ecoff, L., Barone, R. M., et al. Implantable infusion port (Port-A-Cath™). *J. NITA* 6:406–408, 1983.

Gyves, J., Ensminger, W., et al. Totally implanted system for intravenous chemotherapy in patients with cancer. *Am. J. Med.* 73:841, 1982.

Heimback, D. M., and Ivey, T. D. Technique for placement of a permanent home hyperalimentation catheter. *Surg. Gynecol. Obstet.* 143:634–636, 1976.

Hickman, R. Letter to the editor. *Am. J. I.V. Ther.* 3:22, 1976.

Hickman, R. O. Letter to the editor. *Am. J. I.V. Ther.-Clin. Nutr.* 10:3, 1983.

Hoshal, V. L., Jr. Total intravenous nutrition with peripherally inserted silicone elastomer central venous catheters. *Arch. Surg.* 110:644–646, 1975.

Hughes, C. B. and Bryant, J. K. The use of multilumen catheters in acute leukemia patients. *NITA* 7:484–486, 1984.

Lawson, M., Bottino, J. C., et al. Long-term I.V. therapy; a new approach. *Am. J. Nurs.* 79:100, 1979.

Lawson, M., McCredie, K. B., et al. The use of silicone elastomer central venous catheters for intravenous therapy in patients with cancer. *J. NITA* 3:245, 1980.

Maher, M. M., Henderson, D. K., et al. Central venous catheter exchange in cancer patients during total parenteral nutrition. *J. NITA* 5:54–60, 1982.

Niederhuber, J., Ensminger, W., et al. Totally implanted venous and arterial access system to replace external catheters in cancer treatment. *Surgery* 92:706, 1982.

Ryan, J. A. Jr., Abel, R. M., et al. Catheter complications in total parenteral nutrition. *N. Engl. J. Med.* 290:757–761, 1974.

Speer, E. Over-wire silicone catheter insertion. *J. NITA* 6:426–427, 1983.

Speer, E. W. One alternative to the intrasil catheter for peripherally induced central venous catheterization. *J. NITA* 7:405–408, 1984.

Stellato, R. A., Gauderer, M. W., et al. Direct central vein puncture for silicone rubber catheter insertion. *Surgery* 90:896–899, 1981.

Vasquez, R. M. Subclavian catheterization using the peel away sheath. *Surg. Gynecol. Obstet.* 153:852–856, 1981.

Warren, J. The multi-lumen subclavian catheter: A new answer to an old problem. *J. NITA* 8:151–156, 1985.

Wilson, J. M. Right atrial catheters (Broviac and Hickman): Indications, insertion, maintenance, and protocol for home care. *J. NITA* 6:23–27, 1983.

REVIEW QUESTIONS

1. Which catheter material is the least thrombogenic?
2. Which catheter design has a high risk of catheter embolism?
3. A catheter with an introducer and guide wire allows for the insertion of a _____ catheter.
4. Totally implanted pumps are designed for _____ , _____ , and _____ ambulatory therapy.
5. Blood for which laboratory tests should not be drawn through a catheter that has been flushed with heparin or has heparin as a solution additive?
6. Before drawing any blood specimens, the nurse must accurately identify the patient by _____ .
7. Because sterile technique is required for accessing a totally implanted infusion device, the use of _____ becomes an important part of all procedures.
8. When accessing a totally implanted infusion device, how many skin preps should be performed?
9. When refilling an implanted pump, septum penetration may be confirmed by _____ .

CHAPTER 20

Intravenous Administration of Drugs

Ada Lawrence Plumer

Not so long ago the subcutaneous and the intramuscular routes were preferred for the parenteral administration of drugs. With the success of and increase in intravenous therapy, the practice of including drugs in infusions grew. Today intravenous therapy is used extensively for drug administration.

ADVANTAGES

The venous route for drug administration offers pronounced advantages which are given below.

1. Some drugs cannot be absorbed by any other route; the large molecular size of some drugs prevents absorption by the gastrointestinal route, while other drugs, unstable in the presence of gastric juices, are destroyed.
2. Certain drugs, because of their irritating properties, cause pain and trauma when given by the intramuscular or subcutaneous route and must be given intravenously.
3. The vascular system affords a method for providing instant drug action.
4. The intravenous route offers a better control over the rate of administration of drugs; prolonged action can be provided by administering a dilute infusion intermittently or over a prolonged period of time.
5. The vascular route affords a route of administration for the patient who cannot tolerate fluids and drugs by the gastrointestinal route.
6. Slow intravenous administration of a drug permits termination of the infusion if sensitivity occurs.

HAZARDS

In spite of the advantages offered by the venous route, there are certain hazards which are not found in other forms of drug therapy:

1. The possibility of incompatibilities when one or more drugs are added to the intravenous solution.
2. Speed shock (a systemic reaction to a substance rapidly injected into the bloodstream).
3. Vascular irritations and subsequent hazards.
4. Rapid onset of action with inability to recall a drug once it has entered the bloodstream.

INCOMPATIBILITIES

The number of possible drug combinations, provided by the ever-increasing production of drugs and parenteral fluids, is astronomical. With the increase in drug combinations comes an increase in potential incompatibilities. How and why incompatibilities occur and how best to avoid them are problems confronting all those involved in compounding intravenous additives. However well we know the chemical action of one group of drugs, our knowledge falls short when many groups are combined into complex compounds. The nurse, confronted with these problems, faces increased responsibility.

Many hospitals have set up pharmacy-centralized intravenous additive programs. This places the responsibility for prescription compounding with the department best qualified to assume it. The pharmacist is best able to predict or to detect incompatibilities and is alert to prescribed errors. The greater opportunity for sterility and accuracy when drugs are prepared in the pharmacy is obviously an advantage.

However, if such a pharmacy-centralized intravenous additive program is lacking, the responsibility is often left with the nurse. The pharmacist must be directly available, alerting him or her to possible chemical incompatibilities, communicating with various manufacturers on specific pharmaceutical problems, and providing information on certain drugs. An in-service program should be instituted, supplying an approved list of drugs for administration and acquainting the nurse with reactions, contraindications, dosage, stability, and compatibilities.

The individual who mixes and compounds intravenous drugs must be alert to the hazards of drug therapy. Since incompatibilities are a complication of prime consideration in the preparation of solutions, the nurse should have an acquaintance with the concepts involved in this hazard.

Compatibility charts are available but generally show only physical incompatibilities. Even chemical compatibility charts may be useless because of differences in the drug formation from one manufacturer to another or because of changes made by one manufacturer. The order of mixing drugs, the quantity of the drug and the solution, room temperature, and light contribute to incompatibilities not noted on the chart. Incompatibilities are not always obvious, as chemical changes may occur which do not produce a visible change.

Chapter 20 | Intravenous Administration of Drugs

Precipitation may occur when one or more drugs are added to parenteral solution [15]. It does not always occur at the time the solution is prepared, which increases the problem of intravenous administration. Some drugs, stable for a limited period of time, degrade and may or may not precipitate as they become less therapeutically active. If administered intravenously, solutions containing insoluble matter carry potential danger of embolism, myocardial damage, and effect on other organs such as the liver and the kidneys.

CHEMICAL INTERACTIONS

The most common incompatibilities are the result of certain chemical reactions [15].

1. *Hydrolysis* is the process in which water absorption causes decomposition of a compound. In preparing solutions of salt, the nurse should understand that certain salts, when placed in water, hydrolyze, forming a very strong acid and a weak base, or a weak acid and a strong base. Since pH is a significant factor in the solubility of drugs, the increased acidity or alkalinity from hydrolysis of a salt may result in an incompatibility if another drug is added. *Example:* The acid salt sodium bicarbonate when placed in water hydrolyzes to form a strong alkali (sodium hydroxide) and a weak and unstable acid (carbonic acid). Many organic acids are known as weak acids since they ionize only slightly [14].

2. *Reduction* is the process whereby one or more atoms gain electrons at the expense of some other part of the system [14].

3. *Oxidation* is the corresponding loss of electrons occurring when reduction takes place. Antioxidants are often used as a preservative to prevent oxidation of a compound [14].

4. *Double decomposition* is the chemical reaction in which ions of two compounds change places and two new compounds are thus formed [14]. A great many salts act by double decomposition to form other salts and probably represent the largest number of incompatibilities. *Example:* Calcium chloride is incompatible with sodium bicarbonate; the double decomposition results in the formation of the insoluble salt calcium carbonate.

Classification of Incompatibilities

Incompatibilities may be divided into three categories:

1. *Therapeutic.* An undesirable reaction resulting from overlapping effects of two drugs given together or close together.
2. *Physical.* According to Endicott [4], "The term 'physical incompatibility' is somewhat misleading but has come to be accepted as a physical or chemical interaction between two or more ingredients which leads to a visible change in the mixture which can be readily observed." A visible change may not occur with many chemical reactions. The physical change may be [15]:

a. Gas formation, such as occurs when carbonates are placed in acid. (Sodium bicarbonate in acid forms carbon dioxide gas.)
   b. Color change, such as occurs when riboflavin in vitamin B complex and methylene blue form a green color.
   c. Precipitation, occurring when compounds are insoluble. (Acid salts in alkali cause free base to precipitate; base salts in acid cause free acid to precipitate.)
3. *Chemical.* A chemical change is classified here as a change in drug compounds which is not readily observed. Since it may go undetected it has a greater capacity for causing biological effects.

pH AND ITS ROLE IN THE STABILITY OF DRUGS

Since pH plays an important role in the solubility of drugs it may be well to define it. pH is the symbol for the degree of concentration of hydrogen ions or the acidity of the solution. The weight of hydrogen ions in 1 liter of pure water is 0.0000001 gm, which is numerically equal to 10^{-7}. For convenience, the negative logarithm 7 is used. Since it is at this concentration that the hydrogen ions balance the hydroxyl ions, a pH of 7 is neutral. Each unit decrease in pH represents a tenfold increase in hydrogen ions.

It appears likely that the largest number of incompatibilities may be produced by changes in pH [13]. Precipitation occurs when a compound is insoluble in solution. The degree of solubility often varies with the pH. A drastic change in the pH of a drug when added to an intravenous solution suggests an incompatibility or a decrease in stability. Solutions of a high pH appear to be incompatible with solutions of a low pH and may form insoluble free acids or free bases. A chart denoting the pH of certain drugs and certain solutions to be used as a vehicle is helpful in warning of potential incompatibilities.

Factors Affecting Stability or pH

Many factors may affect the stability or pH of drugs:

1. *Parenteral solutions.* Some commonly prescribed drugs precipitate when added to intravenous solutions. Over 90 different infusion solutions, along with their pH, are listed by one company alone. Differences in the physical and chemical properties of each of these solutions may affect the stability of any drug introduced. A compound soluble in one solution may precipitate in another. Sodium ampicillin deteriorates in acid solutions. This drug, when added to isotonic sodium chloride at a concentration of 30 mg per milliliter, loses less than 10 percent activity in 8 hours. However, when it is added to 5% dextrose in water, usually a more acid solution, its stability is reduced to a 4-hour period.

   Another factor affecting the stability of drugs is the broad pH range (3.5–6.5) of dextrose solutions allowed by the United States Pharmacopeia (U.S.P.). "A drug may be stable in one bottle of dextrose 5 percent in water and not in another" [3].

2. *Additional drugs.* One drug may be compatible in a solution, but a second additive may alter the established pH to such an extent as to make the drugs unstable [11].
3. *Buffering agents in drugs.* An important consideration in the stability of drugs is the presence of buffers or antioxidants which may cause two drugs, however compatible, to precipitate. For example, ascorbic acid, the buffering component of tetracycline, lowers the pH of the product and therefore may accelerate the decomposition of a drug susceptible to an acid environment.
4. *Preservatives in the diluent.* Sterile diluents for reconstitution of drugs are available with or without a bacteriostatic agent. The bacteriostatic agents usually consist of parabens or phenol preservatives. Certain drugs, including nitrofurantoin, amphotericin B, and erythromycin, are incompatible with these preservatives and should be reconstituted with sterile water for injection.
5. *Degree of dilution.* Solubility often varies with the volume of solution in which a drug is introduced. For example, tetracycline HC, mixed in a small volume of fluid, maintains its pH range over 24 hours. However, when added to a large volume (1 liter), it degrades after 12 hours, becoming less therapeutically active.
6. *Period of time solution stands.* Decomposition of substances in solution is proportional to the length of time they stand. For example, sodium ampicillin with the high pH of 8–10 becomes unstable when maintained in an acid environment over a period of time.
7. *Order of mixing.* The order in which drugs are added to infusions often determines their compatibility.
8. *Light.* Light may provide energy for chemical reactions to occur. Therefore certain drugs, such as amphotericin B and nitrofurantoin, once diluted must be protected from light [11].
9. *Room temperature.* Heat also provides energy for reactions. After reconstitution or initial dilution, refrigeration prolongs the stability of many drugs.

VASCULAR IRRITATION

The hazards of intravenous therapy can be reduced by adequate precautions (see Chapter 16).

Vascular irritation is a significant hazard of drugs intravenously administered. Any irritation that inflames and roughens the endothelial cells of the venous wall allows platelets to adhere; a thrombus is formed. Thrombophlebitis is the result of the sterile inflammation. When a thrombus occurs, there is always the inherent danger of embolism.

If aseptic technique is not strictly adhered to, septic thrombophlebitis may result from bacteria introduced through the infusion cannula and trapped in the thrombus. This is much more serious, as it carries with it the potential dangers of septicemia and acute bacterial endocarditis.

Preventive Measures

The following precautions must be observed to diminish the potential hazards of vascular irritation:

1. Veins with ample blood volume should be selected when infusing hypertonic solutions or solutions containing irritating compounds.
2. The cannula should be appreciably smaller than the lumen of the vein. A large cannula may occlude the lumen, obstructing the flow of blood; the solution then flows undiluted, irritating the wall of the vein.
3. The venipuncture should be performed at the distal end of the extremity to allow each successive puncture to be executed proximal to the previous. Hypertonic solutions, when allowed to flow through a traumatized vein, cause increased irritation and pain.
4. Veins in the lower extremities are susceptible to trauma and should be avoided.
5. Isotonic solutions should, when possible, follow hypertonic solutions to wash irritating substances from the veins.
6. The rate of infusion may contribute to the irritation. (1) In a large vein, slow administration permits greater dilution of the drug with the circulating blood. (2) In a small vein lacking ample circulating blood, a slow drip prolongs the irritation, increasing the inflammation.
7. Prolonged duration of an infusion increases the risk of phlebitis. After a 24-hour period the danger increases. Periodic inspection of the injection site to detect developing phlebitis is important. After 72 hours the injection site should be changed.
8. Precautions should be observed to avoid administering solutions containing particulate matter by
   a. Proper reconstitution and dilution of additives.
   b. Inspection of parenteral fluids before administration.
   c. Use of freshly prepared solutions.
   d. Use of a set with a filter when danger of precipitation exists.
   e. Periodic inspection of solutions containing additives.
   f. Avoidance of administration of cloudy solutions unless affirmed by the manufacturer.

RESPONSIBILITY OF THE HOSPITAL COMMITTEE

The pharmacy and therapeutic's committee which deals with problems concerning therapeutic procedures should:

1. Provide the nurse with an approved list of medications that may be added to parenteral solutions.
2. The approved drug list should be updated as new drugs are added to the hospital formulary rather than as a result of an annual review of policies.

3. Delineate the types of fluids that may be administered.
4. Provide an in-service program to acquaint the nurse with reactions, contraindications, dosage, and effects.

THE PHYSICIAN'S RESPONSIBILITY

The physician writes and signs all orders for intravenous fluids and drug solutions. In each case the doctor should specify the rate of flow either as milliliters per hour or the approximate length of time of administration of the infusion.

It is the physician who is responsible for administering intravenously all medications not on the list approved for nurses. In some hospitals, this may consist of certain types of drugs such as:

1. Those that may produce a severe immediate reaction.
   Example: Nitrogen mustard, iron preparations, and other drugs in which the possibility of anaphylaxis is of prime concern.
2. Those whose dose is dependent upon the response of the patient and which are to be injected directly into the vein.
   Example: Epinephrine — dilution permits slow infusion and minimizes occurrence of reactions.
3. Those whose extravasation may result in necrosis.
   Example: Levarterenol bitartrate. Infiltration of this drug may lead to severe sloughing of the tissues. It increases the blood pressure by producing peripheral venous restriction, resulting in ischemia of the skin.

THE INTRAVENOUS NURSE'S RESPONSIBILITY

The following tasks are the responsibility of the intravenous nurse, who:

1. Checks the doctor's book for all complete orders of intravenous therapy. If a doubt exists regarding the compatibility or safety of a drug, the physician or pharmacist should be consulted.
2. Compounds only the drugs on the authorized list.
3. Labels solution, indicating patient's name, drug, dose, date, time prepared, expiration date, and the nurse's signature.
4. Delivers compounded, labeled solution to patient's unit, substantiating identification of patient and compounded solution. The nurse is legally responsible for all drugs and solutions that he or she prepares and administers.
5. Questions patient regarding sensitivity to drugs that may cause anaphylaxis. If a question of sensitivity exists, the drug should be administered by the physician.
6. Initiates the infusion and adjusts the rate of flow. No coercion should be used on rational, adult patients. If the patient refuses the infusion, the nurse should notify the physician in charge of the patient.

7. Observes patient for a short time following initial administration of drugs that may cause anaphylaxis.

THE ATTENDING NURSE'S RESPONSIBILITY

The nurse in attendance is responsible for maintaining the infusion and through periodic inspection:

1. Regulates and maintains the prescribed rate of flow.
2. Observes the injection site for any developing complications before serious damage occurs. If phlebitis or infiltration occurs, the cannula is removed.
3. Hangs consecutive containers of intravenous fluid, inspecting compounded solutions for precipitation.
4. Discontinues intravenous therapy, taking care to prevent hematomas from occurring by applying firm pressure over puncture site for at least 2 minutes, or longer if necessary.

NURSES' INTRAVENOUS ADDITIVE STATION

A specially equipped additive unit creates an environment of safety for the preparation of parenteral admixtures. This unit should provide the following:

1. *Isolated clean area.* Medications should be prepared in an area that permits complete concentration, because distraction increases the potential risk of human error.

    As traffic generates airborne contamination, an isolated area provides a better opportunity for sterility. The air in the typical hospital includes tiny contaminating particles, such as dust, lint, medication, and spores, in constant motion. These particles provide lodgment on which airborne bacteria thrive. The increased activity of bed-making, sweeping, and other functions increases the number of airborne particles and provides an environment that interferes with aseptic technique and may contribute to contamination [1].

2. *Laminar flow hood.* Some additive stations are equipped with a laminar flow unit to provide a clean work area where aseptic techniques can be performed. The concept of such a unit was evolved in 1961 and defined by Federal Standard 209a [2] as "air flow in which the entire body of air within a confined area moves with uniform velocity along parallel flow lines, with a minimum of eddies." These units, available in small bench models, play an important role in eliminating the hazard of airborne contamination of intravenous solutions.

3. *Proper illumination.* Adequate light permits visualization of particulate matter. Black and white backgrounds aid in the visual

Chapter 20 | Intravenous Administration of Drugs

detection of these foreign substances. Laminar flow units provide illumination by fluorescent light [3].

4. *Supplies.* A complete stock of equipment should be available, including
   a. Parenteral solutions and administration sets.
   b. Syringes and needles, including filter aspiration needles for glass ampules.
   c. Commonly used intravenous additives.
   d. Diluents:
      (1) Sterile bacteriostatic water injection, U.S.P.
      (2) Sterile water injection, U.S.P.
      (3) Normal saline injection, U.S.P.
   e. Container for the proper disposal of needles and syringes
5. A list of drugs and drug combinations approved for intravenous administration by nurses should be posted.

PREPARATION OF INTRAVENOUS SOLUTIONS AND ADDITIVES

Extreme care in the preparation of solutions diminishes the risk associated with intravenous therapy.

1. *Aseptic technique is imperative.* Bacterial and fungal contamination of drug products and parenteral solutions must be avoided.
2. *Proper dilution of lyophilized drugs is essential.* Two special cautions to assure complete solubility in the reconstitution of drugs must be observed.
   a. The specific diluent recommended by the manufacturer should be used.
   b. The drug should be initially diluted in the volume recommended.
3. *Introduction of extraneous particles into parenteral solutions must be avoided.* Fragments of rubber stoppers are frequently cut out by the needles used and accidentally injected into solutions [8]. Large-bore (15-gauge) needles are practical for use in the nurses' station and appear to have fewer disadvantages than the smaller needles.
   a. Smaller needles may encourage particles which may be difficult to see on inspection.
   b. The small particles may be of a size capable of passing through the indwelling cannula.
   c. Filter aspiration needles, used when preparing admixtures can remove particles.

A solution that on inspection contains fragments of rubber must be discarded.

Procedure in Compounding and Administering Parenteral Solutions

The following steps should be carried out in the preparation of solutions for infusion:

1. Inscribe order for drug additive directly from original order to medication label.
2. Substantiate drug orders with the drug product and the parenteral solution.
3. Inspect solution for extraneous particles.
4. Check drug product for
   a. Expiration date: Outdated drugs should not be used, as loss of potency or stability may have occurred.
   b. Method of administration:
      (1) Intramuscular preparations are not usually used for intravenous administration; they may contain certain components such as anesthetics or preservatives not meant for administration by the vascular route.
      (2) Some are packaged in multiple-dose vials which may contribute to contamination.
      (3) The dosage by the intramuscular route may not coincide with that for intravenous use.
5. With an accepted antiseptic, clean rubber injection site of both the drug product and the diluent.
6. Use sterile syringe and needle.
7. Reconstitute according to manufacturer's recommendation.
8. Check diluted drug for complete solubility before adding to parenteral solution.
9. After adding to solution, invert solution container to mix the additive completely.
10. Clearly and properly label solution container with:
    a. Name of patient.
    b. Drug and dosage.
    c. Date and time of compounding.
    d. Expiration date.
    e. Signature.
11. As an added precaution to prevent errors, recheck label with used drug ampoules before discarding ampoules.
12. Inspect solution for precipitates; if any precipitates are present, discard the solution.
13. Deliver parenteral solutions to patient's unit; substantiate identity of patient with solution prepared.
14. Perform venipuncture (see Chapter 12).

Chapter 20 | Intravenous Administration of Drugs

15. Observe patient for a few minutes following the initial intravenous administration of any drug that may cause anaphylaxis.
16. Use added cautions in administering drugs, the fast action of which could produce untoward reactions:
    a. Controlled-volume set
    b. Microdrip
    c. Electronic control instrument

General Safety Rules

The following safety rules for preparation and intravenous administration of drugs by nurses should be adhered to at all times:

1. Nurses will, upon written order, prepare and administer only those solutions, medications, and combinations of drugs approved in writing by the pharmacy and the therapeutics committee.
2. No intravenous infusion should be given that is cloudy, discolored, or contains a precipitate.
3. All intravenous infusions must be used or discarded within 24 hours of the time the container is opened.
4. Any question regarding chemical compatibility or the relative safety of any drug added to an intravenous infusion should be directed to the director of the pharmacy.

INTERMITTENT INFUSION

"Piggyback" infusions have become popular as a result of the increase in the number of intravenous drugs requiring by-the-clock administration. This technique allows drugs to be given on an intermittent basis through a slow keep-open infusion. The secondary container, containing a single-dose additive, or a multiple-dose admixture connected to a controlled-volume set, is piggybacked through the injection site of the primary infusion. At the desired time, the initial infusion is clamped off and the prescribed dose of medication administered. An in-line check-valve set, which automatically allows the primary infusion to flow when the secondary bottle empties and prevents air from entering the line, may be used.

When using a primary tubing with a back check valve, one can avoid spraying room air with the secondary drug solution and thus losing a portion of the ordered dosage by connecting the secondary container *without* flushing secondary tubing. After connection and taping, lowering the secondary tubing will allow the fluid from the primary container to fill the secondary tubing. This is important to prevent room contamination with antibiotics and cancer chemotherapeutic agents.

Equipment

The following equipment is used:

Intravenous container with admixture

Intravenous administration set (controlled-volume set, if desired)

1-inch 20-gauge needle

Antiseptic (isopropyl alcohol) swabs

Tape

Procedure

The following steps should be adhered to in administering piggyback infusions:

1. Wash hands.
2. Substantiate the identity of the patient and the admixture.
3. Attach the sterile administration set to the fluid container.
4. Suspend the bottle and flush the tubing to clear the set of air.
5. Clamp off the infusion.
6. Scrub the injection site with an accepted antiseptic. Strict adherence to aseptic and antiseptic technique is imperative.
7. Attach a sterile 1-inch 20-gauge needle to adapter of administration set. A longer needle may accidentally puncture the tubing. Small-bore needles are susceptible to breakage, with risk of the needle shaft's entering the infusion.
8. Insert the needle, up to the hub, in the injection site.
9. Tape the needle securely. In-and-out motion of the needle potentially increases the risk of contamination.

THE HEPARIN LOCK

The heparin lock provides a ready route for the intermittent administration of medications. It consists of a small-vein needle with a short length of plastic tubing to which is permanently attached a resealable injection site or over-the-needle intermittent catheter (INT) with an injection cap. To maintain its patency when the cannula is not in use, a dilute solution of heparin is injected in sufficient volume to fill the cannula and the tubing.

The heparin lock saves the patient the trauma of multiple punctures, conserves veins, offers freedom of motion between infusions, and provides a minimal amount of fluid to the patient on restricted intake.

One of the disadvantages of the heparin lock is the necessity for constant vigilance in order to prevent the fluid container from running empty. Once the container runs dry, venous pressure causes the blood to back up in the cannula and tubing, and a clot forms. A clot is an excellent trap for bacteria, whether the bacteria enter through the cannula or migrate from an infection in a remote area of the body. Irrigation may embolize small infected cannula thrombi, providing a potential focus for septicemia. After each infusion the small-vein needle or the INT must be *immediately* flushed with heparin to maintain its patency.

To maintain patency of the cannula and at the same time not interfere clinically with manifestations of altered clotting factors such as the prothrombin and thromboplastin times, 10 units sodium heparin in 1 ml normal saline has been documented [7] and is now the dosage that is usually used to maintain the heparin lock.

Heparin Lock Flush Solution, U.S.P. is available in prefilled syringes, each milliliter containing 10 or 100 U.S.P. units heparin sodium in Tubex.* It may be necessary to flush the heparin lock with a compatible fluid before and after heparin is used; some medications are incompatible with heparin. DO NOT FLUSH WITH STERILE WATER. Water, which is hypotonic, causes hemolysis if given intravenously.

Equipment

The following equipment is used:

Povidone-iodine

Antiseptic (isopropyl alcohol)

Small-vein needle containing a resealable injection site, or an intermittent catheter with an adapter cap that contains an injection port

Syringe and needle for injecting heparin

Sodium heparin injection, U.S.P.

Procedure

Prepare and insert the heparin lock as follows:

1. Put on gloves.
2. With syringe and needle draw up prescribed dose of heparin and expel air from the unit.
3. Scrub the injection site of the small-vein needle or the intermittent catheter with povidone-iodine for 30 seconds.
4. Inject the heparin, through the injection site of the small-vein needle or intermittent catheter, in order to expel the air and fill the lumen of the cannula.
5. Leave syringe and needle attached to the heparin lock.
6. Select the vein. Take special precaution to definitely differentiate the vein from an aberrant artery. Signs of a probable aberrant artery include: (a) pulse, (b) thick tough wall, (c) bright red blood, and (d) excruciating pain on venipuncture or on injection of medication. Inadvertent arterial injections of some medications can result in arteriospasm with impairment of the circulation and gangrene.
7. Make venipuncture.
   a. Scrub the skin site vigorously for 60 seconds with 70% isopropyl alcohol.
   b. Perform the venipuncture using the cannula which has been prepared as a heparin lock.

---

*Wyeth Laboratories, Philadelphia, Pa.

c. With the syringe, already attached, aspirate slightly to check for a blood return. Inject the remaining dosage (prescribed) of heparin and remove the syringe and needle.

d. Tape heparin lock securely.

e. Apply antimicrobial agent and dressing to the site.

f. Indicate the date of insertion, the size of the cannula, and the operator's initials near the dressing.

The following points should be emphasized:

1. The infusion set should be changed every 24 hours. Separate infusion sets must be used for the administration of containers of compounded fluids which are incompatible.
2. The needle on the set should be replaced for each intermittent infusion.
3. The heparin lock should be changed every 48–72 hours.
4. The heparin lock must be flushed immediately on termination of the intravenous piggyback infusion.
5. Remove gloves. Wash hands.

THE INTRAVENOUS PUSH

The intravenous push is the direct injection of a medication into the vein. It may be administered through the injection site in the intravenous tubing, the heparin lock, or a cannula.

The terms *I.V. push* and *bolus* can be confusing and can lead to dangerous misconceptions resulting in too rapid an injection of a medication [10]. Certain drugs, such as radiopaque dye used to visualize the cardiac chamber, must be injected as a bolus (bolus defined as a discrete mass) [10]. Most medications ordered as an I.V. push or bolus must be administered slowly, anywhere up to 30 minutes depending on the drug. Rapid injection increases the drug concentration in the plasma, which may reach toxic proportions, flooding the organs rich in blood — the heart and the brain — and resulting in shock and cardiac arrest. The rate of administration, included with the order of the medication, can reduce any misconceptions and prevent the potential risk of a life-threatening reaction from too rapid administration of the drug.

Because the I.V. push allows instant increased drug levels in the blood, it offers immediate relief to the patient. Nurses in many special care units are trained and authorized to administer specific I.V. pushes. In the past the I.V. push was restricted to the intensive care unit, where the patient was monitored and where a potential crises might arise requiring its immediate use in the absence of a physician. Today, more and more nurses are administering I.V. push injections.

Many drugs, given as I.V. injections, can be potentially dangerous to the patient. The nurse must understand the action of the drug and assess the patient's condition before administering the medication.

Decreased tolerance to the drug can result from factors in the patients' condition [9] such as:

1. Decreased cardiac output.
2. Reduced renal flow or poor glomerular filtration.
3. Diminished urinary output.
4. Pulmonary congestion.
5. Systemic edema.

Greater dilution of the drug and a longer injection time can prevent drug accumulation, reduce irritation to the vein due to a low pH, and allow time to assess the patient's response and detect early reactions. Use of the manufacturer's recommended diluent is most important, for different drugs require different diluents.

Reactions

Knowledge of the expected therapeutic effects of the medication, the recommended dosage range, the side-effects, and the toxic symptoms is essential.

Side-effects may manifest themselves in gastrointestinal distress such as nausea and vomiting, and diarrhea; in allergic skin reactions; and in central nervous system dysfunction [9].

Major reactions may consist of respiratory distress, anaphylaxis, cardiac arrythmias, and convulsions.

Reactions must be detected and reported at once so that proper treatment can be administered.

Antidotes

Nurses who administer I.V. pushes should have a knowledge of various antidotes and their use.

Emergency supplies of antidotes should be readily available. Many are available in prefilled syringes for emergency use. Tubex sterile cartridge needle units, with accurately machine-measured doses, provide a closed-injection system ready for instant use [12].

Available antidotes may consist of [12]:

1. Lidocaine hydrochloride (Xylocaine) for ventricular arrhythmias. Useful in certain conditions of hyperactivity.
2. Epinephrine (Adrenalin) for relief of hypersensitivity reactions, respiratory distress due to bronchospasm, and cardiac arrest following anesthesia reaction.
3. Diphenhydramine hydrochloride, U.S.P. (Benadryl) for allergic skin manifestations.
4. Diazapam (Valium) for convulsions.
5. Trimethobenzamide hydrochloride (Tigan), an antiemetic agent.

IMPORTANT CHECKPOINTS IN THE ADMINISTRATION OF I.V. INJECTIONS

The Drug

1. Understand the expected therapeutic effect of the medication.
2. Know the recommended dosage range and the length of time required for administration.

3. Understand the side-effects and toxic symptoms which can occur.
4. Be knowledgeable in the use of the proper antidote and its location.

The Patient

1. Make positive identification of the patient. Do not rely on the patient's verbal identification of himself or herself.
2. Ascertain allergy history.
3. Assess the patient's condition and be aware of any factors which can effect the drug action.
4. Know what medications the patient is receiving; be aware of therapeutic incompatibilities that may occur between any other medication the patient is receiving and the I.V. push medication.
5. Watch for the patient's response during and after the injection.

Preparation of the Medication

1. Check and doublecheck the order with the drug label.
2. Check the expiration dates of the drug and of the diluent.
3. Use the drug manufacturer's recommended diluent.
4. Clarify any questions or doubts that may arise with the patient's physician.

The Injection

1. Make sure that the cannula is within the vein.
2. Make sure that the drug is compatible with the I.V. solution if it is administered through a primary line. If incompatible, clamp the set and flush the injection port with compatible fluid. DO NOT USE STERILE WATER.
3. Ascertain the compatibility of the medication with heparin when a heparin lock is used. If incompatible, flush the lock before and after the I.V. injection with a compatible fluid.
4. Administer the medication at an evenly divided rate over the length of time recommended by the manufacturer, using a watch with a second hand.
5. Chart the medication, time administered, dosage, time span for administration, any required flushing, the patient's response, and your initials.

The Hospital

Any hospital that authorizes nurses to administer I.V. injections should provide:

1. Written policies for the I.V. injection of medications by nurses.
2. A list of drugs with the recommended dosage range and rate of administration for each drug.
3. A list of drugs that may be incompatible with I.V. injection medications.
4. A list of patient-care units where the I.V. injection is allowed.
5. A list of nurses authorized to administer I.V. injections.

6. An inservice educational program that includes information on the major reactions of the medications, their antidotes, their proper usage, nursing implications for use of drugs, and assessment/monitoring of patients.

REFERENCES

1. Abbott Laboratories. *The Abbott Clean Air Center,* North Chicago, Ill., 1969.
2. Davies, W. L., and Lamy, P. P. Laminar flow. *Lippincott's Hosp. Pharm.* 3:3, 1968.
3. Edward, M. pH — An important factor in the compatibility of additives in intravenous therapy. *Am. J. Hosp. Pharm.* 24:442, 1967.
4. Endicott, C. J. Workshop on parenteral incompatibilities. *Am. J. Hosp. Pharm.* 23:599, 1966.
5. General Services Administration. *Clean Room and Work Station Requirements: Controlled Environment* (Federal Standard 209a). Washington, D.C., 1963.
6. Fonkalsrud, E. W., Pederson, B. M., Murphy, J., and Beckerman, J. H. Reduction of infusion thrombophlebitis with buffered glucose solutions. *Surgery* 63:280, 1968.
7. Hanson, R. L., Grant, A. M., and Majors, K. R. Heparin lock maintenance with ten units of sodium heparin in one milliliter of normal saline solution. *Surg. Gynecol. Obstet.* 142:373, 1976.
8. Ho, H. F. Particulate matter in parenteral solutions. *Drug Intell.* 1:7–25, 1967.
9. McGill, D. Giving I.V. push. *Nursing 73* (3):15–18, June 1973.
10. Miller, A. J. "Bolus" injection (letter). *J.A.M.A.* 248:831, 1982.
11. Pelissier, N. A., and Burgee, S. L. Guide to incompatibilities. *Lippincott's Hosp. Pharm.* 3:15, 1968.
12. *PDR (Physicians Desk Reference).* (39th ed.) Oradell, N.J.: Medical Economics Co., 1985, pp. 625, 698, 1480, 1485, 2288.
13. Provost, G. E. Prescription compounding by nurses in hospitals. *Am. J. Hosp. Pharm.* 23:595, 1966.
14. Sackheim, G. L., Lehman, D. D., and Schultz, R. M. *Laboratory Chemistry for the Health Sciences* (3rd ed.). New York: Macmillan, 1978, pp. 70, 71, 79.
15. Webb, J. W. A pH pattern of I.V. additives. *Am. J. Hosp. Pharm.* 26:31–35, 1969.

REVIEW QUESTIONS

1. What are the advantages of using the venous route for the administration of drugs?
2. List the potential hazards when drugs are administered by the venous route.
3. Incompatibilities are not always obvious because chemical changes may occur which do not produce a visible change. True or false?
4. What are the chemical interactions that cause the most common incompatibilities?
5. What process causes certain salts, when placed in water, to decompose, thereby altering the pH — a factor significant in the solubility of drugs?
6. Name three categories into which incompatibilities may be divided.
7. Solutions with a high pH appear to be incompatibile with solutions with a low pH and may form insoluble free acids or free bases. True or false?
8. List the factors that may affect the pH of drugs when they are added to parenteral solutions.
9. Give three precautions to be observed in order to diminish the potential hazards of vascular irritation.

10. What is the responsibility of the nurse in administering drugs that may cause anaphylaxis?
11. What special cautions must be observed to reduce the risk of introducing extraneous particles into parenteral solutions?
12. What added cautions should be observed when administering fast-action drugs, which can produce untoward reactions?
13. All parenteral solutions must be used or discarded within 24 hours of the time the container is opened. True or false?
14. What are the advantages of a heparin lock?
15. In order to maintain patency, the small-vein needle must be flushed with heparin immediately before and immediately after each infusion. True or false?

CHAPTER 21

Total Parenteral Nutrition — Nursing Practice

Rita Colley □ Vickie Phillips Duty

Provision of nutrients by vein, in amounts sufficient to achieve anabolism, is called total parenteral nutrition (TPN); this therapy is also referred to as intravenous hyperalimentation (IVH) or, simply, hyperalimentation. Although some clinicians do not use these terms interchangeably, in this chapter we treat the terms *TPN* and *IVH* as synonymous.

HISTORY

Development of TPN began in the early 1960s in the Harrison Department of Surgical Research at the University of Pennsylvania Hospital. A young surgical resident, Stanley Dudrick, devised a central venous system of feeding that resulted in the normal weight gain and growth of beagle puppies who were fed solely by vein. Dudrick's fruitful animal experiments quickly led to human application: he successfully hyperalimented a severely ill infant who was unable to sustain herself with any type of gastrointestinal feeding due to small bowel atresia. Dudrick's accomplishments astounded the medical community and he began to receive referrals, starving adult patients who probably would not have survived without TPN [12].

In less than two decades TPN has evolved from this modest beginning into a sophisticated field of therapeutic intervention that has its own specialists, a large body of established knowledge, and organized clinical departments in hospitals throughout the world.

The purpose of this chapter is to give a brief overview of TPN and to provide general guidelines for nursing practice. The route of intravenous (I.V.) nutritional intervention addressed in this chapter is the subclavian or jugular approach to the central venous system. Other methods of providing TPN, such as the peripheral lipid system, which employs the use of less concentrated glucose and daily I.V. fat, and the antecubital approach to the central venous system, for the hypertonic glucose system, are also mentioned but not covered as fully because they are not yet as common in the United States.

INDICATIONS

A nutritional deficit often exists in hospitalized patients. Nurses are familiar with the isotonic I.V. fluid regimens prescribed for many patients — those awaiting surgery, those unable to eat postoperatively, those undergoing multiple days of testing that requires "N.P.O." preparation, or those who are not eating well in the hospital for other reasons. The critical question should always be the same, "Does lack of nutritional support jeopardize the patient's well-being?" The answer, of course, depends upon many variables. These include the patient's nutritional status before disease or injury, the severity of the current illness or trauma, the patient's age, the degree of catabolism, and the anticipated length of time that the patient will be without gastrointestinal feeding.

The specific indications for nutritional support are as vast as the number of clinical conditions that prevent a patient from utilizing the gastrointestinal tract for maintenance or achievement of anabolism. Some of the common indications for parenteral nutrition include gastrocutaneous fistulas; short bowel syndrome; acute renal failure; trauma; large burns; inflammatory bowel disease; pancreatitis; prolonged ileus; large nitrogen losses from infected wounds, fistulas, or abscesses; respiratory failure; sepsis; and in some experimental cases, hepatic failure and cancer [13].

When parenterally nourishing patients with any of the above conditions the clinical approach is disease- and patient-specific and often complex. Some of the indications require unique solutions that are not yet commercially available, e.g., a solution formulated for hepatic failure. Professionals caring for the patient receiving TPN should fully understand the specificity of the many solutions and therapeutic approaches now possible.

SOLUTIONS

Types

Hyperalimentation is now available to patients in a wide variety of solution types. Most patients receive commercially available solutions that contain crystalline amino acids of varying composition. These synthetic amino acids have largely replaced the protein hydrolysate solutions that were the "first generation solutions" of TPN therapy. The synthetic amino acids consist of highly usable essential and nonessential amino acids and generally permit better utilization of infused nitrogen than the protein hydrolysates did because there is less nitrogen wastage during protein metabolism [13].

A solution formulated specifically for the treatment of renal failure is also available. This solution consists of only essential amino acids and is an intravenous modification of the Giordano-Giovanetti diet [1].

Another solution is particularly for the treatment of hepatic failure. The amino acids in this formulation consist of decreased aromatic amino acids and increased branched-chain amino acids. Although widely used in Europe and Japan, this formulation is available only in an experimental form in the United States.

Experimentation has also begun in the use of a solution enriched with large amounts of branched chain amino acids [13] developed to treat patients with overwhelming sepsis.

Fat emulsions are a separate entity and will be discussed in a separate section.

Solution Content

In order to supply protein-sparing, or "energy" calories, the solutions are admixed with large amounts of dextrose and final concentrations commonly range from 20% to 47% dextrose. If the proper calorie-to-nitrogen ratio is not provided, it is impossible to achieve positive nitrogen balance. As more has been learned about I.V. nutritional requirements, it has become clear that this ratio changes with different disease states and is not fixed for a particular patient but is dependent on changing clinical status. The currently accepted calorie-to-nitrogen ratio is 150–250 gm of nonprotein calories per gram of nitrogen [13]. TPN solutions also contain vitamins, electrolytes, minerals, and trace elements in varying amounts to meet the patient's specific nutrient requirements.

Preparation

Because hyperalimentation solutions cannot be sterilized terminally (they "caramelize" if autoclaved), they should be prepared in the pharmacy with stringent aseptic technique. The solutions should be mixed under a laminar flow hood by a pharmacist or trained technicians who are supervised by a clinical pharmacologist. The use of headgear, masks, and sterile gloves is desirable.

All additives should be placed in the dextrose-amino acids mixture at the time of initial mixing. Solution containers should be examined for integrity (bottles for cracks and bags for small punctures), and the solution should be inspected against a strong light to ascertain the presence of particulate matter or turbidity that could indicate bacterial contamination.

The intravenous tubing should be inserted into the bottle under the laminar flow hood. These procedures should be done as close to the time of infusion as possible and not more than 24 hours beforehand. Prepared solutions should be refrigerated until use.

Many institutions cannot practice the ideal method of solution preparation just described. Some adaptations of technique are acceptable and others are not. It is acceptable to prepare the solutions using a completely closed system in a clean environment. Commercially available solution kits are supplied with a closed transfer system of intravenous tubing to facilitate sterile preparation. Prepared solutions must be sealed with a sterile, airtight, waterproof cap.

It is not acceptable to have total parenteral nutrition solutions prepared by an inexperienced, untrained person. An active nurses' station, a utility room or area proximal to the bedpan flusher, and a clean, but breezy designated intravenous admixture area are unacceptable. Proper education in techniques and rules of preparation can eliminate solution contamination and admixture incompatibilities.

At some medical centers, basic solution formulations are prepared with alternative solution mixtures also available. The alternative solutions contain additional salt, insulin, or potassium in any desired combination. Further modifications can be made by adding other elements when necessary [23]. Solutions tailor-made for each patient might sound ideal, but they are inconvenient and expensive when there is a large volume of patients in the hospital. Individualized solutions are also unnecessary for providing proper nutritional formulas, as long as adequate choice exists among the alternatives offered.

Administration

As mentioned earlier, TPN solutions are highly concentrated and contain large amounts of dextrose. These hypertonic solutions must be delivered into a wide-diameter blood vessel so that they may be rapidly diluted and not become sclerotic to the vein. Therefore, the only veins acceptable for catheter tip location are the superior vena cava, the innominate vein, and the intrathoracic subclavian vein. The ideal location for the catheter tip is the middle of the superior vena cava.

Early attempts to administer TPN solutions often employed the antecubital approach to the superior vena cava with the use of polyvinylchloride catheters. These long catheters were frequently associated with painful thrombophlebitis, venous thrombosis, and sometimes, sepsis. Recently, reports have suggested that antecubital catheters made of silicone elastomer are an acceptable alternative to the conventional subclavian or jugular catheter. While early reports suggest that these silicone catheters are less thrombogenic than other materials used, extensive research is needed to determine their true antithrombogenicity and complication rate [5]. Subclavian or internal jugular percutaneous venipuncture remains the approach of choice for most clinicians. The external jugular vein is, however, usually too narrow to be easily cannulated.

CATHETER INSERTION

Patient Considerations

Before the subclavian vein catheterization procedure is begun, the nurse should explain to the patient what is about to occur. Proper teaching beforehand seems to increase patient tolerance and markedly decrease the level of pain experienced during the procedure. It is helpful to tell the patient the following beforehand [8]:

1. The patient will be placed in the Trendelenburg position. (Say, "We will place you in a head-down position. This is so the doctor can find your vein easily, because it fills up more when you are in this position.")

2. The doctor will be wearing a mask, gown, and gloves, and all personnel at the head of the bed will also wear masks. (Say, "We all have some bacteria naturally occurring in our mouths, and wearing masks will prevent infection during this procedure. It is quite routine.")

3. The patient will be draped surgically. (Say, "Small sterile towels will be placed around the area where the catheter is to be inserted. Your face will be turned away and loosely covered, but you will be able to breathe normally and see clearly.")

4. The doctor will place a small towel roll along the vertebrae to hyperextend the neck and elevate the clavicles. (Say, "This raises your

shoulder blades and puts them out of the doctor's way. When the needle is placed beneath your collarbone to puncture the vein, your shoulders must be elevated. It is easier for you if your neck and shoulders are supported.")

5. The patient will be prepped with surgical technique. (Say, "The doctor will wash you with some strong-smelling solutions, applied with large gauze pads held by tongs. The solutions are acetone, which smells like ether, iodine, and alcohol — three very effective cleansers.")

6. The anesthetic will be administered a few minutes before the catheterization and will probably hurt. (Say, "The doctor will give you an injection of Xylocaine, which is a lot like Novocaine and it will help to numb your shoulder. A lot of patients have said this is the most unpleasant part of the whole procedure; the Xylocaine stings, somewhat like a bee sting, until it starts to work.")

7. The search for the subclavian vein produces a bizarre sensation, causing a lot of pressure, and sometimes pain. (Say, "When the doctor searches for your vein with the needle, you will have been given Xylocaine, but you will probably feel a strange sensation, a pressure inside your chest. Everybody feels this; there is nothing wrong. It is just a new experience to have anything from outside of you inside your chest.")

When this teaching is done in a calm, matter-of-fact way, it usually results in a nontraumatic experience for the patient. If it is not done, the patient experiences something totally foreign which he or she cannot anticipate. Nurses should also realize that, because of the operating-room aura of the procedure, the patient might possibly fantasize that emergency surgery was performed without warning. Patients can easily misinterpret the catheterization. It is important to elicit feedback as you teach, so that you can assess the patient's level of understanding and eliminate his or her fears.

Patients should be told also that only a very thin tubing, the catheter — "about one-third the size of regular intravenous tubing" (demonstrate this) — remains inside and that the needle is removed immediately. The patient often wonders about catheter removal at the end of therapy and is relieved to know that this is a quick, simple, and painless procedure. (Say, "It is not anything like having the catheter inserted; we just snip one suture outside of you and slide the narrow tubing out.")

If the patient seems to be especially apprehensive, even after the preinsertion teaching has been done, suggest to the doctor that an analgesic or psychotropic medication be given to the patient.

Certain comfort measures can reduce the fear and isolation instigated by an invasive procedure such as catheterization. The nurse should hold the patient's hand during the procedure. If the nurse is familiar with the equipment and has assembled it ahead of time, he or she is free to support the patient while the doctor places the catheter. Remember to maintain eye contact with the patient.

It is the nurse's responsibility to take an active role in assuring sterile technique, thereby protecting the patient. This means that if a glove becomes contaminated, the nurse should quickly give the doctor a fresh pair. In other words, the nurse should take the initiative in maintaining asepsis.

Catheterization should be performed only by an experienced doctor. The inside-the-needle catheter is placed in the standard method of subclavian venipuncture. When the needle is open to the air, before and during the threading of the catheter, the patient is asked to perform the Valsalva maneuver (forced expiration with a closed glottis). This maneuver is a precaution against possible air embolism and is easily accomplished by instructing the patient to "take a deep breath and hold it, bearing down and straining slightly." If the intubated patient is unable to do this, the nurse may produce the Valsalva maneuver by carefully maintaining inspiration with a manual resuscitation bag.

After the catheter is placed, the needle is withdrawn and covered with a plastic guard to prevent accidental puncture of the catheter. One suture is placed at the catheter insertion site. This prevents in-and-out motion of the catheter, which could introduce skin organisms into the puncture wound, and also helps prevent accidental dislodging of the catheter. Because of the potential complications and discomforts associated with the procedure, repeated, unsuccessful attempts to catheterize a specific vessel are unjustified.

Implantable vascular access devices are frequently used for highly irritating drugs or when there is need for a long-term vascular site (Chapter 19).

Immediate Postcatheterization Management

After the catheter has been sutured, the routine dressing is applied (see Dressing Change Procedures below). A chest roentgenogram is taken immediately. Only isotonic solution should be infused at a slow keep-open (10–20 ml per hour) rate until the chest x-ray confirms central venous location [24]. It is the nurse's responsibility to receive and document the initial chest x-ray result. After it has been confirmed that the catheter tip is located in the superior vena cava or the innominate or intrathoracic subclavian vein, infusion of the initial hyperalimentation solution may be started.

It is unacceptable to have the catheter tip located in the heart, the inferior vena cava, or any extrathoracic vessel. Atrial rupture, valvular damage, myocardial irritability, and cardiac tamponade are some of the possible complications that have been reported when catheter tips are located in the heart. Although the inferior vena cava has a wide diameter, it is contraindicated for catheterization because it has been associated with catheter-induced thrombosis and occlusion [9]. Extrathoracic veins are too narrow and will become sclerosed if used for TPN administration.

Technical Complications

Complications are infrequent, but placement of a subclavian catheter can trigger serious events. The nurse should be particularly alert for signs of respiratory distress, pain, a slowly increasing hematoma, or any unexplainable symptom. Some of the possible complications following a subclavian puncture are listed below [17].

Pneumothorax
Pleural puncture may occur inadvertently due to anatomical proximity of the lung to the subclavian veins. Sharp chest pain or decreased breath sounds may be present, or the pneumothorax may be evident only radiographically. Treat-

ment is based on symptoms. Sometimes a chest tube is indicated, although smaller pneumothoraces often resolve spontaneously.

Hemothorax
The subclavian vein or adjacent vessels may be traumatized during venipuncture, possibly causing slow, constant bleeding into the thorax. This is particularly worrisome if the patient has a bleeding disorder. Symptoms and treatment are the same as those for pneumothorax.

Hydrothorax
The catheter may transect the vein and locate in the thorax, causing intravenous solutions to be infused directly into the chest. Symptoms and treatment for this complication are also like those for pneumothorax.

Inadvertent Arterial Puncture
It is possible to inadvertently enter an artery during attempted venipuncture. This is usually not a problem if the error is clinically observed and the patient is treated immediately. Punctured arteries must receive direct pressure for at least 5 full minutes, timed by the clock, in order to stop bleeding. If the patient has a bleeding disorder or platelet abnormality, direct pressure must be applied for an even longer period of time. Therefore, one must be on the alert for a rapidly expanding hematoma, signs and symptoms of tracheal compression or respiratory distress, or a combination of these. If these symptoms occur, direct pressure must be placed on the arterial site and the doctor must be called immediately.

Brachial Plexus Injury
A tingling sensation in the fingers, pain shooting down the arm, or paralysis of the arms may indicate brachial plexus injury. This is a rare complication of subclavian catheterization. The treatment is symptomatic and may not always resolve the injury. Physical therapy is indicated for paralysis.

Thoracic Duct Injury (Chylothorax)
The thoracic duct is enlarged in cirrhotic patients because of alterations in lymph flow. Therefore, it may be entered accidentally during catheter placement. A left-sided subclavian puncture should therefore be avoided in cirrhotic patients whenever possible.

Sheared Catheter with Distal Embolization
During the process of threading the catheter through the needle, the catheter should never be pulled back for redirection. The entire unit should be removed and a new catheter should be used. If the catheter is pulled back against the needle, it may shear off and embolize. In such cases, cardiac catheterization, with snaring of the catheter embolus under fluoroscopic control, may be necessary [4].

AIR EMBOLISM

Air embolism is a potential danger whenever the central venous system is open to the air. The exact amount of air necessary to cause death remains controversial, but Flanagan et al. have calculated that 100 ml of air can pass through a 14-gauge needle (subjected to a 5 cm water gradient) in *1 second* [14]. This, of course, reemphasizes the need for air embolism precautions — Trendelenburg position and performance of the Valsalva maneuver — during placement of the catheter. Signs and symptoms vary with the severity of the air embolism and may include dyspnea, apnea, hypoxia, disorientation, tachycardia, hypotension, or a precordial murmur. Severe neurologic deficits, including hemiplegia, aphasia, seizures, and coma, have reportedly been associated with air embolism. Coppa et al. in a recent review article attribute the pathophysiology of the neurologic deficit associated with air embolism to direct access of air into the cerebral circulation in most situations. Immediate treatment is aimed at preventing obstruction by air of the right ventricular outflow tract. The patient should be placed in the left-lateral, head-dependent position, and direct intracardiac needle aspiration of air may be necessary [11].

Air embolism can also occur during I.V. tubing change either because of accidental disconnection of tubing junctions or through a tract left after catheter removal. Therefore, air embolism precautions during tubing change and catheter removal are essential, as is the proper securing of tubing junctions. Catheter removal should be followed immediately by placement of an occlusive dressing, such as ointment or petroleum jelly, gauze that is left on for at least 48 hours until the tract is totally healed. Rather than placing the patient in the Trendelenburg position, it is sufficient to have the patient flat in bed during these procedures. The Valsalva maneuver is always necessary, however.

DRESSING CHANGE PROCEDURES

There are many procedural variations of catheter site care that are effective and practical. The following procedure [10], based on the original method of JoAnn Grant and Stanley Dudrick, is still widely used [17].

A sterile dressing-change kit is brought to the bedside and unopened until ready for use. Prepackaged kits are efficient since they eliminate collecting and preparing material in an unclean area and provide the correct equipment. If procedural instructions are enclosed in the kits, they provide the additional advantage of a teaching aid.

Method

Before the procedure is begun, the bedside table is cleansed with an antiseptic solution. The nurse then puts on a mask and washes his or her hands before beginning the dressing change. A mask should also be worn by the patient unless doing so will compromise his or her respiratory function. The nurse also wears sterile gloves and uses a sterile clamp to hold the solution-wet swabs.

First, the nurse scrubs the catheter insertion site with acetone, a defatting agent. Acetone should be applied repeatedly until the prepping sponges come away free of debris. The second prepping solution applied is tincture of iodine, used because of its antifungal as well as antibacterial properties. It is applied

Chapter 21 | Total Parenteral Nutrition — Nursing Practice

for 2 minutes, timed by a watch, and allowed to air dry before removal. Third, alcohol is applied continuously until all the iodine which may cause irritation or burning if left on the skin, is removed. The alcohol should be allowed to air dry naturally without fanning or blotting.

The method of prepping used should emphasize the "clean-to-dirty" technique (see Figure 21.1). The area should be prepared in concentric circles, beginning at the catheter insertion site and moving out to the periphery (see Figure 21.2). A sponge that has touched the periphery should never be returned to the center. Careful attention must be given to cleaning the catheter and all its parts.

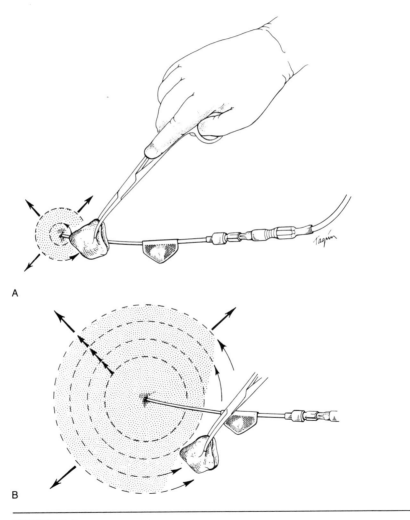

FIGURE 21.1
(A) Preparation of catheter site for change of dressing. (B) Antiseptic solution is applied in concentric circles, starting at the site of catheter insertion and moving out toward the periphery ("clean-to-dirty" technique).

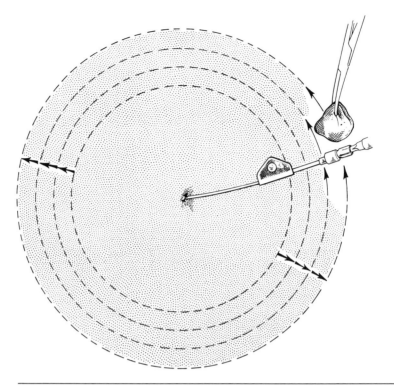

FIGURE 21.2
The prepared area of the catheter site extends to the middle of the catheter hub.

Topical antimicrobial ointment is applied to the catheter insertion site (see Figure 21.3). The site is then covered with two small gauze sponges; the needle and part of the inside-the-needle catheter are left partially uncovered. The exposed skin is sprayed with tincture of benzoin, which toughens the skin and prevents breakdown of tissue (see Figure 21.4), and allowed to dry. Some catheters are left in for a long time, but even with dressing changes every 48 hours, there will be little trouble with skin irritation if the skin has been carefully protected.

Dressing material is handled so that the side touching the patient's skin is not touched by the nurse (see Figure 21.5). The dressing is placed over the sponges in an air-occlusive manner, and the edges are sealed with tape.

A slit piece of tape is placed up under the catheter hub (see Figure 21.6) to ensure occlusion of the dressing and to allow the nurse easy access to the hub when it is time to change the intravenous tubing. All tubing junctions are firmly sealed with tape to prevent accidental separation (see Figure 21.7). The intravenous filter is anchored to the dressing to eliminate traction on the catheter insertion site (see Figure 21.8).

The hyperalimentation dressing is changed every 48 hours, or 3 times a week; the dressing should be changed immediately, however, if it becomes contaminated or wet. If the seal is broken, the dressing should not be reinforced; it should be changed. If the patient has a draining wound or is in a high hu-

Chapter 21 | Total Parenteral Nutrition — Nursing Practice

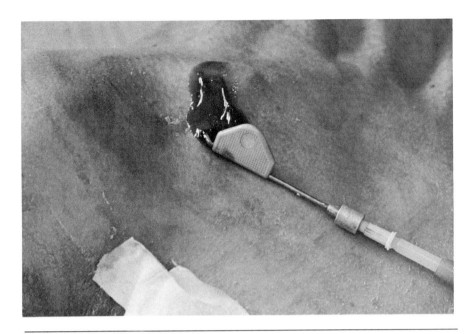

FIGURE 21.3
A subclavian catheter with topical iodophor ointment.

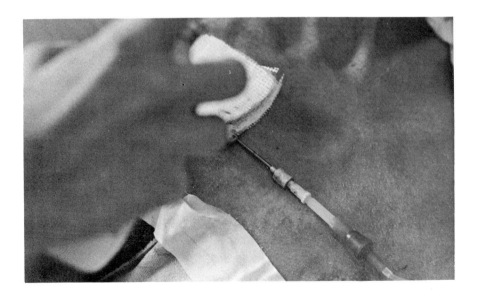

FIGURE 21.4
The catheter insertion site is covered with two small gauze sponges. The needle (or part of the intracatheter) is left partially uncovered. The surrounding skin is being sprayed with tincture of benzoin.

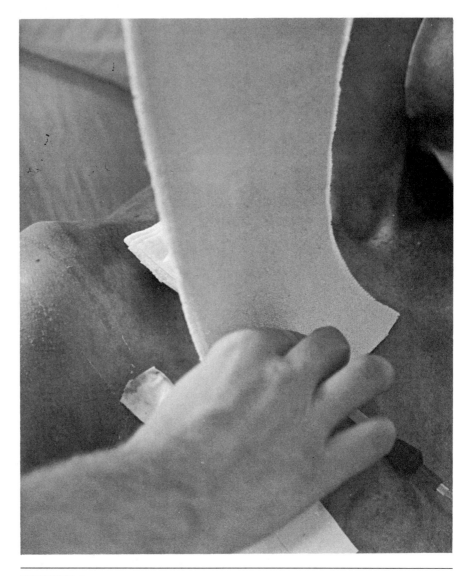

FIGURE 21.5
Elasticized adhesive bandage is placed over the sponges in an air-occlusive fashion.

midity area such as that caused by an oxygen face mask, or if the dressing is likely to become wet for any reason, the dressing is waterproofed. Sterile plastic drapes, similar to those used in the operating room, are placed over the completed dressings to waterproof them.

Materials
New dressing materials now available offer more alternatives for providing patient comfort and safety. One type is a transparent, adhesive-backed drape that provides sterile protection from the environment while it allows vapor to

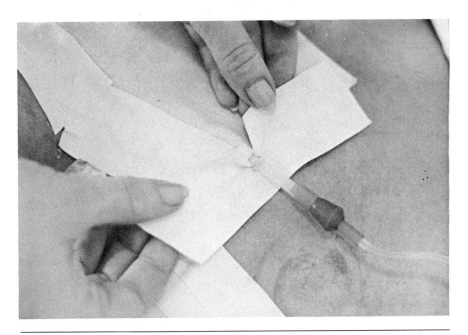

FIGURE 21.6
Adhesive tape placed on the edges of the elasticized bandage and a slit piece of tape placed up under the catheter hub helps ensure air occlusion.

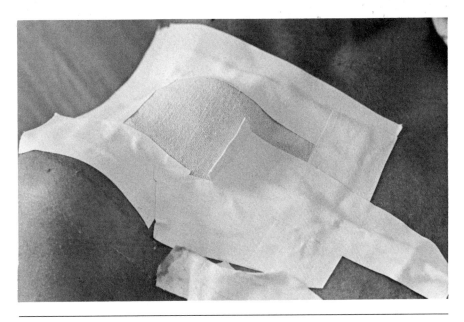

FIGURE 21.7
All tubing junctions are firmly sealed with adhesive tape to prevent accidental separation of tubing and catheter.

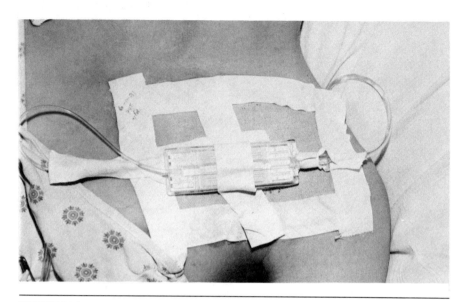

FIGURE 21.8
Tape securely anchors filter, and dressing is completed.

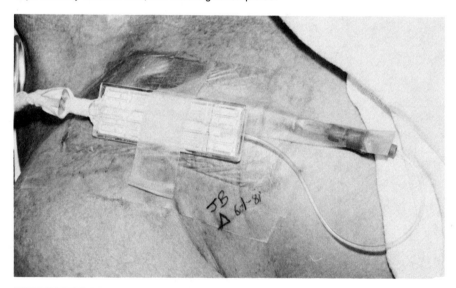

FIGURE 21.9
Op-site, a thin, transparent waterproof dressing, is useful for patients who have tracheostomies or are in a humid environment.

escape (see Figure 21.9). This is particularly useful for patients who perspire a great deal and is also convenient to apply to hard-to-dress areas such as jugular lines. Another dressing favored by patients is a soft, ultra-thin layer which is sponge-like and water resistant (see Figure 21.10). This dressing has proven to be comfortable, and we have found it to be advantageous for patients sensitive to other dressing materials.

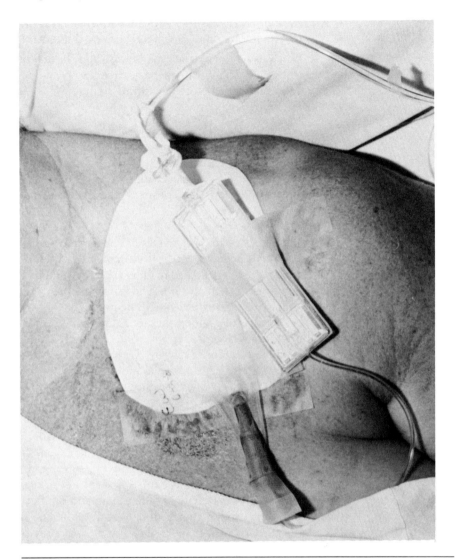

FIGURE 21.10
Microfoam, a soft sponge-like dressing material, is especially comfortable for patients with sensitive skin.

Some useful hints about the dressing are as follows:

1. If the patient is sensitive to acetone as a defatting agent, alcohol may be substituted. Alcohol's value as a prepping agent is now under consideration [21].

2. If the patient is iodine-sensitive, povidone-iodine solution may be used. When povidone-iodine is applied, it should not be removed with alcohol as this can cause skin irritation. It should air dry and remain on the skin.

3. If tincture of benzoin irritates the patient's skin, or if it is

contraindicated as it is with some of the newer dressing materials, try other adhesive sprays such as those used frequently in stoma care.

4. When using the plastic type of dressings, be aware that they sometimes tear easily. Therefore, the basic dressing should be protected with additional tape before anchoring the filter or the junction-securing tape to the dressing.

When the procedure is completed, the nurse notes it in the patient's chart. Any relevant condition is mentioned and the appropriate plan of care is outlined. If erythema, edema, skin ulceration, or drainage exists action must be taken immediately. If skin ulceration or purulent drainage is present, the doctor should order appropriate cultures, and the catheter should be removed immediately.

Certification

One method of "certifying" nurses to change TPN dressings is practiced at the University of Cincinnati Medical Center. Preparation for certification entails witnessing a dressing change, reading the hyperalimentation literature, and attending an orientation session. The nurse then changes a dressing under the supervision of one of the hyperalimentation nurses or someone else who is authorized to certify. When the procedure has been performed satisfactorily, the nurse achieves certification. Some clinicians feel strongly that dressing changes should be done only by the hyperalimentation nurses. This is most desirable; when it is not possible, however, a method of certification may be helpful in ensuring rigidly controlled, standardized care.

INTRAVENOUS TUBING AND FILTER CHANGE

The intravenous tubing and filters should be changed every 24 hours. It is most efficient to standardize the time of tubing, filter, and container changes for when the current day's supply expires and the next day's solutions have arrived in the clinical area. By changing the tubing and filter at the same time that the new container is hung, an additional break in the line is eliminated.

If a filter is used, its porosity should be 0.2 micron or less to effectively retain bacteria, fungi, and particulate matter. Many filters now available also have the ability to eliminate air. The method of filling the filter varies with different brands and is included on package instructions.

There is *always* the risk of contamination when intravenous tubing is changed. Therefore, precautions must be taken. One method of tubing change we have found helpful is as follows: gently grasp the inside-the-needle catheter hub using a clamp for leverage, carefully rotate out the in-use intravenous tubing, and quickly replace the old with the new tubing. If the distal tip of the tubing has touched anything other than the inside of the catheter hub, it is contaminated and should be replaced. If changing the intravenous tubing is difficult, a small sterile sponge placed beneath the catheter hub will help to prevent accidental contamination of the intravenous tubing. This is an important step in maintaining asepsis.

During an intravenous tubing change, the patient should be lying flat in bed. When the catheter is open to the air, the patient should be instructed to perform the Valsalva maneuver. This maneuver enhances positive pressure of the central vessels, thereby decreasing the chance of accidental air embolism.

INFECTION CONTROL

Catheter-related sepsis remains the most dreaded complication TPN therapy. In the early years of hyperalimentation, extraordinarily high rates of therapy-associated infection were reported. A number of studies followed, documenting acceptably low rates of sepsis correlated with careful adherance to aseptic technique and rigid implementation of therapy protocol [16].

As more accurate and sensitive indicators of catheter sepsis are developed, new challenges to interpretation of some previous findings are presented. In other words, better techniques allow us to diagnose instances of catheter-related sepsis that would have been attributed to a different source a few years ago. The simple fact that it requires 3 blood cultures taken within a 24-hour period to obtain a *99 percent* chance of confirming *existing* bacteremia raises skepticism about previous diagnoses [28]. New techniques should also encourage development of a standard definition of catheter-related sepsis throughout the specialty field.

Clearly defining catheter-related sepsis has implications for nursing because the sepsis is usually caused by organisms at the catheter insertion site that migrate along the catheter, rather than from in-line contamination. In addition to the routine nursing responsibilities of proper dressing maintenance, nursing staffing patterns must be considered. During a staff shortage or when personnel unfamiliar with correct catheterization techniques are responsible for dressing maintenance, catheter care suffers. As previously mentioned, this lower-quality care correlates with a statistically significant increase in catheter-related sepsis.

Ideally, we want to be able to assess the effectiveness of our care and prevent *avoidable* complications. Nurses are also primarily responsible for obtaining the updated data that provides more sensitive and accurate diagnostic indications of catheter-related sepsis. This data is partially derived from the results of semiquantative cultures of catheter insertion sites and catheter tips [2].

Nutritional intravenous lines should be placed specifically for administration of hyperalimentation. Nurses should infuse TPN solutions only through a new catheter placed exclusively for this purpose. The nutritional intravenous system should not be used for central venous pressure monitoring, withdrawal of blood, "piggyback" infusions of medication, or intravenous bolus injection of drugs [25].

Nurses play an important quality-control role because they are often first to witness an in-use violation, which renders the catheter unacceptable for hyperalimentation therapy. At some medical centers a method of surveillance has been initiated that encourages staff nurses to call the hyperalimentation team and report any such violations. The doctors on the hyperalimentation team then rule that the catheter is unacceptable for TPN administration. This method of watchfulness seems to ensure inviolate catheters and has worked fairly well. If a staff attempts to adopt such a method of surveillance, it is important that the persons involved realize that this is crucial for patient safety and that sources of information remain anonymous.

Teaching programs should constantly remind staff that hyperalimentation patients are very susceptible to infection, especially fungal sepsis. This keeps the general level of staff awareness high. Every 3 months there can be a hyperalimentation workshop, an 8-hour day devoted to discussing the correct principles of care, open to attendance by interested nurses from other hospitals.

A study of 200 patients at the Massachusetts General Hospital [26] demonstrated that when routine standards of catheter care were upheld by general-duty nurses and staff doctors, the catheter infection rate was 3 percent. On the other hand, in patients whose catheter care deviated from the standard protocol even once, catheter infection rate was 20 percent, or 7 times greater. This finding is statistically significant and demonstrates that nursing care greatly influences the safety of the patient.

Bjornson et al. have documented a similar finding by demonstrating a relationship between a threshhold number of organisms at the insertion site and colonization of the catheter [3].

Certain steps should be taken by the nurse when a hyperalimentation patient experiences a temperature elevation. All patients should have their temperature taken carefully every 6 hours, avoiding axillary temperatures whenever possible, since they are usually inaccurate. Any elevation in temperature should be a warning, i.e., if a patient's usual temperature is 97.8°F (36.5°C), a reading of 99.6°F (37.5°C) could indicate fever. Generally, we consider a fever to be a reading of 100°F (37.7°C) orally or 101°F (38.3°C) rectally. Certain drugs and disease states suppress the normal febrile response and affected patients must be assessed individually.

When an afebrile patient has a dramatic and unexpected temperature elevation, a temperature spike, the entire I.V. system should be changed immediately, including the catheter. The system should be cultured to rule out solution contamination. A new container of hyperalimentation should be hung through new tubing. If new TPN solution is unavailable, 20% dextrose in water, with insulin when appropriate, may be substituted to avoid rebound hypoglycemia. A complete "fever work-up," including a thorough history, physical examination, and culturing should be done. If there is no other obvious source for the fever, the catheter should be removed and cultured. Immediate removal of the catheter is necessary because a dramatic, unabating temperature spike in a patient without an obvious reason for it could implicate the catheter and possibly result in septic shock if the source is not removed.

Typically, catheter sepsis presents as a low-grade fever for several days, progressing gradually to a high fever. Again, a complete fever work-up is necessary, although therapeutic intervention varies with clinical findings and laboratory results [6]. In all cases of suspected sepsis, the nurse should immediately notify the doctor when fever presents and should participate in the thorough culturing necessary to determine the etiology of the fever. Thorough culturing includes urine, sputum, wound drainage, feces, blood, and invasive line sites. If possible, semiquantitative cultures of skin sites around catheter insertion sites and catheter tips should be done. Semiquantitative counts of organisms at the skin site or on the catheter tip yield important information that helps prevent the misinterpretation of "skin contamination, not catheter sepsis" when results are positive. For example: *Staphylococcus epidermidis* is a common skin contaminant of bacterial cultures, but it can also be a dangerous pathogen. If the skin site is growing abundant and unexpected numbers of this organism, infection is to be suspected. On the other hand, without the semiquantitative technique, results are merely qualitative, that is, positive or negative, and not very useful as a diagnostic indicator.

Whether to continue therapy or remove the catheter is the doctor's decision and varies with the patient's clinical status, culture results, and the nature of the offending organism. Some doctors now leave TPN catheters in when gram-negative bacteremia exists, treating the patient with the appropriate antibiotic. In an attempt to eradicate the septicemia before pulling the line, gram-positive bacteremia and fungemia require catheter removal and treatment as indicated before reinstitution of TPN therapy. Many hyperalimentation patients are compromised hosts and are particularly susceptible to fungal infection. Whenever this possibility exists, it is necessary to differentiate between colonization and deep tissue invasion, for example, of invasive candidiasis. Hyperalimentation should not be administered to a patient with deep tissue fungal invasion.

METABOLIC CONSIDERATIONS

The first principle of metabolic support in TPN therapy is the correct provision of all nutrients. Support solutions contain glucose, amino acids, electrolytes, minerals, vitamins, and trace elements. Intolerance to or insufficient amounts of any of these solution components can result in deficiency states or metabolic aberrations.

The nurse should be aware of the signs and symptoms that accompany fluid and electrolyte imbalance and vitamin and trace element deficiency and toxicity. Most commonly, however, metabolic complications of TPN therapy are associated with glucose imbalance.

In most adults, the maximum rate of glucose utilization is between 0.8 to 1.0 gm glucose per kilogram of body weight per hour. This means that some patients can tolerate constant intravenous infusion of the large glucose load found in hyperalimentation solutions without the assistance of exogenous insulin. As the highly concentrated glucose infusion is initiated, a pancreatic beta cell response occurs, creating the frequently found increased serum insulin levels. Initial infusions should begin slowly, usually at an approximate rate of 60–80 ml per hour for the average-weight adult. A gradual increase in flow rate, approximately 25 ml per hour per day, allows the pancreas to establish and maintain the increased insulin production necessary.

Glucose tolerance may, however, be compromised by sepsis, stress, shock, hepatic and renal failure, starvation, diabetes, pancreatic disease, and administration of some medications, particularly, certain steroids, diuretics, and tranquilizers. Age is another variable: the elderly and the very young are particularly susceptible to glucose intolerance. For these patients, administration of exogenous insulin often is necessary. Conversely, when the patient's illness induces a hypermetabolic state, and daily caloric utilization is accelerated, glucose tolerance may exceed 0.8–1.0 gm per kilogram per hour [24].

URINARY GLUCOSE MEASUREMENT

Urine should be tested for sugar and acetone content every 6 hours around the clock [10]. During the initial period of hyperalimentation, as glucose tolerance becomes established, glycosuria is not uncommon. Glycosuria should not be allowed to persist without clinical evaluation and treatment. Urinary sugar content greater than 2+ requires a serum glucose test to determine the exact concentration of sugar present. Because 4+ urinary sugar is an open-ended value, the serum glucose level should be measured immediately whenever this condition exists.

Treatment is directed to the cause of the glucose intolerance. Some patients require a reduction in initial infusion rates and then proceed to tolerance which never requires exogenous insulin during therapy. Others require administration of insulin as needed.

Glycosuria may exist secondary to hypokalemia since potassium deficiency can cause glucose intolerance. The etiology of this disorder remains unclear, but it demonstrates the need for careful maintenance of the serum potassium level [18].

The nurse should bear in mind that certain drugs render a false positive result when the urinary glucose determinations are done by the copper reduction method (Clinitest). These drugs include the cephalosporins, vitamin C (in high doses), aspirin and other salicylates (in high doses), Aldomet (in high doses), Benemid, injectable tetracycline, Chloromycetin, and Levodopa (in high doses) [18].

In order to avoid false negative readings with the glucose oxidase method (Tes-tape) of determining urinary glucose, the nurse should pay careful attention to a band of color that might appear across a portion of the wet tape, even if the total wet surface has not changed color. The color of the band will demonstrate a true positive test in these cases. The glucose oxidase test may yield both false positive and false negative results when the patient is taking Pyridium; the Clinitest should be used for these patients [18].

Urinary sugar measurements are continued every 6 hours throughout therapy. A patient may become glucose intolerant at any time because of the previously mentioned conditions. Without this testing, hyperglycemia can exist undetected. Remember that glycosuria may be the first sign of sepsis. Serum glucose levels should be determined daily until the maintenance flow rate has been achieved and twice a week and PRN thereafter.

INSULIN ADMINISTRATION

When exogenous insulin is required, the dosage may be based on the urinary sugar level. This presupposes that the doctor has determined the patient's renal threshold and knows the serum correlate for the particular level of glycosuria. Some forms of renal disease (e.g., acute tubular necrosis) render urinary glucose measurements meaningless as an indicator of blood sugar. A person with acute tubular necrosis can have, for instance, a blood sugar over 1,000 mg per 100 ml and yield a negative urinary sugar test.

Regular insulin is usually added directly to the hyperalimentation solution. Controversy still exists about whether insulin recoverability in solution is reliable. Many clinicians think that it adheres to both glass and plastic I.V. solution containers and to I.V. tubing. However, the amino acids in TPN are thought to bind a significant amount of the insulin. Patients have been benefitting from this method of I.V. insulin administration since the advent of TPN therapy. It is preferable to administer insulin through the hyperalimentation solution because it provides a more constant serum insulin level than does periodic subcutaneous administration.

FLOW RATES

TPN solutions should be infused at a constant rate around the clock. The flow rate should be checked every 30 minutes and reset to the rate ordered as necessary. Too-rapid infusion of these highly concentrated dextrose solutions can lead to a hyperglycemic reaction or even hyperosmolar, nonketotic coma. The flow rate should not be adjusted to compensate for past increases or decreases in rate, but always should be reset to the rate ordered. To ensure that the nurse can easily assess the accuracy of flow rates, it is helpful to mark the bottle in hourly time allotments of prescribed fluid volume.

When fluids are administered by unassisted gravity infusion, a double-clamping system fixed to the intravenous tubing provides increased patient protection. A second clamp is applied and set to the desired rate, then the regular I.V. tubing clamp is set. The use of two clamps provides a safeguard, thus preventing a free-flow situation.

It is safer and more accurate to infuse TPN solutions with the aid of a mechanical device. Many types of infusion devices are available, offering the user a wide choice of pumps and controllers. At the University of Cincinnati Medical Center, most TPN solutions are administered by a mechanically assisted gravity system that utilizes controllers. The only TPN patients who require a pump are those who have permanent catheters — the Hickman or the Broviac types. Pumps are necessary for these patients because the external portion of their catheters is long and flexible and may easily kink. Use of positive-pressure apparatus helps to avoid clotting which might otherwise occur in these cases.

When choosing infusion apparatus, it is important that the nurse be aware of the advantages and disadvantages that each machine offers. It is particularly important to avoid pumps that are capable of generating high output pressure which may result in a rupture of the I.V. system, thus creating the potential for air embolism and contamination.

Cost-effectiveness is a factor, but it is also true that "one only gets what one pays for." When less expensive machinery meets all the user's requirements and is safe for the patient, it should be used. When it does not meet these criteria, it should be avoided.

ACCURATE CHARTING

Accurate daily weights, measured at the same time of day, using the same scale, and with the patient wearing the same clothing, are important. Intake and output data should also be scrupulously recorded. Without this information, it is difficult for the physician to calculate and prescribe the proper nutritional needs of the patient.

HYPOGLYCEMIA

Hypoglycemia is chemically defined as a serum glucose level of less than 50 mg per 100 ml. Many patients are asymptomatic at this level and the disorder is identified only during routine blood chemistry studies. If a patient complains of weakness, headache, chills, tingling in the extremities or mouth, cold, clammy skin, thirst, hunger, or apprehension or all of these, he or she may be manifesting initial signs of hypoglycemia. Other symptoms include diaphoresis, decreased levels of consciousness, and changes in vital signs. Hypoglycemia can progress to a seizure disorder if untreated.

Treatment depends on the cause. Hypoglycemia often occurs in the total parenteral nutrition patient whose glucose infusion has been abruptly decreased or terminated. After solution flow interruption, serum insulin levels remain elevated longer than serum glucose levels, and this can cause an insulin rebound phenomenon. If a catheter becomes kinked, the flow rate is decreased. If a patient unknowingly bends the intravenous tubing during position change, the flow rate will decrease and may even stop. This, of course, adds the complication of a clotted catheter, which necessitates catheter change, to the hypoglycemic state.

When a patient is transported to another area of the hospital (e.g., for testing), it is important to ensure continuity of solution flow rate. If a nurse cannot accompany the patient and the patient is unable to accurately regulate the infusion, nursing personnel in the area of destination should be alerted so that they may become responsible for flow rate maintenance. Remember that this is not just another I.V.; if no one is able to assume responsibility for the patient's flow rate, it is unfair to send the patient out of the clinical area.

HYPERGLYCEMIA AND HYPEROSMOLARITY

When the body's ability to metabolize the glucose in TPN solutions is inadequate, hyperglycemia occurs. Initial glucose intolerance has already been discussed. However, unchecked, progressive glucose intolerance can lead to the life-threatening complication of hyperglycemic, hyperosmolar, nonketotic coma. Marked hyperglycemia and glycosuria may lead to an osmotic diuresis accompanied by dehydration, electrolyte imbalance, and a decreasing level of consciousness that can result in a comatose state, leading to death, if untreated. Reversal of this state requires immediate discontinuation of the TPN solution, aggressive fluid and electrolyte replacement, and correction of hyperglycemia by insulin administration and correction of acidosis with bicarbonates [18].

INTRAVENOUS LIPIDS

Until I.V. fat became commercially available in the United States, it was not possible to provide true, *total* parenteral nutrition, because fat is an essential nutrient. There are two principal reasons why I.V. fat is administered: to prevent and/or treat essential fatty acid deficiency (EFAD) and to utilize fat as a major energy source in the nutritional regimen.

EFAD can be detected both biochemically and clinically. Biochemical lesions have been reported as early as 3–7 days following initiation of TPN, although clinical signs seem to take 3–4 weeks of dietary inadequacy before appearing. Biochemical lesions are diagnostic of EFAD and, thus, we now know that this deficiency state may exist in occult form for weeks before becoming clinically evident. Some clinical signs and symptoms of EFAD are dry or scaling skin, thinning hair, thrombocytopenia, and liver function abnormalities.

Because EFAD is associated with decreased ability to heal wounds, adverse effects on red cell membranes, and a defect in prostaglandin synthesis [15] these disorders are ample reasons to be concerned with prevention of this deficiency state.

When fat is used as an energy source, it offers the advantage of high caloric yield, 9 kcal per gm versus carbohydrate's lower value of 4 kcal per gm. Initially, a great deal of controversy surrounded the question of whether fat is as effective a protein-sparing calorie as glucose. Now it is generally considered to be so in a normal and moderately stressed person. However, fat is probably not as efficacious as carbohydrate in the severely stressed or, particularly, septic patient. Thus, the conventional central venous administration of hypertonic glucose and amino acids should probably be relied upon in these patients.

If fat is used as a major caloric source in TPN therapy, the amount of glucose in the system can be decreased and a peripheral vein approach to TPN becomes possible. Fat emulsions 10% are isotonic and therefore not sclerotic to veins. Intralipid 20%* has an osmolarity of 330 mOsm per liter, making it also suitable for peripheral administration.

Although the amount of glucose in this dual system is less than the conventional central vein approach, it is often still hypertonic. When this is so, simultaneous infusion of fat and the dextrose-amino acids solution is controlled better by pumps. Use of pumps ensures constant infusion of prescribed rates and causes dilution of the hypertonic glucose, avoiding sclerosis of the veins.

When the dextrose concentration of a simultaneous infusion is not hypertonic and a gravity flow set-up is used, it is sometimes necessary to hang the fat container slightly higher to allow unimpeded flow. A practical limitation of this approach is that continued venous access often becomes a problem in critically ill patients who require multiple venipunctures.

---

*KabiVitrum Inc. Alameda, Ca.

Fat emulsions available in the U.S. today are:

Intralipid 10% and 20%

Lyposin 10% and 20%*

Travamulsion 10% and 20%†

Soyacal 10% and 20%‡

Practical nursing considerations when administering I.V. fat are as follows:

1. Fat emulsions 10% provide 1.1 calorie per milliliter and have an osmolarity of approximately 280 mOsm per liter.
2. Fat emulsions 20% provide 2.0 calories per milliliter and have an osmolarity of approximately 330 mOsm per liter.
3. Before infusing, inspect the emulsion for separation or an oily appearance. If either of these conditions exists, the fat should not be infused because there may be a disturbance of the emulsion.
4. Be aware that it may be advisable to infuse fat emulsions through a non-PVC I.V. tubing. This is because conventional (PVC) I.V. tubing contains a plasticizer, Diethyl Hexyl Phthalate (DEHP) that is extracted from PVC by fat-containing fluids [22].
5. Nothing should be added to I.V. fat-emulsion containers as this could cause instability of the emulsion. One exception to this practice is mentioned in the Liposyn package insert — that heparin has been shown to be stable when added to this emulsion at a concentration of 1 to 2 units per milliliter.
6. Filters should not be used with I.V. fat as they will clog the filter and/or disturb the emulsion.
7. Refrigeration of fat emulsion is no longer required, but it should not be stored above 25°C/77°F (Intralipid 10% and 20%) or above 30°C/86°F (Liposyn 10%). IV fat should be protected from freezing and discarded if it does.
8. Fat is never to be reused, i.e., stored in partially used containers; it is supplied in single-dose containers. This is an important Infection Control principle when using any single-dose container because fats do not contain preservatives. Also, it has been demonstrated that I.V. fat contaminated with pathogens supports luxuriant growth of some of these organisms.
9. The Center for Disease Control (CDC) recommends that I.V. fat hang no longer than 12 hours [20].

---

*Abbott Laboratories, North Chicago, Ill.
†Travenol Laboratories, Deerfield, Ill.
‡Alpha Therapeutic Corp., Los Angslas, Ca.

10. Fat can be infused as a solo infusion or simultaneously with the dextrose-amino acids solution, through a Y-connector located near the infusion site. Connection at this point, *proximal* to the catheter hub, limits the amount of mixing time with simultaneously infused solutions decreasing the likelihood of interactions.

11. Dosage and infusion rates are dependent upon product concentration, the patient's age, and the stage of therapy. It is extremely important that the nurse be familiar with the manufacturer's current recommendations for use. Initial infusion rates are very slow for a limited period of time and the patient is carefully observed for adverse reactions. Maximum daily dose should not be exceeded, in order to decrease the likelihood of adverse reaction.

12. The patient's ability to eliminate infused fat from the circulation should be observed; lipemia must clear between daily infusions.

13. Administration of I.V. fat is contraindicated in patients with disturbances in normal fat metabolism such as pathologic hyperlipemia, lipoid nephrosis, or acute pancreatitis if accompanied by hyperlipemia.

14. A full product disclosure, the package insert, contains a lengthy listing of precautions and adverse acute and delayed reactions. It is important for the nurse to become aware of these precautions, but it is equally important to follow the correct guidelines for administration and to expect that once this is done, fat administration is usually safe and uneventful.

15. There are distinct warnings applied to I.V. fat administration in premature and small-for-gestational-age infants, reemphasizing the need for careful adherence to the manufacturer's specified guidelines.

HOME HYPERALIMENTATION

Home total parenteral nutrition (HTPN) is a special dimension of TPN therapy (see also Chapter 25). Patients who administer their own parenteral nutrition at home experience fewer and shorter hospitalizations and an improved overall quality of life. Since the advent of TPN has increased survival rates in various disease entities (e.g., mesenteric thrombosis), HTPN can be offered to patients as an alternative to prolonged or, perhaps, life-long institutionalization.

There are as many approaches to the methods of teaching and maintaining patients on HTPN as there are doctors who insert the long-term catheters. We intend to offer background information and an introduction to the philosophy and techniques of HTPN as practiced by the University of Cincinnati Medical Center.

Indications

The course of HTPN may be either temporary, to permit rest of the bowel, or permanent, to provide complete nutrition for the patient who has minimal or nonexistent absorptive capabilities. Some of the conditions which may result in the need for HTPN include Crohn's disease, short bowel syndrome, radiation enteritis, and intestinal fistulas.

History

As the specialty of TPN therapy became increasingly sophisticated, it became evident that some patients requiring TPN can be maintained at home. Once it was established that these patients could tolerate intermittent, or cyclic, TPN infusions, the need for a long-term, convenient access to the central venous system was recognized. The daily heparin-locking of the I.V. system showed that subclavian catheters are not easily maintained with self-care because they are too difficult for the patient to reach. They also do not afford the added protection of a long, subcutaneous tunnel exit. In the late 1960s and early 1970s, arteriovenous (AV) shunts and fistulas were attempted for administration of HTPN but were unsatisfactory because "although patients with bowel disease have normal clotting mechanisms, their blood vessels are in poor condition" [19].

The Tenckhoff catheter, used for peritoneal dialysis, was then redesigned as a right atrial central venous catheter [27] and was the precursor of today's HTPN catheters, commonly known as the Hickman and the Broviac catheters. The Broviac catheter was developed first and has a narrower lumen than the Hickman catheter. The larger bore size of the Hickman catheter allows for blood withdrawal and administration of other medications when necessary. A new catheter, called "the double lumen," which fuses both catheters together has been advantageous to clinicians administering advanced treatments to oncology patients who require multiple blood tests, transfusions, and chemotherapy. The Hickman side is used for withdrawing blood and administering medications, and the Broviac is preserved solely for the infusion of hyperalimentation thus reducing violation of the TPN line.

These catheters are made of soft rubber silicone material, which allegedly decreases thrombosis associated with long-term polyvinylchloride catheters. The length of the catheter allows it to be tunneled subcutaneously to an exit site which permits convenient handling in self-care (see Figure 21.11). Tunneling the catheter may contribute to improved asepsis of the catheter, although placing the catheter exit site in distal proximity to the venous entry has not yet proven to be an effective means of preventing catheter-related sepsis.

Implantable vascular access devices are often replacing external central venous catheters (see Chapter 19).

Catheter Placement

Access to the central venous system is usually done surgically under general anesthesia although some doctors utilize heavy sedation and perform the catheter insertion under local anesthesia. As with any surgical procedure, the patient should be instructed about what to expect postoperatively. The nurse who will be doing the postoperative teaching should help in the selection and marking of the catheter exit site, just as enterostomal therapists participate in the choice of ostomy location. Careful site selection provides the patient with easy access to the site and avoids frustrations such as having to wear the catheter under a bra or belt.

Catheter placement begins with a cutdown of the cephalic, jugular, or subclavian vein. The catheter is then threaded through this entry into the superior vena cava. Correct placement of the tip is confirmed by fluoroscopy or x-ray before the catheter is sutured into place. The extravenous portion of the

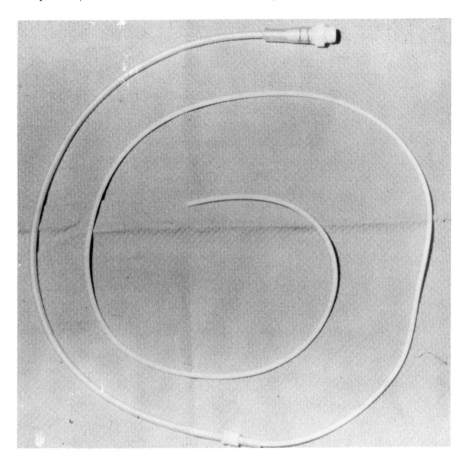

FIGURE 21.11
The Hickman catheter.

catheter is pulled through a subcutaneous tunnel to the predetermined exit site. The exit site is then dressed (see Dressing Change Procedures below).

Postoperatively, the patient may either receive continuous TPN infusions or begin cyclic infusions immediately. The readiness of both the staff and the patient will help the doctor in making this timely decision. Several situations, such as staffing patterns or the patient's progress in recovering from his primary disease, may necessitate maintaining the patient on continuous infusion.

Patient Teaching

Once the decision to employ HTPN has been made, the teaching process should begin immediately. At first, the entire process may be overwhelming to both the patient and his or her family. The patient needs help not only in learning these new and probably totally unfamiliar procedures but also in adapting to a drastic change in life-style. Extra time may be needed at some point in the teaching process for the patient to grieve the loss this change represents to his or her life. Therefore, the teaching process should be open-ended.

In our experience, it has been accomplished in a period ranging from 2 weeks to 2 months.

We begin teaching by having a general discussion with the patient during which the overall plan is explained in detail. If the patient has doubts about being able to perform the procedures, a member of the family or support group is taught. Early involvement of the family is imperative to assure continued and adequate care in the event the patient becomes incapable of caring for him- or herself at some later date. For the purpose of this text, we will assume that the patient performs the procedures independently.

Goals for day-to-day activities concerned with HTPN are delineated in the nursing care plan. At the University of Cincinnati Medical Center, all patients are admitted to the same clinical floor; this fosters continuity of care. The nurses on this unit are supervised and certified to teach the home patients in the same manner that the general staff nurses are trained to change routine TPN dressings.

Methods of instruction are no different from those generally used throughout all of nursing practice. In the beginning someone, usually a family member, reads the procedural step-by-step directions to the patient. These instructions may also be printed in large type on cue cards and propped up so that the patient can read them. Another format some patients like is a tape cassette containing the directions that is operated by a foot pedal during the procedure.

There are six basic components of patient education: (1) the principles of asepsis, (2) solution administration and set-up, (3) starting procedure (including volumetric pump use), (4) discontinuing or heparinizing (capping), (5) site care, and (6) self-evaluation. Each patient is given an individual program of instruction. Procedures are often rewritten many times before the one most suited to the patient's needs is finally adopted. Some patients require steps specified down to the smallest detail, while others perform quite well with more general statements. Following sections describe the basic components of the patient's learning process.

Principles of Asepsis

The patient should thoroughly understand the concepts of asepsis before any of the other teaching steps can begin. This understanding may be achieved in many ways — through the use of books, pictures, descriptions, demonstrations, and repetitive practice sessions. One concept that is reinforced from the beginning is, "If in doubt, throw it out"; guessing is never worth the risk. After procedures have been demonstrated, the patient practices simple techniques while the nurse observes critically. Supplies are left with the patient so that he or she may begin to practice putting on sterile gloves, opening sterile packages, using a syringe, and preparing medications. Before the patient performs the procedures with his or her own catheter, a "practice" catheter may be taped to the skin so that a simulated situation may develop dexterity without risk. Once the patient demonstrates competence in maintaining asepsis, the teaching progresses.

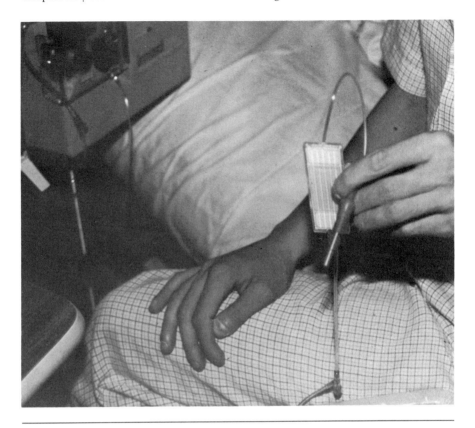

FIGURE 21.12
The patient has just primed the filter with constant awareness of asepsis in order to preserve sterility of the tubing.

Solution Administration and Set-Up

Our patients do not mix their own solutions, as is the pratice in some HTPN programs. Instead, they pick up premixed solution in 2- or 3-liter bags from the outpatient pharmacy 3 times each week. Other necessary equipment includes: a low-pressure volumetric infusion pump, an I.V. administration set, an in-line air-eliminating filter, a sterile cannula, tape, and a clean container to collect solution as it is primed through the tubing.

Solution is inspected for clarity and the bag is checked for leaks and the correct label, including specific contents and correct expiration date. Then the work surface is cleansed with alcohol and the patient puts on a mask and washes his or her hands with soap and water. Next, the solution bag is spiked according to the manufacturer's directions and hung on the I.V. pole. The pump tubing is then primed according to directions, the filter is attached and primed (see Figure 21.12), and a sterile needle cover is placed on the filter's distal Luer tip to protect it from contamination. All I.V. tubing and filter connections without Luer lock fittings are secured with tape to prevent accidental separation. Finally, the tubing is placed so that the patient can easily reach it when it is time to connect it to the catheter.

Starting Procedure (Including Volumetric Pump Use)
After solution priming is completed, the patient prepares the pump by setting the beginning rate and volume to be infused. The usual rate schedule for our patients is 60 ml for the first hour, 200 ml for 8–9 hours, tapered to 80 ml for 1 hour, and 40 ml for the last hour.

A volumetric pump is used that automatically alarms and converts to a keep-open rate when it has delivered the preset volume to be infused. This is critical because an infusion complete alarm that completely stops delivery of solution can cause clotting of the catheter. Patients like the volume-to-be-infused alarm and the automatic conversion to a keep-open rate because it allows them a more restful sleep. They know the machine will alert them when it is time to change the rate and when the infusion is finished, and that it will do this without shutting off and risking a clotted catheter.

An additional safety factor of the alarm-equipped infusion system is the air-in-line detector, which sounds an alarm when a volume of air less than 0.05 ml passes to the distal side of the cassette. It then alerts the patient to clear the air from the line. Further, this pump cannot inadvertently be placed into a free-flow situation, which could overload the patient's system with hypertonic, hyperosmolar solution.

These are significant points to consider when selecting a safe pump for patients' HTPN. Most importantly the pump should be a low-pressure machine which conforms to the specifications of the Broviac or Hickman catheters.

Other equipment needed to start the infusion includes a sterile dressing kit comprising gauze sponges, tape, gloves, scissors, and antimicrobial swabs, a sterile towel, face masks, a rubber-shod or toothless clamp, and a waste receptacle. Our patients use a sterile kit for this procedure; it provides a sterile field and nearly all of the items needed. The hospital may prepackage and sterilize all items used for each procedure. Many manufacturers now express an interest in preparing customized kits. The convenience of this should be carefully weighed against its cost-effectiveness.

The patient begins by washing his or her hands, cleaning the work surface with alcohol, masking, and then rewashing the hands. A sterile field is formed when the kit is opened and any other necessary items such as extra gauze sponges are dropped onto it. The tape anchoring the catheter to the skin is removed and a sterile towel is opened and placed on the lap. Then the tape securing the catheter-cap junction is removed and the junction is carefully dropped onto the sterile towel. It is important to point out that human hands *do not touch* the catheter junction; rather, the catheter is held behind the ridges of the entry port. During the procedure, equipment is always onto a *new* sterile gauze sponge because the catheter and I.V. tubing have contaminated the original sterile towel. New sterile sponges are picked up by one corner, opened lengthwise in the process, and dropped down onto the towel. The catheter junction rests in the fold of the gauze so it may be covered over (see Figure 21.13). This is repeated *every* time the catheter junction is placed down.

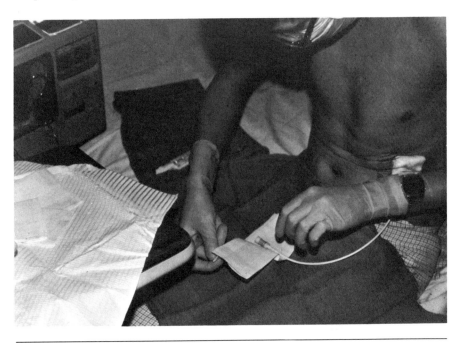

FIGURE 21.13
The patient places the catheter into the center of a new sterile gauze pad, which is now being folded over.

Next, the patient gloves and arranges the materials in the kit. The catheter is picked up behind the ridges and catheter-cap junction is prepped with antimicrobial solution (see Figure 21.14) and allowed to dry for 2 minutes. Then the catheter is placed on a new sterile gauze sponge and firmly clamped with an instrument that is then gently dropped onto the towel edge. The catheter-cap is untwisted, removed, and discarded and the I.V. tubing is then inserted into the catheter and twisted securely to ensure a tight fit. Once again, the junction is dropped onto a new gauze sponge. An important step to prevent clotting from blood backflow follows.

> The clamp is held with one hand while the other hand rests on the "on-off" button of the pump; the catheter is clamped at exactly the same time that the machine is turned off (see Figure 21.15).

Again, the junction is rechecked for security and reprepped as before. Gloves are removed and any excess powder is wiped off the hands away from the sterile field. The catheter tubing junction is not a Luer lock and must be secured by using both crosswise and lengthwise pieces of tape. The patient carefully avoids touching the adhesive back of the tape and places tabs at both ends of the tape so that it can easily be removed. Then the catheter, I.V. tubing, and filter are re-anchored to the patient's skin (see Figure 21.16).

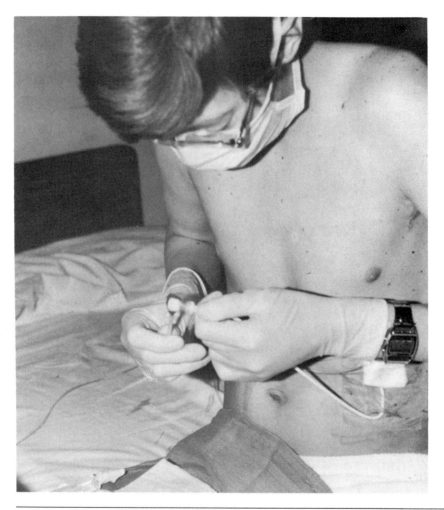

FIGURE 21.14
The patient is prepping the catheter-cap function with antimicrobial solution.

Discontinuing or Heparinizing (Capping)
After the appropriate tapering schedule has been observed, the patient is ready to discontinue the solution and attach the cap and go on to perform activities of daily living such as going to work, school, or on vacation. Supplies used in this procedure are similar to those for in the starting procedure with certain additions: a sterile Luer lock cap, a sterile 6-ml cc Luer lock syringe, an antimicrobial pad, and a unit-dose vial of heparin solution.

The sterile field is prepared as before, with all aspects of asepsis maintained as previously described. Five ml heparin are withdrawn from the prepped vial into the Luer lock syringe, and all air is expelled from the syringe. The needle cover is replaced, the needle removed, and the syringe carefully placed onto the sterile field with the tip pointing inward toward the center

Chapter 21 | Total Parenteral Nutrition — Nursing Practice

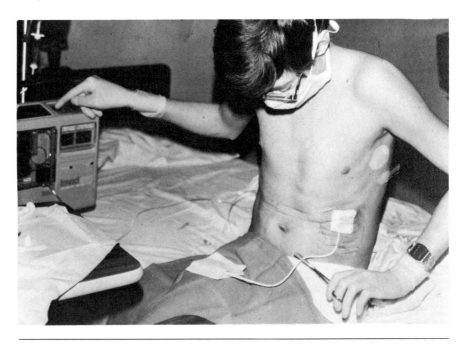

FIGURE 21.15
The catheter is clamped at exactly the same time that the machine is turned off.

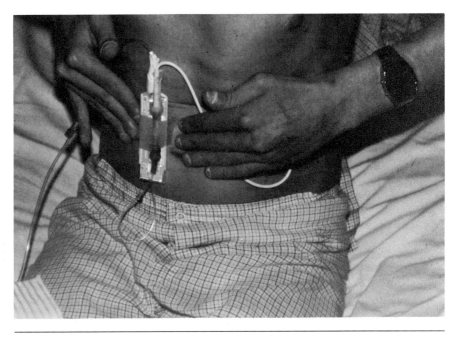

FIGURE 21.16
At the completion of the starting procedure, the patient is anchoring the catheter, I.V. tubing, and filter to his skin.

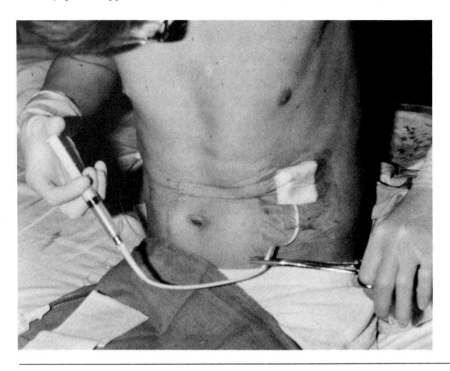

FIGURE 21.17
The patient holds the clamp in place while he gently and slowly injects the heparin solution.

portion of the sterile field. The I.V. tubing–catheter junction is placed on a sterile towel as previously described. After gloving, the Luer lock cap is placed upright so that it may be filled later. The junction is prepped with the same technique described earlier.

Next come two important steps that should be performed almost simultaneously: first the catheter is clamped, and then the machine is turned off without any time delay, to avoid backflow of blood. The patient removes the I.V. tubing and discards it.

After being rechecked to make sure all air has been purged from it, the heparin syringe is then tightly secured to the catheter. Heparin is gently and slowly injected as the catheter is unclamped. The clamp is kept open but in position around the catheter throughout this maneuver in case the syringe dislodges or the catheter ruptures (see Figure 21.17). After 3.5 ml are injected, and before the syringe is empty, the catheter is clamped while the plunger is moving forward. Remaining heparin is used to fill the Luer lock cap, which is picked up cautiously, avoiding contamination of the inside. The *catheter* is placed down into the cap to avoid spilling heparin and to cause displacement of air (see Figure 21.18). This is a Luer lock junction; therefore, the cap must

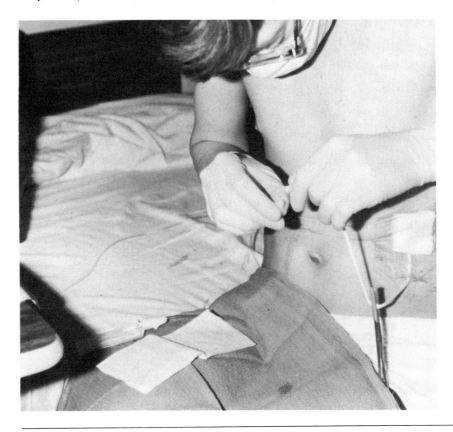

FIGURE 21.18
After the Luer lock has been filled with heparin, the catheter is placed down into the cap to avoid spilling heparin and to displace air.

be screwed on tightly for a secure fit. Lastly, the junction is reprepped and taped as before, and the capped catheter is anchored to the skin.

Site Care
Our patients are taught the same procedure for dressing change as previously described in this chapter, using the material that is best suited and most manageable for them. The dressing change procedure is usually the least threatening procedure for the patient to learn and it often contributes to increased confidence through quick accomplishment. It may be wise to teach this step first once the patient accomplishes mastery of aseptic technique and dexterity in handling the catheter.

Some doctors permit their patients to swim after the exit site is well healed. This process may take up to 6 months. The dressing will usually need to be changed after swimming. During dressing changes, the patient is told to carefully inspect the site for any changes in the skin condition such as redness, irritation, exudate, edema, or any deviation from the normal.

Self-Evaluation

Patients at the University of Cincinnati are taught about potential complications of TPN and the symptoms for each complication. The importance of record keeping and reporting any deviation from the norms they have been taught is understood.

Before being discharged, patients must be able to perform all procedures without prompting or getting corrections from the nurse observer. At home, a daily diary is kept that includes the following:

1. Daily weights.
2. Daily temperatures.
3. Daily urinary sugar and acetone.
4. Condition of site at dressing change.
5. Eating habits and amounts of food intake.
6. Any problems or unusual occurrences during infusion.

This record helps the patient to monitor his or her own progress and has proven to be an excellent report upon return to the clinic for follow-up visits.

Upon discharge, patients are given a letter which summarizes this daily routine. In addition, they are given the telephone numbers of staff members whom they should contact with any questions or problems. They must know that help is available to them 24 hours a day, 7 days a week. After the patient has been home for a few days, one or more of the members of the hyperalimentation team visit and help with any concerns.

GENERAL CONSIDERATIONS

Patients who are not eating require I.V. fat. They can be taught to administer I.V. fat following their routine cycle on prescribed days. To do this, they must learn how to change from one tubing to the next. A specific procedure is written to include the first stage of the stopping procedure, to the point of clamping the catheter and disconnecting the I.V. tubing; the new I.V. tubing is then inserted and the fat infusion begun by resetting the pump with the new rate and volume to be infused.

Two potential catheter-related problems are clotting of the catheter and catheter breakage. Heparin is injected into the catheter between infusions to prevent clotting. Should a clot develop, however, the patient must notify the physician immediately. The doctor may then instill more concentrated heparin solution at spaced intervals to gently clear the clot. Because added pressure could rupture the catheter, if that is unsuccessful the catheter must be removed [26].

Damage to the catheter is avoided through the use of rubber padded or toothless clamps. Should the catheter be damaged through incorrect use or through an inadvertent error such as accidental cutting during dressing change, the catheter must be clamped immediately between the damaged area and the exit site, and the doctor must be notified immediately. The catheter can then be repaired with kits that are available from the manufacturer [10].

Caring for patients on HTPN affords the nurse the opportunity to give *total* care to one patient. For the nurse, this is an exciting challenge: to help another human being go through the metamorphosis from near-total dependency to a level of independence that allows personal growth and contribution not possible without HTPN.

PSYCHOLOGICAL ASPECTS

Until the 1960s, it was impossible for a human being to survive without eating. The era of TPN has created a new population of patients, who often experience total oral deprivation for prolonged periods of time. The analytically curious will find this concept fascinating. Surely there are psychological ramifications associated with the state of oral deprivation, and someday a better understanding will provide useful information that contributes to a more supportive approach to TPN patients.

What must it be like to gain weight and sometimes grow without swallowing a morsel of food? It must also seem curious to be attached by tubing to a mechanical life-giving nutrient system. Although it is true that medical personnel frequently refer to a TPN catheter as "the lifeline," it is equally common for patients to use this terminology spontaneously; an apt analogy is the umbilical cord. Further, the necessity of an artificial feeding system also creates a forced dependency state that has emotional and psychological components.

In many ways, the topic, "Psychological Aspects of TPN Therapy," creates more questions than it provides answers. On the other hand, there are some practical considerations that should help the nurse to provide a more supportive approach to these patients.

Certain elements of emotional support seem basic and necessary to the person receiving TPN [10]. None is presented as absolute fact, but does represent some of the experience of one nurse who has known more than 8,000 patients receiving hyperalimentation therapy. The expressed needs of these patients make the following issues more than esoteric considerations; they point the way toward a plan of care which should decrease patient anxiety and allay sometimes terrifying fears. Hallucinations of taste and smell have been reported by hyperalimentation patients. As the period of "nothing by mouth" becomes prolonged, this phenomenon seems to increase. Varied stimuli such as television commercials, daydreams, a roommate's meal tray, or even simple conversations about food have been associated with this experience. We noticed it so often that we began to forewarn patients that it is not unusual to imagine one tastes, smells, or even sees food while undergoing hyperalimentation therapy. Although the reasons for these phenomena are unclear, we know that many patients are relieved after being told that somewhat bizarre perceptions are not unusual. Often, patients have already experienced hallucinations and were worried that something was terribly wrong with them. We now recognize that some of these experiences are caused by biochemical deficiency states.

Preoccupation with food is not relegated totally to unconscious stimuli. Patients actually *think* about food and questions such as the following are not uncommon: "Will I be able to eat again?" "If my appetite is gone, why do I still miss food?" "How can they really be sure they are giving me the right diet, with nothing missing?" We do not dramatize all of this, but we are ever alert to the mention of food. It is important to offer support and reassurance to the patient receiving TPN. The nurse should point out that hyperalimentation therapy is not irreversible; in fact, as soon as physical conditions permit, the patient may begin to eat while still undergoing therapy.

Many patients become angry or sleepy at mealtime. It is therefore considerate to locate the patient's room away from the kitchen if possible. The aroma and sight of dozens of meals is often frustrating to one who cannot eat. In fact, some patients have recounted impulses to leap out of bed and grab other patients' meals. Again, this has happened often enough that we now tell patients, in a calm, pleasant fashion, that others have felt this way, and they might also.

We began offering these reassurances to patients with trepidation since there is always the possibility that direct suggestion will put ideas into a person's head. Strikingly, we have not witnessed this. Rather a spontaneous smile of relief and a sheepish admission have often revealed an ongoing experience within the patient as we chatted about this intriguing psychodynamic process.

Because TPN therapy is still new in many hospitals, a great deal of teaching occurs at the bedside, making patients aware that something special is happening to them. Quite often a hyperalimentation team of hospital personnel visits them; this enhances the patients' feelings of uniqueness. There is a tendency for patients to be guarded and protective toward their "lifeline," so it is important for the nurse to encourage as much ambulation as possible. As long as the tubing junctions are secured and the intravenous pole is freely mobile, patients can safely ambulate about the hospital. In fact, active exercise helps prevent the catabolic breakdown of lean tissue mass which often results from inactivity.

The absence of taste is unpleasant physically and psychologically. Some of our patients have enjoyed flavored lip balms or a variety of mouth washes, which at least offer some experience of different tastes. One of our cancer patients had a pitcher of martinis at his bedside; he rinsed his mouth each afternoon and evening. This routine provided the man's family an opportunity to mix their loved one his favorite cocktail, and it afforded the patient some semblance of his normal pleasurable routine.

In addition to considering the aesthetic gratification a variety of tastes will provide, the nurse should carefully plan for consistent, correct mouth care. If the oral assessment is overlooked or adequate mouth care is not provided, the NPO patient may develop parotitis, glossy tongue, inflamed, dry, uncomfortable areas, and oral lesions.

TPN patients are already under a great deal of stress, and being deprived of food often adds to this stress. When the nurse has properly explained total nutrition by vein to the patient and his or her family, however, they are usually quite relieved to know that nutrition has not been ignored. In some countries and in primitive societies, it is common practice for the family to carry food to a hospitalized relative. In the United States we often become so involved in providing highly technical therapy that we forget about this basic concern. It is quite usual, after a family teaching session, for a relative to remark, "Oh good, I couldn't figure out how he'd ever get well without getting enough food." This concept is simple and logical, but until the 1960s and Dudrick's work, many patients did not get well because they could not eat.

In summary, explanation of the procedures, feedback for ascertaining whether one's message has been perceived as intended, reassurance to the patient, and careful planning for managing treatment greatly help the patient receiving TPN.

FUTURE TRENDS

In its initial phase, TPN has been recognized as an exciting new method of therapeutic intervention that has helped many patients and saved many lives. Many health professionals — particularly those associated with this rapidly developing, successful field — have also benefited.

Disease-specific solutions are now emerging, enhancing opportunities to influence disease outcome in new ways. Existing therapy will also be improved as nutritional biochemistry advances and better ways to define complete intravenous nutrition requirements are realized.

In all phases of TPN, nurses are immensely important because they provide both a great deal of the support and most of the day-to-day care that these patients require. Specifically, the ever-present nurse is usually the one who makes the initial observations that result in necessary changes in the patient's treatment plan.

As the specialty evolves, nurses must keep their knowledge current with advances in the field. But, equally important, nurses must preserve the simple attention to basic principles of care that characterizes nursing practice associated with TPN.

HYPERALIMENTATION NURSING STANDARDS OF PRACTICE

The following standards have been adopted by the National Intravenous Therapy Association, Inc. (NITA). They are professional nursing standards that serve as guidelines of practice and were developed by NITA's Special Interest Group (SIG) on hyperalimentation. Their application is limited to the adult, nonburned patient receiving central venous TPN in the hospital. Subsequent standards that apply to other patients receiving parenteral nutrition will be written by the SIG.

Credentialling is available for nutrition support nurses through their own association.

Professional nursing standards are not absolutes; they are guidelines, appropriate for every nurse's practice, and are constantly subject to investigation and improvement as the specialty evolves.

As you examine these standards, consider that they exist to protect both the patient's and nurse's rights and therefore warrant compliance.

Director

Rita Colley, R.N., Former Clinical Nurse Specialist/Administrative Director, Hyperalimentation Unit, University of Cincinnati Hospitals, General Division, Cincinnati, Ohio.

Committee Members

Laurie Appleby, R.N., Clinical Nurse, Nutritional Support Unit, Peter Bent Brigham Hospital, Boston, Massachusetts.

Elizabeth Ayello, M.S., R.N., Clinical Nurse Specialist-Surgery, Booth Memorial Medical Center, Flushing, New York.

Julia S. Garner, R.N., M.N., Chief, Consultation and Training, Hospital Infections Branch, Bureau of Epidemiology, Center for Disease Control, Atlanta, Georgia.

JoAnn Gough, R.N., I.V. Therapy Supervisor, Pharmacy Department, Virginia Mason Hospital, Seattle, Washington.

Michelle M. Maher, R.N., Clinical Research Nurse-T.P.N., National Institute of Health, Bethesda, Maryland.

Kate Persse, R.N., Assistant Director for Infection Control Utilization Review, Sandlewood Hospital, Hawthorne, California.

Jeanne M. Wilson, R.N., B.S., Hyperalimentation Nurse Clinician, Nutritional Support Unit, Massachusetts General Hospital, Boston, Massachusetts.

Advisors

Josef E. Fischer, M.D., Christian R. Holmes Professor of Surgery, Chairman, Department of Surgery, University of Cincinnati Medical Center, Cincinnati, Ohio.

Carl H. Iseman, Associate Administrator, University of Cincinnati Hospitals, General Division, Cincinnati, Ohio.

Eli Studebaker, R.N., Director, Invasive Therapy Services, Grant Hospital of Chicago, Chicago, Illinois.

Catherine J. Sullivan, M.Ed., Senior Administrative Assistant, Department of Surgery, University of Cincinnati Medical Center, Cincinnati, Ohio.

Philosophy

The National Intravenous Therapy Association (NITA) upholds the belief that only registered professional nurses who have completed the basic educational requirements adopted under the Standards of Education of the Association shall practice parenteral nutrition intravascular (PNIV) nursing.

As professionals concerned with assessing, establishing, delivering, evaluating, and improving the quality of care, we have a responsibility to control our PNIV nursing practice and to evaluate the competency of the PNIV nurse and the quality of nursing practice.

Utilization of the nursing process, with special emphasis on intervention, is the basis of the holistic approach in providing PNIV nursing.

PNIV nursing encompasses education, management, technology, consultation, research, quality assurance and legalities as provided in health care facilities and in the community.

It is NITA's belief that the quality of care received by a patient in relation to his TPN therapy improves significantly when the care is given by a PNIV nurse. Moreover, the risk associated with this therapy is also reduced. The Association also believes that this care is further improved when practiced with other health care professionals concerned in the delivery of this specialized care.

Introduction

NITA has established the following nursing standards of practice as a model for those practicing PNIV nursing:

Standards

I. *Education*
   A. For NITA recognition to practice PNIV nursing, the registered professional nurse must complete the educational requirements as set forth by the Association. Education is fundamental to preparation for nursing practice in the art and science of parenteral nutrition.
   Continuing education and staff development is essential to sustain and advance PNIV nursing. Sharing this knowledge with other collaborative disciplines improves care.
   B. In keeping with the holistic approach to patient care, it is the registered professional nurse's responsibility to educate the patient and significant others who are involved in delivery of this PNIV specialty. Education and the patient's comprehension is documented, communicated to the appropriate person(s), and stored in a retrievable and accessible system.
   C. Effectiveness of teaching methods will be continually assessed and periodically evaluated by the registered professional PNIV nurse.

II. *Practice*
   Collaboration with other health care professionals provides a comprehensive approach to the PNIV nursing management of the patient. The registered professional nurse uses a holistic approach to the patient. The nursing process is the primary tool for delivery of PNIV nursing.

III. *Management*
   The PNIV nurse is the specialist in the management of PNIV nursing. Other management decisions that establish criteria for care and services delivered to patients receiving parenteral nutrition need PNIV nursing input to achieve optimal outcome.

IV. *Consultation*
   The PNIV nurse is an essential consultant to the health care profession, the community, and related industry. The constant and dominant themes of this consultation are patient advocacy and delivery of optimal PNIV care.

V. *Technology*

Sophisticated technology related to PNIV nursing is continually advancing. The PNIV nurse should continuously evaluate regimens and products used in this nursing specialty.

VI. *Research*

Research is an inherent component of PNIV nursing. Through research and its dissemination, the art and science of this nursing specialty will be advanced.

VII. *Quality Assurance*

All PNIV nurses are responsible for quality assurance as it relates to this specialty. The components of PNIV nursing associated with quality assurance and with monitoring the desired outcome must be identified. The patient receiving PNIV nursing must be guaranteed the highest level of care.

Assessment

The purpose of a nutritional assessment is to identify patients whose nutritional status is or may be potentially compromised. Observation and interview are the primary tools used to collect the data necessary for this assessment.

Recommendations of Practice

1. The nursing history should include a general overview of the patient's nutritional status and practices and should include the following:

    a. Admission weight and height

    b. Normal weight

    c. Recent weight loss

    d. Amount or frequency of oral intake

    e. Recent change in dietary intake or habits

    f. Food preferences — personal, ethnic, and religious

2. Physical assessment could include the following:

    a. Observation of condition of hair, nails, skin, mucous membrane, teeth, and mouth

    b. Body systems — pertinent to nutritional assessment

    c. Simple lab values: complete blood count with differential, serum albumin, serum transferrin

3. In the absence of a dietitian (or designated person) who performs a detailed and specific nutritional assessment on patients who are candidates for intravenous (IV) IV nutritional support, it may be the responsibility of the parenteral nutrition intravascular (PNIV) nurse to complete the assessment. This should include those parameters as established by individual institutional protocol for the administration of total parenteral nutrition (TPN).

4. Continuous nutritional assessments should be made at regular intervals and after any significant change in the patient's clinical status. This provides a monitor of any improvement or deterioration in the patient's nutritional status.

Infusates

The purpose is to insure safe initiation of the prescribed solution or emulsion. If possible, solutions should be admixed within a laminar flow unit (LFU) under pharmacy supervision according to hospital policy. The use of a closed transfer system is acceptable if an LFU is unavailable.

Recommendations of Practice

1. Refrigerate solution at 4°C until use.
2. Verify solution label with prescribed order and check expiration time and date.
3. Inspect solution container to insure the integrity of the container (i.e., that bottles are not cracked and bags are not punctured). Solution should be inspected for clarity to prevent infusion of possible contaminants or precipitates, and emulsion should be inspected for turbidity.
4. It is not recommended that IV fat be filtered.
5. Compatibility of solution ingredients must be authorized by the pharmacy or supported by published reference before admixing occurs.
6. The nurse should be familiar with manufacturer's current directions for infusates.
7. Amino acids/dextrose solution containers are to be discarded after 24 hours. Fat emulsion containers should not be hung for more than 12 hours.
8. When fat is infused simultaneously with an amino acids/dextrose solution, the fat should be infused as close to the catheter insertion site as possible (usually through a "Y-tube" connection) in order to prevent prolonged contact with the amino acids/dextrose solution. This should aid in preservation of the emulsion's stability.

Special Considerations

1. In the absence of a vacuum, a solution container should be covered with a sterile, air-tight, waterproof cover after admixture.
2. When admixing occurs outside the pharmacy, hospital policy should be strictly observed, practicing absolute aseptic technique.

Catheter Placement

The purpose is to provide a safe and effective mechanism for delivery of hypertonic nutrient solutions via the central venous system (CVS).

Recommendations of Practice

1. The nurse should know that the commonly accepted sites of vascular access to the CVS are the subclavian and internal jugular veins.
2. Isotonic solution should be infused at a slow flow rate until radiologic confirmation of the correct catheter tip position within the superior vena cava is documented.
3. Catheter placement should be explained to the patient, including the purpose and goal, a step-by-step description of the procedure, patient positioning, anti-air-embolism precautions, and possible discomforts.

4. The nurse should take an active role in maintaining asepsis while assisting the physician during catheter placement.
5. The nurse should be able to assess the patient's status for common complications and to intervene appropriately during and following catheter placement. The nurse should also assist the physician and help plan intervention should this be necessary.
6. The patency and position of the central venous (CV) catheter should be evaluated after catheter placement. Evaluations of patency and position should also continue throughout therapy.

Special Considerations

1. CVS catheter tip location other than the superior vena cava is occasionally used. These locations include the intrathoracic subclavian vein, innominate vein, and occasionally the right atrium for silastic catheters only.
2. Supplies should be conveniently located during CV catheter insertion to facilitate asepsis, to increase organizational efficiency, and to eliminate unnecessary delay if additional supplies are required. A "hyperalimentation cart" that contains all necessary supplies is an example of this.
3. Air embolism is a life-threatening complication that is potentially avoidable. A patient is at risk for air embolism when the CVS is open to the air during catheter placement or tubing changes, because of accidental disruption, and during and after catheter removal.

    The patient should be placed in the Trendelenburg position during CVS catheter placement and placed flat in bed performing the Valsalva maneuver (taking a deep breath and also bearing down while maintaining inspiration) during the appropriate times at catheter placement, tubing changes, and catheter removal.*

    The nurse should be able to recognize signs and symptoms of air embolism and know how to intervene when this complication occurs.

Catheter Site Care and Dressing Change

The purpose of PNIV catheter site care and dressing change is to provide regular, standardized catheter site inspection, site care, and to apply a sterile partial/total occlusive dressing. These measures should reduce or prevent the complication of catheter-related sepsis.

Recommendations of Practice

1. Catheter site care and dressing change should be performed every forty-eight to seventy-two hours and immediately if the dressing becomes soiled, wet, or loose.
2. Aseptic technique should be maintained during this procedure. The catheter insertion site should be scrubbed with a 1% to 2% iodine solution or tincture that is removed with 70% alcohol, or scrubbed

---

*Colley, Rita, Total Parenteral Nutrition. In Sally Millar, Leslie K. Sampson, Sister Maurita Soukup, and Sylvan Lee Weinberg (Eds.), *Methods in Critical Care: The AACN Manual*. Philadelphia: Saunders, 1980, pp. 417–440.

with a povidone-iodine solution and allowed to air dry. If the scrub is to be followed by application of a topical ointment, iodophor is the ointment of choice.* Then a sterile partial/total occlusive dressing should be applied.

Special Considerations:

1. An occlusive, waterproof dressing should be applied when a patient has a tracheostomy, burns, open wounds, or fistulas near the catheter site, or is in a high humidity environment.
2. Hair removal and use of a skin protector agent may be indicated.

Intravenous Administration Set Change

The purpose is changing the IV administration set is to prevent or minimize sepsis related to the IV delivery system.

Recommendations of Practice

1. To prevent air from entering the CV catheter system when the CV catheter is opened to the air, the system must be occluded with a clamp between the opening and the patient, or the patient must be flat in bed performing the Valsalva maneuver. This change must be done aseptically and quickly.
2. Tubing junctions should be secured by an appropriate method such as taping the junctions, with a Luer lock, or with junction clasping devices.
3. The IV administration set should be changed every 24 hours.
4. An appropriate method of indicating the date of change of the administration set should be employed.
5. Changing of the IV administration set should be carried out in a routine, standardized manner, preferably at the time the first solution container of the new day is hung.

Special Considerations

1. When using tape to secure junctions, minimal amounts should be used so that the tape can be removed easily when necessary.
2. If a filter is used, an air eliminator, in-line final IV filter, that is bacterial and particulate retentive, is preferred.

Infection Control

To minimize catheter-related sepsis, infection control is integrated into many aspects of TPN therapy including catheter placement, catheter care, solution preparation, and tubing change. Early recognition of the signs and symptoms of sepsis, as well as awareness that the patient may be a compromised host, will maximize the prevention of sepsis and insure appropriate intervention in a timely manner.

---

*Maki, D. G., and Band, J. D. "Study of Polyantibiotic and Iodophor Ointments in Prevention of Vascular Catheter-related Infection." U.S. Department of Health and Human Services, Public Health Service, International Conference on Nosocomial Infection. Madison, Wis.: University of Wisconsin, 1980, p. 36.

Recommendations of Practice

1. The patient's temperature should be measured and recorded at least three times per day. Any unusual change in temperature or the presence of fever should be reported and documented.
2. The CVS must not be violated by delivering piggy-back medications or bolus injections of medications, measuring CV pressure, or withdrawing blood through the catheter except at the time of catheter removal.
3. The nurse should be aware of the potential indicators of catheter-related sepsis and of appropriate nursing interventions. These indicators may include the following:
   a. Sudden increase in temperature
   b. Unexplained glucose intolerance
   c. Hypothermia
   d. Hemodynamic instability
4. Routine mouth care is advocated to promote oral hygiene and prevent complications such as parotitis.

Special Considerations

1. Collaboration with the hospital's infection control personnel is advocated strongly.
2. The only exception to not violating the CV catheter system is made for the administration of IV fat emulsion. However, even this violation of the system's integrity must be approved by hospital policy.

Metabolic Aspects

The nurse must know the metabolic implications of administering the nutritional components of TPN to recognize and maximize the benefits and minimize the risks and potential complications associated with this therapy.

Recommendations of Practice

1. Urine should be tested for glucosuria at least every six hours.
2. Daily weights should be obtained.
3. Daily intake and output should be charted.
4. Prescribed infusion should be maintained consistently at the designated flow rate.
5. Time-strip labels should be attached to each solution container used.
6. Active physical exercise should be encouraged to promote protein anabolism.
7. Vital signs should be monitored every eight hours.
8. The patient's skin turgor should be observed.
9. Dependent/generalized edema should be immediately recognized and reported.

10. Physical and mental changes should be observed and noted.
11. Radiological confirmation of correct catheter tip position must be known before initiating TPN solution.
12. The initial infusion of TPN solution should be increased only in gradual systematic increments in flow rate/volume to help avoid glucose intolerance.
13. The routine discontinuation of TPN solution involves gradual and systematic decrease in flow rate/volume to minimize the risk of rebound hypoglycemia. Occasionally there are indications for more rapid weaning. However, this increases the risk of hypoglycemia. Furthermore, when the TPN solution has been abruptly discontinued, the nurse should reassess the patient's acute/short-term need for alternative carbohydrate delivery.

Special Considerations

1. If metabolic aberrations occur, the nurse should be cognizant of the abnormal serum levels of glucose, electrolytes, vitamins, and/or trace elements that are relative to proper management.
2. Electronic infusion devices should be considered for the maintenance of a consistent rate of infusion.
3. A microdrip administration set may be considered when delivering low-volume infusions by mechanically unassisted gravity flow.
4. The presence of infection, stress, steroids, and other drugs may predispose the patient to glucose intolerance.
5. Certain drugs may interfere with accurate results and interpretations of urinary glucose tests.

Catheter Removal

The purpose is to discontinue the CV catheter in a safe and effective manner.

Recommendations of Practice

1. The nurse, as dictated by hospital policy, will remove the CV catheter using aseptic, no-touch technique.
2. Anti-air embolism precautions must be taken during this procedure.
3. A sterile occlusive dressing must be placed immediately over the catheter site for at least 48 hours and/or until the site is healed. Placing iodophor ointment over the skin tract should also help prevent air embolism by aiding in occlusion of the tract.
4. To ascertain complete removal of the catheter, the nurse will assess the length of the discontinued catheter and inspect visually the tip for smoothness.

Special Considerations

1. The nurse, as dictated by hospital policy, will culture the catheter appropriately in a routine, standardized manner, using aseptic, no-touch technique. This practice should be especially encouraged when

the catheter is suspected of being contaminated or when the patient has an unexplained fever.

2. A semi-quantitative method* of catheter culture is recommended.

REFERENCES

1. Abel, R. M., Beck, C. M., Abbott, W. M., Ryan, J. A. Jr., Barnett, G. O., and Fischer, J. E. Improved survival from acute renal failure after treatment with intravenous essential L-amino acids and glucose: Results of a prospective double-blind study. *N. Engl. J. Med.* 288:695–699, 1973.

2. Bjornson, H. S., Bjornson, A. B., Altemeier, W. A., Colley, R., and Fischer, J. E. Association between the number of microorganisms present at the catheter insertion site and the development of catheter-related infection in burned patients. Cincinnati, Ohio: University of Cincinnati College of Medicine, Department of Surgery.

3. Bjornson, H. S., Bjornson, A. B., Colley, R., and Fischer, J. E. Association between the numbers of microorganisms present at the catheter insertion site and the colonization of the central venous catheter in patients receiving total parenteral nutrition (TPN). Cincinnati, Ohio: University of Cincinnati Medical Center, Department of Surgery.

4. Block, P. C. Transvenous retrieval of foreign bodies in the cardiac circulation. *J.A.M.A.* 224:241, 1973.

5. Bottino, J., McCredie, K. B., Groschel, D. M., and Lawson, M. Long-term intravenous therapy with peripherally inserted silicone elastomer central venous catheters in patients with malignant diseases. *Cancer* 43:1937–1943, 1979.

6. Bower, R. H. A logical approach to catheter sepsis. Presented at the 9th Annual N.I.T.A. Convention, Boston, March, 1981.

7. Colley, R. Nursing in Parenteral Nutrition. In J. M. Greep, P. B. Soeters, R. I. C. Wesdorp, C. W. R. Phaf, and J. E. Fischer (eds.), *Current Concepts in Parenteral Nutrition.* Hague, Holland: Martinus Nijhoss Medical Division, 1976, pp. 85–95.

8. Colley, R., and Fischer, J. E. *Understanding Hyperalimentation: A Patient's Guide.* Cincinnati: Berman Printing Co., 1981.

9. Colley, R., and Phillips, K. Helping with Hyperalimentation. *Nursing '73,* July 1973.

10. Colley, R., and Wilson, J. M. Meeting patients' nutritional needs with hyperalimentation. *Nursing '79,* May–August, 1979.

11. Coppa, G., Gouge, T. H., and Mofstetter, S. R. Air embolism: A lethal but preventable complication of subclavian vein catheterization. *J.P.E.N.* 5(2):166–168, 1981.

12. Dudrick, S. J., and Rhoads, J. E. Total intravenous feeding. *Sci. Am.* 226:73–80, 1972.

13. Fischer, J. E. Nutritional support in the seriously ill patient. *Curr. Probl. Surg.* 17(9):482–510, 1980.

14. Flanagan, J. P., Gradisar, I. A., Gross, R. J., and Kelly, T. R. Air embolus — a lethal complication of subclavian venipuncture. *N. Engl. J. Med.* 281:488–489, 1969.

15. Freund, H., Floman, N., Schwartz, B., and Fischer, J. E. Essential fatty acid deficiency in total parenteral nutrition. *Ann. Surg.* 190:139, 1979.

16. Goldmann, D. A., and Maki, D. G. Infection control and total parenteral nutrition. *J.A.M.A.* 223:1360, 1973.

17. Grant, J. N. Patient care in parenteral hyperalimentation. *Nurs. Clin. North Am.* 8:165, 1973.

18. Grant, J. P. *Handbook of Total Parenteral Nutrition.* Philadelphia: Saunders, 1980, pp. 128–130.

---

*Rhame, Frank S., Maki, Dennis, G., and Bennett, John V. Intravenous Cannula-Associated Infections. In John V. Bennett and Philip S. Brachman (Eds.), *Hospital Infections.* Boston: Little, Brown, 1979, pp. 433–442.

19. Guidelines for Prevention of Intravascular Infections. Department of Health and Human Services, Hospital Infections Branch, Bacterial Diseases Division, Center for Infectious Diseases. NITA 5(1):39–50, 1982.
20. Maki, D. G. Growth properties of microorganisms in lipid for infusion and implications for infection control. (Abstracts of Original Papers, 7th Annual Education Conference, A.P.I.C., June 25, 1980.)
21. Maki, D. G., and MacCormick, K. N. Acetone "defatting" in cutaneous antisepsis. Abstracts of Original Papers, 7th Annual Education Conference, *A.P.I.C.*, June 25, 1980.
22. Nursing guide to dual-energy TPN administration. Berkeley, Calif.: Cutter Medical, Cutter Laboratories, 1981: Package insert for liposyn 10% fat emulsion. Abbott Laboratories, North Chicago, Ill.
23. Physicians' Order Form, Parenteral Nutrition Standing Orders, University of Cincinnati Hospitals, General Division, 1980.
24. Protocol for Parenteral Nutrition Patients. University of Cincinnati Hospitals, General Division, 1978.
25. Ryan, J. A., Jr. Complication of Total Parenteral Nutrition. In J. E. Fischer (ed.), *Total Parenteral Nutrition*. Boston: Little, Brown, 1975, pp. 55–100.
26. Ryan, J. A., Abel, R. M., Abbott, W. M., Hopkins, C. C., Chesney, T., Colley, R., Phillips, K., and Fischer, J. E. Catheter complications in total parenteral nutrition: A prospective study of 200 consecutive patients. *N. Engl. J. Med.* 290:757, 1974.
27. Scribner, B. H. History and development of home parenteral nutrition. *Home Parenteral Nutrition,* ASPEN symposium. New York: Pro Clinica, 1981, pp. 6–8.
28. Washington, J. A. II. Subject review, blood cultures, principles and techniques. *Mayo Clin. Proc.* 50:91–98, 1975.

REVIEW QUESTIONS

1. Intravenous fat must be refrigerated until use. True or false?
2. Acceptable catheter tip location(s) for a polyvinylchloride subclavian catheter placed to administer central hyperalimentation include _____ , _____ , and _____ .
3. For central venous hyperalimentation patients, air embolism precautions should be taken during _____ , _____ , and _____ .
4. In order to have 99 percent confidence of confirming existing bacteremia, how many blood cultures should be obtained within a 24-hour period?
5. Catheter-related sepsis in total parenteral nutrition patients most commonly occurs due to _____ .
6. In most adults, maximum rate of glucose utilization is between _____ gm to _____ gm of glucose per kilogram of body weight.
7. Name the drugs that (in high doses) may render a false-positive result when the copper-reduction method is used to measure urinary glucose determinations.
8. Name some clinical signs and symptoms of essential fatty acid deficiency.
9. Intravenous fat emulsions 10% are _____ .
10. It is common for NPO (nothing by mouth) hyperalimented patients to dream about food and feel obsessed by thoughts of it. True or false?
11. The most serious result of inadvertent rapid infusion of TPN solution is _____ .

12. Immediate treatment of air embolism is aimed at prevention of _____ .
13. In the event of suspected air embolism, the patient should be placed in what position?
14. The course of home TPN may be temporary or permanent. Name 4 conditions that may result in the need for HTPN.
15. Name two potential emergency situations for the patient receiving HTPN.
16. Name two reasons why an NPO patient might smell and taste food.
17. For the renal failure patient, I.V. TPN is similar to what diet?

CHAPTER 22

Intravenous Cancer Chemotherapy Administration

Suzanne Adelman Miller

The use of cancer chemotherapeutic agents for the treatment of malignant disease spans a period of approximately 4 decades. Active nursing involvement in the intravenous (I.V.) administration of these agents spans barely 15 years. The I.V. therapist who works with the oncology patient receiving chemotherapy must not only be technically skilled and knowledgeable in the preparation and delivery of these agents, but must be able to adequately educate the patient and the patient's family, monitor the patient for toxic reactions, and provide continuity of care.

NURSE PREPARATION

Training

The majority of nurses administering cancer chemotherapy agents today have received their training through on-the-job experience. Although this is changing, few centers currently have comprehensive training programs leading to I.V. certification in chemotherapy administration. If our goal is to provide consistent, high-quality care to the patient receiving cancer chemotherapy agents, nurses should receive comprehensive and standardized educational programs to ensure patients' safety. The Oncology Nurses Society, which was established in 1975, now offers credentialling in this specialty. Areas for inclusion in programs leading to chemotherapy certification are outlined below.

    I. Audiovisual component
       A. Historical overview of cancer chemotherapy
       B. Cell cycle
       C. Cellular kinetics
       D. Indications for use
       E. Drug actions and classifications
       F. Drug development and investigative trials
       G. Therapeutic intent with combined modality therapy
       H. Side-effects associated with cytotoxic agents

I. Drug calculation, preparation, and storage
   J. Normal dose ranges
   K. Drug administration techniques*
 II. Classroom lecture
   A. Individual facility policy statement
   B. Legal aspects
   C. Nursing management of side effects
   D. Educational materials and teaching strategies
   E. Drug administration techniques
   F. Drug calculation and reconstitution
   G. Charting
III. Individual nurse packet
   A. Nurse qualifications
   B. Policy and procedures
   C. List of drugs for nurse administration (approval by the pharmacy and therapeutics committee)
   D. Samples of written patient education tools
   E. Nomogram
   F. Math test
   G. Pretest
   H. Class evaluation
   I. Bibliography
   J. Selected reprints
IV. Clinical experience
   A. Drug calculation
   B. Drug preparation
   C. Drug storage
   D. Drug administration
   E. Appropriate charting
   F. Patient teaching and follow-up

Recertification should occur on an annual basis to update the nurses' knowledge of new cytotoxic agents in use and new methods of drug delivery. Also, an annual refresher course will assure that nurses are practicing therapy in a consistent manner.

The mechanics of delivering I.V. cancer chemotherapy agents safely is only one aspect in caring for the cancer patient receiving cytotoxic agents. In addition, the nurse specializing in medical oncology should possess a solid foundation of knowledge relevant to the specialty. Suggested areas for inclusion in basic oncology nursing education programs follow.

 I. Pretherapy patient evaluation
   A. Performance status
   B. Nutritional status

---

*Audiovisual programs on I.V. administration techniques of cancer chemotherapeutic agents are available through Adria Labs, Inc., Dublin, Ohio ("Chemotherapy Administration Techniques") and Bristol Labs, Syracuse, N.Y. ("Cancer: Chemotherapy and Care, I and II," 1981).

Chapter 22 | Intravenous Cancer Chemotherapy Administration

    C. Hematological assessment
    D. Psychosocial assessment
    E. Systems review
        1. Cardiac
        2. Renal
        3. Hepatic
        4. Pulmonary
        5. Gastrointestinal
    F. Diagnostic evaluation
II. Treatment selection
    A. Histology
    B. Location, size
    C. Prior therapy
    D. Therapeutic intent
        1. Cure
        2. Palliation
        3. Adjuvant
    E. Drug calculation, scheduling, and dose modifications
    F. Treatment response
III. Pharmacology
    A. Drug classifications
    B. Cellular kinetics
    C. Drug interactions
    D. Drug delivery (route, rate)
IV. Complications and toxicities
    A. Short-term
        1. Alopecia
        2. Gastrointestinal
        3. Bone marrow
        4. Allergic
        5. Psychosocial
        6. Phlebitis/extravasation
    B. Long-term
        1. Genetic
        2. Oncogenetic
        3. Immunosuppression
        4. Reproductive
        5. Psychosocial
    C. Specific organ toxicities
        1. Cardiac
        2. Renal
        3. Pulmonary
        4. Hepatic
        5. Gastrointestinal
        6. Neurologic
        7. Dermatologic
        8. Reproductive

V. Nursing care
  A. Early detection and prevention of complications
  B. Delivery of expert care
  C. Patient and family education
  D. Psychosocial support (newly diagnosed, remission, recurrence, terminal)
  E. Follow-up support needs

It should be emphasized that the therapist working in this specialized field should continue to update his or her knowledge. The frequent addition of new chemotherapy drugs and refinement of current oncologic practices accentuate the need to remain current in the practice of oncology nursing.

Legal Implications

A thorough understanding of legal implications as outlined in Chapter 2 is essential for the nurse who administers I.V. fluids and drugs. Additional legal safeguards pertinent to cancer chemotherapy include:

1. The therapist should not administer cancer chemotherapy agents unless informed consent has been obtained. "If consent has not been obtained, the hospital or institution may be held liable if treatment is administered. Failure to obtain a patient's consent may constitute 'battery.' Battery may be defined as any physical contact of a patient without his permission" [8].
2. The therapist should have in writing a clear statement of the lines of supervision.
3. The therapist should have defined what the standards of care are at the employing facility, what the scope of duty includes, and what "reasonable care" means in the particular area of practice.
4. The therapist should receive adequate training and supervision in I.V. fluid and drug administration before approaching the patient who is to receive chemotherapy. Written documentation of this training in the therapist's personal file is an added safeguard.

While some may feel that unnecessary paperwork is being created, it is to the therapist's benefit to have defined in writing the scope of practice for each setting where he or she practices. The therapist should also explore the current medical liability insurance covering his or her practice. Most large facilities provide adequate coverage for care administered while the nurse is on duty. However, independent practitioners or those working in physicians' offices may need to obtain their own malpractice insurance. Unfortunately, as nurses assume greater responsibility in cancer chemotherapy administration, there will be an increased incidence of nurses involved in litigation proceedings. By taking care to assure that the therapist is functioning within an adequate legal framework, it is hoped that litigation will be avoided.

PATIENT EDUCATION

While the intent of this chapter is not to focus on teaching strategies and methods of communicating vital information regarding side-effects and toxicities associated with cancer chemotherapy, several prefatory points to the discussion of I.V. administration techniques must be included.

Pretreatment

The patient should be provided with written educational materials before chemotherapy is initiated. A thorough review of the side-effects with patient interventions should be covered. Allowance should be made for an extended learning period if necessary. A library for patients should be available for those seeking additional information.

The patient and family should be given the opportunity of touring the area where the chemotherapy agents will be administered. Meeting the I.V. therapist who will be administering the treatment can often allay fears. A meeting with the dietitian may be profitable to those patients who need nutritional counseling.

A brief discussion of the chemotherapy procedure and administration technique can be covered and a nursing assessment of the patient's fears, concerns, and comprehension can be noted. Some facilities complete a written nursing history and assessment at the first visit.

Treatment

A review of the possible side-effects and toxicities associated with the patient's individual treatment program is essential at the time of the first treatment and with each successive treatment. High anxiety levels can impede the learning process, so efforts to allay patient's fears should be made at each treatment.

A drug and food allergy history should be obtained and recorded before the first treatment. At this time, the therapist can review what medications the patient is currently receiving. Frequently oncology patients take medications for symptom control (e.g., pain and nausea) or for secondary problems that are disease-related (e.g., infection, hypercalcemia, or hyperuricemia). In addition, patients may be on drugs for medical conditions not related to the diagnosis of cancer (e.g., hypertension or arthritis). Multiple-drug therapies increase the complexities of patient management. The therapist should report all information learned about the patient's drug history to the physician so that the possibility of adverse drug interactions can be considered before cytotoxic agents are administered.

A general time schedule of the anticipated therapy program may help some patients who plan to continue work or school. Most chemotherapy treatment programs are of 6- to 12-month duration, and knowing this may help patients plan ahead.

Posttreatment

The patient should be instructed not to travel alone. Pretreatment with antiemetics may cause drowsiness, and the cancer chemotherapy agents may cause nausea and vomiting or systemic reactions that are difficult to manage when traveling alone.

The nurse should call the patient after the first treatment and with any successive treatment where potential problems are expected. The patient's response to treatment, his or her concerns and adjustments, and comprehension of the drug program to be taken at home can be discussed. Confirm the patient's return appointment and assure him or her that any problems arising meanwhile can be discussed over the phone or medical assistance may be obtained if necessary.

Patient Involvement

Experience indicates that patients' acceptance of and response to treatment are more favorable when they are actively involved in the therapy program. In administering cytotoxic agents, the nurse should actively solicit the patient's help in assessing vein status. The wise therapist will listen to the patient who says, "The nurse tried 3 times unsuccessfully to give me my medicine in that vein last week." In addition to providing patients with a sense of control, the therapist is acknowledging a respect for the patient's knowledge of his or her body. The fact that patients frequently sense inner changes occurring in their bodies can be used to the therapist's advantage. Many patients who have received chemotherapy in the past can detect a coolness along the venous pathways as intravenous solutions and drugs are infused. Likewise, many patients can detect early extravasation before the therapist is able to do so. For that reason, the nurse should alert the patient to signs of extravasation if necrotic agents are being infused. These may include pain, burning, stinging, a feeling of tightness, tingling, numbness, or any unusual sensation not experienced previously in the area being infused.

Several chemotherapy agents are associated with localized and generalized anaphylactic reactions, and when reported early and treated promptly, their course can be reversed or minimized. Patients are encouraged to report symptoms of generalized tingling, shortness of breath, light-headedness, or chest pains. The therapist should employ sensitivity in imparting this information to the patient, and the patient's overall anxiety level should be assessed prior to initiating a teaching program.

In recommending that patients be encouraged to be active participants in the treatment program, the therapist creates the possibility that some patients may attempt to direct their care. Patient attempts at intimidation with statements such as, "This is the vein you must use today," or "I'll only give you one try, then you've got to go find someone else," should be anticipated. Undoubtedly, the impact of these comments on the therapist's feelings of self-confidence are not realized by the patient. Several minutes spent explaining the process of venous selection to the patient may prevent a recurrence of the situation.

MEDICATION PREPARATION

Increasingly, health-care facilities are utilizing the skills of pharmacists to order, store, reconstitute, and dispense cytotoxic agents. It is highly advised that chemotherapeutic agents be prepared in a Class II Biological Safety Cabinet [5]. If the nurse must reconstitute the drugs without the assistance of a pharmacist, the following guidelines should be followed:

1. Always recheck the medication order against the chart or with the doctor. A safe policy states that the nurse must check the written prescription against the written physician's order. Using the formula given below, calculate the dose on paper.

    The physician has ordered doxorubicin hydrochloride (Adriamycin) administered. The vials are supplied in 10-mg and 50-mg sizes.

$$\text{Formula:} \quad \frac{\text{have}}{\text{mix}} \times \frac{\text{want}}{\text{desired}}$$

or

$$\text{Doxorubicin:} \quad \frac{50\text{-mg vial}}{25 \text{ ml diluent}} \times \frac{45 \text{ mg}}{\times \text{ ml}}$$

$25 \times 45 \qquad\qquad\qquad\qquad\qquad = 1{,}125 \text{ ml}$

$1{,}125 \text{ ml} \div 50 \text{ mg} \qquad\qquad\qquad = 22.5 \text{ ml}$

Give 22.5 ml

Check your conclusion with a colleague. Errors in drug names (e.g., vinblastine and vincristine look similar when written), dosages (e.g., a decimal point may be incorrectly placed, illegibly written, or omitted so that a normal dose of 9.0 mg may be interpreted as a lethal 90 mg), or administration times can be potentially toxic or lethal.

2. Prepare the cytotoxic agents in a quiet area without interruptions. Although many cancer chemotherapy agents are expensive, the cost factor should not receive priority over patient safety. If the nurse is interrupted during the preparation process and, upon returning, has any doubt as to the drug or dose about to be administered, the drug should be discarded. In addition, many feel that nurses who prepare chemotherapy should take self-protective measures to avoid skin and mucous membrane contamination with cytotoxic agents (Figure 22.1). Some nurses appear to show more sensitivity to skin contamination than others do. Since available information on the long-term problems that may arise in drug handlers is lacking, the nurse would be wise to take precautionary measures in avoiding skin contamination [13]. Exercise safety with the use of body protection technique.

3. Review the package insert before preparing the drug. Valuable information regarding the solution to be used for reconstitution, stability, incompatibilities, and storage and administration precautions are included with all commercially available cancer chemotherapeutic agents. A meeting with the pharmacy department can establish a mechanism for reporting cracked vials, cloudy solutions, and those considered to be contaminated.

4. As they are filled, label all syringes with the drug's name and dose (Figure 22.2). Most cytotoxic agents are clear in color and are more easily confused if unlabeled. If a clear drug infiltrates or if a reaction occurs, the nurse needs to know which agent is implicated. The ability to check the drugs, dosages, and routes of administration as listed on the syringes against the written prescription just before their administration is an additional safeguard.

5. A wise policy to follow is to administer only medications you prepare or watch being prepared, except for drugs prepared by a pharmacist. The nurse who administers drugs can be held accountable for any error

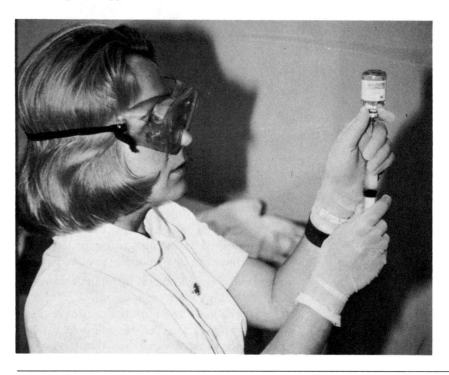

FIGURE 22.1
Glasses and gloves protect the nurse from possible skin and eye contamination if the vial should crack or the needle separate from the syringe. A gown may also be worn. Note that the nurse's hand is placed between the vial's stopper and her face.

that results from a wrong dose or drug being administered if not prepared by a qualified pharmacist.

INTRAVENOUS TECHNIQUE

The nurse who administers cancer chemotherapy agents should previously have participated in and passed an intravenous therapy program at the employing facility. Techniques for venous selection and procedure for performing a basic venipuncture are covered in Chapter 12. Several points pertaining to I.V. cancer chemotherapy administration warrant reemphasis.

An adequate assessment of the patient's venous status should be obtained before each treatment. Discussing with the patient any problems experienced since the last treatment is also helpful. Both arms should be examined for bruises, inflammation, or phlebitis, and these areas should be avoided (Figure 22.3). The examination of both arms also gives the therapist a baseline reference point should changes occur during treatment. If veins are obscure, moderately warm water may be run over the patient's hands and forearms, or warm compresses may be applied to the bedridden patient. Some therapists have used a hair dryer, taking care to avoid sustaining second-degree burns. The shirtsleeves should be rolled up to allow full view of both arms during the entire treatment. This permits visualization of early localized reactions with compar-

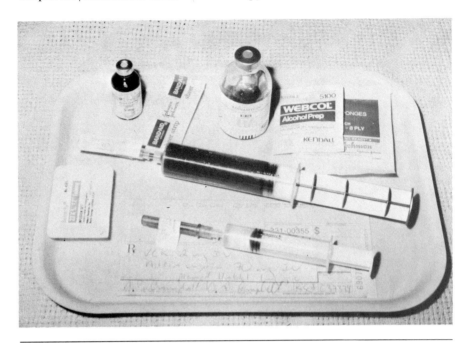

FIGURE 22.2
The tags on the needles list the drug, dose, and milliliters contained in the syringes. This is to be checked against the prescription before being administered.

ison of the untreated arm. Watches or tight jewelry on the treated arm should be removed prior to vein cannulation. Tight jewelry may constrict the venous pathway, impeding the smooth flow of drugs along the venous network.

The arms should be alternated, if possible, with each treatment. Vascular irritation is associated with the I.V. administration of cancer chemotherapy agents, and phlebitis can often be minimized when I.V. sites are rotated. Less frequent use of either arm permits time for resolution of potential venous irritation. Patients can be helpful by remembering which arm was treated last. If not informed of this procedure and if treated by various therapists, the patient may choose to have all treatments in one arm for personal preferences, thus increasing the possibility of phlebitis.

Sterile venipuncture techniques should be thoroughly understood and practiced by the nurse. In addition to the precautions and suggestions found in Chapter 16, the therapist must realize that oncology patients on cancer chemotherapy agents often are leukopenic as a result of treatment and therefore more susceptible to a direct route for contamination to spread systemically. Not infrequently, the nurse will meticulously swab the I.V. site only to unconsciously tap the site one more time with a finger to assure successful cannulation.

Venipunctures should proceed from the proximal point (hand) to the distal point (forearm). If an unsuccessful venipuncture has been attempted on the forearm or if blood drawing was performed and a successful site then established in the hand of the same arm, the possibility exists that the drugs can

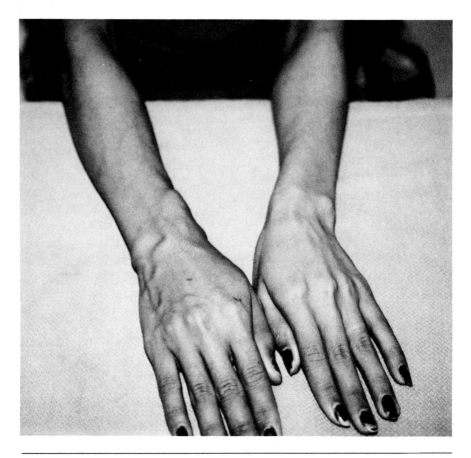

FIGURE 22.3
Both hands and arms should be examined prior to vein cannulation to note existing phlebitis, bruises, or inflamed areas.

leak out of the previous unsuccessful venipuncture site and into the surrounding tissues. If the drug is known to be a sclerosing agent, tissue necrosis can occur. Our nursing practice policy is not to use the antecubital fossa. Many physicians and nurses have strong preferences for using either the hand or the antecubital fossa. The pros and cons of using these areas are listed in Exhibit 22.1. Many therapists prefer to cannulate the forearm because of the morbidity associated with the hand or antecubital fossa. The therapist who is new to a facility should review the established policy before beginning to administer cytotoxic agents.

Despite the therapist's degree of technical competence, occasional situations arise where the therapist may have difficulty locating a vein. An arbitrary limit of three unsuccessful venipunctures is suggested before the nurse seeks the assistance of a co-worker. Repetitive venipunctures will undoubtedly increase the anxiety level experienced by both the patient and nurse, and this may decrease the chance of successfully cannulating a vein.

A preexisting I.V. site should not be used to administer cancer chemo-

Chapter 22 | Intravenous Cancer Chemotherapy Administration

EXHIBIT 22.1
Pros and Cons of Chemotherapy Administration in the Antecubital Fossa

Factors Against Use of This Site:

1. Important anatomical structures, such as median nerves and brachial arteries, are located in this area. If extensive tissue necrosis occurs in this area, the possibility of amputation exists. At a minimum, extensive tissue necrosis could necessitate long, expensive and psychologically traumatic reconstructive efforts.
2. Prolonged infusions restrict arm mobility as elbow flexion must be limited during infusion.
3. Veins in the antecubital fossa are traditionally used for blood specimens. Repetitive needle insertions and infusions of chemotherapeutic agents could fibrose this area and precluding successful blood sampling that is often necessary.
4. Early subcutaneous infiltration is often more difficult to visualize due to the amount of subcutaneous fat and tissue present in this area.

Factors For Use of This Site:

1. Larger diameter veins permit the use of large gauge needles and more rapid administration of sclerosing chemotherapeutic agents. More rapid drug infusion permits the high blood flow to more quickly dilute the chemotherapeutic agent. Some theorize that the less the chemotherapeutic agent is in contact with the wall of the vein, the less chance phlebitis will occur.
2. Some feel this area is preferred over the dorsum of the hand which is a particularly morbid area should extravasation occur. If extensive drug infiltration occurs in the hand, severe contractures of the metacorpophalangeal and wrist joints as well as damage to the underlying tendons and neurovascular bundles can occur.

Source: From Miller, S. A. *Oncol. Nurs. Forum* 7(4): Fall 1980. Reprinted with permission.

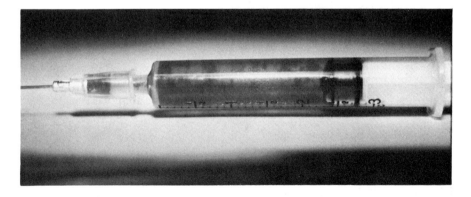

FIGURE 22.4
Obvious precipitation resulting from the combination of doxorubicin HCl (Adriamycin) and heparin sodium.

therapy agents. Frequently these intravenous solutions contain admixtures which may be incompatible with cytotoxic drugs. Figure 22.4 shows an obvious precipitate when doxorubicin and heparin sodium were combined. In addition, the possibility exists that venous irritation and phlebitis may result. If the existing intravenous line is the only site available for chemotherapy administration, the following precautions must be observed.

1. The dressing should be completely removed and vein patency assured by the therapist prior to treatment.
2. The tubing must be changed before and after chemotherapy if the I.V. container contains admixtures.
3. Approximately 50–100 ml normal saline must be infused prior to and after treatment as a flush. The nurse must ascertain that the additional fluid volume is compatible with patients who are on volume restrictions.

An extremity with compromised circulation should not be used to administer cytotoxic agents. Stagnant or sluggish blood flow through the venous system can potentiate a local reaction and delay the chemotherapy from reaching the general circulation. Compromised circulation can exist in extremities with (1) an invading neoplasm, (2) existing phlebitis, (3) varicosities, (4) the side of a previous mastectomy, (5) an immobilized fracture, (6) extensive bruises, or (7) inflamed areas.

Most chemotherapy programs can be administered to patients on an outpatient basis. When treating an outpatient, the small-vein needle is the needle of choice (Chapter 12). Often therapists are forced to cannulate veins in elusive areas such as between the knuckles on the hands or the cephalic vein as it arches over the bones on the radial wrist. Because of the positioning of these veins, the therapist may elect not to tape the needle to the skin so as to not dislodge the needle. The nurse should understand that the short bevel of the needle may be dislodged from the vein with a force of I.V. push or infused medications. For that reason, the wings of the small-vein needle should always be secured to the skin no matter how short a time span is anticipated for an infusion. When securing the needle to the skin, the tape should be applied so that the needle insertion site and the immediate surrounding area are visible for inspection. A common site of extravasation is just above the needle insertion site and, if occluded from visual inspection, an infiltration can go unnoticed.

Before cytotoxic agents are administered, the vein's patency should always be first tested with normal saline. If fragile veins burst or if the needle has perforated the wall of the vein, normal saline can be absorbed without causing damage to the surrounding tissue. Infusion of normal saline is exceedingly important before administering cytotoxic agents through a heparin lock or a permanent-type central venous catheter. If doxorubicin were administered via either of these routes and the line was not adequately flushed, drug incompatibilities could occur (see Figure 22.4). Approximately 2–5 ml normal saline should also be infused between drugs when several drugs are to be administered to ensure that chemical interactions do not occur from drugs being mixed together. Likewise, after all chemotherapy agents have been administered, approximately 20–50 ml normal saline should be infused as a final flush to ensure that the drugs have been washed out of the peripheral veins and to clear the needle and tubing of any remaining drug which could cause tissue irritation as the needle is removed.

Apply slow, even pressure when giving drugs by I.V. push. If resistance is encountered, the drug infusion should be stopped and a possible cause sought.

If the bevel of the needle is against the wall of the vein, a careful repositioning may resolve the problem. Small-gauge needles will be met with more resistance, and if the therapist continues to apply force to the plunger, the patient may complain of pain or venous spasm. Additionally, a fast, forceful infusion of push medications can cause some patients to experience nausea. The possibility also exists that a forceful push may cause a weak-walled vein to burst.

After completion of the chemotherapy treatment, remove cannula using a dry, sterile sponge; apply pressure to the site with the extremity elevated until bleeding stops, approximately 3–5 minutes; apply dressing to the site. With thrombocytopenia being a common side effect in oncology patients today, blood leakage into the subcutaneous tissues can occur from a nonhealing venipuncture site. The resulting hematoma may be painful, unsightly, and preclude the future use of that site until there is resolution. In addition, patients should be cautioned not to carry heavy purses or briefcases with their treated hand.

VENOUS FRAGILITY

Despite the skill of the nurse and the use of appropriate administration techniques, patients will occasionally experience problems unique to the administration of cytotoxic agents.

Elderly, poorly nourished, and debilitated patients are often predisposed to having fragile veins. The unskilled therapist may unknowingly cause painful and unsightly hematomas that prevent future use of veins until healing occurs. If a patient has fragile veins, the therapist should attempt to cannulate the vein without the use of a tourniquet since tourniquet distention and rapid engorgement may cause the wall of the vein to rupture when the tourniquet is released. A second nurse may apply gentle hand pressure above the venipuncture site to effect distention. Other alternatives that be used to distend veins include applying moderate heat or having the patient pump or clench the fist. Gravity flow may be maximized by having the patient dangle the hand and arm. Light tapping of the site with the therapist's finger may also be used to effect venous distention without the use of a tourniquet.

With all maneuvers patients with fragile veins should be approached cautiously with adequate time being allowed by the therapist to effect an adequate venipuncture at the first attempt.

LOCALIZED ACUTE ALLERGIC REACTIONS

Localized allergic reactions, commonly referred to as "flare," are often associated with the administration of doxorubicin hydrochloride; reactions should, however, be anticipated in any patient receiving intravenous cytotoxic agents. The first appearance may be that of erythema along the venous pathways. Blotchiness, hivelike urticaria, or the rapid appearance of welts may also occur as the first sign noted (Figure 22.5). The patient may complain of itching, stinging, or an increased sensation of heat in the area. Some feel that the reaction is due to an intercellular release of histamines which increases cell membrane permeability. Increased cellular permeability may permit drug leakage

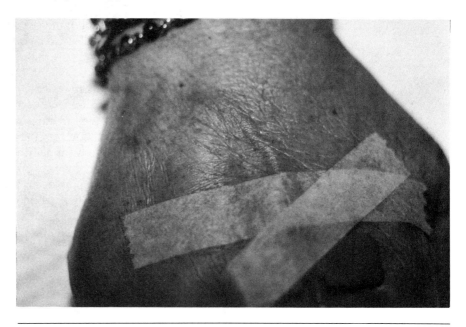

FIGURE 22.5
Rapid occurrence of venous dilatation and erythema from a localized allergic reaction.

into the subcutaneous tissues. Vogelzang [19] suggests that other possibilities include drug interactions or contaminants or a molecular extravasation through the vascular endothelium.

Preventative measures include additionally diluting the chemotherapy agent either by adding the drug to 100–200 ml of solution or by administering the drug piggyback.* A chart similar to Table 22.1 may assist the nurse unfamiliar with rates and methods of administering cytotoxic agents.

Should a localized allergic reaction occur many practitioners feel that, to prevent chemical cellulitis, the drug should be discontinued and a new venipuncture site established. Before removing the intravenous needle, the administration of additional fluid not containing drugs should be infused in an attempt to resolve the erythematous reaction. The medications listed below are suggested to treat localized sensitivity reactions. All require a physician's order prior to their administration.

Hydrocortisone sodium succinate (Solu-Cortef).   Slow I.V. push, 50–200 mg, antiinflammatory agent

Benadryl.   I.V. push, 50 mg, antihistamine

Cimetidine.   Slow I.V. push, 300 mg, histamine antagonist

Long-term studies with possible tissue biopsies may be necessary to determine the extent and significance of localized allergic reactions.

---

*Piggyback refers to a method of infusion through the sidearm of the I.V. tubing while additional diluent is infusing.

VENOUS SPASM

Several cytotoxic agents are associated with complaints of severe pain or spasm along the venous pathway. Carmustine (BiCNU) is diluted with absolute alcohol and may be the offending agent. The breakdown products from photodegradation of dacarbazine (DTIC) may be responsible for the acute local burning associated with the use of this drug [1].

Mechlorathemine hydrochloride (Mustargen) can also cause pain, especially in patients who have received chemotherapy over extended periods. While the administration of these agents should alert the therapist to the possible occurrence of this problem it should be mentioned that *any* agent is capable of causing venous pain in the patient at any time. In addition, venous spasm or pain can also occur if a small-gauge needle is used and the treatment is administered by forceful pushing on the plunger of the syringe. Measures suggested for alleviating venous pain or spasm include

1. Slowing the drug infusion rate.
2. Additionally diluting the drug.
3. Applying either warm or cool compresses to the arm during infusion. Unfortunately, the use of either warm or cool maneuvers at this time is empirically decided. Some patients will respond to one approach and some to the other. The therapist is reminded to take care that second-degree burns do not occur with temperature alteration maneuvers.
4. Administering Xylocaine 1% — ¼ ml (3 ml total) PRN. A physician's order and an allergy history should be obtained before administering the drug.

PHLEBITIS

Chemical phlebitis is a risk associated with the administration of most intravenous cancer chemotherapy agents. With many treatment programs involving the combination of two or more cytotoxic agents, the risk is increased. Early phlebitis can be associated with pain, erythema, occasional limb edema, and a sensation of warmth in the affected extremity (Figure 22.6). As the acute symptom subsides, the venous pathways may retain a dark bluish to brown discoloration for some time (Figure 22.7). Often associated with this are complaints from the patient of restricted arm use. Acute phlebitis reactions can interfere with the patient's routine daily living activities and interrupt usual sleep patterns. Noninvestigational drugs* frequently associated with causing phlebitis are listed on page 459, following Table 22.1.

---

*Noninvestigational drugs are included because accumulated clinical experience has demonstrated their safety and known toxicities. Commercial availability of cancer chemotherapy drugs occurs when the Federal Food and Drug Administration is satisfied that efficacy has been demonstrated in various malignancies and that safe limits for administration have been defined.

TABLE 22.1
Selected List of Cancer Cytotoxic Agents That Can Be Administered by Registered Nurses

Drug	A. Method of Administration* B. Rate of Administration†	Concentration A. Size Vial B. Solution Used C. Resulting Concentration	Drug Ranges
Bleomycin sulfate (Blenoxane)	A. Piggyback Direct B. < 1 min	A. 15-U ampule B. Reconstitute w/ bacteriostatic H_2O C. 5 U/ml	10–20 U/m²/ 1–2 ×/wk
Cytarabine Ara C Cytosar-U Cytosine	A. Piggyback Direct Bottle B. < 5 min	A. 100 mg vial, add 2 ml 500 mg vial, add 10 ml B. Bacteriostatic H_2O^- benzyl alcohol preservative C. 50 mg/ml	1–3 mg/kg/day 100–500 mg/m²/ 5–10 days
Dactinomycin Cosmegen Actinomycin D	A. Piggyback Direct B. 2–5 min	A. 500 mcg/1.1 ml vial B. Sterile H_2O U.S.P. C. 0.5 mg/ml	2 mg/wk/× 3 wks 15–30 mcg/kg/wk 500 mg/5 × daily
Daunorubicin HCl (Daunomycin) (Cerubidine)	A. Piggyback Bottle B. < 10 min	A. 20 mg vial, add 4 ml B. N.S. preservative-free C. 5 mg/ml	30–60 mg/m²
Doxorubicin HCl (Adriamycin)	A. Piggyback Bottle B. < 10 min	A. 10 mg vial, add 5 ml 50 mg vial, add 25 ml B. N.S. preservative-free C. 2 mg/ml	30–120 mg/m²
5-Fluorouracil (5-FU)	A. Piggyback Direct B. 1–5 min	A. 500 mg/10 ml (premixed ampule)	10–15 mg/kg/wk 400–500 mg/m² 3 × daily/Q3 wks

Indications	I.V. Administration Precautions	Side-Effects
Head and neck, skin, lymphoma, sarcoma, penis, testes, cervix, anus, rectum, lung	Generalized anaphylaxis (test dose lymphoma pts 2 U × 2 doses) Tylenol 10 grains and Benadryl 25–50 mg PO pretreatment	Fevers and chills Hyperpigmentation Pulmonary fibrosis (total dose not to exceed 400 U)
Head and neck, lymphoma, leukemias		Nausea and vomiting Diarrhea Myelosuppression Stomatitis Abdominal pain Hepatic dysfunction Fever, arthralgias, rash
Melanoma rhabdomyosarcoma, choriocarcinoma, Wilms', Ewing's, testicular	Tissue necrosis if infiltrated	Nausea and vomiting Myelosuppression Diarrhea Stomatitis Alopecia Pigmentary changes of skin
AML ALL	Localized urticaria Extreme vessicant (tissue necrosis if extravasated) Vein pain, phlebitis	Nausea and vomiting Myelosuppression Red urine (1–2 days after injection) Alopecia Stomatitis Cardiotoxicity (total dose not to exceed 500–600 mg/m^2) Pigmentary changes of nails Skin rash
Breast, bladder, thyroid, lung, ovary, all sarcomas, lymphomas, neuroblastomas, Ewing's	Localized urticaria Extreme vessicant (tissue necrosis if extravasated) Vein pain, phlebitis	Nausea and vomiting Red urine (1–2 days after injection) Stomatitis (3–4 days after injection) Alopecia (1–2 wks after) Myelosuppression (1–2 wks after) Cardiotoxicity (total dose not to exceed 550 mg/m^2) Pigmentary changes of nails
Stomach, colon, breast, bladder	Check ampule for precipitation	Nausea and vomiting Stomatitis Diarrhea Dermatitis Photosensitivity Mild alopecia Myelosuppression

TABLE 22.1
(continued)

Drug	A. Method of Administration* B. Rate of Administration†	Concentration A. Size Vial B. Solution Used C. Resulting Concentration	Drug Ranges

Methotrexate sodium (Mexate)
 	
Amethopterin
	A. Low dose piggyback
	    Direct
	B. 1–2 min
		A. 20 mg/2 ml
		    50 mg/5 ml
		    100 mg/10 ml
		B. NaCl
		C. 10 mg/ml
			Low dose
			25–40 mg/m²/wk

Mithramycin (Mithracin)	A. Piggyback Bottle B. 1–5 min	A. 2,500 mcg/4.9 ml B. Sterile H₂O	25–50 mcg/kg QOD (oncologic use) 25 mcg/kg (hypercalcemia)
Mechlorethamine HCl Mustargen Nitrogen mustard	A. Piggyback B. 5–10 min	A. 10 mg/10 ml B. Sterile H₂O C. 1 mg/1 ml Additionally dilute 0–5 mg/20 cc N.S. 6–10 mg/40 cc N.S.	6 mg/m²
Thiotepa (Thiophosphoramide)	A. Piggyback Direct B. < 1 min	A. 15 mg/1.5 ml B. Sterile H₂O C. 10 mg/ml	0.5 mg/kg/ Q 1–4 wks 6 mg/m²/ × 4 days Q 2–4 wks
Vinblastine sulfate (Velban)	A. Piggyback Direct B. 1–2 min	A. 10 mg/10 ml B. Bacteriostatic-benzyl alcohol preserved N.S. C. 1 mg/ml	4–20 mg/m²

Vincristine sulfate (Oncovin)	A. Piggyback
	    Direct
	B. 1–2 min
		A. 5 mg/10 ml (2 mg/ml)
		    1 mg/10 ml (1 mg/ml)
		B. Own diluent
			0.4 mg–1.4 mg/m²/ wk (total one × dose not to exceed 2.0 mg).

*Method of administration:
Piggyback. Given through the side arm of a free-flowing I.V. solution.
Direct. Given by direct push through a winged scalp vein needle (< 1 min → 5 min).
Bottle. Given additionally diluted in 100–200 cc solution.

†Rate of administration determined by:
1. Total one-time dose
2. Prior systemic patient reactions (check previous nurse's notes)
3. Individual localized patient sensitivity (check previous nurse's notes)
4. Size of vein cannulated
5. Needle size

Indications	I.V. Administration Precautions	Side-Effects
Leukemia, lymphoma, head and neck, breast, colon, lung, sarcoma, ALL, Burkitt's, choriocarcinoma, ovary, multiple myeloma		Nausea and vomiting Diarrhea Stomatitis Myelosuppression Dermatitis
Testicular, stomach, thyroid, glioblastoma	Tissue necrosis if infiltrated	Nausea and vomiting Myelosuppression Anorexia Diarrhea
Hodgkin's disease, lung	Severe tissue necrosis, if infiltrated Thrombophlebitis *Caution:* Chemical burns occur if skin contact and mucous membrane contact occur. Flush immediately w/water	Severe nausea and vomiting Myelosuppression
Lymphoma, breast, ovary, bladder		Nausea and vomiting Myelosuppression Headaches
Lymphoma, breast, testicular, renal cell carcinoma, choriocarcinoma, CML	Tissue necrosis, if infiltrated Thrombophlebitis	Nausea and vomiting Constipation Alopecia CNS and peripheral neuropathies including numbness and myalgias Myelosuppression Stomatitis
Lymphoma, breast, ALL, lung, Ewing's, Wilm's, neuroblastoma	Tissue necrosis, if infiltrated Thrombophlebitis	Nausea and vomiting Constipation Alopecia CNS and peripheral neuropathies including numbness and myalgias Myelosuppression Stomatitis

Source: Prepared by Suzanne Miller, Division of Medical Oncology, Department of Medicine, and Fred Nishioka, Registered Pharmacist, Stanford University Medical Center, Stanford, Calif. From M. Arnold, Storage and stability guide for parenteral antineoplastic agents requiring reconstitution. *Infusion* 4:52–55, 1980. R. Dorr and W. Fritz, *Cancer Chemotherapy Handbook,* New York: Elsevier North-Holland, 1980. M. Knobf, K. Lewis, D. Fischer, W. Schneider, and D. Welch, Cancer chemotherapy treatment and care. New Haven, Conn.: Comprehensive Cancer Center, 1979. B. Lum, F. Torti, and S. Carter, Handbook of NCOG protocol: Chemotherapy agents. Palo Alto, Calif.: Northern California Oncology Group.

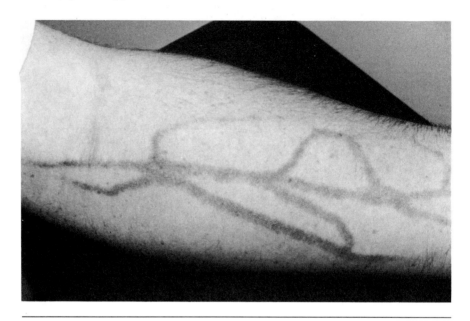

FIGURE 22.6
Acute phlebitic reaction photographed 1 week after Mustargen and vincristine were administered.

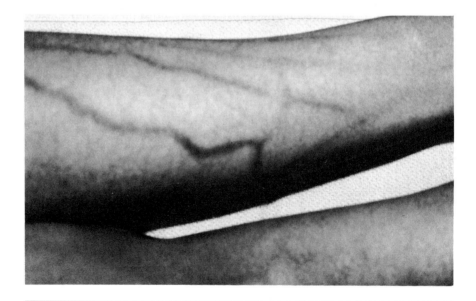

FIGURE 22.7
As the acute symptoms of phlebitis resolve, the venous pathways retain a dark color for some time. If possible, chemotherapy infusions should be avoided in these veins until there is resolution.

Actinomycin D

Dacarbazine

Daunomycin

Doxorubicin HCl

Mechlorethamine hydrochloride

Mitomycin-C

Vinblastine

Vincristine

Extreme caution should be taken by the therapist to prevent the occurrence of phlebitis. Should phlebitic reactions occur in both arms, I.V. chemotherapy treatment may need to be discontinued pending resolution of the problem (Figure 22.8). Inability to aggressively treat growing disease with I.V. cytotoxic agents may jeopardize the patient's chances for long-term disease control. When possible, nonsclerosing agents in the same drug category are substituted for the offending agent. Occasionally a patient will display phlebitic reactions to any I.V. drug administered.

In addition to the preventive measures suggested in Chapter 20, section Vascular Irritation, to diminish the possible occurrence of phlebitis, the therapist may elect to adopt the following measures:

1. Administer hydrocortisone sodium succinate (Solu-Cortef), 50–100 mg, slow I.V. push. It is empirically suggested that half of the total dose be administered pretreatment after ascertaining vein patency and the remaining half after the final flush has been administered and just before the needle is removed. A physician's order is necessary before this drug can be administered.
2. Additionally dilute the agent. Reducing the drug concentration may lessen the occurrence of phlebitis.

Unfortunately, some patients will develop phlebitis despite the most cautious effort of the therapist to prevent its occurrence. Repetitive needle insertions necessary for blood sampling and the administration of multiple intravenous chemotherapy agents increase the possibility that phlebitis and thrombosis will occur. Therapeutic measures that may be indicated once phlebitis has occurred include

1. Elevation of the affected extremity.
2. Application of topical heat.
3. Administration of systemic analgesics (with a physician's order).

Ideally, the venous status should be assessed prior to the patient's receiving any chemotherapy treatments. If the veins are deep and difficult to visualize or palpate with tourniquet distention, or if the peripheral veins are extremely small, several options should be considered as an alternative to inserting a needle with each chemotherapy treatment.

1. Heparin lock (see Chapter 20)

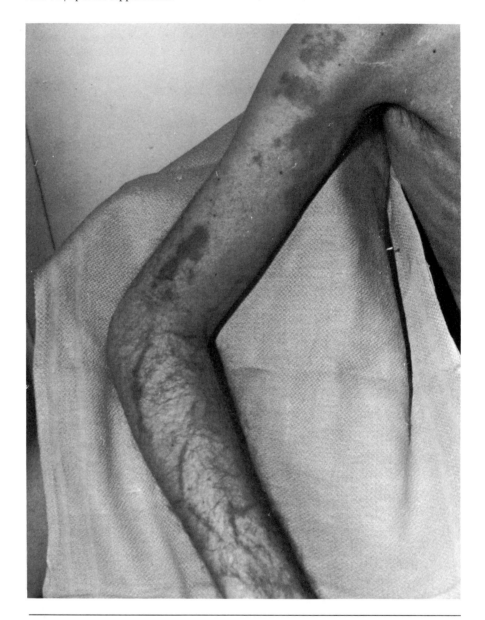

FIGURE 22.8
Repetitive chemotherapy administrations of Mustargen and vincristine produced bilateral phlebitis. Subsequent treatments substituting Cytoxan for Mustargen as an alkylator in the drug combination also produced phlebitis. Treatments were discontinued until the acute reaction subsided.

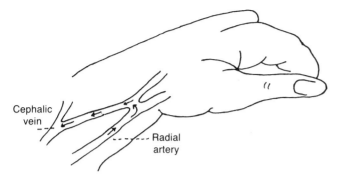

FIGURE 22.9
An arteriovenous fistula. The most common type involves joining the radial artery and the cephalic vein.

2. Central venous pressure line
3. Arteriovenous fistulas
4. Hickman catheters

Arteriovenous Fistulas

With its introduction in 1966, the arteriovenous fistula was primarily intended for gaining vascular access to patients needing long-term hemodialysis [12]. The procedure involves creating an anastomosis between the artery and the vein. The most common type involves establishing a connection between the radial artery and the cephalic vein (Figure 22.9). The advantages and disadvantages of establishing an arteriovenous fistula for chemotherapy access are listed below.

Advantages
1. The dilated venous system permits easier visualization and access for chemotherapy administration.
2. There is less pain associated with needle insertions when using winged small-vein needles, commonly used for chemotherapy administration.
3. Once the fistula is healed, patients are permitted a great deal of freedom in showering, swimming, and participating in sports.

Disadvantages
1. A patient's prognosis and expected response to therapy are often difficult to determine prior to chemotherapy initiation. Medical oncologists are often reticent to subject a patient to unnecessary surgery if long-term survival is uncertain. The greatest chance for a successful surgical procedure is before veins become fibrosed from the administration of cytotoxic agents.
2. The 2- to 4-week delay necessary for vessel maturity to be established may be unacceptable for patients with rapidly growing neoplasms.
3. Blood backflow from high arteriovenous pressure may prevent intravenous infusions (drip) of chemotherapeutic agents from being administered.
4. Infection and hemorrhage, while uncommon, should be considered as a possibility in patients receiving myelosuppressive cytotoxic agents. The

extremity should be monitored for erythema, swelling, and excessive tenderness.

5. Surgical reversal of the procedure may be necessary after chemotherapy treatments have been completed if the appearance and noticeable "thrill" are bothersome to the patient.

Before administering chemotherapy via an arteriovenous fistula, the therapist should discuss nursing care aspects with specialists in nephrology who have accumulated experiences working with fistulas for patients on renal dialysis. The therapist should

1. Understand the surgical procedure.
2. Realize the consequences of short-term and long-term complications.
3. Plan nursing interventions to prevent complications.
4. Explain the care and precautions to the patient, and provide written educational materials as patient participation is essential.
5. Understand the additional hazards — extravasation, hemorrhage, and infection — when working with patients receiving cancer chemotherapeutic agents.

This brief review is intended only to expose the nurse to the possible utilization of arteriovenous fistulas for chemotherapy access. A more thorough review of the literature is recommended [9, 10, 18].

The Hickman Catheter

A more recent development pioneered in the mid-1970s is the Hickman catheter (see Figure 21.11, p. 415). This indwelling right atrial central venous catheter is a modification of the Broviac catheter commonly used for total parenteral nutrition. Advantages of using the Hickman catheter include the following:

1. The patient's peripheral venous system is preserved.
2. Blood products, nutritional products, antibiotics, analgesics, antiemetics, and cytotoxic agents may be administered through this line.
3. The patient is spared the psychological trauma of repetitive and often traumatic attempts at venous cannulation.

Disadvantages are as follows:

1. Clotting may occur as a result of improper or inadequate irrigation or an inadequate filling of the catheter with heparinized normal saline.
2. Infection may occur if aseptic techniques are not taught and adhered to by the staff and patient. Patients who are discharged with a Hickman catheter should be shown how to care for the catheter in the hospital with return demonstrations given to the nurse until patient technique is adequate. The patient's family is included in the teaching-learning process. A detailed written procedure should also be given to the patient to follow at home.
3. Air embolism can occur if the catheter clamp and Luer lock screw cap

are not in place. All connections should be taped as an additional safeguard. Adequate patient instruction should prevent this from occurring.

4. Severing of the catheter, although infrequent, reemphasizes the need to discuss its prevention with the patient. A smooth-surfaced catheter clamp should always be on hand and the patient given instructions as to how to manage this problem [2].

Implantable Vascular Access Devices

The development of the vascular access devices that can be completely implanted affords a method for treatment involving highly irritating drugs or the need for a long-term vascular site. The risk of infection is reduced, there is no need for external catheter care, and the potential risk of drug infiltration and vein sclerosis from irritating drugs is reduced (see Chapter 19).

GENERALIZED ANAPHYLACTIC REACTION

The therapist should be prepared for the occurrence of an anaphylactic reaction at any time, with any drug, in any patient. Considering this will forewarn and prepare the therapist for the possibility. Before initiating treatment, the therapist should understand the facility's policy for the administration of cytotoxic agents. Knowledge of the procedure for initiating emergency care and awareness of the location of an emergency cart are essential for the therapist who administers cytotoxic agents. For example, some hospital policies state that the nurse may not administer cancer chemotherapy agents without a physician being present. In addition, many institutions do not permit nurses to administer investigational drugs until their safety has been established and approval has been granted by the pharmacy and therapeutics committee. The rationale for this practice is that investigational drugs do not have the years of accumulated experience that are available with commercially available drugs. Since documented clinical experience is lacking, many policymakers feel that unknown side-effects cannot adequately be assessed and managed by nurses.

In anticipating the possibility of anaphylaxis, the nurse should continuously monitor the patient for signs of flushing, shaking, sudden agitation or anxiety, nausea, vomiting, urticaria, hypotension, generalized pruritus, throbbing in the ears, palpitation, paresthesias, or any respiratory distress (wheezing, coughing, shortness of breath, or an asthma-type reaction). If undetected, a generalized anaphylactic reaction could cause convulsions and cardiopulmonary arrest.

Prior to initiating therapy, the nurse should position the patient so that the reclining position can easily be managed if necessary (Figure 22.10). The therapist will find it most difficult to treat an anaphylactic reaction if the patient is seated at a table without a bed nearby. In addition, an emergency cart with the following appropriate medications should be readily available as well as the stethoscope and sphygmomanometer.

Epinephrine (Adrenalin)

Diphenhydramine hydrochloride (Benadryl)

Dopamine HCl (Intropin)

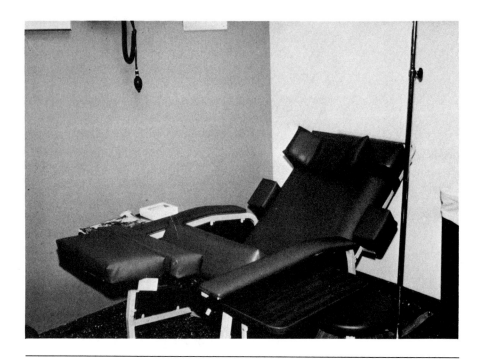

FIGURE 22.10
Should generalized anaphylactic reactions occur, a reclining chair is capable of supporting the patient. Note a wall-mounted sphygnomanometer.

Levarterenol bitartrate (Levophed)

Isoproterenol hydrochloride (Isuprel)

Sodium bicarbonate

Aminophylline

Hydrocortisone sodium succinate (Solu-Cortef)

Some facilities initiate a "standing order" sheet for each patient signed at treatment initiation by the responsible physician (Exhibit 22.2). This valuable time-saving procedure permits the therapist to initiate emergency treatment until physician assistance arrives.

The therapist should also obtain a baseline blood pressure reading prior to treatment. If the patient is normally hypotensive, establishing a normal blood pressure reading will be useful if symptoms of shock occur. Also, the baseline reference point of the patient's mental status should be observed by the therapist. The presence of metastatic brain disease or other mental alterations, if not noted early, can be misleading for the therapist who is attempting to determine if early symptoms of anaphylaxis are being manifested (e.g., agitation, anxiety, speech disorders, and mental confusion).

Regardless of whether a patient displays a mild reaction such as generalized pruritus or sustains a complete cardiovascular collapse, the therapist should be prepared to:

EXHIBIT 22.2
Routine Standing Orders

Routine Standing Orders for the Patient Receiving Cancer Chemotherapeutic Agents

Patient: _____ Drug Allergies: _____

Medical Record #: _____ Physician: _____

Date: _____

1. Patient should/should not (circle one) have scalp hypothermia/tourniquet used.

2. The orders listed below will be initiated for the prevention or reduction of nausea or vomiting:
   Compazine: 10 mg PO q4h PRN
   Compazine*: 10 mg IM q4h PRN
   Compazine: 25 mg rectal suppository q4h PRN
   Torecan: 10 mg IM q6h PRN
   Torecan*: 10 mg IM q6h PRN
   Torecan: 10 mg rectal suppository q6h PRN

3. The orders listed below will be initiated any time *Bleomycin* is administered:
   Benadryl: 25 mg PO ×1 if not vomiting
   Benadryl*: 25 mg PO ×1 if vomiting and if platelet count over 50 K
   Benadryl: 25 mg IV push if vomiting and platelet count under 50 K
   Tylenol: 600 mg PO ×1

4. The orders listed below will be initiated for the reduction of local vein discomfort due to the administration of IV DTIC, BiCNU or Streptozotocin: Xylocaine 1% (IV) ¼ cc PRN up to a total of 3 cc during the administration of the chemotherapeutic agent to titrate relief of local vein pain.

5. The orders below will be initiated to minimize the adverse reactions of extravasation of drugs causing tissue necrosis:

Nitrogen Mustard:	⅙ molar Sodium Thiosulfate 1 cc subcutaneous multiple injections around the periphery and into the site of extravasation.
Vincristine or Velban:	Wydase 1 cc (150 U.N.F.) subcutaneous multiple injections around the periphery and into the site of extravasation.
Adriamycin:	NaHCO$_3$ 4 cc IV and/or subcutaneous and Solu-Cortef 50 mg IV and/or subcutaneous according to department protocol.

6. The order below will be initiated to prevent or reduce local vein inflammation due to irritating and sclerosing drugs:
   Solu-Cortef 25–50 mg IV before and/or after drug therapy.

*Platelet count must be at least 50 K to administer IM injections.

Source: Stanford University Medical Center Oncology Day Care Center, Stanford, Calif.

1. Recline the patient safely and quickly.
2. Administer basic CPR resuscitative measures.
3. Maintain a patent I.V. line for emergency drug administration.
4. Provide reassurance to the patient.
5. Administer appropriate drugs as ordered.
6. Monitor the patient until the reaction subsides.

Prevention of anaphylaxis is a goal with the administration of all cancer chemotherapeutic agents. The therapist should be aware of the agents known to cause anaphylaxis and be prepared to administer those agents as recommended in the product brochure.

1. *Bleomycin sulfate (Blenoxane).* The package insert recommends treating lymphoma patients with 2 units or less with the first 2 doses [3].
2. *Cisplatin (Platinol).* No specific recommendations for dose attenuation or length of time of administration [16]. Suggestions for symptom management are listed in the product brochure.
3. *Asparaginase (Elspar).* "Desensitization should be performed before administering the first dose of Elspar on initiation of therapy on positive reactors, and on retreatment of any patient in whom therapy is deemed necessary after carefully weighing the increased risk of hypersensitivity reactions" [15].

In addition, an allergy history should be obtained and charted even though it is presumed to have been done by the physician. Precautionary measures to use when potential anaphylactic reactions are possible might include:

1. Test dosing.
2. Antihistaminic, steroidal, and/or antiinflammatory/antipyretic pretreatment.
3. Uninterrupted dosing to prevent a significant buildup of reactive antibodies [6].

EXTRAVASATION

"The treatment of local infiltrations of cancer chemotherapy agents is controversial. No treatments have well-documented efficacy" [6]. Controlled clinical trials are undoubtedly lacking in this area because of the low number of accruable patients treated by skilled therapists and because of the ethical issues associated with a control or no-treatment arm. It is often difficult, in fact, to ascertain that an infiltration actually has occurred. No trained therapist would knowingly permit an infiltration of sclerosing agents to continue to the point of being frankly obvious. Therefore, justifications of studies involving patients have been ethically and morally difficult to defend. Because of the particularly morbid effect of doxorubicin hydrochloride (Adriamycin) on tissues, the majority of studies on extravasation have been conducted using this drug. To date, only preclinical studies have been conducted using the animal model systems. "Those studies are themselves in question because when attempts have been made to recreate a standard type of tissue necrosis model in pigs, mice, rabbits and dogs, there has been a wide range of variability of necrosis from the same dose of a given drug [doxorubicin hydrochloride]" [4].

Consequences The consequences to the patient of extensive tissue necrosis are numerous. Areas to be considered include the following:

1. *Pain.* Extensive necrotic areas frequently require narcotics for pain control. Often patients are unable to sleep.

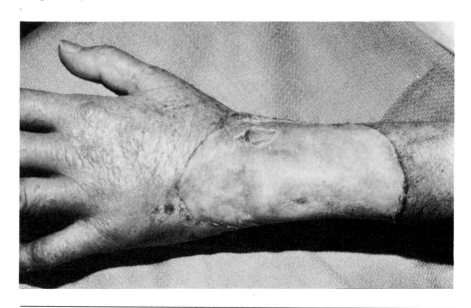

FIGURE 22.11
The patient is a piano teacher, thus hand concealment is not possible.

2. *Physical defect.* Patients may be unable to work for months. If they are employed in areas where public exposure is great, the cosmetic defect may have a severe emotional impact (Figure 22.11).

3. *Cost.* In most instances, patients bear the financial responsibility for the lengthy and numerous hospitalizations and extensive plastic surgery procedures that may be necessary. If patients are debilitated, additional time may be required and secondary medical problems may occur (Figure 22.12 A, B).

4. *Disease control.* Valuable time may be lost if patients are unable to continue medical treatments to control the disease process. Myelosuppression from previous chemotherapy treatments may cause a necrosed area to become secondarily infected, thus lengthening the interval before which chemotherapy treatments can be reinitiated.

5. *Time.* Patients who are employed or attend school may be unable to do so until healing occurs. The inability to sustain oneself financially may be an additional hardship for the entire family.

6. *Psychological impact.* The 5 points above emphasize that this is a difficult time for the patient. Communication between the therapist and patient may be strained because of the therapist's own feelings of guilt.

Prevention

Undoubtedly, years of experience in administering cytotoxic agents will perfect the therapist's technique. However, despite the skill of the therapist, extravasation of tissue-sclerosing agents can occur. This statement is underscored in an effort to allay the inevitable anxiety experienced by nurses who administer

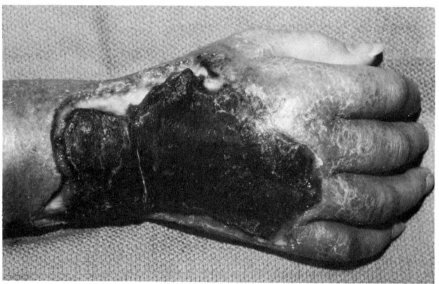

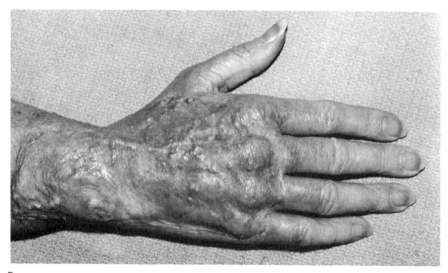

FIGURE 22.12
(A) Tissue necrosis from doxorubicin hydrochloride (Adriamycin) extravasation. Wide excision of the necrotic tissue and reconstructive plastic surgery were necessary. (B) The same patient after extensive debridement of involved soft tissues and tendons with skin-grafted flap. Further reconstructive surgery will be necessary to permit full extension of the hand.

Chapter 22 | Intravenous Cancer Chemotherapy Administration

cytotoxic agents. The emphasis should be on the perfection of I.V. techniques, anticipating and planning for the possibility of extravasation and detecting and treating *early* suspected infiltration. While there is no guarantee that extravasation will not occur, there should be a reasonable degree of assurance that the *extent* of involvement will be minimal.

Patient Education

The patient must be informed of the possible consequences when cancer chemotherapy agents are being administered. "Informed consent" is a necessity. Knowledge of the possibility of extravasation constitutes an essential part of informed consent. Of course, such information should be conveyed in a sensitive manner so as to allay unnecessary fears. Naturally, the unconscious or irrational patient should not have cytotoxic agents infused without a therapist being in constant attendance. The rational and cooperative patient may report stinging, burning, pain at the cannula insertion site, or any unusual sensation. It should be emphasized, however, that extravasation can occur in the absence of these reported symptoms.

General Precautions

In administering cytotoxic agents, the therapist should understand and follow the suggestions given below:

1. *Anticipate the possibility of extravasation.* Before initiating treatment, the therapist should know which agents, listed below, are capable of producing tissue necrosis.

   Dactinomycin (Cosmegen)

   Dacarbazine (DTIC)

   Daunomycin

   Doxorubicin (Adriamycin)

   Mechlorethamine HCl (Mustargen)

   Mithramycin (Mithracin)

   Mitomycin (Mutamycin)

   Vinblastine (Velban)

   Vincristine

   A conveniently posted chart listing vesicant agents and their recommended antidotes should be available (Table 22.2). In addition, the antidotes should be readily available for administration. Several studies suggest that delay in administering antidotes may increase the severity of local tissue reaction [11, 17]. The policy for the application of heat or ice as used by the nurse's facility should be understood (Exhibit 22.3). If standing orders are available, they should be signed by the individual physician and placed in the chart. Planning ahead can often minimize the severity of damage to the subcutaneous tissues.

2. *When in doubt, stop the infusion of the chemotherapy agent.* If there is any doubt in the nurse's mind that the cancer chemotherapy agent is not infusing properly, then the drug should *immediately* be discontinued. There is general agreement that the greater the amount of extravasation into the subcutaneous tissues, the more severe is the local

TABLE 22.2
Recommended Antidotes for Treating Extravasation of Vesicant Agents

Extravasated Drug	Recommended Antidote	A. Route for Administration B. Preparation C. Theoretical Action
Mechlorethamine HCl (Mustargen)	Sodium thiosulfate 10%-⅙ molar 1 gm/10 ml (product brochure recommendation)	A. SQ B. Add 4 ml of antidote to 6 ml sterile H_2O for injection C. Chemical neutralization, decreases DNA bonding
Vinca alkyloids	Hyaluronidase (Wydase) 150 U.N.F. (1 ml–150 N.F. — product brochure recommendation)	A. SQ B. Premixed vials C. Enhances absorption and dispersion of infiltrated drug
Daunomycin HCl (Adriamycin)	Sodium bicarbonate injection, U.S.P. 8.4%–50 mEq (1 mEq/ml) 4.2 gm (84 mg/ml)	A. SQ B. Premixed vials C. Alters the environmental pH, disrupts the DNA-doxorubicin linkage
Other potential vesicant agents	Hydrocortisone sodium succinate	A. I.V., SQ B. Varies with manufacturer's brand C. Antiinflammatory effect

EXHIBIT 22.3
Use of Heat and Ice for Extravasations

I. Heat
   A. The desired effect is to:
      1. Increase blood supply and increase the dispersion of the enzyme Hyaluronidase (Wydase) into the subcutaneous tissues.
      2. Promote healing after the first 24 hours by increasing blood supply.
      3. Enhance the absorption of the vessicant agent (theoretical effect of vasodilation).
   B. Opponents of the use of heat feel that vessicant agents injure the cells' metabolic mechanisms. Heat increases metabolic demands and therefore may decrease cellular destruction.*

II. Ice
   A. The desired effect is to:
      1. Decrease the blood supply and decrease the absorption of drugs into the subcutaneous tissues.
      2. Constrict peripheral veins which decrease blood supply to the area and thereby minimize localized pain.
      3. Decrease the absorption and diffusion of the vessicant agent, thereby resulting in local tissue "pooling" (theoretical effect of vasoconstriction).
   B. Proponents of the use of a cooling maneuver feel that ice decreases many enzymatic reactions and decreases the destructive effect of released white cell components (e.g., lysozymes). Ice also slows cellular metabolic rates and may improve survival of marginally injured tissues.*

Personal communication: V. Hentz, M.D., Plastic Surgery, Stanford University Medical Center, Stanford, California. In Miller, S. A. *Oncol. Nurs. Forum* 7(4): Fall 1980. Reprinted with permission.

tissue destruction. If veins are at a minimum, the therapist may elect to replace the drug with normal saline and infuse sufficient quantities while watching for signs of extravasation.

3. *Infuse at least 5–10 ml normal saline before cytotoxic agents are administered to ascertain vein patency.* Only when the therapist is sure beyond a doubt that the solution is infusing into the vein and not into the subcutaneous tissues should cytotoxic agents be administered. Additional infusion of normal saline may be necessary to satisfy the therapist. Once again, if there is any doubt about needle placement at any time during the drug infusion, normal saline should be infused or the venipuncture site changed.

4. *The therapist should be aware of a slow leak or insidious infiltration.* If the needle punctures the posterior wall of the vein, chemotherapy agents could leak into the deep subcutaneous tissues. If small-gauge needles are used and if a large amount of subcutaneous fat is present, this infiltration could remain unnoticed for some time. This reemphasizes the need to initially assess the venipuncture site and immediate surrounding skin for comparison. Some therapists outline the suspected area of infiltration with a pen, and watch for the outlined area to change in dimension while infusing normal saline.

5. *The therapist should be available to monitor the flow rate and check the blood flow frequently.* When administering drugs by I.V. push* the therapist should pull back on the plunger of the syringe approximately every 3–4 ml to note blood backflow. Although a good blood return does not guarantee that extravasation has not occurred, any change in blood backflow should be investigated. Repositioning of the needle may be necessary if the bevel is against the wall of the vein. A national study on I.V. therapy practices conducted over a 12-month period revealed that infiltration was reported as the most frequently seen complication (68 percent of the 7,000 responders) [14]. While the study did not indicate the types of I.V. solutions infused, this alarming statistic emphasizes the need for frequent observation (every 2–3 minutes), especially when vesicant agents are being infused. Nurses who work on inpatient units with additional patients to care for, frequently are not permitted the time to return to a patient's room every 2 to 3 minutes to monitor chemotherapy infusions. For that reason, many facilities have written policies that infused vesicant agents are not permitted unless the nurse is in constant attendance.

6. *A replacement nurse should have a thorough orientation.* Patients appreciate the security of knowing that when their regular nurse leaves a replacement nurse is qualified to assume their care. Introducing the patient to a replacement nurse is a courtesy often forgotten but greatly appreciated by the patient. The replacement nurse should take the time

---

*Push refers to an injection directly into the vein through the tubing of a needle.

to examine the I.V. site, check for vein patency, and review the chemotherapy drugs and rate of infusion. Both nurses should feel comfortable with the transition, and it should be accomplished in an unhurried atmosphere. The replacement nurse does not have a baseline pretreatment reference point for comparison and, if the I.V. site has not been examined closely with the nurse who initiated the procedure, uncertainties can later occur.

7. *A patient should not be permitted to leave the treatment area when vesicant agents are being infused.* Hospitalized patients frequently have diagnostic studies and therapies scheduled that occur during the time that chemotherapy is being administered. When patients are gone from the unit for extended periods and when physical maneuvering is expected, the possibility for needle dislodgment exists. In general, the larger the volume of drug extravasated, the greater the degree of tissue necrosis. Knowing this, the nurse should be cautioned against sending the patient away from his or her close supervision. If it is absolutely essential that the patient leave the treatment area, the cytotoxic agents should either be temporarily discontinued and normal saline substituted pending the patient's return, or the nurse should accompany the patient to supervise the drug infusion.

The last general precaution should be kept foremost in the therapist's mind.

8. *If there is ever any doubt that the cytotoxic agent may not be infusing properly, it should be discontinued and a new site established.* This may seem difficult to defend in patients with a scarcity of veins for whom venipuncture is difficult and painful. However, when vesicant agents are being administered, there should be no hesitancy in restarting the I.V. if doubt exists to the vein's patency.

Treatment

It was mentioned previously that many early infiltrations are difficult to detect. A point bearing reemphasis is that if extravasation is *suspected* when vesicants are being administered, it should be treated as a *presumed* extravasation. General guidelines to follow when vesicants have extravasated are outlined below. Recommended antidotes are found in Table 22.3. At this time, clinicians are not in agreement as to the best method of managing suspected infiltrations. Management techniques are empirically suggested based on personal experience, the literature, and reports from other experienced clinicians. Controlled prospective clinical studies will be necessary to determine the efficacy of those agents in preventing tissue necrosis. In addition, there is a need to devise a method of determining (1) whether infiltration has actually occurred and (2) the exact amount of extravasated drug. The ethical issues involved in assessing these two points clinically emphasizes the complexity of the problem.

Charting

The therapist should be reminded that for medicolegal purposes and to facilitate memory recall, charting should be completed as soon after the extravasation as possible. Not infrequently, potential litigation does not reach the

TABLE 22.3
Suggested Guidelines for the Treatment of Extravasation Associated with Vesicant Agents

Procedure	Rationale
1. Stop the infusion.	1. To prevent further drug leakage into the subcutaneous tissues.
2. Aspirate back remaining drug in the needle and tubing by drawing back on the syringe.	2. To remove any residual drug.
3. Superimpose normal saline.	3. To dilute the extravasated agent.
4. Administer by I.V. push sodium succinate (Solu-Cortef) 50 mg through the existing winged small-vein needle (physician's order needed).	4. To minimize inflammation.
5. Administer by I.V. push suggested antidotes, (physician's order needed). (See Table 22.2.)	5. To intentionally extravasate the antidote via the same route as the extravasated drug.
6. Remove the winged small-vein needle.	6. To facilitate step number 7. The site can no longer be used as an I.V. route.
7. Administer suggested antidotes (see Table 22.2) SQ with multiple punctures into the suspected extravasation site.	7. Direct infiltration of the antidote into area of greatest concentration.
8. Elevate extremity.	8. To minimize swelling.
9. Apply heat or ice.	9. See Exhibit 22.3.
10. Apply topical antidotes.	10. To minimize surface (skin) inflammatory and erythematous reactions.
11. Obtain a plastic surgery consult.	11. Early plastic surgery intervention with wound debridement is mentioned by several authors when doxorubicin HCl has extravasated [4,17]. When doxorubicin was initially introduced clinically, the necrotic ulcers from extravasation were followed without debridement. The ulcers showed no tendency to heal spontaneously. It is believed that doxorubicin attaches to the DNA molecule and causes cell death. It is thought that the drug is then released to attach to adjacent living cells with further cellular destruction. Early excision is advised to stop this progression.
12. Document in writing in official patient record.	12. To enhance later recall and for medicolegal purposes.
13. Call the patient.	13. To follow symptomatology and ensure that appropriate interventions are initiated.

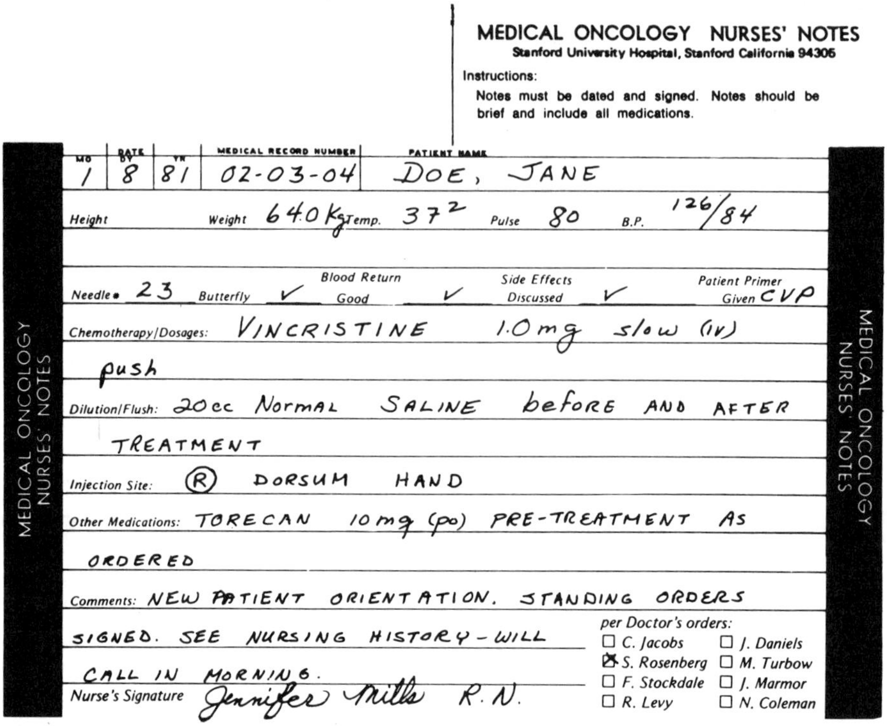
MEDICAL ONCOLOGY NURSES' NOTES
Stanford University Hospital, Stanford California 94305
Instructions:
Notes must be dated and signed. Notes should be brief and include all medications.

MO	DAY	YR	MEDICAL RECORD NUMBER	PATIENT NAME
1	8	81	02-03-04	DOE, JANE

Height — Weight 64.0 Kg Temp. 37[2] Pulse 80 B.P. 126/84

Needle # 23 Butterfly ✓ Blood Return Good ✓ Side Effects Discussed ✓ Patient Primer Given CVP

Chemotherapy/Dosages: VINCRISTINE 1.0 mg slow (iv) push

Dilution/Flush: 20cc Normal SALINE before AND AFTER TREATMENT

Injection Site: (R) DORSUM HAND

Other Medications: TORECAN 10 mg (po) PRE-TREATMENT AS ORDERED

Comments: NEW PATIENT ORIENTATION. STANDING ORDERS SIGNED. SEE NURSING HISTORY - WILL CALL IN MORNING.

Nurse's Signature Jennifer Mills R.N.

per Doctor's orders:
☐ C. Jacobs ☐ J. Daniels
☒ S. Rosenberg ☐ M. Turbow
☐ F. Stockdale ☐ J. Marmor
☐ R. Levy ☐ N. Coleman

MEDICAL ONCOLOGY NURSES' NOTES

FIGURE 22.13
Essential information pertaining to each chemotherapy treatment is recorded on the medical oncology nurses' notes. The nurses' note reflects a new patient treatment. Information pertaining to an extravasation would be recorded in the "comments" section.

courts until several years after the incident. While the therapist is permitted to review the medical documents, the situation will more readily be recalled if charting is complete and recorded in detail at the time of the incident. Our facility includes the charting listed below:

1. Facility's Nurses' Notes (Figure 22.13)
2. Extravasation Record (Figure 22.14)
3. Incident Report

REFERENCES

1. Baird, G. M., and Willoughby, M. L. N. Photodegradation of dacarbazine. *Lancet* 2:681, 1978.
2. Bjeletich, J., and Hickman, R. The Hickman indwelling catheter. *Am. J. Nurs.* 80:62–65, 1980.
3. Bleomycin sulfate product brochure. Syracuse, N.Y.: *Bristol-Myers* October, 1978.
4. Bowers, D., and Lynch, J. Adriamycin extravasation. *Plast. Reconstr. Surg.* 61:86–92, 1978.
5. Cancer Chemotherapy Guidelines and Recommendations for Nursing Education and Practice. Oncology Nursing Society, 1984.

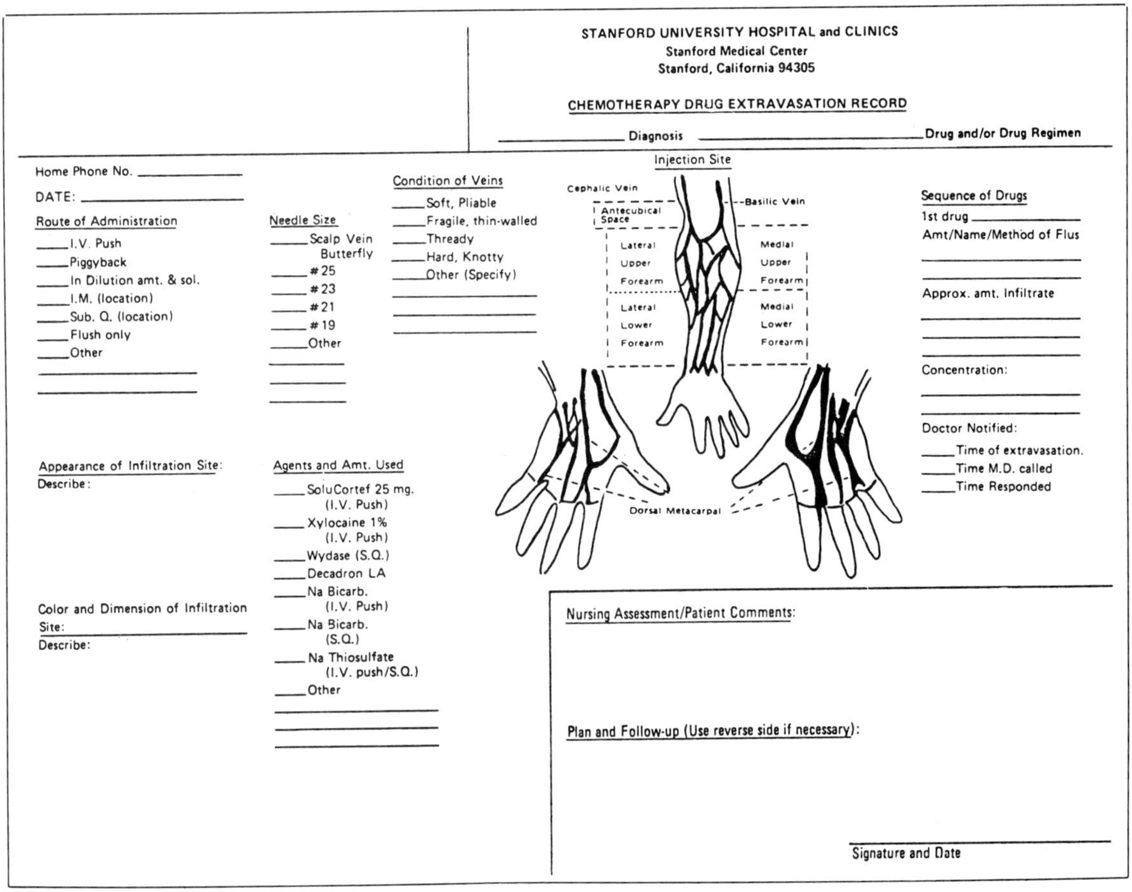

STANFORD UNIVERSITY HOSPITAL and CLINICS
Stanford Medical Center
Stanford, California 94305

CHEMOTHERAPY DRUG EXTRAVASATION RECORD

__________ Diagnosis __________ Drug and/or Drug Regimen

Home Phone No. __________

DATE: __________

Route of Administration
____I.V. Push
____Piggyback
____In Dilution amt. & sol.
____I.M. (location)
____Sub. Q. (location)
____Flush only
____Other

Needle Size
____Scalp Vein Butterfly
____#25
____#23
____#21
____#19
____Other

Condition of Veins
____Soft, Pliable
____Fragile, thin-walled
____Thready
____Hard, Knotty
____Other (Specify)

Injection Site

Sequence of Drugs
1st drug __________
Amt/Name/Method of Flus

Approx. amt. Infiltrate

Concentration:

Doctor Notified:
____Time of extravasation.
____Time M.D. called
____Time Responded

Appearance of Infiltration Site:
Describe:

Agents and Amt. Used
____SoluCortef 25 mg. (I.V. Push)
____Xylocaine 1% (I.V. Push)
____Wydase (S.Q.)
____Decadron LA
____Na Bicarb. (I.V. Push)
____Na Bicarb. (S.Q.)
____Na Thiosulfate (I.V. push/S.Q.)
____Other

Color and Dimension of Infiltration Site: __________
Describe:

Nursing Assessment/Patient Comments:

Plan and Follow-up (Use reverse side if necessary):

____
Signature and Date

FIGURE 22.14
Extravasation Record used at Stanford University Hospital and Clinic. From Miller, S. A. *Oncol. Nurs. Forum* 7 [4]: Fall 1980. Reprinted with permission.

6. Dorr, R., and Fritz, W. *Cancer Chemotherapy Handbook*. New York: Elsevier North-Holland, 1980, p. 109.
7. Dorr, R., and Fritz, W. *Cancer Chemotherapy Handbook*. New York: Elsevier North-Holland, 1980, p. 115.
8. Dorr, R., and Fritz, W. *Cancer Chemotherapy Handbook*. New York: Elsevier North-Holland, 1980, p. 745.
9. Haimov, M. Vascular access for hemodialysis. *Surg. Gynecol. Obstet.* 141:619, 1975.
10. Hall, N. Arteriovenous access. *N.I.T.A.* 3:214–216, 1980.
11. Ignoffo, R., and Friedman, M. Therapy of local toxicities caused by extravasation of cancer chemotherapy drugs. *Cancer Treat. Rep.* 7:17–27, 1980.
12. Irwin, B. Hemodialysis means vascular access . . . and the right kind of nursing care. *Nursing '79*, 9:48–53, 1979.
13. Knowles, S., and Virden, J. E. Handling of injectible antineoplastic drugs. *Br. Med. J.* 281:589–591, 1980.
14. Kurdi, W. Report on intravenous therapy national survey. *Nursing '81*, 11:80–82, 1981.

15. L-Asparaginase product brochure. West Point, Pa.: Merch Sharp & Dohme, June, 1979.
16. Platinol product brochure. Syracuse, N.Y.: Bristol-Myers, August, 1979.
17. Rudolph, R., Stein, R., and Pattillo, R. Skin ulcers due to Adriamycin. *Cancer* 38:1087–1094, 1976.
18. Tellis, V. A., Veith, F. J., Gaberman, R. J., Freed, S. Z., and Gliedman, M. L. Internal arteriovenous fistula for hemodialysis. *Surg. Gynecol. Obstet.* 132:866, 1971.
19. Vogelzang, N. Adriamycin flare: A skin reaction resembling extravasation. *Cancer Treat. Rep.* 63:2067–2069, 1979.

BIBLIOGRAPHY

Burkhalter, P., and Donley, D. *Dynamics of Oncology Nursing.* New York: McGraw-Hill, 1978.

Cline, M. J. *Cancer Chemotherapy.* Philadelphia: Saunders, 1971.

Marino, L. *Cancer Nursing.* St. Louis, Mo.: Mosby, 1981.

Pratt, W., and Ruddon, R. *The Anticancer Drugs.* New York: Oxford University Press, 1979.

REVIEW QUESTIONS

1. The goal in administering intravenous chemotherapy is to provide _____ care to each patient.
2. If treatment is administered to a patient without his or her informed consent, the therapist may be held liable for _____ .
3. List four reasons why patients should be educated about and become active participants in their I.V. chemotherapy treatment program.
4. If there is any doubt that I.V. cancer chemotherapy agents are not infusing properly, the therapist should _____ .
5. List six essential points to consider before establishing a venipuncture site on a patient who is to receive I.V. anticancer drugs.
6. List four methods to affect vein distention without using a tourniquet.
7. List four alternatives available for establishing a patent venous pathway for each I.V. chemotherapy administration.
8. List six precautions the therapist should take when preparing and mixing I.V. chemotherapy agents for administration.
9. In general, a preexisting I.V. site should be used to administer I.V. cytotoxic agents. True or false?
10. Before administering I.V. chemotherapy, what precautionary steps should the therapist take in anticipating and preventing anaphylactic reactions?
11. Extravasation is always preventable. True or false?
12. List nine potentially vesicant agents.
13. The best method for treating extravasations is _____ .
14. List six reasons why extravasation should be avoided.
15. Charting an extravasation should be completed soon after the occurrence because _____ and _____

CHAPTER 23

Intraarterial Therapy

Faye Cosentino

INTRAARTERIAL ACCESS

The growth of I.V. therapy as a specialty nursing service coincided with the increasingly common practice of performing arterial punctures. Through technical advancement of blood analyzers it was now possible to obtain measurements of blood levels and pressures of carbon dioxide and oxygen as well as bicarbonate blood levels because the lungs had eliminated carbon dioxide from and added oxygen to arterial blood. Since arterial blood supplies all body tissues, medical practitioners recognized the advantages gained for diagnosis and assessment of treatment if this blood analysis were performed on arterial rather than venous blood. It soon became apparent that arterial punctures could be safely performed. The next step was the placement of indwelling arterial catheters to allow for multiple drawings of arterial blood specimens and/or continuous arterial pressure monitoring. Many institutions recognized that I.V. nurses already possessed venipuncture expertise and therefore were the best qualified personnel to perform arterial punctures.

GENERAL CONSIDERATIONS

Methods and Purposes	An arterial puncture may be performed with a syringe and needle for a one-time sample of arterial blood for ABG measurement or by insertion of an indwelling catheter to obtain serial or daily ABG samples and constant arterial pressure monitoring.
Sites	The *radial artery* is usually considered the site of first choice because (1) it is very superficial and easiest to enter, (2) its location at the wrist makes it easy to stabilize for a quick entry, (3) if thrombosis should occur, the ulnar artery will, by collateral circulation, supply blood to the entire hand (shown by the

Allen's test), and (4) it is easy to apply a postpuncture pressure dressing at this site.

Second, and third site choices vary according to institution and personal preferences.

The *ulnar artery* is usually much deeper and more difficult to stabilize than the radial artery, so although it may be larger it is usually not the first choice as an entry site. Further, most authors will agree that if the radial artery has been entered the ulnar artery of the same arm should not be used.

The *brachial artery* at the antecubital fossa frequently lies deep, close to nerves and tendons, and is difficult to stabilize. If thrombosis should occur in the brachial artery, blood supply to the forearm and hand may be compromised (Figure 23.1).

The *femoral artery* located midway between the anterior superior spine of the ilium and the symphysis pubis (Figure 23.2) is the largest accessible artery and is easily palpated, stabilized, and entered. However, it is difficult to maintain with intact dry sterile dressings and digital pressure is required for postpuncture pressure. If postpuncture thrombosis should occur in the femoral artery a limb- or life-threatening condition may result.

ONE-TIME ARTERIAL BLOOD GAS SAMPLING

Patient Preparation Steps for patient preparation ABG sampling include the following:

1. The physician's order should include the fraction of inspired oxygen (FIO_2) or, room air fraction of oxygen (21% O_2), and the patient should be at this steady state continuously for 15–20 minutes prior to drawing the blood sample.
2. Unless a postexercise sample is ordered, the patient should be at rest for this period of time.
3. The patient's position can result in varied ABG measurements. A supine position may result in more difficult breathing than would sitting upright. The most comfortable position for the patient should be used for all blood sampling procedures.
4. The procedure must be fully explained to the patient because anxiety and fear can cause hyperventilation and alteration of the blood values.
5. The person performing the arterial puncture should be competent because undue trauma will cause pain, often leading to hyperventilation by the patient and resulting in alteration of the blood values.

Equipment The laboratory requisition form should have all the usual information plus the oxygen status of the patient, time of day (for serial drawings), and, if the patient is on a respirator, all pertinent settings. In some institutions, the patient's temperature and hemoglobin count are also required.

ABG blood samples can be drawn with existing hospital equipment.

Chapter 23 | Intraarterial Therapy

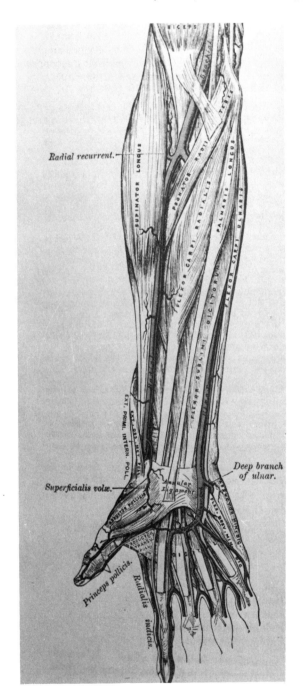

FIGURE 23.1
Anatomical location of radial, ulnar and brachial arteries. Courtesy of Gray, H. *Anatomy, Descriptive and Surgical.* New York: Crown, 1977.

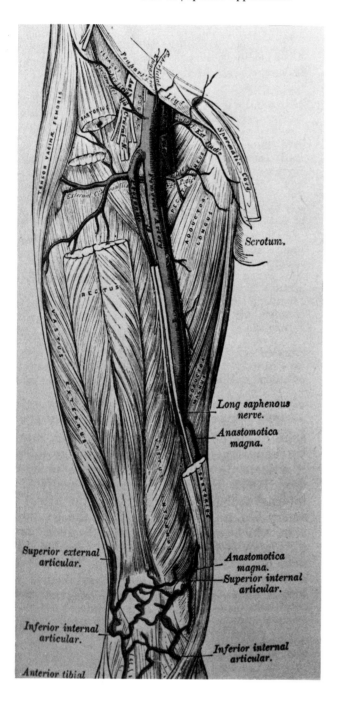

FIGURE 23.2
Anatomical location of the femoral artery. Courtesy of Gray, H. *Anatomy, Descriptive and Surgical.* New York: Crown, 1977.

Needed supplies are as follows:

>   Airtight syringe (2 ml–10 ml)
>
>   Appropriate size needles (2)
>   a. for radial or brachial artery: 25 gauge × ⅝ inch or 22 gauge × 1 inch
>   b. for femoral artery: 22 gauge × 1½ inch or 20 gauge × 1½ inch
>
>   Heparin 1 ml (1,000 U.S.P. units/ml)
>
>   Alcohol swab
>
>   Iodophor prep
>
>   Sterile 2 × 2 inch sponge
>
>   Rubber stopper or syringe cap
>
>   Labeled container with ice (paper cup or emesis basin)
>
>   1 inch adhesive tape

To heparinize syringe, attach needle other than one to be used for puncture to syringe, cleanse top of heparin vial or neck of ampule with alcohol swab, and open ampule. Withdraw 1 ml heparin into syringe, draw plunger back and forth several times to coat plunger with heparin, and rotate plunger to eliminate dry spots. To eliminate any air bubbles, hold syringe with needle upright and gently tap sides of syringe, or turn syringe with needle pointed downward and *slowly* invert syringe upright. Discard needle used for heparinization, and place and *secure tightly* needle selected for arterial puncture. With syringe in inverted position, push plunger up and expel all excess heparin. *The only heparin remaining should be in the dead space of the needle and on the walls of the syringe.* Excess heparin or air bubbles will alter the resultant ABG values.

An ABG kit is commonly used for this procedure. Such kits have become quite inexpensive and contain, except for ice and tape, all equipment needed to perform a one-time arterial puncture. If the kit contains a heparinized prefilled syringe, remove syringe cap, place and secure appropriate size needle, wet inner walls of syringe with heparin, and expel excess heparin with the same method used for a syringe that is not prefilled. Most ABG kits contain a plastic bag for the iced blood sample. An ABG blood sample that has not been immediately placed in ice can have faulty results since red blood cells will continue to metabolize O_2 and give off CO_2.

Procedure

Radial Puncture

As with any invasive procedure, begin by donning gloves. Check the site for a palpable pulse and take precautions to monitor the condition of skin, surrounding tissues, and any previous arterial puncture marks.

Perform Allen's test to assure the adequacy of collateral circulation. Locate and compress both the radial and ulnar arteries; blanching of the hand shows successful compression (Figure 23.3). Release only the ulnar artery pressure; good color should return to the entire hand. If this does not occur, another site for the puncture must be selected.

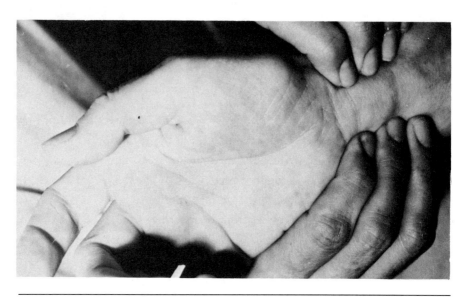

FIGURE 23.3
To perform Allen's Test, locate and compress both the radial and ulnar arteries.

A rolled towel may be placed under the wrist, causing hyperextension of the hand to stretch and stabilize the artery. The skin is prepped with iodophor, wiping with the circular method and allowing at least a 30-second contact time with the intended puncture site. Gloves should be worn.

A local anesthetic is not always necessary for an arterial puncture with a needle. With it, the chances for a quick, successful entry are less, and the anesthetic does not help the discomfort of arterial entry. However, if a difficult entry is anticipated or multiple attempts are necessary, a local anesthetic injected at the intended entry site will eliminate skin discomfort.

To perform the radial puncture, palpate artery and align two or three fingertips along the direction the artery follows. Hold syringe no higher than a 30° angle with the needle pointed directly toward the artery. With one smooth step, quickly enter skin and artery. Artery pressure will usually cause the blood to spontaneously pulsate back into the syringe (Figure 23.4). If blood pressure is low or the syringe not free flowing, it may be necessary to withdraw *gently* upon the plunger. If strong traction is applied to draw the blood faster, the chances of arterial spasm, blood hemolysis, and air contamination are all increased. The blood return will stop when the level of the automatic shutoff is reached. If a shutoff feature is not available, 1–2 ml blood is sufficient for the blood gas analyzer.

The 2 × 2 inch sterile sponge is folded to form a pressure point and, immediately following the quick withdrawal of the needle and syringe, is applied with digital pressure to the puncture site. Taking precautions not to encircle the entire wrist, the pressure dressing is firmly secured with tape.

If a syringe cap is to be used, remove the needle from the syringe and

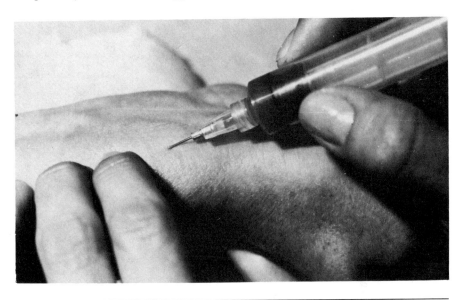

FIGURE 23.4
Performing radial artery puncture. (Pulsator syringe, Concord Laboratories, Inc., Keene, N.H.) Revised recommendations call for gloves to be worn.

attach the cap quickly and securely. If a rubber stopper is to be used, stick the needle tip into the center of the stopper. Roll the syringe back and forth between the hands for 5–10 seconds to ensure mixing of the blood and heparin. The unit is then placed in the iced container and taken immediately for analysis. A small amount of cold water added to the ice provides for even, cold distribution and facilitates placement of the sample so that all the blood in the barrel is in contact with iced water.

Femoral Puncture
The femoral artery is usually easily palpated with the patient in supine position. If the patient is very obese, assistance may be needed to hold the abdomen away or the patient's buttocks may be placed on an inverted bedpan.

Wearing gloves, prepping of patient's skin, and finger prepping are done in the same manner as for a radial artery puncture.

The following two different techniques may be utilized to perform a femoral arterial puncture:

1. The artery is located and "fixed" between two fingers, allowing pulsation to be felt on both fingers but at the same time allowing enough room between them for the needle entry. The syringe and needle are held almost straight down. When the puncture is made in this manner, care must be taken not to pierce through the other wall of the artery (Figure 23.5).

2. The entry may be performed with the same techniques used for a radial artery puncture. Two or three fingertips are placed along the direction

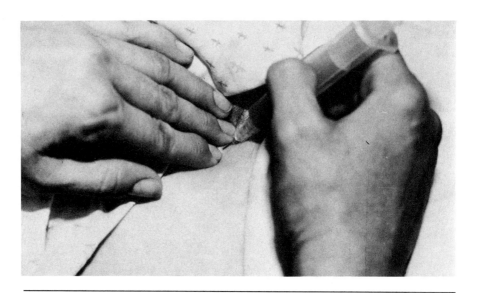

FIGURE 23.5
Performing femoral artery puncture. (Pulsator syringe, Concord Laboratories, Inc., Keene, N.H.) Revised recommendations require gloves to be worn.

of the femoral artery, and the syringe and needle are held no higher than a 30° angle. This method must be used for femoral artery catheter placement and, if used for a one-time needle and syringe sample, there is less chance of artery perforation.

Regardless of the method used, when pulsation is strong it will be relayed up through the needle and syringe as the needle touches and penetrates the artery. The walls of the femoral artery are usually very thick and resistant to puncture, so feeling pulsations can be a good needle tip placement guide. When the artery is entered, the blood will usually pulsate back into and fill the syringe without any traction being applied upon the plunger.

When the needle and syringe are removed, digital pressure is needed since a pressure dressing with tape is difficult to maintain in the femoral artery area.

The care of the blood sample is the same as that outlined for a radial artery puncture.

Postprocedure Patient Care
If the oxygen status of the patient has been altered *only* for the blood sampling, presampling status should be resumed as soon as the blood specimen is drawn.

The pressure dressing should be maintained long enough — usually 5 minutes is sufficient — to prevent excessive seepage of blood into the tissues. The pressure dressing must not be so restrictive as to cause blanching or severe restriction of venous blood in the hand. It should be removed when bleeding has stopped and not left on indefinitely. *If the patient is receiving anticoagulation therapy, digital pressure must be used for all arterial punctures. Personal observation and digital pressure must be maintained until all signs of bleeding have stopped or massive hematomas may result.*

Chapter 23 | Intraarterial Therapy

PLACEMENT OF AN INDWELLING ARTERIAL CATHETER

Serial or Daily ABG Sample Drawing

Frequently, serial or daily ABG sample drawing is necessary. To avoid multiple punctures it may be advisable to place an indwelling catheter to obtain the blood samples.

The *radial artery* is usually the site of first choice because it is the easiest to enter, easiest to maintain with intact sterile dressings, and allows the patient the greatest freedom of movement. It is imperative that Allen's test be performed before placing any indwelling catheter in the radial artery because the long-term placement with decreased blood flow will increase the risk of thrombosis.

The *brachial artery* may be the site given first choice because it is the largest artery in the arm. However, its use requires splinting of the elbow to prevent movement and displacement of the catheter.

The *femoral artery* may be the least favorable site because of the extreme difficulty in maintaining sterility of the site with intact dressings and the limits of mobility placed upon the patient.

When inserting any indwelling arterial catheter, extra precautions must be taken to do a thorough hand washing. Skin prepping in this instance may include an acetone defatting as well as a complete iodophor prep. In some institutions, sterile gloves are mandatory for this procedure and should always be used by those practitioners without expertise where probing is anticipated.

A local anesthetic may be injected at the insertion site, especially if an 18-gauge or larger catheter is being used. It is preferable that only experienced personnel perform this procedure because a successful entry with the first attempt is highly desirable since the availability of suitable arteries is limited.

Catheter Insertion And Sample Drawing

Catheter with Obturator

When using a catheter with obturator, follow the procedure outlined below.

1. Wearing gloves, insert catheter at a 30° angle, utilizing the same techniques as those used to perform venipuncture of a superficial vein without a tourniquet (Figure 23.6).

2. As the catheter tip touches and enters the artery, pulsation can be felt up through the catheter. The artery walls are thicker and more resistant to entry than vein walls, making this procedure quite painful if not done quickly and with expertise.

3. When the artery is fully entered, blood will pulsate back into the stylet; the catheter is then fully advanced (Figure 23.7).

4. To maintain a sterile field while removing the stylet and placing the obturator, an iodophor swab or sterile 2 × 2 inch sponge may be placed under the catheter hub.

5. To facilitate the stylet–obturator change, the arterial blood flow may be temporarily shut off, either by digital pressure at the catheter tip or by adequate placement of a tourniquet proximal to the insertion site.

6. After the obturator is removed from its protective shield, the stylet is

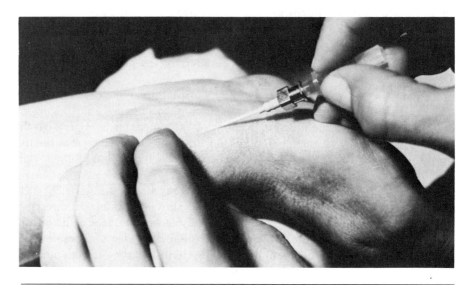

FIGURE 23.6
Inserting catheter into radial artery. (Jelco catheter, Critikon, Inc., Tampa, Fla.)

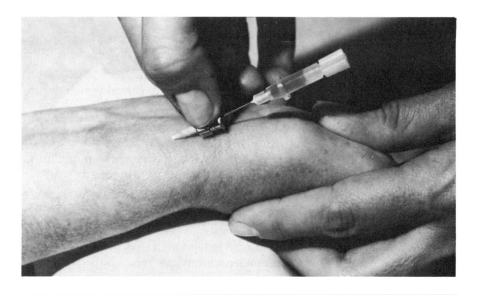

FIGURE 23.7
Advancing catheter into radial artery. (Jelco catheter, Critikon, Inc., Tampa, Fla.)

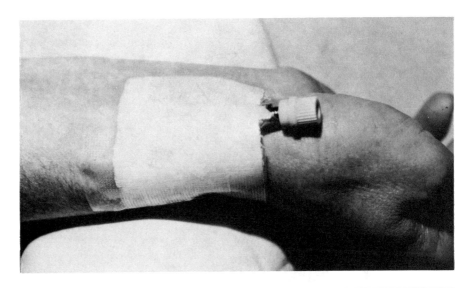

FIGURE 23.8
Catheter with obturator in radial artery. (Jelco catheter-obturator, Critikon, Inc., Tampa, Fla.)

removed from the catheter, obturator is inserted and locked by twisting in place, and arterial pressure is released.

7. Apply antimicrobial ointment and sterile 2 × 2 inch dressing to the insertion site and firmly secure with tape. Take care not to encircle the wrist and cause a tourniquet effect, which could compromise circulation to the hand.
8. Label the arterial entry, and include the date and time of insertion and the initials of the person performing the procedure on the dressing (Figure 23.8).
9. Chart the procedure stating the date, time, type and gauge catheter used, insertion site, any patient reactions, and name of person performing procedure.

Arterial Blood Gas Sample
When an ABG sample is needed:
1. Wearing gloves, prepare heparinized syringe without needle.
2. Apply digital or tourniquet arterial pressure.
3. Place iodophor swab or sterile 2 × 2 inch sponge under catheter hub.
4. Remove obturator.
5. Connect heparinized syringe to catheter hub.
6. Release arterial pressure.
7. Allow syringe to fill with required amount of blood.
8. Reapply arterial pressure.

488 Part VI | Specific Applications

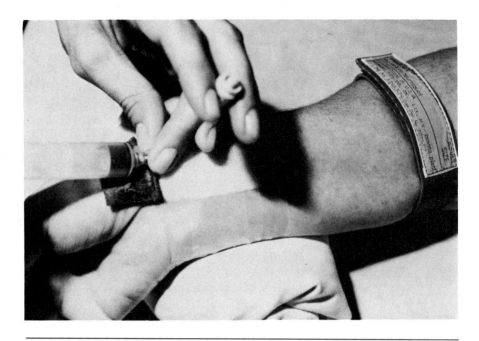

FIGURE 23.9
Drawing ABG sample from catheter with obturator. Revised recommendations call for gloves to be worn. (Jelco catheter-obturator, Critikon, Inc., Tampa, Fla.)

9. Remove syringe from catheter.
10. Insert and lock new sterile obturator.
11. Release arterial pressure.
12. Cap syringe and treat sample as for a one-time puncture for ABG specimen (Figure 23.9).

PRN Catheter (Heparin Lock)
When using a heparin lock, observe the following method:

1. Wearing gloves, insert catheter using same techniques used for catheter with obturator.
2. Pressure to stop arterial blood flow is not needed because there is no stylet–obturator change.
3. Flush catheter with dilute heparin solution.
4. Dressing, documentation at site, and charting are the same as for catheter with obturator.

Arterial Blood Gas Sample
When an ABG sample is needed:

1. Wearing gloves, prepare (a) heparinized syringe with 1 inch × 22 gauge needle for the blood sample, (b) plain syringe with 1 inch × 22 gauge needle for withdrawal of dilute heparin in heparin lock, and (c) syringe and needle

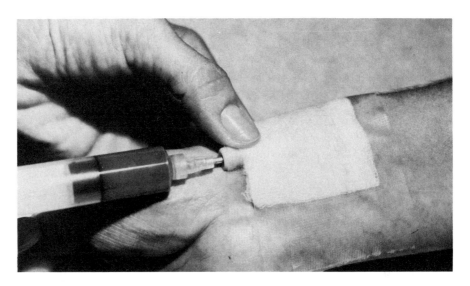

FIGURE 23.10
Drawing ABG sample from PRN catheter. (Jelco intermittent-injection cap. Critikon, Inc., Tampa, Fla.)

with dilute heparin solution for flushing the catheter after drawing the ABG sample.

2. Cleanse injection site of catheter with antiseptic.
3. Securely anchor catheter hub with free hand to prevent excessive pressure at insertion site and insert needle with plain syringe. Withdraw and discard approximately 0.5 ml of blood with dilute heparin from catheter.
4. Re-cleanse injection port and insert needle of syringe heparinized for ABG sample. Allow syringe to fill with enough blood for sample (see Figure 23.10). Remove syringe with needle.
5. Re-cleanse injection port and, still maintaining secure anchorage of catheter hub, insert needle of syringe with dilute heparin and flush catheter. Remove syringe and needle.
6. Treat blood sample in the same manner as for one-time puncture for ABG specimen.

When entering any PRN catheter with a needle, *extreme care must be taken to use a needle short enough that the needle tip cannot pass beyond the catheter hub* into the catheter itself. If the needle tip does enter the catheter, the catheter can be pierced and broken off by the needle tip with a resultant catheter embolus. The needle gauge must be small enough to allow postpuncture closure of the entry site, otherwise leakage of blood and risk of contamination are increased.

Aftercare of Patient

Close site monitoring, including the following steps, is required after placement of any type indwelling arterial catheter:

1. Observe the site for thrombosis of the artery, hematoma formation, perforation of artery, and catheter kinking or dislodgement.
2. Check the hand for adequate blood supply by noting color and temperature.
3. Maintain secure, clean, and intact dressings.
4. Avoid undue stress at insertion site by using the unaffected arm for blood pressure monitoring and venipunctures.

CONSTANT ARTERIAL PRESSURE MONITORING

Placement of Catheter

Constant arterial pressure monitoring requires placement of an indwelling arterial catheter. This procedure allows for

1. Continuous systolic, diastolic, and mean arterial pressure readings.
2. An assessment of the cardiovascular effects vasopressor/vasodilator drugs during the treatment of shock.
3. Simultaneous drawing of arterial blood for ABG measurements.

A cardiac monitor with a module for measuring arterial pressure is required. The monitor is connected by cable and a transducer to a special I.V. set-up. The I.V. system consists of a 500-ml bag of normal saline solution which has been heparinized (usually 500 units/500 ml) to inhibit catheter clotting and thrombus formation at the catheter tip. The bag is connected to an I.V. tubing and placed inside a pressure infusor bag with a gauge and inflation bulb, the same one used to pump blood transfusions. Some institutions prefer microdrip tubings, but air bubbles are more persistent with this size drip. Other hospitals prefer macrodrip tubings; this size drip allows a larger volume of fluid to be infused. The I.V. tubing is connected by a high-pressure extension tubing, a continuous flush attachment, and three-way stopcocks to a transducer dome. The entire system is flushed. *All connections must be secured and all air bubbles eliminated.* The transducer is covered with the dome and secured on a plate attached to an I.V. pole at the level of the patient's right atrium (see Figure 23.11). Each manufacturer provides detailed instructions for this set-up, which should be read and carefully followed.

Any indwelling catheter may be used for this procedure and the insertion is the same as that shown for serial or daily ABG sample drawing. The catheter is connected to the primed I.V. tubing by placing an iodophor swab or sterile 2×2 inch sponge under the catheter hub, applying digital or tourniquet arterial pressure distal to the site, removing stylet, connecting and securing tubing adapter, and releasing arterial pressure. The pressure infusor bag is inflated to 300 mmHg to automatically deliver a designated volume, depending on the drip size, of fluid per hour.

Antimicrobial ointment and a sterile dressing are applied to the insertion site and securely taped. The site is labeled to clearly denote an arterial entry,

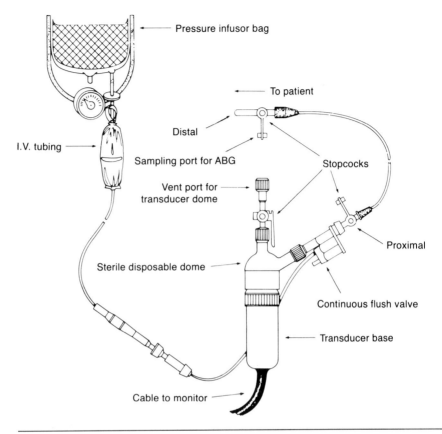

FIGURE 23.11
I.V. system for arterial pressure monitoring.

date, time, type and gauge of catheter, and initials of person performing the insertion. A short handboard may be required to limit wrist motion. If restraints are necessary they should be applied around the handboard, not the patient's wrist, as this could cause arterial pressure interference and increase the risk of catheter kinking or dislodgement.

Aftercare
Aftercare of the insertion site is the same as that for an indwelling catheter placed for serial or daily ABG drawing.

Arterial Blood Gas Sample
When an ABG sample is needed a sampling port provides for an easy arterial access. Sampling may be performed with the use of syringes and needles or, to minimize the number of port punctures into a latex port, a pediatric vacuum tube holder (22 gauge × 1 inch needle) and pediatric specimen tubes may be used.

Syringe and Needle Method
The syringe and needle method is performed as follows:

1. Prepare an empty 3 ml syringe with 22 gauge × 1 inch needle and a heparinized syringe and needle for the ABG sample.
2. Swab injection latex port with antiseptic.
3. Insert needle of empty syringe into port.
4. Turn stopcock ON between catheter and injection port, OFF between catheter and transducer.
5. Allow syringe to fill to rid line of I.V. fluid and blood mixture.
6. Remove and discard filled syringe.
7. Cleanse injection port.
8. Insert needle of heparinized syringe into injection port and allow syringe to fill to the appropriate level.
9. Remove syringe and needle.
10. Turn stopcock back to operating position and flush tubing until it is clear of blood.

If the injection port is the type which has a cap without a latex entry site, the syringes are used without needles and a new sterile cap must be replaced on the port, after each sample drawing.

Pediatric Vacuum Tube Method
For the pediatric vacuum tube method, use the following steps:

1. Swab injection port with antiseptic.
2. Insert needle connected with pediatric vacuum tube holder and a plain vacuum tube into injection port.
3. Turn stopcock ON between catheter and injection port.
4. Fully insert tube into holder and allow to fill with I.V. fluid and blood mixture (Figure 23.12).
5. Remove and discard filled tube.
6. Insert heparinized tube and allow to fully fill.
7. Remove filled heparinized tube (ABG sample) and place in ice.
8. Insert plain vacuum tube, turn stopcock back to operating position, and allow it to fill, rinsing port free of blood. Remove and discard filled tube and holder.
9. Flush remainder of tubing until clear of blood.

The blood specimen is gently rotated to ensure mixing of blood with heparin, placed in a labeled iced container, and sent immediately for analysis.

Malfunctions and Complications

Malfunctions
Common malfunctions occurring in arterial pressure lines include the following:

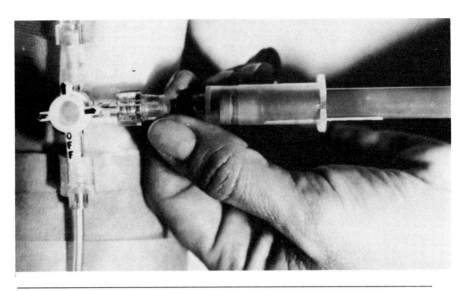

FIGURE 23.12
Drawing ABG sample from continuous pressure monitoring stopcock, using pediatric vacuum holder and tube. (Veroject holder and tube, Kimble-Terumo, Elkton, Md.)

1. Air bubbles in the system can cause distorted wave patterns. Care must be taken during the original set-up that all air bubbles are eliminated and all connections tightly secured. During each manipulation of the system, caution must be taken that air is not allowed to enter the line.

2. Near-exsanguination has been reported from disconnection of the line with the catheter remaining in the artery. Here again, care must be taken that *all* connections are secure during the original set-up and at frequent intervals thereafter to avoid this serious malfunction.

3. A "damped" pressure tracing, almost flat, will result if the catheter tip lies against the artery wall or the catheter becomes kinked. Secure catheter hub taping, intact dressings, and proper application of restraints can all help prevent this malfunction.

4. Catheter clotting occurs if the pressure infusor bag is allowed to fall below 300 mmHg. The pressure must be periodically checked to assure that it is properly maintained.

5. If the height of the transducer is zero reference point, an abnormally high or low reading will result if the transducer is not maintained at the same level. If the transducer used is the type placed with a plate on an I.V. pole not attached on the bed, the transducer will not remain at the level of the right atrium when the bed is raised or lowered and abnormal readings will result. One method used to avoid this malfunction is to tape a note on the control switch of an electric bed or place on the crank of a manual bed.

Complications

Certain complications related to arterial pressure lines are as follows:

1. The incidence of thromboses, hematomas, pseudoaneurysms, and prolonged arterial spasms may be reduced by the therapist's exercising expertise during catheter insertion and by careful monitoring of insertion sites.

2. Infection is an important threat. Arterial pressure monitoring has been related to as high as 13 percent of reported outbreaks of nosocomial bacteremia. Incidences of contaminated transducers, transducer domes, and flush solutions have all been well documented. Sterilizing the transducer after each use, using disposable domes, and changing the entire monitoring system except for the catheter every 2 days have all been shown to reduce infection rates. As with any invasive procedure, thorough hand washing prior to insertion and maintaining of aseptic techniques during set-up of the entire system, during insertion, and during all manipulations of the line is mandatory.

SWAN GANZ CATHETERS

Although the insertion sites for Swan Ganz catheters are veins, they are included in arterial access because they enter the pulmonary artery and measure arterial pressures. CVP (central venous pressure) lines give assessment only of right heart pressure. Swan Ganz catheters, however, give assessment of both right and left heart pressures so they are frequently used for diagnosis and management of treatment in heart failure resulting from myocardial infarction and cardiogenic shock. In the treatment of cardiogenic shock the Swan Ganz catheter not only serves as a guide for I.V. therapy administration, a site for this administration, and evaluation of any therapeutic drugs given but also provides information regarding the cause of shock.

Basic Swan Ganz catheters have double or triple lumens. Catheters are approximately 110 cm in length and come in sizes 5 Fr., 6 Fr., and 7 Fr. Each has a balloon tip which is inflated with 0.8 ml–1.5 ml of air, depending on the size and manufacturer. A double-lumen catheter contains a larger port, which is connected to an I.V. system and monitor to measure pulmonary artery wedge pressure (PAWP), and a smaller port, with a two-way stopcock for inflation and deflation of the balloon. Triple-lumen catheters contain a third proximal port, which is connected to another I.V. system and may be used to monitor right atrial pressure.

The *I.V. system* contains a heparinized bag, pressure infusor bag, pressure tubings with stopcocks, and transducer with cable connected to a monitor. This equipment is the same as that used for arterial monitoring except that for Swan Ganz catheters the lines may be coded in blue to differentiate them from arterial lines, which may be coded in red.

Insertion

The Swan Ganz catheter may be inserted either percutaneously or by cutdown in any accessible vein large enough to allow passage of the catheter. As the catheter is threaded and the tip passes the superior vena cava, inflation of the

Chapter 23 | Intraarterial Therapy

balloon will allow normal blood flow to assist catheter advancement. The tip enters the right atrium and passes through the tricuspid valve, entering the right ventricle. It then passes through the pulmonic valve into the pulmonary artery (Figure 23.13). Use of a cardiac monitor is essential during this insertion because the pattern shows definite changes with each advancement, thus providing a guide for tip location (Figure 23.14) and simultaneously allowing for patient monitoring throughout the procedure. The catheter tip placement must be confirmed by x-ray the same as any CVP catheter.

PAWP, which reflects left heart pressure, is measured intermittently by inflating the balloon to its recommended level. Care should be taken not to overinflate or to inflate too frequently. The usual recommendation is to inflate every four hours with the pressure maintained no longer than 1–2 minutes.

Complications

Possible complications of Swan Ganz catheters include:

1. Cardiac arrhythmias may occur during insertion. Lidocaine and defibrillation must be immediately available. Serious arrhythmias during insertion are extremely rare when the procedure is done by an experienced person.
2. Catheter knotting may be seen with the 5 Fr. and occurs when the catheter is advanced too far for the chamber whose pressure is being registered.
3. Balloon rupture in a patient without intracardiac shunting of blood usually is not a hazard except for the very severe possible result of embolization from the balloon fragments.
4. Pulmonary damage may result from pulmonary artery blood flow obstruction due to peripheral migration of the catheter to a wedged position. This is preventable with constant monitoring and by following recommendations regarding frequency and duration of balloon inflation.
5. Infection is always possible with any indwelling catheter. Adequate sterilization of all reusable equipment (e.g., transducer), use of disposable equipment whenever possible, strict adherence to aseptic techniques during insertion and during all subsequent manipulations of the line, adequate I.V. system changes down to the catheter, and maintenance of sterile intact dressings have all been shown to lower the risk of bacteremia.

ARTERIAL BLOOD GAS PARAMETERS

The purposes of arterial blood gas interpretation are to cope with respiratory imbalances, specifically, to diagnose, regulate oxygen therapy, and assess all other therapy — and metabolic imbalances — in particular, to diagnose and assess the effectiveness of the therapy.

To interpret ABG (arterial blood gas) values it is necessary to understand the physiological, chemical, and physical processes that influence each parameter.

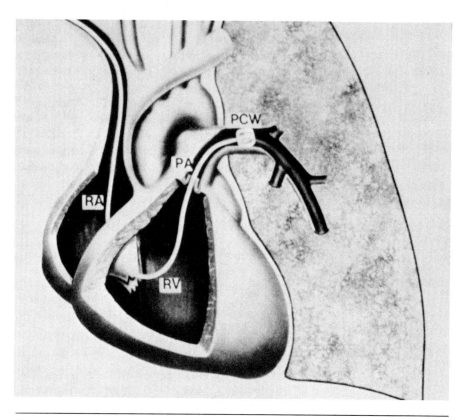

FIGURE 23.13
Insertion of Swan Ganz catheter through the right atrium (RA), into right ventricle (RV), up into pulmonary artery (PA), with the tip wedged in a pulmonary capillary (PCW). Courtesy of American Hospital Supply Corporation, Edwards Laboratory, Santa Ana, Calif.

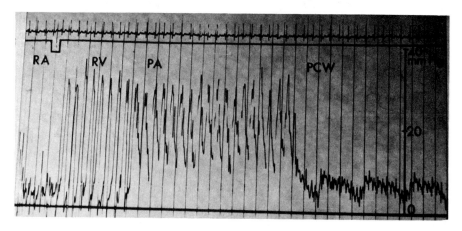

FIGURE 23.14
Monitor strip reading during passage of Swan Ganz catheter. Pattern seen when catheter tip in right atrium (RA), right ventricle (RV), pulmonary artery (PA), and pulmonary capillary wedge (PCW). Courtesy of American Hospital Supply Corporation, Edwards Laboratory, Santa Ana, Calif.

Chapter 23 | Intraarterial Therapy

pH

pH is the parameter that refers to the degree of acidity or alkalinity of the blood. It is not an absolute measurement, but shows an approximation of hydrogen (H^+) concentration. The pH scale is as follows (numbers are inversely related to the degree of acidity): (1) the range compatible with life is roughly 6.8–7.8; and (2) the normal range lies between 7.35–7.45. A pH increase represents a decrease in acidity and a pH decrease represents an increase in acidity; a pH decrease of 0.3 shows a doubling of hydrogen concentration. Blood pH 7.10 has twice the hydrogen concentration of blood pH 7.40.

Blood pH is directly proportional to the ratio of carbonic acid (CA) to bicarbonate (HCO_3^-). When there is 1 part CA to 20 parts HCO_3^-, the resultant pH is 7.35–7.45. If only CA increases or only HCO_3^- decreases, the ratio becomes closer (1 part CA : 5–16 parts HCO_3^-) and acidosis results. Conversely, when only CA decreases or only HCO_3^- increases, the ratio widens (1 part CA : 25–50 parts HCO_3^-) and alkalosis results.

Carbonic acid or bicarbonate changes per se produce no toxic effects; it is the ratio alteration and resultant pH change that interferes severely with enzyme activity.

Hydrogen

Cell metabolism produces hydrogen (H^+), which combines with bicarbonate (HCO_3^-) to form carbonic acid ($H_2CO_3^-$). This breaks down into water (H_2O), which is excreted by the kidneys, and carbon dioxide (CO_2), which is excreted by the lungs.

Because waste products of metabolism are mainly acidic, people are by nature acid-producing animals. The body generates and processes 15,000–20,000 mEq hydrogen (H^+) daily. The majority (99.8%) is nonfixed or volatile acid, which means it can change into gaseous form. The remainder (0.2%) is fixed or nonvolatile.

Body processing of hydrogen is accomplished without any appreciable change in blood concentration by elimination of volatile acid as carbon dioxide (CO_2) by the lungs, by excretion and reabsorption of fixed acid and bicarbonate (HCO_3^-) by the kidneys, and by chemical buffering.

Buffers

A buffer is a solute which resists pH change when acids or bases are added. The buffer base consists of bicarbonate and all nonbicarbonate buffers. The bicarbonate buffer system cannot buffer volatile acids but does buffer approximately 75 percent of all the fixed acid generated by the body. The nonbicarbonate buffer system (Buf^-) consists primarily of proteins, hemoglobin, and phosphate. It buffers volatile, nonfixed, acids.

Bicarbonate

The primary metabolic parameter bicarbonate (HCO_3^-) may be reported as CO_2 content, CO_2 combining power, CO_2, or standard bicarbonate, any of which refers to the same factor. HCO_3^- is measured by concentration and reported as mEq/liter. It is universally related to the quantity of fixed acid *excess* and therefore is more a controlled than a controlling factor.

Sources of fixed acids are: (1) organic and inorganic dietary acids; (2) lactic acid as a by-product of cell metabolism without oxygen; and (3) keto acids as by-products of cell metabolism without glucose or insulin.

The normal excretion rate of fixed acid by the kidneys is 50 mEq each day. However, the excretion and reabsorption of both hydrogen and bicarbonate can be greatly increased or decreased by body demands.

The normal HCO_3^- range is 24 ± 3 mEq per liter. The minimal stated as being compatible with life is 1 mEq/liter, the maximal is 48 mEq per liter.

Base Excess

The parameter base excess (BE) is the sum total in concentration of all the buffer anions (HCO_3^- and Buf^-) in a sample of whole blood, equilibrated with a normal PCO_2 (40 mmHg). As BE is equilibrated with a normal PCO_2, it is not affected by primary respiratory imbalances.

Normal BE is 48 ± 3 mm per liter, but is reported as plus or minus zero with zero representing 48 mm per liter. In metabolic acidosis BE is minus; in metabolic alkalosis BE is plus.

Because BE is not relevant in respiratory imbalances and because of the apparent contradiction of saying the base *excess* is *minus*, this parameter is not used in many institutions.

Physics of Gas

So far we have discussed parameters that are measured by concentration. The two respiratory parameters measured by pressure (intensity) warrant a brief review of the physics of gas.

Gas has *volume*, which refers to the space the gas occupies and is measured in centimeters (cc). Gas has *pressure*, which is measured mathematically as force per unit area by noting height to which force can support a column of mercury, and is expressed in mmHg (millimeters of mercury). Gas has *temperature*, which is generated by gas molecules in constant motion and is measured in degrees centigrade (C) or Fahrenheit (F).

Dalton's law regarding the behavior of gas in a mixture, as applied to oxygen in the atmosphere (room air), tells us the following:

1. The total pressure of the gas mixture equals the sum of the partial pressures of each gas, or P_{atm} (total pressure of atmosphere) = PO_2 (partial pressure oxygen) + PN_2 (partial pressure nitrogen) + PCO_2 (partial pressure carbon dioxide).
2. Each gas acts independently, as if it alone occupied the total space.
3. Each gas contribution to the total pressure depends solely upon the percentage of the total gas it occupies. The contribution of oxygen to the total atmospheric pressure is 21 percent. (Other variables not discussed here can exist.)
4. The partial pressure of each gas is dependent upon the number of molecules existing in the fixed space. At high elevations, because the number of oxygen molecules is decreased, the partial pressure of oxygen (PO_2) will be decreased.
5. Each gas is unaffected by any changes in other gas molecules. The partial pressure of oxygen (PO_2) will not increase or decrease because the partial pressure of carbon dioxide (PCO_2) is increased or decreased.

Partial Pressure Carbon Dioxide

PCO_2 (partial pressure carbon dioxide) reflects the adequacy of alveolar ventilation. It is the primary respiratory parameter.

CO_2 is eliminated by the lungs at the same rate formed by the tissues, and at the same time maintains constant blood levels.

Arterial PCO_2 is inversely related to the level of ventilation. With hypoventilation, carbon dioxide is retained and the PCO_2 elevates; with hyperventilation, carbon dioxide is blown off and the PCO_2 decreases.

PCO_2 normal range is 40 ± 4 mmHg. The minimal value stated as compatible with life is 9 mmHg, with the maximal value 158 mmHg.

Partial Pressure Oxygen

PO_2 (partial pressure oxygen) is also an intensity factor, measured in mmHg. It tells how fast and for how long oxygen will pass from blood into tissue. PO_2 is usually not a direct influence in acid–base balance.

Normal PO_2 values are oxygen- and age-dependent.. When the FIO_2 (fraction of inspired oxygen) is 21 percent (room air) and the patient is 60 years of age or under, the PO_2 should be at least 80 mmHg. With each 10-year advance in age, the normal PO_2 will decrease by 10 mmHg. If the PO_2 is 50 mmHg or below in a patient under 60 years of age, respiratory failure is present. A PO_2 between 50 and 75 mmHg reflects moderate hypoxemia.

Hypoxemia

Hypoxemia is insufficient oxygenation of the blood and can be measured directly by the PO_2. Hypoxia is insufficient oxygenation of the tissues; it cannot be directly measured but is presumed, if the P_vO_2 (partial pressure oxygen, venous blood) is 30 mmHg or below. To avoid hypoxia when hypoxemia is present, either the cardiovascular system must increase the rate of tissue perfusion or the hemoglobin content must be elevated.

Shunting is frequently a cause of hypoxemia. *Shunting* is any impediment in the blood transport system that results in blood not coming in contact with oxygen. This can be seen in vascular lung tumors, a right-to-left intracardiac shunt, or capillary shunting where pulmonary capillary blood comes in contact with totally unventilated alveoli (dead space).

Oxygen Saturation

O_2 Sat (oxygen saturation) is the parameter that tells the amount of oxygen taken up by hemoglobin when fully saturated. It is a quantity factor and is measured in percentage (%). It may also be called $PO_2\%$.

The normal adult values are 96–97% under 65 years and 95–96% in older patients. Oxygen saturation (O_2 Sat)

1. Depends upon PO_2. When the pressure exceeds a certain value the amount of oxygen taken in no longer increases.
2. Is altered by pH. If PO_2 remains constant, O_2 Sat will decrease when the pH decreases, and increases when the pH increases.
3. Is altered by temperature. If the PO_2 is constant, O_2 Sat will decrease when the temperature increases and increase when the temperature decreases.

Part VI | Specific Applications

This tells us that hyperthermia causes metabolic acidosis and hypothermia causes metabolic alkalosis. In hypothermia, the oxygen need is decreased but the oxygen is bound so tightly to the hemoglobin that the ability to deliver it is greatly decreased. Inhalation of carbon dioxide (CO_2) may be used to cause acidosis and release the bound oxygen.

Chemoreceptors

Chemoreceptors located peripherally in aortic and carotid bodies and centrally in the brain play a role in body responsive changes to abnormal PCO_2 and PO_2 values. Chemoreceptors signal the brain to stimulate or depress ventilation, according to body needs. The response to an elevated PCO_2 is greater than a decreased PO_2 because PCO_2 elevation is a danger signal of respiratory failure. At high altitudes where oxygen supply is lowered, oxygen need is greater than PCO_2 constancy; the chemoreceptors stimulate hyperventilation to obtain more oxygen, but this hyperventilation results in a decreased PCO_2.

ABG Normal Values (at sea level)

pH: 7.35–7.45
PCO_2: 36–44 mmHg
PO_2: 80–90 mmHg
O_2Sat: 95–96%
HCO_3^-: 22–26 mEq per liter
BE: ± 3

FOUR PRIMARY ACID–BASE IMBALANCES

Metabolic Acidosis

Metabolic acidosis is a process resulting from an excess of fixed acids or a primary HCO_3^- deficit.

The primary causes are

1. Increased production of fixed acids.
   a. Keto-acids, as seen in diabetic acidosis or starvation, where glucose and insulin are unavailable for cell metabolism.
   b. Lactic acid, as seen in cardiopulmonary failure when oxygen is unavailable for cell metabolism.
2. Failure of kidneys to excrete fixed acid.
3. Primary bicarbonate deficit.
   a. Severe diarrhea.
   b. Bowel or biliary fistula.

This is a metabolic imbalance because HCO_3^- is the parameter primarily affected. Acidosis is present because the carbon dioxide level has not changed, but the decrease in HCO_3^- has caused the ratio to go closer than 1 part acid to 20 parts base. It can be anywhere between 1 : 16 and 1 : 5, depending upon the degree of HCO_3^- deficit. As pH is dependent upon the acid-base ratio, and this ratio has now narrowed, acidosis is present. BE is minus because there is not enough HCO_3^- to buffer the fixed acid.

ABG Values in Metabolic Acidosis

pH: <7.35
HCO_3^-: <22 mEg/liter
PCO_2: normal (40 ± 4 mmHg)
BE: < −3

If the metabolic acidosis is of renal origin, the kidneys cannot respond. If it is of nonrenal origin, the kidneys will increase the excretion of hydrogen and increase the reabsorption of HCO_3^-. This response is slow, but, once started, can be maintained for weeks or months.

The chemoreceptors are sensitive to the increase in hydrogen and will stimulate compensatory hyperventilation to blow off carbon dioxide (CO_2) decreasing the PCO_2 <40 mmHg to obtain an acid–base ratio closer to normal (1 : 20) needed for a normal pH. This compensatory respiratory response is prompt and predictable — it will occur within minutes but becomes less effective with time. The limit of compensatory hyperventilation is when the PCO_2 reaches 12 mmHg.

After the kidneys and lungs have responded, HCO_3^- will increase to a level closer to normal, PCO_2 will decrease, and the acid–base ratio will come closer to 1 : 20 with a resultant pH closer to normal. Compensation thus occurs.

With bicarbonate administration, HCO_3^- will revert to normal, and the lungs will stop hyperventilation. Therefore PCO_2 will revert to normal, resulting in a 1 : 20 acid–base ratio and allowing a normal pH (7.35–7.45). Correction thereby is achieved.

Metabolic Alkalosis

Metabolic alkalosis is a process resulting from a decrease in body content of fixed acids or a primary HCO_3^- excess. The primary causes are

1. Excessive loss of fixed acids by
   a. Prolonged vomiting,
   b. Gastric suctioning,
   c. Potassium (K^+) deficit.
2. Primary HCO_3^- excess by
   a. Excessive administration of sodium bicarbonate or sodium citrate,
   b. Chloride (CHl^-) deficit, where HCO_3^- increases to maintain cation–anion balance,
   c. Sodium (Na^+) deficit, with HCO_3^- excretion dependent upon sodium.

This is a metabolic imbalance because the primary parameter affected is HCO_3^-. Alkalosis is present because the acid–base ratio has widened to 1 part acid : 25–50 parts base. This ratio results in a pH elevation; since there is an excess of HCO_3^- the BE is plus.

ABG Values in Metabolic Alkalosis

pH: >7.45
HCO_3^-: >26 mEg/liter
PCO_2: normal (40 ± 4 mmHg)
BE: >+3

Whether the kidneys respond to metabolic alkalosis depends upon several factors. An increase in HCO_3^- causes the excretion of HCO_3^- to increase, provided there is no deficit of chloride or potassium. If a chloride depletion is present, HCO_3^- will be reabsorbed as the accompanying anion for sodium. Because a HCO_3^- increase is usually accompanied by (1) an increase in sodium, (2) a decrease in chloride, and (3) a potassium deficit, HCO_3^- is not excreted but reabsorbed.

Compensatory respiratory response to metabolic alkalosis is quite variable. The degree of hypoventilation that occurs depends upon the causing factors. Regardless of the cause, hypoventilation as a compensatory response will rarely be sufficient to bring the PCO_2 above 55 mmHg because an elevated PCO_2 will cause the chemoreceptors to stimulate breathing to prevent respiratory failure.

When the lungs and kidneys do respond, some compensation will occur. HCO_3^- will decrease, PCO_2 will increase, and the acid–base ratio will come closer to 1 : 20; thus the pH will decrease to a level closer to normal.

Correction occurs with the administration of solutions containing chloride and potassium.

In the assessment and treatment of respiratory imbalances, ABG measurements are an absolute clinical necessity because ventilation is reflexed in PCO_2 and oxygenation in PO_2. Furthermore, acute respiratory failure may occur with slight changes in pulse, blood pressure, or alertness until cardiopulmonary collapse occurs.

Respiratory Acidosis

Respiratory acidosis is always caused by CO_2 retention due to hypoventilation. This is rarely seen without hypoxemia (PO_2<60 mmHg). The causes of hypoventilation include

1. Anesthesia, narcotics.
2. Central nervous system (CNS) disease such as polio, spinal cord lesions.
3. Severe hypokalemia.
4. Intrathoracic collection of blood, fluid, or air.
5. Pulmonary diseases.
    a. Restrictive (congestive heart failure, tumors, atelectasis).
    b. Obstructive (bronchitis, emphysema, asthma, or foreign body).

This process is respiratory because the PCO_2 is the primary parameter involved. Nonfixed, volatile, acid (PCO_2) is in excess but the base (HCO_3^-) is normal. The acid–base ratio is closer than 1 : 20; it is between 1 : 5 and 1 : 20, resulting in acidosis.

ABG Values in Respiratory Acidosis

>   pH: <7.35
>   PCO$_2$: >44 mmHg
>   HCO$_3^-$: normal (24 ± 2 mEq per liter)

As the lungs are always the primary cause of respiratory acidosis, they cannot play any role in compensation. Renal compensation is always slow in onset but very effective once started: generation and reabsorption of HCO$_3^-$ will increase, excretion of H$^+$ will increase, and the excretion of CHl$^-$ will increase, resulting in a chloride deficit.

With renal response, HCO$_3^-$ will elevate above normal, and PCO$_2$ will remain unchanged. The acid ratio will be closer to 1 : 20, allowing for some compensation, with a pH closer to normal.

Correction of respiratory acidosis is possible only by correction of the pulmonary cause. Chloride solutions are usually given to treat the chloride deficit.

Respiratory Alkalosis

Respiratory alkalosis is always caused by a CO$_2$ deficit due to hyperventilation. Factors causing hyperventilation include

1. Chemoreceptor response to hypoxemia. The chemoreceptors sense the decrease in oxygen and send a message to the brain to stimulate ventilation. This hyperventilation results in CO$_2$ being blown off, thus decreasing PCO$_2$. This is normal at high altitudes.
2. Respiratory response to metabolic acidosis. This response can persist for several hours or days after correction of the metabolic acidosis, due to higher levels of hydrogen excess in cerebrospinal fluid and the fact that chemoreceptors are more responsive to cerebrospinal fluid than to blood.
3. CNS malfunctions (trauma, infection, brain lesions).
4. Anxiety, pain, fever, shock.
5. Anemia, carbon monoxide poisoning.
6. Epinephrine, salicylates, and progesterone.
7. Improper mechanical ventilation. Any patient with chronic obstructive pulmonary disease (COPD) who is overcorrected by mechanical ventilation so that the PCO$_2$ decreases faster than 10 mmHg per hour will have respiratory alkalosis.

This hyperventilation process is respiratory because PCO$_2$ is the primary parameter affected. Alkalosis is present because CO$_2$ is decreased and the HCO$_3^-$ is normal resulting in an acid-base ratio between 1 : 25–50. This ratio results in a pH above 7.45.

ABG Values in Respiratory Alkalosis

>   pH: >7.45
>   PCO$_2$: <36 mmHg
>   HCO$_3^-$: normal (24 ± 2 mEq/liter)

Because the lungs are the primary cause of respiratory alkalosis, they cannot respond for compensation. Renal response occurs after several hours or days. The kidneys will decrease excretion of H^+, increase excretion of HCO_3^-, and increase excretion of H^+. However, the urine cannot become more alkaline than pH 7.0. This renal response will create some *compensation*. HCO_3^- will decrease below 24 mEq per liter. The acid–base ratio will come closer to 1 : 20, allowing the pH to come closer to normal.

Correction of respiratory alkalosis can be obtained by administering chloride solutions to replace the bicarbonate ion load. However, the buffering capacity of the plasma has been compromised as a result of the alkalosis and any additional insult to the balance will be poorly tolerated.

MIXED ACID–BASE IMBALANCES

In the hospital setting, 2 or more primary imbalances may coexist in the same patient. The following combinations sometimes occur:

1. Metabolic acidosis and metabolic alkalosis appear in a patient with diabetic acidosis who is vomiting.
2. Metabolic acidosis and respiratory acidosis show up in a patient with severe pulmonary edema, followed by cardiogenic shock.
3. Metabolic acidosis and respiratory alkalosis are seen in a patient with both kidney and liver failure.
4. Respiratory acidosis and metabolic alkalosis appear in a patient with chronic respiratory insufficiency who is on a salt-poor diet and taking diuretics.
5. Respiratory alkalosis and metabolic alkalosis are usually seen as a result of mechanical overventilation.

Respiratory acidosis and respiratory alkalosis cannot coexist because a person cannot hypoventilate and hyperventilate at the same time.

ACKNOWLEDGMENT

Special thanks to Lawrence B. Annes, M.D., Assistant Professor of Medicine, New York Medical College; Attending Cardiologist, Lawrence Hospital of Bronxville, N.Y., for his contributions to this chapter.

BIBLIOGRAPHY

Betson, C. The nurse's role in blood gas monitoring. *Cardiovasc. Nurs.* 7:6, 1971.

Broughton, J. *Understanding Blood Gases*. Reprint no. 456. Madison, Wisc.: Ohio Medical Products, 1971.

Cosentino, F. Intra-arterial access. *J. NITA* 3:5, 1980.

Cosentino, F. Arterial blood gas interpretation. *J. NITA* 4:4, 1981.

Demers, R., and Meyer, S. Fundamentals of blood gas interpretation. *Respir. Care* 18:2, 1973.

Gambino, S. *Blood pH, PCO_2, Oxygen Saturation and PO_2*. Chicago: American Society of Clinical Pathologists, 1967.

Gardner, R. Catheter-flush system for continuous monitoring of central arterial waveform. *J. Appl. Physiol.* 13:3, 1978.

Gray, H. *Anatomy, Descriptive and Surgical.* (Revised American edition from the 15th English edition). New York: Crown, 1977.

Hathaway, R. The Swan Ganz catheter: A review. *Nurs. Clin. North Am.* 13:3, 1978.

Maki, D., and Band, J. Septicemia From disposable pressure-monitoring chamber domes. *Chest* 74:5, 1978.

Pressure monitor called important bacteremia threat. *Hosp. Trib.* 14:12, 1980.

Shapiro, B. *Clinical Application of Blood Gases.* Chicago: Year Book, 1977.

Swan, H., and Ganz, W. Use of balloon flotation catheters in critically ill patients. *Surg. Clin. North Am.* 55:501–520, 1975.

REVIEW QUESTIONS

1. Two methods used *only* for drawing arterial blood gas samples are _____ and _____.
2. The artery usually considered site of first choice for drawing a one-time sample of blood for ABG measurement is the _____.
3. The physician's order for ABG sampling should include _____ and _____.
4. The only heparin remaining in an heparinized syringe should be in the dead space of the needle because _____.
5. A blood sample drawn for ABG measurement is immediately placed in ice because at room air the red cells will continue to _____ and _____.
6. Strong traction upon the plunger of the syringe to withdraw ABG samples faster can increase the chances of _____, _____, and _____.
7. In a patient receiving anticoagulation therapy, the drawing of an ABG sample must include _____.
8. Before insertion of any indwelling catheter in the radial artery, Allen's test is done to _____.
9. During the initial set-up and any manipulations of the I.V. system used for constant arterial pressure monitoring, extreme care must be taken to secure all connections. This is done to prevent _____ and _____.
10. When measuring pulmonary artery wedge pressures (PAWP) with a Swan Ganz catheter, care must be taken not to _____ and _____.
11. Blood pH is directly proportional to the ratio of _____.
12. The primary metabolic parameter in ABG values is _____.
13. The primary respiratory parameter in ABG values is _____.
14. The ABG parameter that reflects ventilation is _____.
15. The ABG parameter that reflects oxygenation is _____.
16. ABG values within the normal range are _____, and _____, and _____.
17. At the onset of metabolic acidosis, parameters that will be *decreased* are _____, _____, and _____.
18. Metabolic alkalosis is caused by _____.
19. At the onset of respiratory acidosis, _____ will be *increased*.
20. Respiratory alkalosis is always caused by _____.

CHAPTER 24

Unique Features of Pediatric Intravenous Therapy

Betsy Cohen Teitell

This chapter focuses on features of I.V. therapy that are unique in dealing with pediatric patients. A major subdivision between neonates and general pediatrics is outlined, since these two groups have vastly different intravenous requirements. In this chapter, patient monitoring, including equipment, procedures, and techniques will be discussed for each type of I.V. therapy. Nursing responsibilities for each therapy will also be analyzed.

PRELIMINARY CONSIDERATIONS IN PEDIATRIC I.V. THERAPY

How do a pediatric patient's needs differ from those of an adult? An adult's bodily circumference alters relatively little from the onset of adulthood through the remainder of life, whereas a child's bodily circumference must accommodate more than a threefold increase in length and approximately a twentyfold increase in weight between birth and adolescence [1]. Thus, a child's stress levels and basal metabolic rates are exceedingly higher than an adult's. A more subtle area of concern is the child's developmental needs, which require patience, education, and understanding from the I.V. therapist. A full comprehension of the stage of development a child is in according to his or her age enables the health care team to provide appropriate, nonthreatening care. Furthermore, understanding a child's developmental stage enhances the staff's ability to recognize that children's needs vary markedly, not only by stress levels but by growth and developmental levels.

Some common reasons for intravenous therapy in the pediatric patient include the following:

1. *Maintenance of fluid and electrolyte balance.* The younger the child the greater the risk not only of fluid and electrolyte imbalance, but also of fluid overload and congestive heart failure. Rehydration of a child with diarrhea may seem routine, but complexities can arise even in a

child who requires fluid for rehydration when experiencing respiratory distress, altered electrolyte balance, or other complications. In this type of situation manipulations according to actual fluid restriction are made.

2. *Antibiotic therapy.* The most common pediatric disease requiring antibiotic therapy is sepsis. Even before a child who displays the symptomatology of sepsis (i.e., increased heart rate, irritability, temperature spikes) is actually diagnosed, prophylactic I.V. antibiotics are routinely administered while a complete sepsis workup is in progress (e.g., urine cultures, throat cultures, blood cultures, wound cultures, etc.). If the sepsis workup reveals a positive blood culture, the I.V. antibiotics are continued for a complete 10-day course of therapy. If the sepsis workup is negative, the prophylactic I.V. antibiotics are discontinued.

3. *Nutritional support.* Administration of I.V. nutrition begins via a peripheral or central line. These nutrients provide calories essential to meet the demands of the growing child. A section on this important form of I.V. therapy follows later in this chapter.

4. *Insulin drips.* Juvenile diabetes occurs generally in the pediatric age group. Infusions of I.V. insulin, primarily in the low-dose form given by syringe, is a new method which has been favorably reported.

5. *Anticancer drugs.* Most chemotherapy or anticancer drugs required for treating childhood cancers use the I.V. route because of its efficacious absorption. There are many more different I.V. protocols designed for the child with cancer compared to the adult, primarily since most childhood cancers are unique to children (e.g., Wilms' tumor, neuroblastoma, and retinoblastoma). Precision in regulating the specific I.V. chemotherapy along with monitoring I.V. clearance is crucial in this group because of the incremental risk of fluid overload, electrolyte imbalances, and chemotherapy side-effects.

Obtaining Venous Access

Let us now analyze sites appropriate for I.V. therapy, including the usual route for administration. Depending on the child's age, a site for administering I.V. drugs is typically more difficult to find than in an adult. Both hydrational status and previous I.V. therapy may be used as predictors of difficulties in obtaining an intact venous access. In the child, the site selected for I.V. therapy should involve minimal risk and allow maximum efficiency and safety [2].

When selecting the optimal site for I.V. therapy, there are certain basic strategies to follow. The best site in the young infant through the toddler is the head, since the scalp has an abundant supply of superficial veins (Figure 24.1). The bilateral superficial-temporal veins just in front of the pinna of the ear, or the metopic vein which runs down the middle of the forehead, are generally easy to find and involve minimal patient risk. Other favorable peripheral I.V. sites include the hand, foot, or antecubital fossa [3]. Once venous access has been obtained, the next strategy involves stabilization of the I.V.

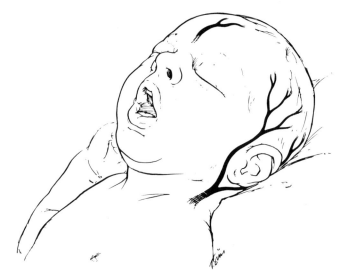

FIGURE 24.1
Sites for scalp vein infusions. Courtesy of B. Teitell, Children's Medical Center, Dallas, Texas.

Stabilizing the I.V.

Stabilization is essential, primarily in the younger child whose level of comprehension concerning the importance of not manipulating the I.V. site is minimal. All I.V.s placed in the head are taped in a U-shaped chevron pattern, and the extension tube is looped into a coil so that if the child pulls on the I.V. the tension of the pull will affect the coil, not the I.V. site. A small, open-ended paper cup is placed on top of the site to act as a protective covering (Figure 24.2). Second-choice sites requiring stabilization include the hand (Figure 24.3) and the arm, both of which generally require armboard support. The advantage of this type of stabilization is that it restricts the child's range of movement, thereby decreasing the risk of dislodgement of the I.V. needle. The third and least favorable site, which also demands stabilization, is the foot, primarily the saphaneous vein. Venous accessibility in the foot is not only more difficult, but it results in mobility restriction from the stabilizing legboards and sandbags that are used to keep young children, especially under age 2, from manipulating the needle (see Figure 24.4).

General I.V. insertion techniques will not be discussed in this chapter (see Chapters 12 and 19). The technique of I.V. insertion for neonatal therapy and hyperalimentation will be included, however, because these procedures are unique for children.

Fluid Requirements

Let us now advance to the area of fluid requirements during I.V. therapy. At what rate should I.V.s be administered to the child? Obviously, the answer to this question is determined by the child's stature and metabolic rate. The amount of fluid required for maintenance levels depends very much on insensible water loss from lungs, skin, urine, and stools and from metabolic expenditures from both internal or external stress levels.

Chapter 24 | Unique Features of Pediatric Intravenous Therapy 509

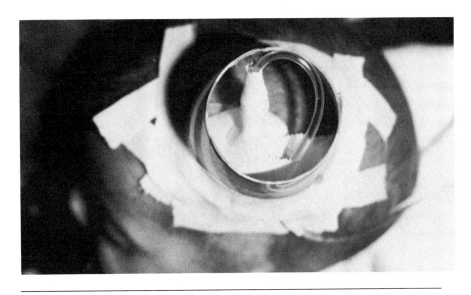

FIGURE 24.2
Example of scalp vein infusion displaying stabilization using paper cup and chevron U-shaped taping.

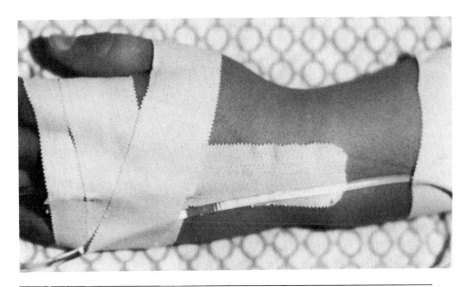

FIGURE 24.3
Example of site for I.V. therapy in the hand of an adolescent.

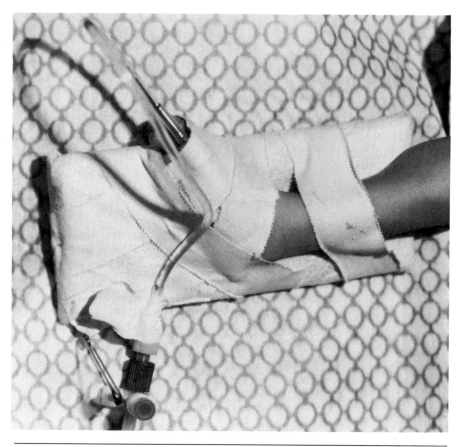

FIGURE 24.4
Example of site for I.V. therapy in foot, displaying footboard stabilization.

Assessing Fluid Needs

Before deciphering fluid requirements, familiarization with the 3 different methods for assessing 24-hour maintenance fluids is crucial: namely, the meter square, caloric, and weight methods. The methods listed below are according to the guidelines from Graef and Cone [3].

1. *The meter square method* has an arbitrary estimate of requirement of 1,500–1,800 ml fluid per square meter. The advantage of this method is its simplicity; its disadvantage is in the accessibility of a visual nomogram.
2. *The weight method* uses the child's weight in kilograms to estimate fluid needs. The advantage of this method also is its simplicity; the disadvantage is that it is less accurate in the patient who weighs more than 10 kg [3].
3. *The caloric method* calculates that the usual expenditure of fluid is approximately 150 ml for every 100 calories metabolized. This method

too is simple, but not totally accurate unless actual calorie requirements and energy intake are continuously assessed.

Graef and Cone [3] recommend using the weight method of 100–150 ml per kilogram for estimating fluid requirements in the child who weighs below 10 kg; they further recommend using the square meter method in children weighing more than 10 kg.

The methods just discussed only address maintenance replacement according to insensible losses and do not address the additional metabolic expenditures that require further replacement therapy. For example, the most common cause of incremental fluid and caloric needs is temperature elevation. An increase in temperature elevation by 1°C increases the child's caloric needs by 12 percent. Conversely, a child who is hypothermic has a caloric decrease of 12 percent per degree Celsius, which decreases his or her fluid requirements.

Other conditions that affect incremental fluid requirements include gastrointestinal losses, small intestinal drainage, and ongoing diarrhea. The physician and the nurse should assess the entire metabolic situation before prescribing the amount and type of I.V. therapy a child needs. A precise intake and output record is the most valuable assessment tool for determining fluid requirements. When abnormal losses occur via the kidneys, it is wise to determine the extent of the loss and replace it rather than estimate according to the previously mentioned methods [15]. To ensure accuracy in judging fluid needs, most children receiving I.V. therapy are on strict intake and output, including diaper weighing.

Accurate intake requires precision in I.V. administration. It is paramount that the rate of I.V. fluids be delivered at a constant rate. Even the smallest error can cause serious problems, especially in the compromised child. Rates in pediatrics generally vary from 5 to 80 ml per hour depending on the size of the child. Adolescent fluid requirements are similar to those for adults, ranging from 100 to 175 ml per hour.

I.V. INSERTION

Equipment

Essential equipment required for performing the pediatric I.V insertion consists of the following:

1. I.V. tubing with an inline calibrated chamber on a child with a prescribed fluid rate of less than 100 ml per hour to monitor rate more accurately and to prevent fluid overload.
2. The smallest container of solution that will last 24 hours.
3. Stabilization equipment (e.g., footboards, armboards, paper cups).
4. An extension tubing and a three-way stopcock if I.V. medications are ordered.
5. Cleansing material for the aseptic venipuncture consisting of povidone-iodine, alcohol swabs, and sterile gauzes.
6. Adhesive tape and a cling dressing for securing and protecting the I.V. site.

7. An I.V. pole on which to hang the solution.

8. An infusion pump for specific rates in the small child. Whether to use a pump is a nursing judgment. Each patient's individual fluid and electrolyte requirements must be fully assessed. It is difficult to arrive at an arbitrary figure for requisitioning for pumps, so wise nursing judgment must be used. If a child's rate is less than 15 ml per hour, it may be difficult to monitor and may require an infusion pump. In a fluid-restricted child, a pump may be needed for precision even when the rate is as high as 100 ml per hour.

9. A plastic cannula or winged small-vein needle, depending on the accessibility of the vein and the estimated duration of therapy. In pediatrics, the average-size needle ranges from a 21-gauge to a 25-gauge, depending on the size of the child and the size of the vein.

Surgical Cutdown If routine vein accessibility is extremely difficult, a surgical cutdown performed by the surgical team may be indicated. The 2 most common cutdown sites include the saphanous vein of the foot and/or the radial vein in the forearm. Since this procedure requires venous laceration or minor surgery, the site must be cleaned subsequently with antiseptic solution of povidone-iodine and povidone-iodine ointment at least biweekly to prevent local infection.

EMOTIONAL CONSIDERATIONS

What other considerations are essential to maintain the highest caliber of care in children? Even though children of varied ages and intellectual capacities all receive similar I.V. therapies, pre- and post-I.V. therapy education must be given, taking these variables into account. A child's capacity for understanding the significance of I.V. therapy, including the importance of not manipulating the I.V. site, usually occurs between the ages of 3½ to 5 years depending on the individual child. Explanations of all procedures must be disclosed to both the child and the parent. Parents provide a great deal of emotional support by their presence, most likely representing security, during the time of the actual I.V. insertion. Presence of parents may prevent excessive I.V. sticks caused by the movement of frightened and hyperexcitable children surrounded by strangers in the unfamiliar hospital environment.

Establishing Trust To gain insight into the problems of establishing trust, the practitioner should recognize the child's point of view. A thought-provoking question for practitioners is, "How can I expect the child to totally trust me while I am about to hurt him or her by performing a venipuncture?" Usually it is best to tell the child that the venipuncture will hurt, but only for a short time. Define the term *time* not by minutes — since young children will not understand this — but by comparison to other procedures, e.g., "The actual I.V. puncture takes about the same time as it takes me to take your vital signs, get you a glass of orange juice, or for you to finish your dinner." Inform the child that even though this therapy may be painful initially, it should make him or her feel better similar to before the illness. Always be honest with a child. Allow the child the op-

Chapter 24 | Unique Features of Pediatric Intravenous Therapy   513

portunity to cry. If possible, let the child participate in the therapy; a child's ability to rip tape, open alcohol swabs, and hold tubing may be as good as many assistants'.

Play Therapy

Play therapy, consisting of practicing I.V. therapy on a doll, is an ideal teaching strategy that allows emotional preparation through acting out. It may not, however, always be practical due to the urgency of I.V. therapy or the availability of dolls. When it is pragmatic, nurses certainly can participate in this form of play therapy for teaching purposes, or they may seek such assistance from the child-life workers.

Use of Restraints

In younger children, especially those in the toddler group, great care must be taken to protect the I.V. site. In general, restraints are seldom used at children's medical centers because it is not only very confining but also creates a sense of frustration and mistrust in the child. Only on a rare occasion, with an extremely uncooperative child, may restraints be used.

Establishing Rapport

Another very important aspect of I.V. therapy is establishing rapport with the family and child through good communication. Communication differs with all age groups according to their intellectual level. Adolescents in particular, require a great deal of individual attention and allowance for their independent nature versus their dependent situation. Adolescents feel grown up and desire the opportunity to assess their disease status; they deserve the opportunity to participate in the decision-making aspect of their care. Adolescents are easily hurt when criticized. They feel that they are grown up but lack the experience and knowledge of the adult [10]. Therefore, educational techniques practiced with adolescents should encompass a commonsense approach, permitting each adolescent an opportunity to deal with intravenous therapy to the best of his or her ability. Overexpectation and performance pressure from the I.V. practitioner can result in emotional conflicts and depression in this age group.

NEONATAL I.V. THERAPY

This section deals with the unique I.V. requirements of the youngest group of children, generally below 2 months of age. Fluid requirements for optimal management of low-birth-weight infants can only be achieved by closely monitoring their intake and output, typically on intake and output sheets. If the infant's fluid requirements are not met, a number of physiological and metabolic states may occur, including evidence of weight loss in association with hyperosmolality, hypernatremia, and increased hematocrit and bilirubin, as well as evidence of metabolic acidosis, dehydration, and frequently, multiple apnea spells. Conversely, administration of excess fluid, either intravenously or occasionally as a result of respiratory support systems, can be associated with edema, patent ductus arteriosus, congestive heart failure, and even bronchopulmonary dysplasia [8] in the neonate.

Factors Affecting Fluid Requirements

How do fluid requirements differ in a neonate? Actual water requirements vary between a newborn, a low-birth-weight infant, and a high-risk infant. The exact amounts of calories, water, and electrolytes required depend upon the newborn's gestational age, body stores, and metabolic rates. The smaller and more immature the infant is, the greater is the total body water content. For example, the water content of a 28-week gestational age infant is 85 percent of total body weight, as compared to the term infant, whose water content is only 70 percent [7]. To arrive at specific fluid requirements all of these factors are accounted for, and a strict intake and output is maintained.

Other factors that affect fluid requirements in the neonate include many therapeutic devices affecting metabolic rates. For example, radiant warmers and single-walled incubators may be effective in maintaining the infant's temperature, but this temperature elevation in turn increases the infant's insensible fluid losses. Phototherapy, though effectively used in the treatment of hyperbilirubinemia in the neonate, will increase insensible fluid losses and cause water requirements to be greater [6]. These various losses must be included when determining fluid replacement.

Major Reasons for Neonatal I.V. Therapy

Let us now progress to discussing the major reasons for I.V. therapy in neonates. The categories are as follows:

1. *Maintenance of fluid and electrolytes balance.* Since their fluid requirements are greater proportionately due to their higher percentage of total body water, infants are at greater jeopardy for both fluid overload and dehydration. Also, electrolytes must be followed closely by laboratory tests to determine whether the neonate is in a state of isotonic versus hypertonic dehydration.

2. *Management of antibiotic therapy.* Neonates are generally at greater risk of becoming septic, possibly due to an acquired congenital disorder resulting in intestinal obstruction, immaturity in lung compliance resulting in respiratory distress syndrome, or immaturity of gastrointestinal tract resulting in necrotizing enterocolitis. All these problems mandate antibiotic coverage by the I.V. route due to the neonates' immature gastrointestinal system and decreased tolerance to the systemic effect of the infection.

    Total parenteral nutrition (TPN) in neonates may be used to decrease the risk of infection due to immunosuppression. Administration of both antibiotics and TPN to a neonate poses many fluid restrictions and is a very difficult task. Therefore, guidelines have been developed for administering antibiotics and TPN separately, with consideration given to the smallest volume safe to dilute and administer antibiotics in. Table 24.1 gives specific guidelines for fluid conservation in the infant according to the specific type of antibiotic administered. These guidelines should help both nurses and physicians determine the best approach to maintain antibiotic coverage while maintaining nutritional status and preventing fluid overload.

3. *Nutritional support.* Because of their immature gastrointestinal systems, infants tend to malabsorb more nutrients and have less

TABLE 24.1
Minimum Dilutions and Maximum Flow Rates for Antibiotics

Drug	Minimum Diluent*	Concentration of Initial Dilution*	Final Maximum Concentration for I.V. Use†	Maximum Rate of Administration‡		
				mg/min	cc/min	cc/hr
Amikacin §		50 mg/cc; 250 mg/cc	2.5 mg/cc	17	6.8	408
Gentamicin		10 mg/cc; 40 mg/cc	1.6 mg/cc	3	2	120
Kanamycin		75 mg/2 cc; 500 mg/2 cc	5 mg/cc	17	3	180
Tobramycin		10 mg/cc; 40 mg/cc	1.6 mg/cc	4	2.5	150
Ampicillin	125 mg vial–1.2 cc 250 mg vial–1.0 cc 500 mg vial–1.8 cc 1 gm vial–3.5 cc	125 mg/cc 250 mg/cc 250 mg/cc 250 mg/cc	135 mg/cc	100	0.74	45
Carbenicillin	1 gm vial–2.0 cc 5 gm vial–9.5 cc	400 mg/cc 400 mg/cc	50 mg/cc	33	0.66	40
Ticarcillin	1 gm vial–2.0 cc 3 gm vial–6.0 cc	400 mg/cc 400 mg/cc	50 mg/cc	33	0.66	40
Cefamandole	1 gm vial–3.0 cc		100 mg/cc	333	3.3	200
Clindamycin		150 mg/cc	6 mg/cc	30	5	300
Keflin	1 gm vial–4.0 cc		100 mg/cc	333	3.3	200
Methicillin	1 gm vial–1.5 cc	500 mg/cc	20 mg/cc	200	10	600
Nafcillin	500 gm vial–1.7 cc 1 gm vial–3.4 cc	250 mg/cc 250 mg/cc	33 mg/cc	100	3	180

Source: Prepared by and for Children's Medical Center, Dallas, Tex., Feb. 1981.
*Based on manufacturer's suggestions as stated in package inserts.
†Based on usual adult dose and minimum volume of infusion recommended to manufacturer.
‡Based on usual adult dose, minimum volume of infusion, and minimum time of infusion recommended by manufacturer.
§Package insert for Amikacin states above values for infants.

reserves than older children. Therefore I.V. supportive nutrition, discussed later in this chapter, may be used.

Umbilical Catheterization

Most sites for neonatal I.V. therapy are similar to those for children discussed earlier in this chapter. However, there are 2 additional, unique sites used for the neonate: first, the umbilical vessels, and second, the central line, which will be discussed in the section on nutritional therapy.

Umbilical catheterization is common practice in many neonatal and intensive care units in the treatment of acutely ill infants. This mode of therapy provides an easy route for I.V. administration. However, there are many undesirable risks such as thrombosis, embolism, vasospasm, vascular perforation, infection, and hemorrhage. To prevent these complications, a specially designed umbilical catheter with the following features should be selected.

1. Flexibility.
2. Relatively rigid walls for accurate pressure monitoring.

3. A single end-hole to avoid clotting in the tip.
4. Smoothness of the tip to prevent perforation of the vessel wall during catheter insertion.
5. Radiopaqueness to radiographically visualize the location of the tip of the catheter.
6. Small capacity so that only a small amount of blood need be withdrawn to clear the catheter for blood sampling.
7. Size from 3.5 to 5 Fr. catheter.

Arterial Versus Venous Catheterization

Let us now examine the difference between arterial and venous umbilical catheterization. Within minutes of birth, the umbilical arteries normally constrict; delays in the process, however, occur in states of hypoxia and acidosis. The vast majority of infants are catheterized in the first day of life since catheterization is generally not possible past the fourth day of life.

The procedure for umbilical catheterization begins with the surgeon's preparation for asepsis including hand washing, gloving, masking, and gowning. This step precedes the preparation of the umbilical stump with an iodine solution, followed by cleansing with alcohol, and subsequently draping the sterile field and exposing the umbilical area. Dissection begins at the umbilical cord around 1.5 cm from the skin until the umbilical vessels are identified. Two thick-walled, pinpoint-sized arteries are easily distinguishable from a large thin-walled vein. The heparinized catheter is passed through either the umbilical artery or vein, depending on the type of therapy desired.

Arterial catheterization accomplishes 5 goals: (1) blood sampling, (2) measurements of arterial pressures, (3) parenteral or antibiotic therapy in the vascularly compromised child, (4) exchange transfusions, and (5) arterial pH and blood gases. Venous umbilical catheterization accomplishes 4 goals, including (1) and (3) above as well as providing a means for a direct measurement of central venous pressure and a route for the infusion of TPN [7].

Placements differ between the umbilical venous route and the arterial route. Ideally, the tip of the umbilical venous catheter should be positioned in the inferior vena cava near the right atrium in good position for central venous pressure and TPN administration. Comparatively, the umbilical arterial catheter is best positioned above the level of aortic bifurcation in good position for arterial measurements and exchange transfusions.

Once the catheter is placed correctly and is confirmed radiographically, a suture may be placed superficially through the stump tying it firmly to the catheter for anchorage [6]. The catheter is generally connected to a three-way stopcock for pressure monitoring, blood drawing, and fluid administration. When fluid administration is not necessary, the line may be heparinized. It is of the utmost importance to maintain patency of the indwelling catheter, for blood clots can otherwise form. Irrigation with 1 unit of heparin per milliliter I.V. fluid should be done daily.

Increased thrombosis when administering fluids through an umbilical artery has been reported; therefore this mode of therapy should be used with caution. The nursing assessment for pending complications should include the following:

1. Examine buttocks to detect blanching caused by arterial spasms.
2. Closely monitor the umbilical line with Luer lock attachments to prevent disconnection of the tubing with resultant hemorrhage.
3. Closely monitor peripheral edema, unequal femoral pulses, and respiratory distress, which could indicate emboli formation.
4. Perform daily dressing changes with the application of povidone-iodine ointment to decrease the risk of sepsis.

If complications arise, report them immediately to the appropriate physician so immediate medical attention can be provided. Early intervention can reduce the risk of morbidity and mortality when using the umbilical access for I.V. therapy.

Because of the risks of complications when using the umbilical vessel for intravenous therapy, many physicians now prefer to use an alternate site, like the scalp or hand.

TOTAL PARENTERAL NUTRITION

This section addresses a life-saving form of I.V. therapy. Total parenteral nutrition, or TPN, is becoming one of the most important therapeutic parameters in the successful management of certain pediatric diseases. The widespread use of TPN has sustained numerous children while their gastrointestinal tracts develop enough absorptive capacity to tolerate basal caloric requirements.

Retrospectively, one of the most intriguing aspects about TPN is its unusual history, which can be traced back more than 300 years to Sir Christopher Wren's first attempt to inject ale, wine, or opium into the veins of dogs, using a prototypic hypodermic syringe made from a pig's bladder and a goose quill. The first sophisticated attempt at intravenous feeding was Claude Bernard's successful infusion of sugar solutions into animal veins about 200 years later. By the end of the nineteenth century, intravenous infusion of sugar and saline solutions into humans was commonplace [11]. Many attempts were made to increase the caloric density of I.V. nutrition through higher concentrations of dextrose solution. Helfrich and Abelson (1944) even made early attempts to combine glucose and protein. Although they were not totally successful their ingenuity credits them with the first conceptual model of TPN therapy. However, the paucity of successful I.V. nutrition therapy stemmed from two culprits: (1) hypertonicity of the infusate, resulting in frequent transfers of the peripheral I.V. sites because of thrombophlebitis; and (2) when problem (1) existed, insufficient calories were provided [5].

A major breakthrough in parenteral feedings occurred in the late 1960s when Stanley J. Dudrick and his colleagues at the University of Pennsylvania began to report their first experiments with central venous hyperalimentation. The success of Dudrick's early experiments with subclavian catheters, supplying hypertonic glucose, amino acids, vitamins, and minerals to beagle puppies, led to further success with human infants and adults who could not be fed adequately by the enteral route because of severe gastrointestinal disorders. Dudrick's initial success using TPN in neonates led to its widespread use in adult surgical patients, followed by its widespread use in high-nutritional-risk cancer patients.

Dudrick devised a simple statement of criteria that differentiates patients who potentially can benefit from TPN therapy into categories. These categories include those patients that (1) can't eat, (2) won't eat, or (3) can't eat enough [13]. TPN should be used only in patients having inadequate gastrointestinal function thereby disallowing feeding by the enteral route (especially since TPN costs are very high).

Composition Requirements

Solutions are generally made by hospital pharmacy staff, and the assembly of tubings and solutions is done under a laminar air hood. The general constituents for TPN — amino acids, a dextrose calorie source, electrolytes, minerals, trace elements, and vitamins — provide amounts of nutrients sufficient to promote growth and maintain a positive nitrogen balance. Nitrogen balance is maintained through the amino acids intake, while calories are obtained by glucose. Intravenous fat preparations are currently used to supply essential fatty acids (2–5% of the total caloric intake). Electrolytes are usually added to the TPN solution in amounts approximately established for oral or intravenous maintenance requirements. Minerals like calcium, magnesium, and phosphorus are incompletely absorbed from the gastrointestinal tract. Therefore, the parenteral needs for minerals are significantly lower than oral needs, and the amounts in the TPN solution rarely exceed half the usual oral amounts. Trace elements may be needed and are now included in commercial solutions, while vitamins are added according to children's recommended daily allowances. (Note: The yellow color of the TPN solution results from the addition of multivitamins.)

Pediatric requirements for I.V. nutrition follow general guidelines. The range of nitrogen requirement is 2.5–4.0 gm per kilogram for the infant and lowers considerably to approximately 0.75–1.5 gm for the adolescent. Most physicians prefer to administer the lower range of nitrogen in non-severely stressed children since not only can a positive nitrogen balance be thus achieved, but complications culminating from the additional higher levels of amino acids also can be decreased. Nonprotein calories are provided by glucose: requirements in the infant generally range from 125 to 150 calories per kilogram per day, whereas the adolescent may require between 1,500 to 3,000 calories per day. As mentioned earlier, electrolytes, vitamins, minerals, and trace elements are provided in accordance with the child's daily requirements. Depending on caloric expenditure based on stress levels, lipids may be provided prophylactically biweekly, or daily to supplement caloric requirements. Administration of piggyback lipids through a nonfiltered system is commonplace in hospital practice today. The lipids must be connected as close to the venous junction as possible, thereby preventing the mixing of the incompatible lipid and hyperalimentation solutions.

Specific Formulas

Two main formulas for TPN have been developed. One is the weaning on solution or peripheral formula called *starter strength*. The second formula consists of a high dextrose and protein concentration and is appropriately labeled *full-strength solution* (see Table 24.2). Due to the hyperosmolality of the full-strength solution, this formula is prescribed only for a large vein perfusion like that of the superior vena cava for central TPN. Additionally, when these stock formulas are unable to provide all of the desired nutrients and electrolytes, individualized formulas are designed. We also include Liposyn or Intralipid 10% peripherally in our daily formula for its caloric value and to prevent fatty-acid deficiency. Occasionally, in the venous-compromised child, this is administered piggyback in the central line.

Indications

Pediatric patients receiving TPN usually fall into 2 major categories: (a) those with either congenital or acquired anomalies of the gastrointestinal tract, or (b) those infants with intractable diarrhea syndromes. The gastrointestinal tract anomalies that generally require TPN include (1) intestinal obstruction (obstruction in the intestinal lumen), (2) gastroschisis (a congenital fissure in the wall of the abdomen that remains open), and (3) necrotizing enterocolitis (necrosis of the small or large bowel due to sepsis or hypoxia). The most dramatic treatment requires major resection of both small and large bowel and TPN may be needed for several weeks, sometimes months [11]. Other pediatric diseases that may require I.V. nutrition include (1) cystic fibrosis, (2) renal failure, (3) congenital heart disease, (4) cancer, and (5) Crohn's disease. With the addition of TPN into their therapy regime, affected children can be expected to gain weight normally with only parenteral nutrients. In addition, TPN supplies enough calories to maintain the positive nitrogen balance required for normal growth and development. (See Chapter 19 for insertion of central venous lines.)

Team Approach to Total Parenteral Nutrition

Because past experiences have demonstrated that higher complications of sepsis occur in patients in institutions without TPN teams, most hospitals have now established the team approach. The TPN, or nutrition, team consists of a physician whose primary responsibility is to oversee the intravenous nutrition program [4], a nurse who assists the physician and other staff in all aspects of the program, a pharmacist who provides aseptic assembly of the TPN solution, and a dietitian who evaluates patients' nutritional intake according to requirements.

When a child experiences one of the aforementioned diseases requiring nutritional support, consults are written to the nutrition team. Determining when TPN is the best therapeutic modality and no other simpler mode of nutritional therapy can be maintained is generally a medical decision. Usually, a consult is written to the nutritional support service requesting that current nutritional status, gastrointestinal functionability, and effectiveness of current nutritional therapy be evaluated. With the assistance of the nutritional support service, the decision of whether to order central venous hyperalimentation can

TABLE 24.2
Routine TPN Stock Solution*

Solution	Starter Strength (ml)	Full Strength (ml)
Amino acid solution (8.5%)	100	165
D/W 50%	125	220
NaCl (2.5 mEq/ml)	5	5
MgSO$_4$ (4 mEq/ml)	2	2
Ca gluconate (0.45 mEq/ml)	9	13
KPO$_4$ (4.4 mEq k/ml) 3 mmol P/ml)	1	1.5
KCl (2 mEq/ml)	3	2
MVI	2	2
H$_2$O	252	89
Total volume	500	500
kcal/ml	0.49	0.86
Glucose concentration	12.5%	22%
Protein concentration	1.7 gm/100	2.8 gm/100

Source: Prepared by and for Children's Medical Center, Dallas, Tex., July 1980.

*Trace elements added: ZnSO$_4$, CuSO$_4$, MnSO$_4$, CrCl$_2$, and Fe^{3+}. Weekly supplementation (IM injection): Vitamin K, Folate, and Vitamin B$_{12}$.

be made and carefully designed orders can be written (see Table 24.3). After writing the routine orders, the surgeon is consulted.

Catheter Insertion Procedure

As for adults, in larger children the catheter is usually inserted percutaneously through the subclavian vein. However, this approach can be extremely dangerous in infants due to the small size of the subclavian vein. Therefore, in children under the age of 5, and especially in infants, catheter placement is done in the operating room under anesthesia. The catheter is usually inserted through the facial vein or the external and internal jugular vein to the superior vena cava (Figures 24.5 and 24.6). After proper placement is verified by chest x-ray, subcutaneous tunneling of the catheter is done — either up the parietal occipital area or down the chest wall to the fourth or fifth intercostal space, depending on the catheter type.* This distal exit site from the original phlebotomy site provides a barrier from infection [9], facilitates catheter maintenance, and provides the child with full-range neck mobility.

Maintaining Sterility of the I.V.

The next area of concern, maintaining sterility, in TPN therapy is the most crucial one. It encompasses the administration and monitoring of TPN therapy. In fact, an efficient and knowledgeable nursing staff is key for implementing and monitoring the TPN regime.

---

*The catheter used may be a cardiac translucent one-way valve catheter or the opaque, Dacron-cuffed Broviac catheter.

TABLE 24.3
Routine TPN Orders

Orders	Baseline	Routine
Chest x-ray	Each time of insertion	1 per wk
Laboratory	Ca, PO$_4$, Mg, BUN, bilirubin (D/T), SGPT, transferrin, protein, electrophoresis, glucose, CBC, Na, K, Cl, CO$_2$, creatinine	Tuesday, Friday 2 per wk: NH$_3$, PO$_4$, bilirubin (D/T), CBC, SGPT, protein electrophoresis Friday Weekly: Ca, PO$_4$, bilirubin (D/T), BUN, Na, K PRN: glucose, Mg, Zn, Cu, Fe, transferrin, platelet, CO$_2$/pH, osmolality
Glucose Tes-Tape	Pre-TPN	q void on infant. q4h on older, stable children $\bar{p}$ 2 (−) urine Tes-Tapes
Dressing changes	N.A.	Monday, Wednesday, Friday (evaluate site chart in nurses' notes)
Laboratory (triglycerides)	N.A.	qd when on continuous lipid. If value > 125 mg/dl, report to physician
Line change outs	Each time of insertion	qd with a 22-micron in-line filter with a Metriset attachment
Solutions	Hang D/W $\bar{p}$ 10% insertion	$\bar{p}$ chest X-ray confirmation begin a stock solution, unless patient requires individualized formula. Orders rewritten daily.
Weight	Pre-weight	Daily
Intake & output	Day of insertion	Daily
Anthropometric measurements	Pre-insertion	Weekly

Source: Prepared by and for Children's Medical Center, Dallas, Tex., May 1981.

Dressing Changes
Since the indwelling subclavian catheter is a long-term foreign body and potential source of infection, the necessity of maintaining sterility of this lifeline cannot be stressed enough. Great care is needed to avoid contamination, because any break in the skin may facilitate the entry of organisms. Therefore, one major responsibility of the nurse is to perform routine aseptic dressing changes on Monday, Wednesday, Friday, and PRN, and daily aseptic tubing changes. If the catheter site is erythematous or purulent, the nurse should culture the site, inform the physician, monitor the culture, and place the patient on a daily dressing regime until the insertion site becomes clean and dry. Silver sulfadiazine has been successfully applied to treat topical catheter site infections of *staphylococcus aureus* and *S. epidermides.*

522 Part VI | Specific Applications

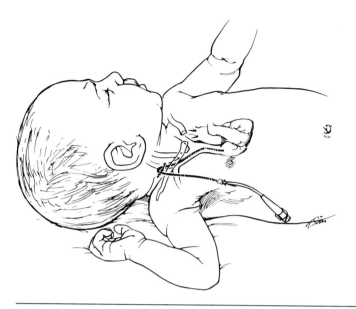

FIGURE 24.5
Example of pediatric infant-size Broviac catheter. Notice the catheter is threaded into the external jugular to the right atrium and tunneled subcutaneously down the chest wall. Courtesy of B. Teitell, Children's Medical Center, Dallas, Texas.

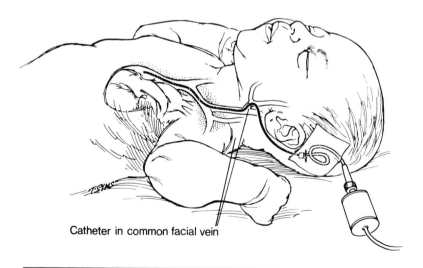

Catheter in common facial vein

FIGURE 24.6
Example of pediatric one-way valve Pudenz Infant Cardiac Catheter. Notice the catheter is threaded into facial vein to the right atrium and tunneled subcutaneously up behind the ear. Courtesy of B. Teitell, Children's Medical Center, Dallas, Texas.

The technique of performing the dressing change is similar to the original design used by Dudrick and associates and is discussed in Chapter 21. Acetone is applied for defatting, followed by a povidone-iodine scrub and application of povidone ointment for its bactericidal effect at the catheter site. The site is then covered with sterile gauze, and occlusive tape is placed on top of the gauze. This format has worked well in the prevention of catheter site infection. Current protocol includes the use of the Clinipad dressing kit, which provides staff with supplies for the organization and expediency needed to perform a quality dressing.

Maintaining Proper Infusion Rate

The second major area of responsibility for the nurse is in the delivery of TPN by a constant and proper infusion rate. The amount and rate of flow are governed by the optimal sugar utilization as determined by the renal threshold and the patient's specific requirements. If too little fluid is given, the sugar will be well below the threshold and the maximum caloric intake will not be reached. If too much solution is given, the renal threshold is exceeded and a sugar spill will be noted in the urine. The infusion rate should be checked frequently, at least every hour. Urine Tes-Tapes should be done after every void in neonates. A positive 2+ urine × 2 or a 3+ or 4+ urine requires immediate nursing intervention. If this occurs, the physician should be notified; a serum glucose may be ordered and the infusion rate may be adjusted and/or insulin may be added, depending on the individual needs of the patient. Infusion pumps serve as helpful aids in monitoring desired rates, especially in the pediatric age group. For this reason, all pediatric TPN patients are placed on infusion pumps.

Patient Assessment

The third area of nursing responsibility is patient assessment. The nurse monitors the patient's physical status on a daily basis and screens, intervenes, and reports abnormal findings of temperature spikes, inappropriate glucose spills, chills, rashes, irritability, decreased level of consciousness, and so forth. Any observable abnormality is immediately reported to the physician.

Providing Psychological Support

The fourth major area of nursing intervention in a child receiving TPN is psychological support. Most TPN patients are infants who are acutely ill and deprived of maternal warmth and comfort. Even though a child on central TPN may be NPO, cuddling and holding the child should assist in meeting maternal needs. Also, allowing parents every opportunity to participate in their child's care is extremely important. First, the nurse should assess the family's level of comprehension about TPN and intervene by offering support in their areas of weakness and insecurities to decrease parental anxiety. As soon as the decision is made to place a child on TPN, it is best to use the preoperative teaching methodology of explaining purpose, procedures, and potential complications. Of course, all further questions can be handled on a daily basis. Permitting this open channel of communication not only supplies parents with the knowledge needed to become involved, but assists them in comprehending the purpose of TPN and why adherence to the protocol of TPN therapy is so important.

Complications

Like all therapies, there are disadvantages to TPN stemming from potential complications. It is essential that every nurse understand the possible complications of TPN therapy, including the symptoms of each specific complication. Complications are subdivided into 3 categories: catheter insertions, postinsertion complications, and metabolic complications.

Catheter Insertions
1. Infection
2. Malposition
3. Vein perforation

Postinsertion Complications
1. Infection
2. Thrombosis
3. Superior vena cava syndrome

Metabolic Complications
1. Hyperglycemia
2. Hypoglycemia
3. Electrolyte imbalance
4. Mineral disorder
5. Hyperammonemia
6. Hyperbilirubinemia

Most of the aforementioned complications can be treated or even prevented. Maintaining high-caliber aseptic techniques when handling the TPN line reduces the potential risk of sepsis. Certain metabolic complications are preventable through close nursing monitoring, although some predisposing metabolic abnormalities may require immediate medical intervention. With the incremental advances in technology and the formation of TPN teams, even the most prominent complication, sepsis, has decreased to very acceptable rates. In the practice of TPN therapy, the catheter sepsis rate in children may rise as high as 10% due to the increased risks and general behaviors of children (e.g., teething children have been known to bite the TPN catheter).

Recommendations for TPN Specialists

A new, and problematic, challenge for TPN nurses arises ironically, from improvements in technology. Numerous brands of I.V. equipment are now available: this poses problems when one nursing unit is accustomed to a certain type of equipment and changes are made. However, changes in technology expand patient tolerance to many nutritional formulas. A further difficulty in the field of pediatric TPN is that it represents a small percentage of the total patient population and manufacturers are thus unlikely to design equipment especially for this small group. So nurses are faced with the dilemma of how to adapt adult equipment to the small child [12].

When deciding which equipment to use, choosing the simplest, most reliable equipment for the specific situation is best. If your current protocol is working well, do not arbitrarily change it. Seek improvements only in problem areas; otherwise unnecessary, continual changes may create a high tension level in the staff, which could affect performance.

In conclusion, specific principles in caring for pediatric patients receiving I.V. therapy have been discussed, as well as the fluid and nutritional requirements and diseases that necessitate pediatric I.V. therapy. By familiarizing nurses with this current information it is hoped that their understanding of the complexities involved in caring for a child receiving I.V. therapy will be deepened.

REFERENCES

1. Blake, F. G., Wright, F. H., and Wachter, E. H. *Nursing Care of Children*. Philadelphia, Pa.: Lippincott, 1970, p. 11.
2. Clarke, T. A., and Reddy, P. G. Intravenous infusion technique in the newborn. *Clin. Pediatr.* 18(9): 1979.
3. Graef, J., and Cone, T. *Manual of Pediatric Therapeutics*. Boston: Little, Brown, 1977.
4. Heird, W. Total Parenteral Nutrition. In Committee on Nutrition (eds.), *Pediatric Nutrition Handbook*. American Academy of Pediatrics, 1979.
5. Heird, W. C., and Winters, R. Parenteral nutrition: Pediatrics. In H. Schneider, C. Anderson, and D. Coursin (eds.). *Nutrition Support of Medical Practice*. New York: Harper & Row, 1977.
6. Kitterman, J., Phibbs, R., and Tooley, W. Catheterization of umbilical vessels in newborn infants. *Pediatr. Clin. North Am.* 17:895–896, 1970.
7. Klaus, M. H., and Fanaroff, A. *Care of the High Risk Neonate* (2nd ed.). London: Saunders, 1979.
8. Levitt, E. Neonatal I.V. therapy. *J. NITA* 3:169, 1980.
9. Meyenfeldt, M., Stapert, J., DeJung, P., et al. TPN catheter sepsis: Lack of effect of subcutaneous tunneling of PVC catheters on sepsis rate. *J.P.E.N.* 4(5), 1980.
10. Sunshine, P. *Feeding the Neonate Weighing Less Than 1500 Grams — Nutrition and Beyond*. Fluid requirements of the low-birthweight infant. Columbus, Mo.: Ross Laboratories, 1980, p. 2.
11. Teitell, B. Cohen. The role of the pediatric TPN nurse with pediatric oncology patients. Paper presented at ASPENS Third Clinical Congress, 1978.
12. Teitell, B. Cohen. What does the future hold for the pediatric nutritional support nurse? *Nutr. Supp. Serv.* 1(3):1981.
13. Third National Cancer Survey. Nutritional Cancer Institute. *Ca — A Cancer Journal for Clinicians*. Published by the American Cancer Society, 27 (1), 1977.
14. Van Eys, S., Copeland, E., Taylor, G., et al. Supportive therapy with curative intent. *State of Curability of Childhood Cancer*. New York: Raven Press, 1980.
15. Watson, E. H., and Lowery, G. H. *Growth and Development of Children*. Chicago: Year Book, 1958.

REVIEW QUESTIONS

1. When assessing the child for I.V. therapy, what needs are generally overlooked?
2. Common reasons for I.V. therapy include _____ , _____ , and _____ .
3. Name the factors that can be used as a guide to predict complexities of I.V. therapy.

4. The first choice for I.V. site in the young infant is the _____.
5. The least favorable site for I.V. therapy in a child is the _____.
6. The best formula for assessing maintenance fluids in the infant is the _____.
7. Name the factors that should be analyzed when estimating fluid requirements in a child.
8. Which sites for I.V. therapy are uniquely used in the neonatal age group?
9. Meningomyelocele is a disease that alters nutrient absorption and may require I.V. nutritional support. True or false?
10. What complication of central TPN most likely would result in immediate removal of the catheter?

CHAPTER 25

Home Intravenous Therapy

Faye Cosentino

Self-administration of intravenous medications in the home is the fastest growing area in I.V. therapy. It has been estimated that home health agencies will increase 15–20% annually, with a 1990 projected annual revenue of $12–15 billion.

Many factors are responsible for this rapid growth. These include the public's desire to take more responsibility for its own health treatment, public outrage at skyrocketing costs of health care, government intervention to stop the rising costs, and the success of the Home Nutritional Program.

Self-responsibility for I.V. administration of medication in the home is a natural spin-off of our "do-it-yourself" society.

People have demanded and received the right to know and have a voice in decisions that will affect their bodies. An obvious question to a "do-it-yourself" society would be "Why can't I do it myself?"

Skyrocketing costs of health care have created a questioning public. "What are they doing with all that money?" "Can't something be done to stop it?"

Government intervention came as a result of public outrage at rising health care costs. In an attempt to stabilize these costs, the reimbursement system was changed. The old method was based on hospital costs. The more the hospital spent, the more it was reimbursed. The new Prospective Payment System (PPS) is based on diagnosis. DRG (Diagnosis Related Group) is a method of payment based according to an average cost of treating a particular diagnosis. If the hospital costs are greater than this amount, no additional monies are received. If the costs are less, the hospital keeps the difference. With this system, the shorter the patient stay the more profitable it is for the hospital.

The success of the Home Nutritional Program has established the fact that patients can be taught to safely administer I.V. admixtures and monitor their care in a home setting. This can be done at a cost far below that required for hospitalization.

HOME I.V. THERAPY PROCEDURES

The majority of I.V. procedures performed in the hospital can be performed in the home. Hemophilic patients giving themselves factor VIII were the pioneers in home I.V. therapy.

Total parenteral nutrition (TPN) was the first complex intravenous procedure to be self-administered in the home (see Chapter 21, section Home Hyperalimentation). The success of this program was a double victory for the patient. It not only gave patients a chance to receive treatment while leading a normal life, but it also proved that nonmedical people can be trained to safely perform highly complex nursing procedures on themselves.

Antibiotic therapy is now a well-established home procedure. Home self-administration of I.V. antibiotics has been life saving for those without hospital insurance coverage.

Chemotherapeutic agents are administered to home patients by various I.V. systems. Nonvesicant chemotherapeutic agents are being administered through peripheral cannulas. Vesicant and nonvesicant agents are being administered by centrally placed catheters, implanted catheters, and implanted pumps.

If home treatment is not available, the amount of precious time spent in the hospital can be devastating to the patient and the family.

Continuous or intermittent self-administration of I.V. analgesics in the home allows terminal patients to stay with their families without pain. Because these patients are not medically stable, a household member must be the primary care giver.

Maintaining fluid balance in elderly patients is also being performed at home. A household member again provides the care.

Long-term I.V. replacement of electrolytes and minerals are also being self-administered in the home.

Transfusions of blood/blood components are now performed on home patients. In many areas of the country, the need for a transfusion does not require a trip to the hospital. A sample of blood is brought to the blood bank for cross-matching. The compatible blood is taken to the home and transfused. This procedure requires continuous nursing supervision. The same guidelines that apply to an inpatient are followed.

Arterial blood gas samples (ABG) are easily drawn on home patients. The sample is placed in ice to prevent a change in values during transportation.

Blood sample drawing for all types of laboratory testing is available in most urban and some rural communities.

PATIENT SELECTION

The criteria used for patient selection plays a major role in the success or failure of a home I.V. therapy program. *Reimbursement* is frequently the most difficult aspect. There is no standard system for third-party coverage for this type of health care.

The ability and willingness to pay any required portion of charges must receive patient consent before any other step is taken. Each individual person's insurance must be thoroughly investigated to determine what will be covered. If home I.V. therapy is covered under a major medical portion, the patient may have to pay the deductible plus 20% of all charges. Approval, on an individual basis, may be obtained from an insurance carrier by stressing the cost-saving factor.

Medical stability is essential if the patient is to perform all required procedures himself or herself. If the patient is not medically stable, but has medical approval for home care, a household member may assume full responsibility for performing all required procedures. A back-up person may be necessary, depending upon each individual situation. If the patient is doing self care and periods of medical instability are expected, a back-up person becomes a necessity. If the primary care provider is a household member, a back-up person is needed to provide periods of relief.

Emotional stability and individual motivation with a desire to be involved in one's own care is essential to the success of the program. Home I.V. therapy is not the program of choice for a suicidal patient or a drug abuser.

The patient's lifestyle must be considered. If the patient is taken out of a controlled hospital environment, will he or she be responsible for avoiding situations which could be detrimental to the cannula or to recovery?

Intellectual ability to learn and peform procedures which require strict following must be assessed. Average intelligence is sufficient for adequate training. Illiteracy may be overcome by audio or audiovisual training programs.

Visual acuity is required for maintaining sterility and avoiding touch contamination of supplies. Magnifying or reading glasses may be required. During admixture, visual acuity is very important to ensure that proper drug dosages are being given.

Manual dexterity is needed to prepare supplies without touch contamination. This becomes very important when the patient must inject a small sterile needle into a small sterile area.

The home setting must be evaluated to assure that the procedures can be followed in its environment. There should be clean dry storage space for supplies. A refrigerator large enough to store admixtures must be available. A clean low-traffic area is needed for procedure preparation. The home should have sufficient space to allow patient privacy while performing procedures. If an electronic instrument on a moving pole is to be used, safe ambulation and availability of electrical outlets must be considered.

PATIENT EDUCATION

A *written medical order* is required to start patient teaching. If a central venous line is to be used, *teaching should start before catheter insertion.* The use of a *check-off teaching sheet,* which lists all training requirements, can be useful to ensure that all required areas have been covered (Exhibit 25.1). Placing the completed sheet on the patient's chart will serve as *training documentation.*

The *home health care company should be notified* to assure that the *identical* supplies and equipment used for training will be supplied for home care. All manufacturers vary the style and recommended usage of their supplies and

EXHIBIT 25.1
Sample Check-Off Teaching Sheet

General Hospital **Hickman Catheter/** **Non-Hyperalimentation** *Primary I.V. Therapist*	Has received item	Has had discussion	Had demonstration	Return demonstration c̄ assistance	Return demonstration c̄ assistance	Return demonstration c̄ assistance	Return demonstration s̄ assistance	Return demonstration s̄ assistance	Return demonstration s̄ assistance	Return demonstration s̄ assistance	Can perform care independently	Back-up person has been taught
1. Patient given copy of Training Manual												
2. Catheter functions and insertion												
3. Activity limitations												
4. Catheter precautions												
5. Complications; causes, signs & symptoms, treatment & prevention;												
a. air embolism												
b. catheter bleed												
c. infection												
d. catheter leak												
e. connection leak												
6. Catheter clamp												
7. Intermittent injection cap												
8. Aseptic techniques												
9. Procedure slides reviewed												
10. Injecting heparin flush												
11. Changing intermittent injection cap												
12. Catheter exit site care												
13. Cutdown site care												
14. Patient received and signed for individual treatment sheet with specific instructions												

Comments

Patient signature _____

EXHIBIT 25.2
Instructions for Connecting Admixture to Peripheral INT Catheter

1. Equipment
    - 1.1 I.V. bag with medication (1)
    - 1.2 I.V. tubing (1)
    - 1.3 1 inch 22-gauge needle (1)
    - 1.4 Povidone-iodine swab (1)
    - 1.5 Strip 1 × 2 inch tape (1)

2. Procedure
    - 2.1 WASH HANDS THOROUGHLY.
    - 2.2 Hang I.V. bag on hook or pole. Remove blue tab.
      DO NOT ALLOW PORT TO TOUCH ANY OBJECT.
    - 2.3 Open I.V. tubing box. Remove tubing. Slide roller clamp up close to drip chamber. Close roller clamp.
    - 2.4 Carefully open needle package and remove protective cover from I.V. tubing needle adapter. Securely, connect needle to tubing.
    - 2.5 Carefully remove tubing spike protective cover and fully insert spike into bag port.
    - 2.6 Squeeze drip chamber. Release and drip chamber will fill *half full* with I.V. fluid.
    - 2.7 Open roller clamp to flush tubing and needle.
      CLOSE ROLLER CLAMP.
    - 2.8 Open povidone-iodine swab and scrub injection cap END for *30 seconds*.
    - 2.9 Carefully remove needle protective cover and insert needle full length into CENTER of injection cap. If any obstruction is felt, DO NOT FORCE THE INSERTION; recheck the needle angle.
    - 2.10 Apply the strip of tape to secure tubing to the arm.
      DO NOT PLACE TAPE OVER THE DRESSING TAPE.
    - 2.11 Open roller clamp to allow 60 drops per minute. Solution will run in over approximately 20 minutes.

---

equipment. The patient should not be expected to translate knowledge of one company's products to that of another.

The person doing the teaching is extremely important to the success of the training program. The *teacher must believe the patient is capable of learning and must believe in the concept of self care*. If not, he or she can unconsciously make sure that the patient does not learn. *One-on-one demonstration and return demonstrations* are essential to the learning process. Audiovisual equipment can be very helpful as a secondary training aid.

The *training program should be broken down into small steps*. After one step is mastered, another is added with the patient continuing to perform the steps previously learned. Choosing a first step which can be easily learned will boost the patient's self-confidence and make the learning process easier.

A written copy of the procedure should be given to the patient. This can be used for reference while learning and after going home (Exhibits 25.2 and 25.3). *Samples of supplies should be given to the patient for examination and practice handling*. Familiarity with the products will enhance learning.

The training program must include all possible complications. *The patient must demonstrate the ability to prevent, recognize, and apply appropriate action if any complication should occur*. The identical training program is used for teaching a household member or back-up person.

EXHIBIT 25.3
Instructions for Discontinuing Admixture and Flushing Peripheral INT Catheter with Heparin

1. Equipment
   1.1 Povidone-iodine swab (1)
   1.2 Heparin flush with holder (1)

2. Procedure
   2.1 WASH HANDS THOROUGHLY.
   2.2 Open povidone-iodine swab.
   2.3 Prepare heparin flush, expel air from unit.
   2.4 Allow solution to run as far down the tubing as it will go and flow stops.
   2.5 CLOSE TUBING CLAMP. Remove strip of tape from arm.
   2.6 Stabilize catheter hub, with one hand, while removing needle and tubing with other hand.
   2.7 Maintaining catheter hub stabilization, cleanse END of cap with povidone-iodine for 30 seconds.
   2.8 Continue to stabilize catheter hub, insert needle of heparin flush unit into CENTER of cap. If any obstruction is felt, DO NOT FORCE THE INSERTION; recheck needle angle.
   2.9 GENTLY inject full dose of heparin.
   2.10 Maintain catheter stabilization, while withdrawing unit from cap.

3. Precautions
   3.1 CHECK I.V. SITE BEFORE PREPARING TO GIVE MEDICATION. Look for any redness or swelling. If present, DO NOT give medication and call I.V. therapist for site change.
   3.2 If during drug administration, fluid runs sluggishly and rate is difficult to maintain, RECHECK I.V. SITE, move tubing clamp to different location on tubing.
   3.3 Be sure to flush needle with I.V. solution, BEFORE CONNECTING TO CATHETER. Air blockage in the needle can cause difficulty in getting I.V. fluid to run.
   3.4 DO NOT FORCE ANY NEEDLE ENTRY INTO INJECTION CAP. If obstruction is felt, recheck needle for proper alignment.
   3.5 When setting flow rate, extreme accuracy is NOT required. Approximation is acceptable.
   3.6 Be careful NOT to touch any equipment part which must remain sterile. If any part is accidentally touched, DO NOT USE that piece of equipment; replace with a sterile piece.
   3.7 After using needles, protect yourself from accidental puncture.
   3.8 Even if no problems are noted, the I.V. site must be changed at least every 3 days, to prevent infection and/or phlebitis.

The *standards of care* for a home patient should be the same as for an inpatient. Both should be in accordance with the National Intravenous Therapy Association (NITA) Standards and the Center for Disease Control (CDC) Guidelines.

A *representative from the home health care company should visit the patient prior to discharge.* An estimated discharge date should be made available to the company.

The importance of keeping supplies and equipment away from the reach of children, and the methods which can be used to dispose of used supplies should be discussed. The patient should be informed as to which supplies and equipment will be provided by the company. If the patient is responsible for any additional items, he or she should be informed by a written list, well before discharge.

DAY OF DISCHARGE

The patient must demonstrate (1) the ability to safely perform all required procedures, and (2) knowledge of the prevention, the recognition, and the appropriate action required for any possible complication, before discharge. If a household member or back-up person is providing care, the same conditions must apply.

The patient consent form must be signed, and the written physician's order must be obtained. The home health care company should be contacted to reaffirm continuation of care and delivery of supplies and equipment. Written instructions for therapy and each required procedure should be sent home with the patient (Exhibit 25.4).

AFTER DISCHARGE

A registered nurse should visit the patient on the day of discharge. All *supplies and equipment should be checked* to assure they are complete and/or functioning properly. An equipment supply list can be helpful (Exhibit 25.5).

The *patient should be observed while performing procedures* to assure that instructions can be followed in the home environment.

The frequency of nursing visits will depend upon physician's order, patient needs, and nursing judgement. A permanent record should be kept of all home visits and telephone contacts with both patient and physician.

A method should be instituted which allows patient documentation of treatment. This can be easily accomplished by a treatment fill-in sheet (Exhibit 25.6).

Physician orders, laboratory results, and monthly reports to the physician are all a part of the permanent record.

MONTHLY REPORT TO THE PHYSICIAN

A monthly report should be sent to the physician. This should include patient compliance with treatments, reeducation required, vital signs, weight, patient progress, emotional status, and proposed nursing plan.

FOLLOW-UP CARE

Home visits should be coordinated with patient procedure time to observe treatments being given. Reassessment of competency can document areas requiring reeducation. The patient and/or care giver should have 24-hour access to appropriate health care professionals. Medical orders should be reviewed and updated routinely. Supplies and equipment should be continuously evaluated and available. Any pertinent observation requiring medical treatment, should be reported to the physician immediately.

EXHIBIT 25.4
Instructions for Therapy

General Hospital I.V. Therapy Department:
Hickman-Catheter/Non-Hyperalimentation
Instructions for Care

1. Your EQUIPMENT HOME SUPPLIER is _____.
   Telephone _____.

2. Your HOME I.V. THERAPIST is _____.
   Telephone _____.

3. NUMBER of NOTCHES to CLOSE YOUR CATHETER CLAMP: _____.

4. HEPARIN FLUSHES:
   Flush catheter(s) *every other day* with _____ cc heparin (_____) units.

5. INTERMITTENT CAP CHANGES:
   Change intermittent injection cap(s) *every 6 days (every third time you flush)*.

6. CARE OF CATHETER EXIT SITE:
   Perform site cleansing and dressing *every day* IMMEDIATELY AFTER BATHING.

7. CARE OF CUTDOWN SITE:
   Perform site cleansing and dressing *every day* IMMEDIATELY AFTER BATHING, until sutures are removed.
   MAKE AN APPOINTMENT WITH DR. _____ to remove sutures and examine site on _____.
   Further instructions as to care of site will be given to you at that time.

8. DO NOT ALLOW ANY PERSON, OTHER THAN THE BACK-UP PERSON TRAINED WITH YOU, TO PERFORM ANY PROCEDURE WITHOUT FIRST DISCUSSING THE SITUATION WITH YOUR PHYSICIAN OR I.V. THERAPIST.

9. REMEMBER, ALWAYS DO A THOROUGH HAND WASHING BEFORE TOUCHING YOUR CATHETER OR PERFORMING ANY OF THESE PROCEDURES.

I have reviewed these instructions and have indicated my understanding by signing on the space below. I have been given a copy to take home with me for use after discharge, and a copy has been retained by the hospital for its records.

_____   _____
Patient signature   Date

_____   _____
Witness   Date

THE ADVANTAGES OF HOME TREATMENT

In most instances, home treatment will be *less expensive* than treatment in the hospital. If the home health care supplier is small, due to low-volume purchasing, supply costs may be very high.

Home treatment *allows the patient to remain in a familiar, comfortable surrounding.* This is very important for the young and the aged. Disorientation and confusion may result from changing the environment of the elderly.

EXHIBIT 25.5
Equipment/Supply List

	Date											
IV Pole												
100 ml 5% D/W												
50 ml 5% D/W												
100 ml 0.9% NS												
50 ml 0.9% NS												
IV Tubing (2C0001)												
20 cc vial NS												
100 U/ml tubex Heparin Flush												
Tubex holder												
Intermittent injection caps												
20 cc syringes												
20 G × 1½" needles												
22 G × 1" needles												
20 G catheters												
22 G catheters												
Swabs povidone-iodine												
Alcohol swabs												
Ointment povidone-iodine												
Sponges 2" × 2" sterile												
Tape												
Clear sterile tape												
Tourniquet												

To prevent overstocking of supplies, call _____ *on morning of delivery date, giving amount of each item needed to replace used supplies.*

Name _____

Address _____

EXHIBIT 25.6
Treatment and Medication Sheet

Name _____   Physician _____

Address _____   Orders _____

Date	Time	Medication	Treatment and Therapist's Notes

In many situations, home treatment *allows the patient to return to normal activities* between treatments. A student may return to classes and receive treatments after school. Some patients may return to work during the day and receive their treatments at night while sleeping.

The *risk of acquiring a nosocomial infection is lessened* with home care. Many nosocomial infections are due to the hospital environment. Lowering hospital contact will lower the risk of acquiring a nosocomial infection.

Self-administered I.V. therapy at home *satisfies the need for responsibility and control of one's own body* at the same time one is receiving necessary medical treatment.

BIBLIOGRAPHY

Antoniskis, A., Anderson, B. C., et al. Feasibility of outpatient self-administration of parenteral antibiotics. *West. J. Med.* 128:203, 1978.

Bergers, R., et al. A home I.V. antibiotic program. *J. NITA* 8:238, 1985.

Daffara, K. The future of health care delivery. *J. NITA* 7:293, 1984.

Dudrick, S. J., O'Donnell, J. J., and Englert, D. M. 100 patient-years of ambulatory home parenteral nutrition. *Ann. Surg.* 199:770, 1984.

Gibson, J. A program for outpatient intravenous antibiotic therapy. *J. NITA* January 1978.

Hergenhahn, B. R. *An Introduction to Theories of Learning.* Englewood Cliffs, N.J.: Prentice-Hall, 1976.

Johnston, J. B., and Davidson, M. R. Use of a mini-infuser syringe pump for the self administration of I.V. antibiotics in the home. *J. NITA* 7:381, 1984.

Knutsen, C., et al. A service-oriented program providing continuity of high-quality care to the home hyperalimentation patient: Hospital without walls. *J. NITA* 7:369, 1984.

Larkin, M. From the editor: Home intravenous care. *J. NITA* 7:10, 1984.

National Intravenous Therapy Association (NITA). Home I.V. therapy nursing standards of practice. *J. NITA* 7:93, 1984.

Neave, L. The use of Intrasil catheters in long-term phlebotomy patients. *J. NITA* 6:423, 1983.

Oncology nurses see DRGs as a challenge for innovation. *Oncology Times* August 1985.

Pelletier, G. Home intravenous antibiotic therapy: A growing concept. *J. NITA* 4:45, 1981.

Pelletier, G. Responding to a need: Home intravenous therapy. *J. NITA* 5:383, 1982.

Poretz, D. M., et al. Intravenous antibiotic therapy in an outpatient setting. *J.A.M.A.* 248:336, 1982.

Sheehan, K., and Gildea, J. Home antibiotic therapy: A less-than-ideal candidate. *J. NITA* 8:157, 1985.

Stiver, H. G., Telford, G. O., et al. Intravenous antibiotic therapy at home. *Ann. Intern. Med.* 89:690, 1978.

Studebaker, E. Home health agencies: Functions and reimbursements. *J. NITA* 8:43, 1985.

Swenson, J. P. Training patients to administer intravenous antibiotics at home. *Am. J. Hosp. Pharm.* 38:1480, 1981.

Terry, J. Home care utilizing Silastic catheters. *J. NITA* 6:348, 1983.

Thomson, S., and Lang, K. The I.V. solution: A home care alternative. *J. NITA* 7:397, 1984.

Weinstein, S. Intravenous therapy within the scope of home health services. *J. NITA* 7:39, 1984.

Weinstein, S. The how-to's of home care. *J. NITA* 8:227, 1985.

Koithan, M. Home total parenteral nutrition: Complications. *J. NITA* 8:231, 1985.

Whatley, K., et al. Developing a patient assessment and teaching program for right atrial catheters. *J. NITA* 7:529, 1984.

Wise, M., and Huff, S. Home I.V. therapy: A hospital-based program. *J. NITA* 8:309, 1985.

REVIEW QUESTIONS

1. Prospective Payment System (PPS) reimbursement is based on _____ .
2. A written _____ is required before patient training starts.
3. One-on-one demonstrations and _____ are essential to the learning process.
4. Choosing a first step that is _____ will boost patient self-confidence and enhance learning.
5. The patient must demonstrate ability to _____ , _____ , and _____ if any complications should occur.
6. Patient _____ must be signed prior to starting home I.V. therapy.
7. The first nursing home visit should be on _____ .
8. Two important reasons for this visit are (1) _____ and (2) _____ .
9. A _____ should be sent to the physician.
10. Any pertinent observation requiring medical treatment should be _____ .

Answers to Review Questions

Chapter 4

1. injury, negligence
2. factual
3. poor doctor-patient relationship, poor communications
4. problem identification, problem evaluation, implementation of corrective action, reevaluation (follow-up), problem minimization or solution
5. structure, process, outcome
6. objective, measurable
7. yes, no, numbers
8. standardization, reliability, validity
9. high negative correlation
10. reevaluation (follow-up)

Chapter 5

1. 24 to 48
2. The tubing a few inches from the cannula is kinked, while the tubing between the cannula and the kinked tubing is pinched and released. If resistance is met, it may be due to a clot obstructing the cannula.
3. Application of heat on the vein directly above the cannula will increase the rate of flow of the infusion.
4. Irrigation may result in (a) propagating a thrombus, which may cause infarction; and (b) embolizing small, infected cannula thrombi, which may cause septicemia.
5. The central venous vein is more likely to have a negative pressure than are the peripheral veins. Negative venous pressure would result in air being pulled into the vein from an open catheter or a loose connection.
6. false
7. false
8. redness, induration, and tenderness

Chapter 6

1. Superficial veins and deep veins unite freely in the lower extremities. A thrombus occurring in the superficial veins may extend to the deep veins and cause a pulmonary embolism.
2. Phlebitis. There may be untoward reactions when toxic concentrations of the pooled medication in the varicosity reaches the circulating blood. A delay in effect of the drug may occur when immediate action is required.
3. An arteriovenous fistula is an anastomosis of an artery and a vein resulting from past penetrating injury of the vein or occurring on a congenital basis.
4. An arteriovenous fistula and the veins draining it are overburdened with high-pressure arterial blood.
5. An aberrant artery is one that is located superficially in an unusual place.
6. Spasm from inadvertent arterial injection of a drug may result in impaired circulation and, possibly, necrosis and gangrene to the related area.
7. tunica media or middle layer
8. change in temperature, mechanical irritation, and chemical irritation
9. heat
10. digital, metacarpal, cephalic, accessory cephalic, basilic, and median veins, median cephalic, and median basilic
11. median cephalic, median basilic
12. A hematoma may readily occur if the patient flexes the elbow to stop the bleeding rather than elevating the arm.
13. epidermis, dermis
14. superficial fascia
15. cellulitis

Chapter 7

1. intracellular, extracellular
2. extracellular
3. electrolytes, nonelectrolytes
4. dextrose, urea, and creatinine
5. Electrolytes are molecules that ionize or break into electrically charged particles called ions when dissolved in water.
6. Normal blood plasma has an osmolality of about 290 mOsm/kg water; it is dependent upon the concentration of sodium, chloride, and bicarbonate.
7. sodium
8. potassium
9. to control water volume by osmotic pressure and to maintain proper acid–alkaline balance
10. pH
11. 7.35 to 7.45
12. carbonic acid — sodium bicarbonate system
13. the carbonic side
14. respiratory acidosis
15. The body attempts to compensate for the increase in carbonic acid by an increase in bicarbonate.
16. Calcium ionization is decreased in alkalosis; calcium ionization is influenced by pH.
17. the bicarbonate side
18. The kidney regulates the amount of cations (hydrogen, ammonium, and

Answers to Review Questions 541

   potassium) needed to combine with the reabsorbed bicarbonate in exchange for sodium ions.
19. Bicarbonate anions increase to replace the loss of chloride anions since, to maintain electrolyte equilibrium, the total number of cations must equal the total number of anions. Thus alkalosis results.
20. bicarbonate
21. uncontrolled diabetes or starvation, which results in excessive accumulations of ketone acids; renal disease, with accumulations of inorganic acids like phosphate and sulphate; diarrhea or intestinal drainage, which produces excessive losses of bicarbonate; intravenous administration of excessive amounts of sodium chloride or ammonium chloride
22. adrenal glands, pituitary glands, parathyroid glands, kidneys, skin, lungs
23. adrenal glands
24. Aldosterone increases the reabsorption of sodium from the renal tubules in exchange for potassium.
25. antidiuretic hormone (ADH)
26. renal failure with potassium retention, excessive or rapid administration of potassium in fluid therapy, or a sudden shift of potassium from intracellular to extracellular fluid as the result of catabolism (as in a crushing injury)
27. Sodium controls the distribution of water throughout the body and maintains a normal fluid balance.
28. 135–145 mEq per liter
29. ADH
30. ADH controls the urinary output as follows: when increased sodium concentration occurs, ADH causes water to be retained, diluting sodium to a normal level; when sodium concentration is decreased, ADH is inhibited, resulting in a loss of water, which raises the concentration of sodium to normal.
31. about 5 mEq per liter
32. normal clotting of the blood and regulation of neuromuscular irritability
33. parathyroid glands
34. diarrhea, problems in gastrointestinal absorption, extensive infections of the subcutaneous tissue, and burns
35. Calcium ionization is increased in acidosis.
36. Magnesium's main role is enzyme activity, contributing to the metabolism of carbohydrates and protein.
37. 100–106 mEq per liter
38. true

Chapter 8

1. to maintain daily requirements, to restore previous losses, to replace present losses
2. the amount of waste products to be excreted and the concentrating ability of the kidneys
3. body surface area
4. maintenance
5. 1,500
6. Glucose supplies calories for energy, spares body protein and minimizes the development of ketosis occasioned by the oxidation of fat stores in absence

of glucose, and improves hepatic function when converted into glycogen by the liver
7. Protein repairs cells, heals wounds, and synthesizes vitamins and some enzymes.
8. vitamin C and B complex vitamins
9. Vitamin B complex metabolizes carbohydrates and maintains gastrointestinal function.
10. Vitamin C promotes wound healing.
11. potassium
12. 1 kg or 2.2 pounds
13. epinephrine, norepinephrine
14. aldosterone, hydrocortisone
15. nonelectrolyte solutions
16. hyponatremia (water excess)
17. restricting the fluid intake
18. water-yielding solutions or nonelectrolyte solutions
19. diuresis
20. nutritional and physiological
21. The infused glucose is stored as glycogen.
22. Vitamin B complex aids carbohydrate metabolism, and vitamin C promotes healing.
23. intravascular to interstitial
24. fluid shift from plasma to tissues, exudate from the burned area, water in the form of vapor at the burned area, and blood lost through the damaged capillaries
25. The lowered blood volume causes a diminished renal flow, increased endocrine secretions contribute to a decrease in urinary output, and ADH causes antidiuresis.
26. When plasma is lost in edema and exudate, sodium is also lost.
27. Loss of bicarbonate ions accompanying the loss of sodium ions as well as from altered aerobic metabolized tissue destruction results in acidosis.
28. to combat hypovolemic shock and prevent renal depression
29. When the fluid shifts back to plasma, excess parenteral fluid can cause circulatory overload and pulmonary edema.
30. interstitial to intravascular
31. the need to decrease fluids because of the edema mobilization that is taking place
32. A decreased red blood cell volume is not apparent until 48 hours after the burn; hemoconcentration is usually present. It is better to provide the colloids, fluids, and electrolytes necessary at this time than to increase the blood volume with red cells until needed.
33. Cellular metabolism of glucose and its conversion into glycogen is prevented; glucose accumulates in the bloodstream (hyperglycemia); glucose spills into the urine (glycosuria); water excretion increases (polyuria).
34. Hyperosmolality of the blood as a result of hyperglycemia causes water to be drawn from the cells. Extracellular fluid deficit results from (a) increased urinary output due to glycosuria and increase in ketone bodies,
(b) vomiting, (c) reduced oral intake, and (d) hyperventilation induced by acidiotic state.
35. decreased renal blood flow caused by low blood pressure
36. Ketosis is the excessive production of ketone bodies in the bloodstream.

Answers to Review Questions 543

37. hyperglycemia, glycosuria, polyuria, thirst, weakness and tiredness, flushed face, rapid deep breathing, acetone breath, nausea and vomiting, weight loss, low blood pressure, and oliguria
38. isotonic solutions of sodium chloride or hypotonic electrolyte solutions
39. There is already an increase in serum potassium concentration due to (a) catabolism (glycogen breaking down into glucose) and (b) retention of potassium due to impaired kidney function resulting from the lowered blood volume.

Chapter 9

1. Osmotic pressure is the drawing power of body fluid determined by the total ion concentration, expressed in milliosmoles and exerted when the concentration of ions between the extracellular fluid and the intracellular fluid differs.
2. true
3. a. 290 mOsm (−50 mOsm) per liter
   b. 290 mOsm (+50 mOsm) per liter
4. hypertonic, hypotonic, isotonic
5. false
6. false
7. 50
8. Dextrose provides calories for essential energy, improves hepatic function, spares body protein, minimizes or prevents ketosis, and causes shift of potassium from the extracellular to the intracellular compartment.
9. hypokalemia, dehydration, hyperinsulinism, and water intoxication
10. 2,500–3,000 ml per day
11. hypernatremia, acidosis, hypokalemia, and circulatory overload
12. severe dilutional hyponatremia and severe sodium depletion
13. to assess the status of the kidneys, to hydrate medical and surgical patients, and to promote diuresis in dehydrated patients
14. They provide more water than is required for excretion of salt.
15. They provide fluid to meet the patient's fluid volume requirement and cellular and extracellular electrolytes in quantities balanced between minimal needs and maximal tolerance of the patient.
16. a. hyperkalemia,
    b. water intoxication
17. Isotonic multiple electrolyte fluids provide replacement for heavy loss of water and electrolytes resulting from severe vomiting, diarrhea, or diuresis.
18. ammonium ions, hydrogen ions, urea
19. alkalizing fluids
20. Oxidation of the lactate ions is necessary to increase the bicarbonate concentration.
21. true
22. true
23. central venous pressure, quality and rate of the pulse, peripheral veins, weight, thirst, intake and output, skin, edema, and laboratory values
24. Divide pounds by 2; 10 percent of this quotient is subtracted from the quotient to obtain the weight in kilograms.
25. The skin over the forehead or sternum in an adult and on the medial aspects of the thighs in pediatric patients is picked up, pinched, and

released; skin that remains in a raised position indicates a deficit in fluid volume.
26. Peripheral edema is detected by finger printing, the process of rolling the finger over the bony prominence of the sternum or tibia.
27. diminished plasma volume due to dehydration
28. patients who receive isotonic fluids around the clock, early postoperative or posttrauma patients, and elderly patients
29. loss of fluid and electrolytes of the same tonicity as plasma through vomiting, diarrhea, or loss of whole blood
30. rapid infusion of hypertonic saline solution
31. Adequate intake of fluids may not be met because of a decrease in thirst stimuli, excess urination from loss of tubular ability to concentrate urine, and a diminished responsiveness to ADH.
32. hypotonic expansion (water intoxication)

Chapter 10

1. surface area of the body, condition of the patient, age of the patient, composition of the fluid, and patient's tolerance to the infusion
2. 3 ml
3. true
4. pulmonary edema
5. pediatric infusion set and infusion pump
6. 8 hours
7. true
8. diuretic
9. 8 ml per square meter of body surface area per minute for 45 minutes
10. a. 2 ml per minute
    b. to test the patient's sensitivity to the protein
11. $\dfrac{\text{gtt/ml of given set}}{60 \text{ (min in hour)}} \times \text{total hourly volume} = \text{gtt/min}$
12. 60 gtt/min
13. height of container, clot in needle, change in position of needle, change in temperature of solution, trauma to vein, and plugged vent

Chapter 12

1. Vasovagal reaction is an undesirable autonomic nervous system response to stress characterized by cold, clammy skin, nausea, vomiting, syncope, and peripheral venous collapse.
2. Retention of fluids, increased blood volume, and increased blood pressure with the threat of pulmonary edema can occur.
3. Explain the procedure to the patient.
   Instill confidence in the patient.
   Alleviate patient's fears.
   Never exceed two punctures in attempting to initiate an infusion.
4. The prominent vein could be sclerosed or in a location impractical for prolonged infusion.
5. Joint motion can result in phlebitis and infiltrations. Irritating drugs and solutions can thrombose veins, rendering them useless.
6. a. Phlebitis and thrombophlebitis with the risk of pulmonary embolism can occur.

Answers to Review Questions 545

  b. Sluggish circulation makes the veins of the lower extremity susceptible to trauma.
7. metacarpal veins
8. suitability of location, condition of the vein, purpose of the infusion, and duration of therapy
9. The venipuncture may be performed by inserting the cannula in the direction of the distal end of the extremity.
10. Differentiate between vein and artery. An artery has a pulse and a thicker, tougher wall, and the blood is brighter red than that in a vein.
11. Digital pressure is applied to disperse the fluid.
12. a. The blood may leak into the tissues before the entire bevel is within the lumen of the vein.
  b. Insert the cannula bevel-down.
13. a. tight enough to stop venous flow and still maintain arterial flow
  b. just below that of the diastolic pressure
14. The vein becomes hard, tortuous, and rolls when pressure from the cannula is exerted on the vein.
15. minimum rate to prevent speed shock when the manually clamped tubing is released
16. To prevent the development of a hematoma, do not apply the tourniquet above the site of a previous puncture.
17. date of insertion; type, length, and gauge of cannula used; and the initials of the operator
18. a. If the venipuncture is unsuccessful, do not reinsert stylet into the plastic cannula.
  b. Make sure the level of the needle is properly protected with the bevel shield. Never pull the catheter back through the needle. Always remove the catheter and needle together.

Chapter 13

1. on the red cells
2. antigens
3. antigens
4. true
5. false
6. true
7. true
8. true
9. CDE antigens
10. antibodies, antigens
11. group AB Rh negative plasma, because it contains neither A nor B antibody and will not react with A or B red cells
12. (a) AB, (b) A or AB, (c) B or AB, and (d) O, A, B, AB
13. group A or group B because O packed red cells contain antibody A and B, which would react with antigen A and B on the recipient's red cells
14. Rh (D) immune globulin
15. hypertonic, circulatory overload
16. true
17. true
18. antibodies, antigens
19. true

Chapter 14

1. Autotransfusion is a method by which a person's own blood is returned to the circulation.
2. Therapeutic phlebotomy is the removal of blood for the treatment of a patient.
3. the amount of blood to be withdrawn
4. acute pulmonary congestion (a less likely reason today because of improved monitoring methods and drugs available), polycythemia, and hemochromatosis
5. vasovagal
6. False. The two recommended procedures for adequate recipient protection are more involved.
7. 50 mm Hg to 60 mm Hg
8. Stop the phlebotomy.
   Lower the head, elevate the feet.
   Loosen restrictive clothing.
   Apply cold compresses to the forehead.
   Administer aromatic spirits of ammonia.
9. Have donor breathe into a paper bag.
10. Decontaminate blood infected with the hepatitis virus according to hospital procedure. The blood may be placed in a water bath in a sealed glass container and autoclaved at 120°C at 15 psi for 60 minutes.

Chapter 15

1. fibrinogen
2. the cells
3. true
4. by using an anticoagulant to prevent the blood from clotting
5. The sample is placed on ice.
6. Glycolysis is the production of lactic acid by the glycolytic enzymes of the blood cells, causing a drop in pH on standing.
7. to prevent escape of carbon dioxide
8. without a tourniquet
9. tests for carbon dioxide and pH
10. Hemolysis is the lysis of cells; it causes serious errors in many tests by allowing the substance being measured to escape into the serum.
11. Never draw blood proximal to an infusion; instead, use the contralateral extremity. Make note of any substance in the infusion that may affect the analysis.
12. by lightly pressing the vein above the needle and allowing it to fill, by using a smaller needle, or by using a syringe
13. Never apply a tourniquet proximal to the puncture site immediately after the venipuncture; use the contralateral extremity.
14. false
15. until the bleeding stops
16. Take care not to spill the specimen on the outside of the container; place, well labeled, in a bag or plastic container.
17. positive identification

Answers to Review Questions 547

Chapter 16

1. inflammation and thrombosis
2. chemical, mechanical
3. Thrombophlebitis denotes thrombosis plus phlebitis, and phlebothrombosis denotes thrombosis with a relatively inconspicuous inflammation.
4. septicemia, acute bacterial endocarditis
5. phlebothrombosis
6. Irritation to the wall of the vein caused by duration of the infusion, composition of the solution, site of the infusion, technique, and method employed are all factors that may contribute to thrombophlebitis.
7. Refrain from using veins in the lower extremities.
   Select veins with ample blood volume when infusing irritating substances.
   Avoid veins in areas over joint flexion.
   Anchor cannula securely to prevent motion.
8. Infiltration predisposes the patient to infection, limits veins, and may result in necroses and gangrene.
9. Examine solutions carefully before administering and dispose of them after they have been opened 24 hours.
   Use sterile technique in adding drugs to solutions.
10. Use adequate filters in the administration of blood and blood components.
    Avoid using veins on the lower extremities.
    Do not use positive pressure to relieve clot formation in the cannula.
11. Use vigilance in preventing vented containers from running dry, especially in the use of Y-type infusions and central venous infusions.
    Instruct the patient to perform the Valsalva maneuver when the central venous catheter is open to air.
12. air embolism
13. Turn the patient on his or her left side, head down.
    Administer oxygen.
    Notify physician.
14. pulmonary edema
15. Maintain rate prescribed while administering fluids.
    Never apply positive pressure to infuse solutions.
    Administer only the amount ordered.
16. Speed shock refers to a systemic reaction that occurs when a substance foreign to the body is rapidly introduced into the circulation.
17. Use special devices that give added protection by preventing large quantities of fluid from being accidentally infused: controlled volume infusion sets, pediatric-type infusion sets, and electronic controllers or pumps. Ascertain that the solution is flowing freely before adjusting the rate of flow.

Chapter 17

1. air, skin, and blood
2. skin
3. no
4. Resident flora are bacteria on the skin that are normally present and relatively constant in a given individual.
5. Transient flora are bacteria picked up by the individual from his or her

environment; they are loosely attached to the skin and vary from day to day in quality and quantity.
6. false
7. hepatitis virus
8. Pathogenic bacteria are capable of producing disease. Nonpathogenic bacteria do not usually produce disease, though bacteria previously considered nonpathogenic have been reported to produce infection.
9. *Serratia* is nonpathogenic, but has been implicated in gram-negative septicemia.
10. Increased use of antibiotics, which are highly effective against gram-positive organisms, has eliminated the competitive inhibition of gram-positive bacteria and allowed the more resistant gram-negative organisms to proliferate.
11. no
12. diabetes mellitus, chronic uremia, cirrhosis, cancer, and leukemia
13. immunosuppressive drugs, corticosteroids, anticancer agents, and extensive radiation therapy
14. pH, temperature, and presence of essential nutrients
15. administration sets, medication sites, cannulas, supplementary apparatus, and containers of fluid
16. 24
17. 48
18. false
19. The injection site should be scrubbed with an accepted antiseptic such as 70% isopropyl alcohol. The needle inserted into the injection site should be securely taped to prevent an in-and-out motion of the needle from introducing bacteria into the infusion.
20. *Serratia*
21. Apply with friction for 1 minute.
22. bactericidal, fungicidal, sporicidal
23. The sustained release of free iodine, which may be necessary for germicidal action.
24. It is carried from patient to patient and used just prior to venipuncture.
25. Mechanical and septic phlebitis may result from motion of the catheter, which irritates the vein and allows bacteria to enter.
26. daily
27. no
28. Septicemia from embolizing small infected cannula thrombi or infection from propagating a thrombus may result.
29. drugs, rubber closure, and glass ampules
30. filters such as a filter aspiration needle, final filters, and filters for blood administration

Chapter 18

1. at the junction of the superior vena cava and the right atrium
2. the patient's right atrium
3. increase central venous pressure, distend the entry vein
4. basilic vein
5. chest x-ray
6. air embolism

Answers to Review Questions

7. placing the patient in a supine position, on the left side, with the feet elevated
8. 15 or more
9. Pressure exerted must not be greater than that recommended for the catheter and/or any device being used.
10. air embolism
11. catheter-related sepsis

Chapter 19

1. silicone
2. inside-the-needle catheter (INC)
3. multiple lumen
4. continuous, low volume, long-term
5. prothrombin time and partial prothrombin time
6. the patient's hospital identification band
7. sterile gloves
8. three
9. injecting 5 ml normal saline, releasing syringe plunger, and allowing solution to return to syringe

Chapter 20

1. Some drugs cannot be absorbed by any other route.
   Instant drug action is afforded by the use of the vascular system.
   The rate of drug administration can be controlled.
   Slow administration permits termination if sensitivity occurs.
   The vascular system affords a route of administration for the patient who cannot tolerate fluids and drugs by the gastrointestinal route.
   Drugs which cause pain and trauma by intramuscular or subcutaneous routes must be given intravenously.
2. potential incompatibilities when drugs are added to intravenous solutions, speed shock, vascular irritations and subsequent hazards, and rapid onset of action with inability to recall the drug once administered
3. true
4. hydrolysis, reduction, oxidation, and double decomposition
5. hydrolysis
6. therapeutic, physical, and chemical
7. true
8. pH of parenteral solutions, additional drugs, buffering agents in drugs, preservatives in the diluent, degree of dilution, period of time solution stands, order of mixing, light, and room temperature
9. Avoid veins in the lower extremities; use a cannula appreciably smaller than the lumen of the vein; and, when possible, follow hypertonic solutions with isotonic solutions.
10. Question patient regarding sensitivity to drugs that may cause anaphylaxis, and observe patient following initial dose of such drugs. If there is a question of sensitivity, the drug should be administered by the physician.
11. Properly dilute lyophilized drugs, use a filter when necessary, and observe the solution for particulate matter before administration.
12. Use a controlled-volume set, a microdrip, or an electronic controller or pump.

13. true
14. A heparin lock conserves veins, provides minimal amount of fluid to the patient on restricted intake, and saves the patient the trauma of multiple punctures while offering freedom of motion.
15. false

Chapter 21

1. false
2. superior vena cava, intrathoracic subclavian vein, innominate vein
3. catheter placement, intravenous tubing change, catheter removal
4. 3
5. organisms at the catheter insertion site that migrate along the catheter
6. 0.8 to 1.0
7. vitamin C, Aldomet, salicylates, and levodopa
8. dry or scaling skin, thinning hair, thrombocytopenia, and liver function abnormalities
9. isotonic
10. true
11. hyperosmolar, hyperglycemic, nonketotic coma
12. air obstruction of the right ventrical outflow tract
13. left-lateral, head-dependent position
14. Crohn's disease, short bowel syndrome, radiation enteritis, intestinal fistulas
15. clotting of the catheter and breakage of the catheter
16. biochemical and psychological
17. Giordano-Gioranetti

Chapter 22

1. consistent and high-quality
2. battery
3. It gives them some sense of control in the situation.
   They accept the treatments better.
   Their anxiety level is reduced.
   They can sense inner changes better than the therapist can.
4. Immediately discontinue the infusion or administration of the drug.
5. Always assess the venous status adequately.
   Avoid the side of a mastectomy, immobilized fracture, or resolving phlebitis.
   Patient education should precede the administration of vesicant agents.
   A baseline reference point of the patient's mental status should be obtained.
   A baseline blood pressure reading should be recorded with drugs known to cause anaphylaxis.
   Sterile technique should be adhered to because patients on cytotoxic drugs often are leukopenic and thus more susceptible to infection.
6. Dangle the hand and arm.
   Apply warm water over the hand and arm.
   Gently tap the site.
   Have another nurse provide moderate hand pressure.

Answers to Review Questions

7. central venous pressure line, heparin lock, arteriovenous fistula, Hickman catheters
8. Double-check the medicine order against the chart.
   Check drug calculations with a co-worker.
   Read the drug's package insert.
   Wear gloves.
   Prepare the drugs without interruption.
   Label all syringes or containers.
9. false
10. Obtain an allergy history.
    Have an emergency cart and drugs readily available.
    Talk with the patient to establish a baseline mental point of reference.
    Take a baseline blood pressure reading.
    Have the patient in a position where he or she can be readily reclined.
11. false
12. doxorubicin, Mechlorethamine, vincristine, vinblastine, daunomycin, dactinomycin, dacarbazine, mithramycin, mitomycin
13. not yet known
14. It is extremely painful to the patient.
    Reconstructive measures are expensive.
    The patient's disease may grow when chemotherapy is not given while awaiting resolution of infections and surgical healing.
    Precious time is lost if the patient is not working or attending school.
    The cosmetic defect may be unacceptable if the patient works in areas where the hands are readily visible.
    The psychological trauma associated with the five points above should be considered in the cancer patient for whom life expectancy may be limited.
15. it is more readily recalled; for medicolegal purposes

Chapter 23

1. syringe and needle, catheter with heparin lock
2. radial artery
3. postexercise or at rest, FIO_2 or room air
4. excess heparin will alter the resultant ABG values.
5. metabolize O_2, give off CO_2
6. blood hemolysis, air contamination, arterial spasm
7. personal observation and digital pressure of puncture site
8. assure adequacy of collateral circulation
9. air bubbles in the line, near-exsanguination
10. overinflate the balloon, inflate balloon too frequently
11. CA to HCO_3^-
12. HCO_3^-
13. PCO_2
14. PCO_2
15. PO_2
16. pH of 7.35–7.45, PCO_2 of 36–44 mm Hg, HCO_3^- of 22–26 mEq per liter
17. pH, HCO_3^-, BE
18. a decrease in body content of *fixed* acids
19. PCO_2
20. CO_2 deficit

Chapter 24

1. developmental needs
2. maintenance of fluid and electrolyte balance, antibiotic therapy, nutritional support
3. hydrational status and previous I.V. therapy
4. head
5. foot
6. weight method
7. age, weight, stress levels, disease status, and temperature spikes
8. umbilical vessels and central line
9. false
10. catheter site edema

Chapter 25

1. diagnosis
2. physician's order
3. return demonstrations
4. easily learned
5. prevent, recognize, and apply appropriate action
6. consent form
7. day of discharge
8. to check that all required supplies and equipment are available, complete, and functioning; to assure instructions can be followed in the home environment
9. monthly report
10. reported to the physician immediately

Index

Aberrant artery, 60–61, 173, 174
ABO blood group system, 191, 192, 193, 194, 240
  patient identification of, 204
  plasma transfusion and, 198–199
  platelet transfusion and, 200
  transfusion reactions and, 207
Accessory cephalic vein, 63
Acetoacetate plus acetone, reference values for, 242–243
Acetone, 403
Acetone breath, 99
Acid(s)
  fixed, 497, 500, 501
  keto, 497, 500
  lactic, 242–243, 497, 500
  uric, 246–247
Acid–alkaline (base) balance 73, 77, 104
  blood measurement of, 233–234
Acid–base imbalances, 73, 74–75, 76, 500–504
Acid-citrate-dextrose (ACD), 195
Acidifying infusions, 116–117
Acidosis, 88
  burns and metabolic, 94
  calcium and, 80
  diabetic, 97–99, 234
  isotonic saline and, 110, 111
  metabolic, 76, 110, 501
  respiratory, 74, 75, 502–503
  sodium bicarbonate and, 116
Actinomycin D, 454–455

Adenosine triphosphate, 195
Administration sets, 51
  outdated, 54, 286
Adolescents, 513
Adrenal glands, 77, 89, 90
  reference values for, 262–263
Adrenalin, 20, 21, 90, 385
Adrenocorticotropin (ACTH), 89–90, 250–251
Adriamycin, 449, 454–455, 466
  antidote for, 470
  plastic surgery and, 473
Age
  and blood coagulation, 196
  and rate of flow, 131
Agglutinins, in red blood cells, 197
Agglutinogens (antigens), 191, 192–193, 207, 211
  hemolysis and, 239
AIDS (Acquired Immune Deficiency Syndrome), 210–211
  blood transmission of, 282–283
Air, as bacteria source, 281, 286
Air-eliminating filter, .022 micron, 53–54, 152, 294, 320
Air embolism, 27, 275, 277
  from blood transfusion, 209–210
  catheterization and, 311, 315, 435
  and fluid level, 53
  Hickman catheter and, 462–463

  infusion pumps and, 155
  positive-pressure infusion sets and, 146
  pumps and, 409
  standards on prevention of, 432
  total parenteral nutrition and, 394, 396
  trapped air and, 53
  tubing changes and, 142–143, 405
  Y-type infusion sets and, 144
Albumin, 236
  human serum, 202
  incomplete antibodies of, 192–193
  reference values for, 246–247
Albumin-globulin ratio and serum protein, 120
Alcohol, 92
  and antidiuretic hormone, 89, 90
  as germicide, 289
  infusion rate of flow and, 132
  postsurgical infusions of, 91
  as prepping agent, 403
Aldolase, 232–233
Aldosterone (mineralocorticoid), 77
  reference values for, 248–249
Alkalizing fluids, 115–116
Alkalosis, 85, 86
  ammonium chloride and, 88
  calcium and, 80
  metabolic, 76, 502
  respiratory, 73, 74, 503–504

Allen's test, 478, 481, 485
Allergic reactions
  to chemotherapy, 451, 452
  patient's history of, 466
  to transfusions, 209
Alpha subunit, 240–241
Alpha-fetoprotein, 260–261
Alpha-1-antitrypsin, 260–261
Altitude, flow rate and, 334
Ambulating patients and infusions, 52
Amethopterin, 456–457
Amino acids, 84, 90
  crystalline, 92
  in parenteral fluids, 390–391
Ammonia, 115
  reference values for, 242–243
Ammonium chloride, 116–117
  alkalosis and, 88
Ampules, contamination and glass, 293
Amylase, 234
  reference values for, 242–243
Analgesics, in home intravenous therapy, 528
Anaphylactic reaction to chemotherapy, 463, 464, 465–466
Anastomosis, arteriovenous, 58–59
Anatomy, 25, 57–64
  vascular, 301, 302, 303–304
Anemia, hemolytic, 241
Anesthesia, 142
  catheter insertion and, 414
Antebrachial vein, median, 63
Antecubital fossa, chemotherapy and, 448, 449
Antecubital veins, 173
Anterior pituitary gland, 90
Anti-DNA antibodies, 260–261
Antibiotics, 144
  decline in asceptic technique and, 284
  gram-negative bacteria and, 283
  need for small-vein needle and, 176
  particulate matter and, 293
  in pediatric intravenous therapy, 507
Antibiotic therapy
  final filters and, 154
  home, 528
  neonatal, 514
  in total parenteral nutrition, 407

Antibodies, 191, 192–193, 207
  anti-DNA, 260–261
  frozen blood and, 198
  incomplete, 240
  saline, (complete), 192–193
Anticancer drugs. See Chemotherapy
Anticoagulants, 195–196, 225
Antidiuretic hormone (ADH), 77, 89, 90, 231
  alcohol and, 92
  burns and, 94
  elderly and, 125
  urinary output and, 79
  water intoxification and, 114
Antidotes
  in chemotherapy, 469, 470
  intravenous push and, 385
Antigens (agglutinogen), 191, 192–193, 207, 211
  and hemolysis, 239
  Human leukocyte (HLA), 192
Antihemophilic factor (AHF), 199
Antinuclear antibodies, 260–261
Antitoxins, drug stability and, 375
Anxiety, nurse, 448
Ara C, 454–455
Armboard, securing of, 178, 181, 183, 184
Arterial blood gases. See Blood gases, arterial
Arterial catheter, indwelling, 485, 487, 488, 489–490
Arterial catheterization, umbilical, 516–517
Arterial pressure monitoring, 490, 491–492, 493–494
Arteriovenous anastomosis, 58–59
Arteriovenous fistulas, chemotherapy and, 59, 461–462
Arteriovenous shunts, 292
Artery(ies), 57
  aberrant, 60–61, 173, 174
  brachial, 478, 485
  femoral, 477–478, 483, 484, 485
  puncture of, 314, 395
  radial, 477–478, 481, 482, 483, 485
  therapy via (see Intraarterial therapy)
  ulna, 478, 481
  umbilical, 515–517
  veins and, 59–60

Ascorbic acid, 242–243
Aseptic techniques. See Sterile techniques
Asparaginase (Elspar), 466
Assault, and battery, 12, 442
Autotransfusion, 214–215
Axillary vein, 302

Bacteria, 407. See also Contamination; Infection
  contamination and infection from, 284–285, 286–291
  factors influencing the survival of, 283–284
  gram-negative, 283, 287–288, 289, 407
  sources of, 281–283
Base excess (BE), 498, 500
  in metabolic acidosis, 501
  in metabolic alkalosis, 502
Baseline blood pressure, 464
Basilic vein, 63, 300, 312
Battery, assault and, 12, 442
Bence Jones protein, 262–263
Bevel of needle, 177, 471
Bicarbonate, 75–76
  in acid-base imbalance, 98
  as blood gas parameter, 497–498
  as cure for metabolic acidosis, 501
Bicarbonate ions, 73, 98
Bilirubin, 236, 242–243
Bleeding time (Simplate), reference values for, 254–255
Blenoxane, 454–455, 466
Bleomycin sulfate (Blenoxane), 454–455, 466
Blood
  autotransfusion of, 214–215
  as bacteria source, 282–283
  bank for, 214
  burns and whole, 95
  cell count of, 120
  contamination of, 211, 349
  cultures of, 230–231
  dextrose as preservative of, 195
  edema and backflow of, 273
  filters of (see Filters, blood)
  frozen, 197–198
  immune response of, 193
  measurement of acid-base balance in, 233–234
  monitoring flow of, 471
  science of (immunohematology), 191, 192–193

sugar level of, 90, 238–239
therapeutic withdrawal of, 215, 216, 218–220
vacuum system of withdrawal, 228–229, 231
whole, 95, 195–197, 225
Blood embolism, 53
Blood gases, arterial (ABG)
handling of, 226
in metabolic acidosis, 501
in metabolic alkalosis, 502
normal values of, 500
parameters of, 495, 477–500
sampling of (see Blood gas sampling)
values in respiratory acidosis, 503
values in respiratory alkalosis, 503
Blood gas sampling, 478, 481, 482, 483, 484
during arterial pressure monitoring, 491
frequent, 485, 487, 488, 489, 490
home intravenous therapy and, 528
Blood group systems. See ABO blood group system; Rh (Rhesus) system
Blood pressure
arterial, 490, 491–492, 493–494
central venous (see Central venous pressure)
chemotherapy and baseline, 464
cuff for measurement of, 177
low, 99
Blood sample collection, 15
antecubital veins and, 173
through central venous catheters, 346–347, 348–352, 362–364
home intravenous therapy and, 528
infection from, 226
median veins and, 63
nurses and, 227
procedures for, 21–22, 24
for therapeutic phlebotomy, 216, 218–220
vein valves and, 59–60
venous, 225–229, 230
Blood sugar level, 90
tests for, 238–239
Blood transfusions
administration of, 23, 204–206

autotransfusion as, 214–215
frozen blood and, 197–198
home intravenous therapy and, 528
instruction in, 30
isotonic saline and, 110
objectives in use of, 195
packed red blood cells and, 197
particulate matter and, 293
plasma and, 198–202
plasma substitute (dextran) in, 203
positive-pressure infusion sets for, 144–145
prewarmed blood and, 148
quality assurance study of, 43–46
reaction to, 207–211
T-type blood component sets for, 149, 150
whole blood in, 195–197
Y-type infusion sets for, 144, 149, 150, 200
Blood typing, 239–241
Blood urea nitrogen (BUN), 85, 120, 236–237, 238
Blood vessels, 59–61, 305. See also Artery(ies); Vein(s)
Blood volume, 242–243, 302, 303–304. See also Central venous pressure
Blood warmers, 148
Body fat, and water, 70, 83
Body fluids, 70–71. See also Blood; Edema; Fluid-electrolyte balance; Specific fluids
composition of, 72–73, 74, 75–76
extracellular compartment for, 123, 124
Body surface area, 85, 113, 133
Bolus injection, 359, 360, 361, 366–367, 384
Bone marrow, 57, 193
Brachial artery, 478, 485
Brachial plexus, injury to, 395
Breath, acetone, 99
Breathing, mouth, 119
Brooke Army Hospital formula, 96–97
Broviac catheter, 414, 462
Bubble oxygenators, 196
Buffers, 73
as blood gas parameter, 497, 500
drug stability and, 375

Burns, 93–95, 96–97
isotonic saline with dextrose and, 111
plasma transfusion and, 198
thirst and, 119
Butler-type parenteral fluids, 113, 126

Calcitonin, 240–241
Calcium, 80, 88
binding of serum, 225
deficit of, 196
laboratory measurement of, 233
reference values for, 242–243
Calcium chloride, 210
Call system of intravenous department, 20
Caloric method of assessing fluid needs, 510–511
Calories
dextrose and, 107
postsurgery and, 91
rate of flow of dextrose infusion and, 131
in total parenteral nutrition, 391
Cancer chemotherapy, intravenous, 466–467, 469–473, 474
allergic reactions to, 451, 452
anaphylactic reaction to, 463, 464, 465–466
antecubital fossa and, 448, 449, 450
antidotes in, 469, 470
arteriovenous fistulas for, 461–462
central venous catheterization and, 304
cephalic vein in, 450
certification for, 439–440
cytotoxic agents in, 454–457
hazards of, 466–467, 469
Hickman catheter for, 462
legal implications of, 443
management problems of, 451
medication preparation for, 444–445, 446
necrosis from, 448, 466, 467, 469, 472
normal saline in, 450
nurse preparation for, 439–442
patient education for, 442–444, 469
pediatric, 507
phlebitis from, 453, 459, 461

techniques in, 446, 447, 448, 449, 450, 451
venous spasm from, 453
Cannula, 52
 anchoring of, 181
 clotting of, 37–38, 133
 insertion of, 60
 instruction in use of, 26
 outmoded, 54
 plugged, 53
 policies on intravenous use of, 18–19
 rate of flow and, 133
Carbamazepine, 242–243
Carbohydrates, 91. *See also* Dextrose; Glucose
Carbon dioxide
 hypothermia and, 500
 laboratory measurement of, 233–234
 partial pressure (*see* Partial pressure carbon dioxide)
 reference values for, 242–243
Carbonic acid, 73, 74, 497
Carbonic acid-sodium buffer, 73
Carbon monoxide, 242–243
Carcinoembryonic antigen (CEA), 260–261
Cardiac surgery, whole blood and, 196
Carmustine, 453
Carotenoids, 242–243
Catheter(s), 166, 167, 171
 burns and venous, 95
 Broviac, 414, 462
 central venous (*see* Central venous catheters)
 clamp to, 317–318
 clotting of, 424, 462, 493
 contamination of, 290
 culturing of, 290–291, 435–436
 cutdown, 186
 dressing changes in, 396–397, 398, 399, 402, 403
 double lumen, 414
 Hickman, 414, 462, 534
 improvements to, 5
 indwelling arterial, 484, 487, 488, 489–494
 indwelling tunneled, 328, 331
 insertion of, 392–395, 414, 520
 nontunneled, 339–340
 with obdurator, 485, 487, 488, 489–490
 radiopaque, 324
 selection of, 175–177
 standards on, 431–436
 subclavian, 394
 Swan Ganz, 494–495
 totally implanted, 353, 355–356, 359
 tubings of, 46–48
 tunneled, 340
 umbilical, 515–517
Catheter embolism, 277, 315, 489
Cells, and immune response, 193
Cellular dehydration, 118–119
 hypertonic contraction and, 125
 hypertonic expansion and, 124
Cellulitis, 64
 chemical, 452
Central venous catheter(s), 169, 170
 blood sample collection through, 229, 346–347, 349–352, 362–364
 cannulation of, 311–312
 complications from, 314–317
 heparin flushing of, 342–343, 344–345
 implantable pumps, 364–365, 366–367
 indwelling tunneled, 328, 331
 injection cap of, 345–346
 insertion sites for, 312–314
 inside-the-needle (INC), 324, 326
 maintenance of, 317–319, 320, 321
 materials, of, 323, 324
 patient preparation for, 310
 with removable introducer, 326, 327
 site care of, 339, 340
 on spool, 328, 330
 totally implanted (*see* Totally implanted catheters)
 totally implanted pump in, 335, 336, 339
 totally implanted venous access device and, 333, 335
 vascular anatomy and, 301, 302, 303–304
Central venous pressure, 304–307
 monitoring of, 117–118, 307, 309–310
Centrifugation, 201
Cephalic vein, 62–63, 300, 313
 in chemotherapy, 450
Cephalin, 237
Certification
 chemotherapy, 439–440
 of total parenteral nutrition dressing, 404
Cerubidine, 454–455
Ceruloplasmin, 242–243
Charting in total parenteral nutrition therapy, 410
Check-valve infusion sets, 143
Chemical interactions, in drug intravenous therapy, 373–374
Chemoreceptors, 500, 501, 502, 505
Chemotherapy, intravenous cancer. *See* Cancer chemotherapy, intravenous
Children. *See also* Pediatric intravenous therapy
 diarrhea in, 506–507, 511, 519
 hypothermia and, 511
 infusion rate of flow and, 131
 pulmonary edema in, 131
 rapport with, 513
 stress of, 506
 superficial veins of, 507
Chloramphenicol, 242–243
Chlorides, 80, 90
 alkalosis and, 85, 88
 as correction for metabolic alkalosis, 502
 laboratory measurement of, 232
 reference values for, 242–243
 as treatment for respiratory acidosis, 503
 as treatment for respiratory alkalosis, 503
Cholesterol, 237, 244–245
Chylothorax, 395
Chylous fluid, 260–261
Circulation, 58, 292
Circulatory overload, 118, 120, 123–124
 from blood transfusion, 209
 hypertonic saline and, 124
 infusion pumps and, 155
 isotonic saline and, 110, 111
 prevention of, 27
Cisplatin (Platinol), 466
Citrate-phosphate-dextrose (CPD), 195, 198
Citrate-phosphate-dextrose-adenine (CPDA-1), 195, 198
Citrate toxicity, 210
Civil law, 11
Clamp
 catheter, 317–318
 clip-type, 318
Clean-to-dirty technique, 397
Clotting, 225
 in cannula, 37–39, 133
 catheter, 424, 462, 493

Index

factors in, 199, 382–383
retraction of, 2
Coagulation
  age of blood and, 196
  as cause of thrombosis, 323
  plasma transfusion and, 198, 199
Coagulation factors, reference values for, 254–255
Colloids, 95, 96, 97
Coma, 410
Complications
  instruction in handling of, 26–28
  of intravenous therapy, 280–281
  of pediatric total parenteral nutrition, 524
  of Swan Ganz catheter, 495
Consent, informed, 442
Containers, fluid, 137–138
Contamination. *See also* Infection(s)
  bacterial, 284–285, 286–291
  blood, 351
  factors contributing to, 284–285, 286–291
  particulate (*see* Particulate matter)
  pumps and, 409
  of skin, 406–407, 445
  tubing changes and risk of, 404
Controlled-volume infusion sets, 144
Controllers, 164, 165
Convulsions, 220
Coombs' test, 211, 240–241
Copper, 242–243
Cortisol, 248–249
Cosmegen, 454–455
Craniotomy, 123
Creatine kinase (CK), 242–243
Creatinine, 71, 237–238
  reference values for, 242–243
Criminal law, 11
Cryoprecipitate, 199–200
Crystalline amino acids, 92
Culturing of catheter, 290–291, 435–436
Cutdown catheter, 186
Cyroprecipitable proteins, 262–263
Cytarabine, 454–455
Cytoglomerator, 197–198
Cytosar-U, 454–455
Cytosine, 454–455
Cytotoxic agents, 454–457. See *also* Cancer chemotherapy, intravenous

Dacarbazine, 453
Dactinomycin, 454–455
Dalton's law, 498
Daunorubicin HCl (Daunomycin), 554–455
  antidote for, 470
Decomposition, double, 373
Dehydration, 121
  burns and, 94
  cellular, 118–119, 124, 125
  diabetic acidosis and, 97–98
  fluid tonicity and, 105
  sodium and, 80
  use of dextrose and, 107, 108
Dehydroepiandrosterone (DHEA), 248–249
Dehydroepiandrosterone sulfate (DHEA-S), 248–249
11 Deoxycortisol, 248–249
Deprivation, oral, 425
Dermis, 64
Dextran (plasma substitute), 203
Dextrose, 71
  as blood preservative, 195
  carbohydrates and, 91
  contamination of, 285
  in hydrating fluids, 112
  hypertonic expansion and, 125
  hyponatremia and, 91, 108
  in hypotonic fluids, 113
  infusion rate of flow and, 131
  in isotonic saline infusions, 111
  low venous pressure and, 118
  pH of, 104
  in water, 106–109
  water intoxication and, 126
Diabetes mellitus, 90
Diabetic acidosis, 97–99, 234
Diarrhea, childhood, 506–507, 511, 519
Diazepam (Valium), 385
Digitoxin, 260–261
Digoxin, 260–261
1, 25-Dihydroxyvitamin D, 252–253
Dilantin, 244–245
Diphenhydramine hydrochloride U.S.P. (Benadryl), 385
Diphosophoglycerate (DPG), 195
Distilled water, 83
Diuretics, 231
Divalent electrolytes, 105
Dopamine, 208
Dorsal digital veins, 61

Double decomposition, 373
Double lumen catheter, 414
Doxorubicin HCl (Adriamycin), 449, 454–455, 466
  allergic reaction to, 451
  antidote for, 470
  plastic surgery and, 473
Dressing changes, 51
  catheter, 396–397, 398, 399, 402, 403
  certification in, 404
  home, 423
  in pediatric therapy, 521, 523
DRG (Diagnosis Related Group), 527
Drug(s)
  addition to infusion systems of, 138
  administration of, 18, 23
  blood transfusions and, 205
  contamination of, 287, 292–293
  education about, 387
  error in, 27
  incompatibilities of, 372–374
  investigational, 10, 463
  parenteral fluids and, 104
  preparation of chemotherapy, 444–445, 446
  rate of flow and administration of, 131
  stability of, 375
Drug intravenous therapy, 379–381, 385–387
  aberrant arteries and, 173
  advantages of, 371
  allergy history and, 443
  arterial irritation in, 60, 63
  dextrose as vehicle in, 108
  hazards of, 372–376
  heparin lock in, 382–384
  instruction in, 28–30
  intermittent infusion in, 381–382
  intravenous push in, 384–385
  laminar flow hood in, 287
  responsibility for, 376–379
  sites for, 141, 142, 143
  syringe pumps and, 156, 157
  vascular irritation in, 60
Duodenal drainage, 260–261

Edema
  blood backflow and, 273
  burns and, 94, 96
  concealment of vein and, 174
  early detection of, 119–120

hypernatremia and, 91
  measurement of serum protein and, 120
  pulmonary (see Pulmonary edema)
  water replacement and, 114
Education
  about catheter insertion, 392–394
  chemotherapy and patient, 442–443, 469
  drug, 387
  home care, 415–416, 417–418, 423–424, 529
  about intravenous therapy, 25–28
  on legal factors, 24–25
  in solution preparation, 391
  total parenteral nutrition therapy and nursing, 429
Elderly
  advantage of home care for, 534
  antidiuretic hormone and, 89, 90
  blood transfusions and, 209
  clip-type clamp and, 318
  dorsal metacarpal veins and, 174
  fluid balance maintenance of, 528
  fragile veins of, 452
  hypernatremia and, 110
  hypertonic contraction in, 125
  hypotonic expansion and, 126
  infusion rate of flow and, 131
  isotonic infusions and, 123
  isotonic multiple-electrolyte fluids and, 114
  loss of sodium and, 127
  metacarpal veins and, 62
  pulmonary edema in, 278
  skin of, 63–64
  thirst and, 119
  water excess and, 90
Electrolyte(s). *See also* Fluid-electrolyte balance; Fluid-electrolyte therapy; *Specific electrolytes*
  composition of, 71–73
  concentration of, 231, 232–233
  definition of, 71
  divalent, 105
  laboratory studies of, 120
  univalent, 105
Electrolyte fluids
  hypotonic multiple, 113
  isotonic multiple, 114, 115, 120
Electrophoresis, 246–247
Elspar (Asparaginase), 466
Embolism
  air (*see* Air embolism)
  blood, 53
  catheter, 277, 315, 489
  pulmonary (*see* Pulmonary embolism)
  from thrombus, 375
Emergency care, in chemotherapy, 463
Emotional considerations, in pediatric intravenous therapy, 512–513
Endocrine homeostatic controls, 88–89
Enzymes, laboratory measurement of, 234–235
Epidermis, 63–64
Epinephrine (Adrenalin), 90, 385
  preparation of, 20–21
Equipment, intravenous
  administration sets for, 139, 140
  blood warmers as, 148
  catheters as, 166, 167, 169, 170
  check valve sets for, 143
  controlled-volume sets for, 144, 145, 146, 147
  controllers as, 164, 165
  filters as, 150, 151
  final filters as, 151, 152, 153, 154, 155
  fluid containers as, 137–138
  home, 535
  infusion pumps as, 155–156
  infusion systems as, 138–139
  instruction in, 25
  intraarterial therapy, 476, 481
  pediatric adaption of adult, 524–525
  for pediatric intravenous therapy, 511
  pediatric sets as, 141, 142–143
  syringe pumps as (*see* Pumps, syringe)
  Y-blood component sets for, 149, 150
Erythroblastosis fetalis, 240
Erthrocyte count, 256–257
Essential fatty acid deficiency (EFAD), 411
Estradiol, 248–249
Ethanol, 242–243
Ethylenediaminetetraacetic acid (EDTA), 225

Euglobin lysis, 244–245
Evans formula, 97
Extracellular body fluid compartment
  contraction of, 123
  definition of, 70
  hypertonic expansion and, 124
Extracellular body fluids
  and acid-base balance, 77
  volume of, 118, 119
Extravasation. *See* Infiltration
Extremities, lower, 173, 271

Fainting, phlebotomy and, 220
Fascia, superficial, 64
Fasting, laboratory tests and, 226
Fasting blood sugar (FBS), 238, 239
Fat
  body, 70, 83
  and home hyperalimentation, 424
  stool, 252–253
  subcutaneous, 471
  for total parenteral nutrition solutions, 411–413
  violation of system and, 434
  water and body, 70, 83
Fat emulsions, 93
Fatigue, diabetic acidosis and, 98
Fears
  alleviation of patient, 25
  of chemotherapy, 443
  of oral deprivation, 425
  risks associated with, 172
Febrile reactions to transfusions, 208–209
Femoral artery, 477–478, 483, 484, 485
Femoral vein, 58–59
Ferritin, 246–247
Fever, 109
  and flow rate, 336
  work-up of, 315–316, 406
Fibrogen, 199
  split products of, 244–245
Filters
  blood, 150, 151, 196–197, 205–206
  changing of, 404
  final, 151, 152, 153, 154, 155
  0.22 micron air-eliminating, 53–54, 152, 294, 318
  particulate matter and, 294, 295
Fistula, arteriovenous, 59, 461–462

Index

Fixed acid, 497, 500, 501
Flares, 451
Flow rates, 130–131, 134
  age and, 131
  of administration sets, 139
  altitude and, 336
  ambulation and, 52
  computation of, 132–133
  fever and, 336
  heart and, 130, 131
  instruction in, 28
  monitoring of, 471
  need for accurate, 164
  need for constant, 156
  need for minimal, 141
  need for rapid, 144, 147
  of parenteral infusions, 130–134
  pediatric, 508, 511, 523
  pump, 336
  of total parenteral nutrition therapy, 409
  of transfusion, 206
  vascular irritation and, 376
  vein selection and, 173, 174
  viscosity of fluid and, 177
Fluid(s). *See* Body fluids; Fluid-electrolyte balance; Fluid-electrolyte therapy; *Specific fluids*
  containers for, 137–138, 178
  hydrating, 112–113
  negative balance of, 128
  nonelectrolyte, 79
  parenteral (*see* Parenteral fluids)
  particulate contamination and, 293
  requirements for, 508, 510–511, 513–514
  tonicity of, 105
Fluid-electrolyte balance
  body fluids and, 70–71, 72–73, 74, 75–76
  calcium and, 80
  disturbances in, 120, 121, 123–127
  home maintenance of, 528
  introduction to, 69–70
  monitoring of, 117–120
  in neonates, 514
  in pediatric intravenous therapy, 506–507
  potassium and, 77–79
  sodium and, 79–80
  tonicity and, 105
Fluid-electrolyte therapy
  burns and, 93–95, 96–97
  diabetic acidosis and, 97–99
  increased use of, 69
  instruction in, 28
  objectives of, 83–85, 88
  surgery and, 88–89, 90–93
5-Fluorouracil (5-FU), 454–455
Folic acid, reference values for, 256–257
Follicle-stimulating hormone (FSH), 250–251
Food, preoccupation with, 425
Frozen blood, 197–198
Fungal sepsis, 406

Gangrene, 58, 60
Gas, physics of, 498
Gases, arterial blood. *See* Blood gases, arterial
Gastric analysis, reference values for, 260–261
Gastric parietal cells, 260–261
Gastric replacement fluids, 115
Gastrin-I, 260–261
Gauge, needle, 177
Glass ampules, 293
Globulin, 246–247
Glucocorticoid secretions, 90, 92
Glucose, 83, 92, 106, 195. *See also* Dextrose; Hyperglycemia; Hypoglycemia
  diabetic acidosis and, 97, 98, 99
  intolerance of, 407–408, 435
  intravenous lipids and, 411
  maintenance therapy and, 84
  in pediatric total parenteral nutrition, 518
  reference values for, 231, 232, 242–243
  tolerance test for, 238–239
  urinary measurement of, 408
Glucose-6-phosphate dehydrogenase, 256–257
Glycerol, 197
Glycosuria, 97, 98
Government
  regulations of, 8–10
  and cost of therapy, 527
Gram-negative bacteria, 283, 287–288, 289, 407
Gram-positive bacteria, 283
Granulocytes, 201–202
Gravity, flow of, 164
Growth hormone, 250–251
Guide wire, catheter, 328

Hand(s)
  in pediatric intravenous therapy, 507, 508
  use of armboard and, 181
  as vein site for chemotherapy, 448, 450
Haptoglobin, 256–257
Head, as site for pediatric intravenous therapy, 507
Heart, 78
  infusion rate of flow and, 130, 131
Heat
  for extravasations, 470
  for vein distention, 446, 451
Hematocrit, 117, 120
  reference values for, 256–257
Hematomas, 63
  from blood sample collection, 227
  fragile veins and, 451
Hemochromatosis, 215
Hemoconcentration, 225
Hemoglobin, reference values for, 256–259
Hemoglobinemia, 208
Hemolysis, 193, 207–208
  agglutinogen and, 239
  intravascular, 193
  reaction in, 204
  and test errors, 225
  transfusion reaction in, 194, 207–208, 211
Hemophiliacs, 199
  AIDS and, 211
Hemothorax, 314, 395
Heparin, 424
  in home total parenteral nutrition, 420, 422, 423
  instructions for home use of, 532
  and prothrombin time testing, 346
Heparin flush
  of central venous catheter, 342, 344–345
  for totally implanted catheters, 353, 355–356
Heparin lock, 414
  for intraarterial therapy, 488, 489–490
  intravenous drug therapy and, 382–384
Hepatitis
  from blood transfusion, 210
  blood transmission of, 282
  fibrogen and, 199

frozen blood and, 198
  plasma and, 198
  plasma substitute and, 203
  venipuncture and, 228
Hickman catheter
  chemotherapy and, 462–463
  for home intravenous therapy, 414, 534
History
  allergy, 466
  of home total parenteral nutrition, 414
  of intravenous therapy, 3–6
  of total parenteral nutrition, 389
HLA antigens, platelet transfusion and, 200
Home intravenous therapy, 527–529, 531, 532–533, 537
  Hickman catheter in, 534
Home total patenteral nutrition (HTPN), 413–414, 415, 528
  patient education in (see Education, homecare)
Hormone,
  follicle-stimulating, 250–251
  growth, 250–251
  luteinizing, 250–251
  parathyroid, 80, 252–253
  thyroid-stimulating, 252–253
HTLV-III (Human T-Cell lymphotropic virus), 210–211, 282
Human leukocyte antigens (HLA), 192
Human serum albumin, 202
Human T-Cell Lymphotropic Virus (HTLV-III), 210–211, 282
Hyaluronidase (Wydase), 470
Hydrating fluids, 112–113
Hydrocortisone (glucocorticoid), 90, 92
Hydrocortisone sodium succinate (Solu-Cortef), 452
Hydrocortisone sodium succinate, 459
Hydrogen
  as blood gas parameter, 497
  in metabolic acidosis, 501
  in metabolic alkalosis, 502
  in respiratory acidosis, 503
  in respiratory alkalosis, 503
Hydrogen ion concentration (pH). *See* pH
Hydrogen peroxide, 340

Hydrolysis, in drug intervenous therapy, 373
Hydrolysates, protein, 92, 132
Hydrothorax, 315, 395
25 Hydroxyvitamin D, 242–243
Hyperadrenalism, 254
Hyperalimentation. *See* Total parenteral nutrition therapy
Hyperglycemia, 97, 98, 256
  from total parenteral nutrition therapy, 410
Hyperinsulinism, 108
Hyperkalemia, 79
  hypotonic multiple-electrolyte fluids and, 114
  packed red cells and, 197
  use of dextrose and, 108
Hypernatremia, 91
  hypertonic saline and, 124
  isotonic saline and, 110, 111
  use of dextrose and, 108
Hyperolmorarity, 410, 519
Hyperparathyroidism, 80, 256
Hypertonic contraction, 125–126
Hypertonic expansion, 124–125
Hypertonic saline, 124, 127
Hyperventilation, 478, 500, 501, 503, 504
Hypoglycemia, 256
  from total parenteral nutrition therapy, 406, 408, 410, 435
Hypokalemia, 78, 93
  isotonic saline and, 110
  use of dextrose and, 108
Hyponatremia, 90–91
Hypoparathyroidism, 256
Hypotension, 118, 305
  pump flow rate and, 336
Hypothermia, 500
  blood transfusions and, 210
  in children, 511
Hypothyroidism, 260
Hypotonic contraction, 127
Hypotonic expansion (water intoxication), 126–127
Hypotonic multiple-electrolyte fluids, 113
Hypoventilation, 256–257, 500, 502, 504
  elevated potassium and, 254
Hypovolemia, 198
  and blood volume, 303
Hypovolemic shock, 196
  plasma substitutes and, 203
Hypoxemia, 499, 502, 503

Ice, for extravasations, 470
Identification, patient. *See* Patient identification
Iodine, 403
IgG antibodies, 193
IgM antibodies, 193
Immune response, 193, 211
Immunoglobulins, reference values for, 262–263
Immunohematology, basic, 191, 192–193
Implantable pumps, 364–365, 366–367
Implantable vascular access devices, 170–171, 394, 463
Incomplete antibodies, 240
Independent practitioners, and malpractice insurance, 442
Indwelling arterial catheter, 485, 487, 488, 489–494
Indwelling tunneled catheter, 330, 333
Infants. *See* Neonatal intravenous therapy; Pediatric intravenous therapy
Infection(s), 290–291
  airborne, 281
  during arterial pressure monitoring, 494
  bacterial, 284–291
  from blood samples, 226
  catheter-related, 315–316
  central venous catheterization and, 311
  from Hickman catheter, 462
  home intravenous therapy and decrease in, 537
  implantable vascular access devices and, 463
  instruction in handling, 26
  neonatal, 514
  small-vein needle and, 288
  Swan Ganz catheter and, 495
  in total parenteral nutrition, 405–407
Infiltration, 272, 273
  from cancer chemotherapy, 466–467, 469–473, 474
  at injection site, 54
  instruction on, 28
Inflammation, 54
Informed consent, 442, 469
Infusion(s)
  acidifying, 116–117
  blood sample collection and, 229, 230

Index

discontinuing, 342–343, 344
intermittent (piggyback), 381–382, 452
maintenance of, 52–55
short-term, 306
standards for, 431
termination of, 55
Infusion pumps, 155–156
pediatric therapy and, 512, 523
Infusion sets
check-valve, 143
controlled-valve, 144
pediatric, 492
positive pressure, 144, 145, 146, 147
Y-type, 144
Infusion systems, 138–139
continuous, 356–357, 358
Injection
bolus, 359, 360, 361, 366–367, 389
lactated Ringer's, 96, 115
Injection cap, catheter, 345–346, 351
Injection ports, 287
Innominate vein, 332
Insertion sites for central venous catheterization, 312–314
Inside-the-needle (INC) catheter, 166, 187, 326, 394, 398
associated risks of, 183–184
cannula selection and, 175
Insulin, 97, 98, 99, 107, 108
administration of, 408–409, 410
in pediatric therapy, 523
reference values for, 240–241
Insulin drips, 507
Insurance
malpractice, 12–13, 31–32, 442
patient, 529
Intermittent (piggyback) infusion for drug therapy, 227, 381–382, 452
Interstitial fluid, 70
Intoxication, water, 108–109, 114, 126–127
Intraarterial therapy, 477–478, 488, 489–490
instruction on, 28
Intracellular body fluid compartment, 70
and acid-base balance, 77
potassium and, 70, 77–78
Intravascular hemolysis, 193

Intravenous cancer chemotherapy. See Cancer chemotherapy, intravenous
Intravenous department
collection of blood samples in, 21–22
directorship in, 16
functions of, 17–21
of Mass. General Hospital, 22–25
organization of, 15–30
parenteral teams in, 15–16
philosophy and objectives of, 16–17
teaching program in, 24–30
Intravenous drug therapy. See Drug intravenous therapy
Intravenous equipment. See Equipment intravenous
Intravenous fluids. See Fluids; Parenteral fluids
Intravenous hyperalimentation. See Total parenteral nutrition therapy
Intravenous nurse, qualifications of, 19
Intravenous push, 384–387, 459, 471
Intravenous therapy
acid-base imbalances and, 500–504
blood gas parameters in, 495, 497–500
blood gas sampling in, 478, 481, 482, 483, 484
constant arterial pressure monitoring for, 490, 491–492, 493–494
equipment for (see Equipment, intravenous)
hazards and complications of, 269–272, 273–278, 280–281
indwelling arterial catheter for, 485, 487, 488, 489–490
instruction in, 25–28
legal implications of, 8–13
Swan-Ganz catheters in, 494–495
techniques of (see Techniques of intravenous therapy)
Introducer, catheter, 326, 328
Investigational drugs, 463
legal implications of, 10
Iontophorsis, 252–253
Iron, 232–233
excess of, 215

Isoenzymes, 232–233
Isotonic contraction, 123–124
Isotonic expansion. See Circulatory overload
Isotonic multiple-electrolyte fluids, 114, 115, 120, 121
Isotonic saline infusions, 83, 110, 111
Isotonic solutions, 431

Jaundice, 259, 260
Jugular vein, 300, 301, 310–311

Keto acid, 497, 500
Ketosis, 98
dextrose and, 107
Kidney(s)
acid-base regulation and, 77
assessing status of, 112–113
bicarbonate concentration and, 75–76
dehydration and, 98
difference in individual, 125
function tests for, 260–261
infusion rate of, flow and, 130, 131
metabolic alkalosis and, 502
potassium and, 85, 93, 231
transplantation of, 198
water and, 83, 126
Kilograms, conversion to, 118

Laboratory test(s), 120, 224, 230–231
of acid-base balance, 256–257
of blood samples, 235–230
of blood sugar, 261–262
of blood typing, 262–263, 264
of electrolyte concentration, 231, 254, 255, 256
of enzymes, 257–258
of liver function, 259–260
normal reference values of, 253, 254, 255
of transaminase, 258–259
Lactated Ringer's injection, 96, 115
Lactic acid, 497, 500
reference values for, 232–233
Lactic dehydrogenase, 234–235
Laminar flow hood, 286, 378, 391, 431
drug preparation and, 287
Law
civil, definition of, 11
criminal, definition of, 11

Lead, 234–235
Legal implications
    for cancer chemotherapy, 443
    instruction in, 24–25
    of intravenous therapy, 8–13
Leukocyte alkaline phosphatase, 258–259
Leukocyte count, 256–257
Leukopheresis, 201
Liability, nurse's personal, 12, 445, 446
Light
    at additive station, 378–379
    drug stability and, 375
Lipase, 234–235
    reference values for, 244–245
Lipids
    intravenous, 411–413
    in pediatric therapy, 518
    reference values for, 244–245
Lithium, 244–245
Litigation, need for charting and, 472, 474
Liver
    blood transfusions and, 210
    citrated whole blood transfusion and, 196
    damaged, 70
    function tests for, 236–237
    gastric replacement fluids and, 115
    toxicity and, 88
Low blood pressure, 99
Lower extremities, 173, 271
Lungs, 502–504
    fluid balance and, 77
Lupus erythematosus (LE), 258–259
Luteinizing hormone, 250–251
Lymphocytes, 198

Macrophages, 193
Magnesium, 80, 244–245
Malaria, 211
Malpractice, 12, 13, 31–32
    insurance for, 442
Management risk, 31–32
Mannitol, 208
Manometer, 307
Manual pressure, 134
Massachusetts General Hospital, 22–24
    burns and, 95, 96–97
    hypotonic multiple-electrolyte fluids and, 113
    infection control and, 406

Mean corpuscular hemoglobin concentration (MCHC), 256–257
Mean corpuscular volume (MCV), 256–257
Mechlorathemine hydrochloride (Mustargen), 453, 456–457, 470
Median vein, 63
Medications. See Drug(s)
Metabolic acidosis, 110, 500–501, 503, 504
    alkalizing fluids and, 115–116
    burns and, 94
    carbohydrates, 91
    excess bicarbonate and, 76
    gastric replacement fluids and, 115
    hyperthermia and, 500
Metabolic alkalosis, 76, 115, 116, 501–502, 504
    carbon dioxide content and, 266–267
    hypothermia and, 500
Metabolic aspects of total parenteral nutrition, 407–408, 434–435
Metacarpal veins, 62, 174, 181
Meter square method, 510, 511
Methotrexate sodium, 456–457
Mexate, 456–457
0.22 micron air-eliminating filter, 53–54, 152, 294, 320
Mineralocorticoid secretions (Aldosterone), 77, 248–249
Mithramycin (Mithracin), 456–457
Mitochondria, 252–253
Mouth breathing, 119
Mouth care, 426
Muscles
    skeletal, 262–263
    smooth, 260–261
Mustargen, 453, 456–457
    antidote for, 470
Myocardium, 304–305

National Intravenous Therapy Association, 6, 9, 13, 16
    micron air-filters and, 152
    over-the-needle catheter and, 175
    standards for total parenteral nutrition, 427–435
Nausea, 99, 220
    chemotherapy and, 443

Necrosis, 58
    alcohol and, 92
    arterial damage and, 60
    from chemotherapy, 448, 466, 467, 469, 472
    dextrose and, 109
    infiltration and, 272
Needle(s), 176
    bevel of, 177, 471
    insertion of, 511–512
    small-gauge, 451, 453
    small-vein (see Small-vein needle)
    steel, 176, 177
    for totally implanted catheters, 351
Negative fluid balance, 92, 125
Neonatal therapy, 513–514, 515–517. See also Pediatric intravenous therapy
Newborns, 195, 196
Nitrogen
    balance of, 92, 391
    blood urea, 85, 120, 246–247
    stool, 262–263
Nitrogen mustard, 456–457
Nitroglycerine, absorption of, 140
Nonelectrolytes, 71, 79
Nonfixed acid, 497
Nonpolyvinylchloride, 140
Nontunneled catheter, 339–340
Norepinephrine, 90
Normal saline
    in chemotherapy, 450
    extravasations and use of, 470
Nurse(s)
    anxiety during chemotherapy and, 448
    blood sample collection and, 224
    chemotherapy preparation by, 439–442
    competency of, 24
    guilt and, 467
    legal status of, 8–13
    liability for drug error and, 445, 446
    monitoring of fluid-electrolyte balance and, 117
    and observation, 12–13
    and patient relationship, 13, 25, 172
    qualifications of intravenous, 293
    replacement, 471–472

Index

and responsibility in
 intravenous therapy, 50–55,
 103, 377–381
risks in drug handling and, 445
responsibility in intravenous
 therapy and, 103
standards for total parenteral
 nutrition therapy and, 427–
 435
transfusions and, 206
Nursing Practice Act, 8
Nutrition, parenteral, 83–85. *See
 also* Total parenteral nutrition
assessment of needs for, 430
dextrose and, 108
neonatal, 514, 515
in pediatric intravenous therapy,
 507
surgery and, 91

Obesity, 114
Observation, as act of nursing,
 12, 52–55
Obturator, catheter with, 485,
 487, 488, 489–490
Oliguria, 99
Oncovin, 456–457
Oral deprivation, 425
Osmolality
electrolytes and, 72–73
formulas for, 106
reference values for, 234–235
Osteomyelitis, 57
Outpatient, cancer, 450
Over-the-needle (OTN) catheter,
 166, 167, 175, 184, 186, 326
for drug administration, 382
Oxidation, 373
Oxygen, 478
partial pressure of, 499, 500
release of, 195
saturation of, 244–245, 499–
 500
therapy of, 495
Oxygenators, bubble, 196

Packed red blood cells, 196, 197
Pain, 466
Palpation of veins, 174
Parathyroid hormone, 80, 252–
 253
Parenteral drug therapy. *See* Drug
 intravenous therapy
Parenteral fluid(s), 18, 390–392.
 See Fluids; *Specific fluids*
acidifying, 116–117

alkalizing, 115–116
blood sample collection and,
 225–226
Butler-type, 113, 126
containers for, 284–285, 286
definition of, 103–104
dextrose in, 106–109
drug addition to, 380–381
drug stability and, 374
electrolytes in (*see* Electrolytes)
flow rate of (*see* Flow rate)
hydrating, 112
hypertonic sodium chloride in,
 111–112
hypotonic multiple-electrolyte,
 113, 114, 115
isotonic sodium chloride in,
 109–111
nutrition in, 83–85
official requirements of, 104–
 106
outdated, 286
particulate contamination of,
 293
rate of flow and composition
 of, 131–132
water and electrolyte balance
 in, 117–120, 121, 123–127
Parenteral nutrition. *See*
 Nutrition, parenteral; Total
 parenteral nutrition therapy
Parenteral solutions. *See*
 parenteral fluids
Parenteral teams. *See* Intravenous
 department
Parenteral therapy. *See* Drug
 intravenous therapy; Fluid-
 electrolyte therapy; Total
 parenteral nutrition therapy
Parkland formula, 96
Partial pressure of carbon dioxide,
 499, 500
in metabolic acidosis, 501
in metabolic alkalosis, 502
in respiratory acidosis, 503
in respiratory alkalosis, 503
Partial pressure of oxygen, 499,
 500
Partial prothrombin time, 346
Partial thromboplastin time
reference values for, 254–255
Particles, limit of, 151
Particulate matter, 104, 291–292,
 379
blood filters and, 196–197,
 294, 295

inspection for, 178
intravenous fluids and, 293
Pathogens, 283
Patient(s)
ambulatory, 52
approach to, 172
blood identification of, 204,
 216, 224, 239
for central venous
 catheterization, 310
consequences of chemotherapy
 for, 466
education of (*see* Education)
fears of, 448
home care and stability of, 529
identification of, 346–347, 364
insurance of, 529
movement during chemotherapy
 of, 472
preparation of, 178–179, 310
rate of flow and condition of,
 130–131
and relationship to nurse, 13,
 32
self-evaluation of, 424
susceptibility to infection of,
 447
Pediatric intravenous therapy,
 506–507, 508, 510–511
emotional considerations, 512–
 513
infusion sets for, 131
infusion systems for, 141
needle insertion in, 511–512
neonatal, 513–514, 515–517
speed shock and, 278
total parenteral nutrition in,
 517–519, 520, 521, 523–525
vacuum tube method for, 492
Penicillinase, 231
Peripheral veins, 117
Personal liability, rule of, 12
pH (hydrogen ion concentration),
 73
as blood gas parameter, 497,
 500
chemical interactions and, 373
of dextrose, 104
drug stability and, 374
laboratory measurement of, 257
in metabolic acidosis, 500, 501
in metabolic alkalosis, 502
propagation of bacteria and,
 283–284
reference values for, 233–234,
 244–245

in respiratory acidosis, 503
in respiratory alkalosis, 503
Phenobarbital, 234–235
Phenytoin (Dilantin), 234–235
Phlebitis, 27–28, 58, 173, 176
  alcohol and, 92
  arm flexion and, 309
  chemical, 453, 459, 461–463
  chemotherapy and, 446, 447
  infusion rate of flow and, 134
  inside-the-needle catheter and, 183
  mechanical, 167, 173
  operator caused, 271
  over-the-needle catheter and, 186
  particulate matter and, 293
  peripheral insertions and, 314
  from vascular irritation, 376
Phlebothrombosis, 173, 270–272
Phlebotomy
  central venous catheterization and, 306
  therapeutic, 214–216, 218–222
Phosphatase, 234–235, 248–249
Phosphate, 80, 195
Phosphorus, 233, 234–235
Physician(s)
  drug intravenous therapy and, 377
  infusion rate of flow and, 134
  standing orders and, 464, 465, 469
Physiology, 25, 57–64
Piggyback (intermittent) drug administration, 277, 381–382, 452
Pituitary gland, 79, 89, 90
Plasma, 70, 198–202
  definition of, 225
  electrolyte determination and, 71–72
  frozen, 96
  frozen blood and, 197
  osmolality of, 73
  packed red cells and, 197
  transfusion of, 198–199
Plasma protein fraction (human), 202
Plasma substitute (dextran), 203
Plastic, 137
Plastic surgery, 467, 473
Platelet(s)
  activation of, 32
  agglutination of, 293
  transfusion of, 200–201

Platelet aggregation, 293
  reference values for, 248–249
Platelet factor 3, 248–249
Platinol, 466
Play therapy, 513
Pneumothorax, 314, 394–395
Polycythemia vera, 215
Polyurethane, 324
Polyuria (water excretion), 97, 98
Polyvinylchloride, 323
Porphyria cutanea tarda, 215
Positive-pressure infusion sets, 144, 145, 146, 147
Posterior pituitary gland, 89, 90
Postprandial sugar test, 261
Potassium, 77–79. See also Hyperkalemia; Hypokalemia
  burns and, 94
  chloride and, 80
  diabetic acidosis and, 98, 99
  errors in measurement of, 225, 226
  excretion of, 90
  hypotonic multiple-electrolyte fluids and, 114
  infusion rate of flow and, 131
  laboratory measurement of, 231, 254
  metabolic alkalosis and, 76, 502
  packed red blood cells, 197
  plasma, 71
  postsurgery and, 93
  reference values for, 236–237
  renal impairment and, 85, 93
  sodium and, 79
  whole blood transfusions and, 196
Potassium chloride, 88
Precipitation, from drug incompatibility, 373, 374
Pregnancy, 194
Preservatives
  drug stability and, 375
  for whole blood, 195–196
Pressure, gas, 498
Pressure cuff, 145–146
Primidone (Mysoline), 236–237
Private-duty nurse, legal status of, 11
Procainamide, 236–237
Professional regulations, 8–13
Progesterone, 238–239
Prolactin, 242–243
Propranolol, 252–253
Prospective Payment System (PPS), 527

Protein
  Bence-Jones, 252–253
  hydrocortisone and, 90
  maintenance therapy and, 84
  reference values for, 236–237
  surgery and need for, 92
Protein hydrolysates, 99, 132
Prothrombin time, 237, 346
  reference values for, 254–255
Psychological aspects
  of chemotherapy, 466
  of pediatric therapy, 523
  of total parenteral nutrition therapy, 425–427
Pulmonary circulation, 58, 77
Pulmonary edema, 278
  blood transfusion and, 209
  burns and, 95
  children and, 131
  hypertonic saline infusion and, 112
  isotonic expansion and, 123
  isotonic fluids and, 114
  phlebotomy and, 215
  vasovagal reaction and, 172
Pulmonary embolism, 26–27, 58, 59, 274–275
  deep-vein thrombosis and, 323
  elevated venous pressure and, 117
Pulse, fluid-electrolyte balance and, 118
Pumps
  implantable, 364–365, 366–367
  infusion, 155–156, 512, 523
  oxygenating, 196
  syringe (see Syringe pumps)
  totally implanted, 335, 336, 339
  in total parenteral nutrition therapy, 409
Push, intravenous, 384–387, 459, 471
Pyrogenic reactions, 201–202
  antidotes and, 385
Pyruvate kinase, 256–257
Pyruvic acid, 236–37

Quality assurance studies, 32–37
  and blood transfusion, 43–46
  and cannula clotting, 37–39
  and catheter tubings, 46–48
Quinidine, 246–247

Radial artery, 477–478, 481, 482, 483, 485
Radiopaque catheters, 324

Index

Rapport, with children in therapy, 513
Recertification for chemotherapy, 440
Red blood cells, 195
Reduction, 373
Reimbursement, of home care costs, 527, 528–529
Renin activity, 252–253
Renocardiovascular system, 77
Resistance, host, 283
Respiratory acidosis, 74, 75, 502–503, 504
　calcium and, 256
Respiratory alkalosis, 73, 74, 503–504
Restraints, in pediatric intravenous therapy, 513
Reticulocyte count, 258–259
Reticuloendothelial system, 193
Rh (Rhesus) system, 192, 193–194, 239
　patient identification of, 204
　platelet transfusion and, 200
Rh $(_o)$ (D) immune globulin, 203
Rheumatoid factor, 260–261
RhoGAM, 203
Risk management, 31–32
"Rule of Nines," 95

Salicylate, 246–247
Saline (complete) antibodies, 192–193
Saline solutions
　bacteria and, 284
　hypertonic, 111–112
　maintenance therapy and, 120, 121
　normal, 450, 470
Salt, hyponatremia and, 91
Saphanous vein, 58, 508, 512
Self-evaluation, patient, 424
Sepsis. See infection(s)
Serum, definition of, 225
Serum protein, compared with albumin-globulin ratio, 120
SGOT (Serum glutamic oxaloacetic transaminase), 235
SGPT (Serum glutamic pyruvate transaminase), 236
Shock
　from burns, 94, 95
　cardiogenic, 305–306, 494
　decreased urinary output and, 119
　diabetic acidosis and, 99
　isotonic saline with dextrose and, 111
　need for baseline blood pressure and, 463
　plasma transfusion and, 198
　prevention of speed, 27, 133
Short-term infusion, 306
Shunting, 499
Shunts, arteriovenous, 292
Silicone, 324
Silver sulfadiazine, 520
Simplate, 254–255
Skeletal muscle, 242–243
Skin
　as bacteria source, 281–282
　contamination of, 406–407, 445
　fluid balance and, 77
　infection and preparation of, 288–290
　layers of, 63–64
　lesions of, 215
　observing changes in, 119
　sterile preparation of, 179, 216, 396–397, 398
SLD (Serum lactic dehydrogenase), 236
Small-gauge needle, 451, 453
Small-vein needle, 176, 473
　cancer outpatients and, 450
　chemotherapy and, 461
　for drug administration, 382
　low rate of infection and, 288
Smooth muscle, 260–261
Sodium, 77, 79–80, 90, 127
　abnormal levels of (see Hypernatremia; Hyponatremia
　burns and, 94
　dehydration, 80
　laboratory measurement of, 231, 232
　in packed red blood cells, 197
　plasma, 71
　potassium and, 78
　reference values for, 246–247
Sodium bicarbonate, 77, 115, 116
　acidosis and, 88
　as antidote to Daunomycin HCl, 470
Sodium chloride, 124
　alkalosis and, 88
　blood transfusion and, 205
　diabetic acidosis and, 99
　hyponatremia and, 124
　hypotonic, 112
　infusions of (see Saline infusions)
　isotonic infusions of, 109–110
　osmolality of, 73
Sodium citrate, 195, 197
Sodium lactate, 88, 116
Sodium succinate, 473
Sodium thiosulfate, 470
Solu-Cortef, 473
Solution administration, home care and, 417–418, 419, 420, 422–423
Solutions, parenteral. See Parenteral fluids
Somatomedin C, 252–253
Spasms, 60, 453
Specimen tubes, labeling of, 347
Speed shock, 278
　prevention of, 27, 133
Spool, catheter, 328, 330
Standing orders, 464, 465, 469
Steel needle, 176, 177
Sterile technique(s)
　at additive station, 378
　AIDS and, 282–283
　of catheter site, 337–338
　central venous catheterization and, 11
　in chemotherapy, 447
　in dressing changes, 396, 397, 398, 400
　for Hickman catheter, 462
　in home care, 417
　injection ports and, 287
　instruction in, 26
　for intravenous drug therapy, 379
　kit for, 418
　for parenteral solutions, 273–274
　patient education in, 416
　in pediatric therapy, 520, 521, 523
　phlebothrombosis and, 271
　standards on, 432–433
　for totally implanted catheters, 351
　and use of intravenous containers, 50
　vascular irritation and, 375
　violations of (see Contamination; Infection[s])
Sterile water, 340
Steroids, 254
Stool fat, 262–263
Stool nitrogen, 262–263
Stopcocks, three-way, 287–288

Streptokinase, 316
Stress
  childhood, 506
  endocrine response to, 88–89
  hypotonic expansion and, 126
  isotonic infusions and, 123
  oral deprivation and, 426–427
  protein deficiency from, 92
  sodium bicarbonate and, 77
  water intoxication and, 114
Subclavian catheter, 394
Subclavian vein, 303
  central venous catheterization and, 312
  insertion into, 186
  search for, 393
Sulfonamide, 246–247
Superficial fascia, 64
Superficial veins, 58–59, 61–63, 173, 174
  in children, 507
Superior vena cava, 304, 414, 431
  dextrose administration and, 109
  for pediatric therapy, 519
Surface body area, 130
Surgery, 91
  access to central venous system and, 414–415
  cardiac, 196
  parenteral therapy and, 88–89, 90–93
  plastic, 467–473
  vein selection and, 173
Swan Ganz catheter, 494–495
Syphilis, 211
Syringe and needle method, 492
Syringe pumps, 156, 157
  volumetric, 158, 159, 160, 161, 162, 163
Systemic circulation, 58
  and particulate contamination, 292
Systemic complications, of intravenous therapy, 273–275, 277–278

Teaching program, in intravenous department, 24–30
Techniques, intravenous
  for anchoring the cannula, 181, 183
  for approaching patient, 172
  and cancer chemotherapy, 447, 448–451
  for cannula selection, 175–177
  for catheter insertion, 183, 184, 186
  for lighting, 177
  for tourniquet application, 177–178
  for vein selection, 173–175 (see also Vein, selection of)
  for venipuncture, 178–181 (see also Venipuncture)
Teflon, as catheter material, 323
Temperature
  change in, 60
  drug stability and, 375
  effect on blood of, 205
  gas, 498
  measurement of, 434
  pediatric elevation of, 511
  proliferation of bacteria and, 284
  as symptom of infection, 406
Testosterone, 240–242
Therapeutic phlebotomy. See Phlebotomy, therapeutic
Thiotepa (Thiophosphoramide), 456–457
Thirst
  cellular dehydration and, 118–119
  diabetic acidosis and, 98
  elderly and, 119, 125
  hypertonic expansion and, 124
Thoracic duct, injury to, 395
Three-way stopcocks, 287–288
Thrombin time, 254–255
Thrombocytes, 200–201
Thrombophlebitis, 269–270, 375. See also Phlebitis
  inside-the-needle catheter and, 183
Thrombosis, 58, 59, 269, 270–272
  arterial, 490
  from chemotherapy, 459
  deep-vein, 316, 323, 324
  in femoral artery, 478
  infusion rate of flow and, 134
  insertion of cannula and multiple infusions and, 174
  rubber silicone and, 414
  from venipuncture, 228
Thrombus
  catheter occlusion and, 316–317
  embolism caused by, 375
Thyroxine-binding globulin capacity, 252–253
Thymol, 237
Thyroid colloid, 260–261
Thyroid-stimulating hormone (TSH), 253–254
Tongue, leathery, 119
Tonicity, parenteral fluid classification by, 104–105
Tort, 11–12
Total parenteral nutrition (TPN), 389–392, 424
  air embolism and, 396
  catheter insertion in, 392–395
  certification in, 404
  dressing procedures in, 396–397, 398, 400, 402, 403–404
  flow rates and, 409
  future trends in, 427
  history of, 389, 517–518
  home (see Home intravenous therapy)
  hyperglycemia and, 410
  hypoglycemia and, 410
  infection control in, 405–407
  insulin administration in, 408–409
  intravenous lipids in, 411–413
  metabolic considerations, 407–408, 434–435
  National Intravenous Therapy Association (NITA) and, 427–435
  neonatal, 514
  pediatric, 517–520, 521, 523–525
  psychological issues in, 425–427
  tubing and filters in, 404–405
  urinary glucose measurement, 408
  volumetric pumps in, 159, 160
Totally implanted catheter, 352, 355–357, 359
  bolus injection and, 359, 360, 361
  drawing blood samples through, 362, 363–364
Totally implanted pump, 335, 336, 339
Totally implanted venous access device, 333, 335
Tourniquet
  application of, 177–178
  in chemotherapy, 451
  hematomas and, 227
  infiltration and, 273
  as source of infection, 289
Training documentation, in home intravenous therapy, 529

Index

Transaminase, 236–237, 235–236
Transcellular body fluid compartment, 70
Transfusion(s). *See* Blood transfusion(s)
Trendelenburg position, 392, 396, 432
  increase of pressure and, 311, 315
Triiodothyronine, 252–253
Trimethobenzamide hydrochloride (Tigran), 385
Tubing, changing of, 320, 404–405
Tubing sets, large bore, 146, 147
Tunicae (layers), of blood vessels, 59–61
Tunneled catheters, 340

Ulnar artery, 478, 481
Umbilical catheterization, 515–517
Univalent electrolytes, 105
University of Cincinnati Medical Center, 404, 409, 413, 424
Urea, blood, 71, 73
Urea nitrogen, blood (BUN), 85, 120, 238
  reference values for, 246–247
Uric acid, 246–247
Urinary output, 119
  antidiuretic hormone and, 79
  burns and decreased, 94
Urine, glucose in, 408
Urokinase, 316

Vacuum system, of blood withdrawal, 228–229, 231
Vacuum tube method, pediatric, 492
Valsalva maneuver, 394, 396, 405, 432, 433
  air embolism and, 275, 310, 311
  dangers of, 315
  tubing changes and, 320
Valves, vein, 59–60
Varicosities, 59, 173, 271
Vascular access devices, implantable, 170–171, 394, 463
Vascular anatomy, 301, 302, 303–304
Vascular irritation, from intravenous drug therapy, 375–376

Vascular route, for particulate matter, 291–292
Vascular system. *See* Artery(ies); Vein(s)
Vasoconstrictors, 57, 50, 172, 470
  stimulation of, 133
Vasodilators, 57, 470
Vasopressors, 90, 208
Vasovagal reaction, 25, 172, 215
Vein(s), 57
  antebrachial, 63
  antecubital, 173
  arteries and, 59–60
  axillary, 302
  basilic, 63, 302, 314
  for blood sample collection, 227
  cephalic, 62–63, 301, 313, 450
  chemotherapy and fragile, 451
  collapse of, 228
  distending of, 26, 446, 451
  dorsal digital, 61
  dorsal metacarpal, 174
  edema and concealment of, 174
  femoral, 58–59
  fragile, 451
  innominate, 332
  jugular, 302, 303, 312–313
  median, 63
  metacarpal, 62, 174, 181
  palpation of, 174
  peripheral, 117
  saphanous, 58, 508, 512
  selection of, 173–175, 392, 444, 507, 515
  superficial (*see* Superficial veins)
  valves of, 59–60
Velban, 456–457
Venipuncture
  basic, 179, 180–181
  blood transfusion and, 206
  for blood withdrawal, 227–228
  hepititis from, 228
  instruction in use of, 26
  policies on, 18
  preparation for, 178–179
  techniques in, 179
Venous catheterization, umbilical, 516–517
Venous pressure. *See* Central venous pressure
Venous spasm, 453
Vesicant agents, antidotes for, 470
Vinblastine sulfate (Velban), 456–457
Vinca alkyloids, 470

Vincristine sulfate (Oncovin), 456–457
Visual acuity, for home intravenous therapy, 528
Vitamin A, 246–247
Vitamin B_{12}, 258–259
Vitamin D, 233, 252–253
Vitamins
  maintenance therapy and, 84–85
  postsurgery and, 93
Volume, gas, 498
Volumetric pumps, 158, 159, 160, 161, 162, 163
  home care and, 418
Vomiting, 99, 220

Warmers, blood, 148
Water. *See also* Body fluids
  body fat and, 70, 83
  dextrose in, 106–108
  distilled, 83
  electrolyte-free, 126
  excess of, 90
  excretion of (polyuria), 97, 998
  intake and output of, 119
  intoxification from, 108–109, 114, 126–127
  maintenance therapy and, 83–84
  replacement of, 114
  sodium and retention of, 79
Weight
  gain in, 124, 127
  ideal vs. actual, 114
  loss in, 99, 125
  need for measuring daily, 114
  sudden shift in, 118
Weight method, and pediatric fluid needs, 510, 511
Whole blood, 225
  transfusions of, 96, 196
Whole blood clot lysis, 254–255
Wrist, 183, 491
  as site for intraarterial therapy, 481, 482
  venipuncture and, 64
Wydase, 470

Xanthomatosis, 237
Xylocaine, 385, 453
Xylose absorption, 241, 242

Y-type blood component sets, 149, 150
  platelet transfusion and, 200
Y-type infusion sets, 144